THE C…
Calorie, Fat & …

BONUS DIET GUIDES & COUNTERS

Weight Control Tips

Eat & Drink Sensibly

- **Eat 2-3 sensible meals daily,** ideally within an 8-10 hour window. Fast for the remaining 14-16 hours (except for water, coffee/tea without milk or sugar).
- **Eat mainly wholefoods** with adequate protein, healthy fats, and ample lower starch vegetables, beans, lentils and nuts.
- **Avoid highly processed foods** with seed oils, refined grains/flour and added sugar (particularly soda and candy).
- **Quench your thirst with water.**

Exercise Daily

- Aim for at least 30 minutes daily – even in 5-10 minute lots. For motivation, find an exercise buddy, personal trainer or join a gym. *(Extra Notes ~ Page 12)*

Reshape Eating Behaviors

- **Keep a Food & Exercise Journal.** A journal helps you see exactly what you eat and drink, and how much you exercise. An excellent motivator and proven weight loss aid.

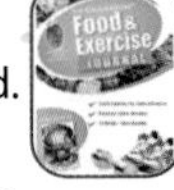

- **Also focus on social and emotional situations** that may trigger compulsive eating. *(Extra Notes ~ Page 14)*

Arrange Moral Support

- Gain the support of workmates, family and friends.
- Get extra professional help and coaching, from your doctor, dietitian/nutritionist, psychologist, personal trainer, or slimming group.

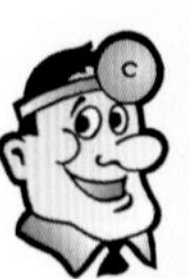

DOCTOR CHECK-UP

Ask your doctor to check your blood pressure, blood sugar and fats levels – even your insulin levels.

Dont wait to develop insulin resistance, prediabetes, or a fatty liver!

HEALTHY WEIGHTS
~ MEN & WOMEN ~
(Over 18 Years)

Based on weights with least risk of disease or death from heart disease, diabetes, stroke and cancer.

Based on Body Mass Index of 20-25

BMI calculated as: $\frac{\text{Weight (kg)}}{\text{Height (m)}^2}$

Height (No Shoes) Ft Ins		Healthy Weight Range (Pounds)
4'7"	~	86-108
4'8"	~	88-110
4'9"	~	92-114
4'10"	~	97-121
4'11"	~	99-123
5'0"	~	101-127
5'1"	~	105-132
5'2"	~	110-136
5'3"	~	112-140
5'4"	~	114-145
5'5"	~	119-149
5'6"	~	123-156
5'7"	~	127-158
5'8"	~	129-162
5'9"	~	134-167
5'10"	~	138-173
5'11"	~	143-178
6'0"	~	145-182
6'1"	~	149-187
6'2"	~	156-193
6'3"	~	158-198
6'4"	~	162-202
6'5"	~	170-211
6'6"	~	172-215
6'7"	~	175-220

Body Fat Distribution & Health

Moderate amounts of body fat do not compromise health. However, excess fat above the hips carries a far greater health risk than fat on or below the hips - better to be a 'pear-shape' than an 'apple-shape'.

Abdominal obesity greatly increases the risk of developing diabetes, heart disease, high blood fats, hypertension, stroke, sleep apnea, arthritis, fatty liver, and some cancers. So-called 'cellulite' carries no extra health risk.

Waist Circumference directly reflects the increased health risk of abdominal obesity. Waist size associated with a higher health risk:

Men ~ Over 40 inches   **Women** ~ Over 35 inches

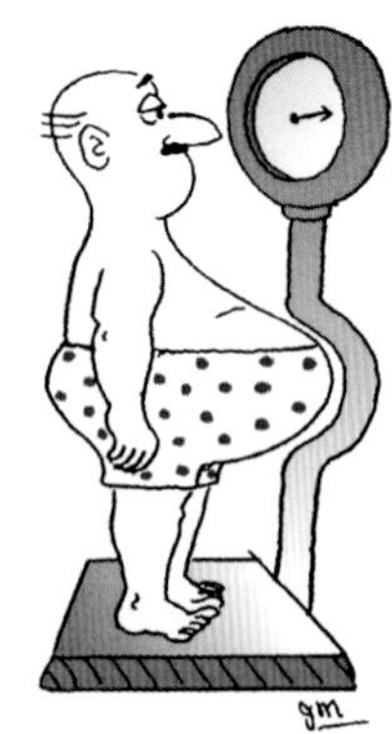

Abdominal obesity greatly increases the risk of ill-health and earlier death.

Body Mass Index (BMI)

BMI is a general (but not specific) indicator of body fatness. Although BMI alone is not diagnostic, the higher the BMI, the greater the health risk of developing diabetes, high blood pressure and heart disease. BMI does not apply to heavily muscled persons. BMI is used in a different way for children.

Check Your BMI: Find your height (no shoes) - look across the row to the weight nearest your own. Then track down to BMI.

Ht	WEIGHT (LBS) ~ ADULTS													
5'1"	100	106	111	116	122	127	132	137	143	148	153	158	185	211
5'2"	104	109	115	120	126	131	136	142	147	153	158	164	191	218
5'3"	107	113	118	124	130	135	141	146	152	158	163	169	197	225
5'4"	110	116	122	128	134	140	145	151	157	163	169	174	204	232
5'5"	114	120	126	132	138	144	150	156	162	168	174	180	210	240
5'6"	118	124	130	136	142	148	155	161	167	173	179	186	216	247
5'7"	121	127	134	140	146	153	159	166	172	178	185	191	223	255
5'8"	125	131	138	144	151	158	164	171	177	184	190	197	230	262
5'9"	128	135	142	149	155	162	169	176	182	189	196	206	236	270
5'10"	132	139	146	153	160	167	174	181	188	195	202	207	243	278
5'11"	136	143	150	157	165	172	179	186	193	200	208	215	250	286
6'0"	140	147	154	162	169	177	184	191	199	206	213	221	258	294
6'1"	144	151	159	166	174	182	189	197	204	212	219	227	265	302
6'2"	148	155	163	171	179	186	194	202	210	218	225	233	272	311
6'3"	152	160	168	176	184	192	200	208	216	224	232	240	279	319
6'4"	156	164	172	180	189	197	205	213	221	230	238	246	287	328
BMI	19	20	21	22	23	24	25	26	27	28	29	30	35	40

BMI Classification:

BMI Below 19
Underweight

BMI 19-24.9
Healthy Weight
(Low Health Risk)

BMI 25-29.9
Overweight
(Moderate Health Risk)

BMI 30-40
Obese (High Health Risk)

BMI Over 40
Morbid Obesity
(Very High Risk)

Interactive BMI Calculator
www.calorieking.com

Calories & Weight Loss

Calories in Food

Calories in food are derived from protein, fat and carbohydrate. Alcohol also provides calories. Vitamins, minerals and water provide no calories.

Calorie Values Per Gram

Fat/Oil	~ 9 Calories
Carbohydrate	~ 4 Calories
Protein	~ 4 Calories
Alcohol	~ 7 Calories

Note that fats have over double the calories of protein and carbohydrate. The higher the fat content of food, the higher the calories.

Sample Calculation

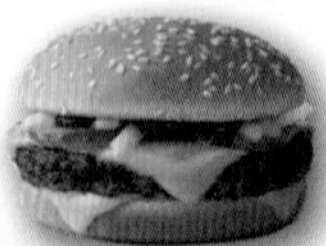

QUARTER POUNDER® WITH CHEESE has 520 calories derived from:

26g Fat (x 9 cals/gram)	= 234
42g Carbohyd.(x 4 cals/gram)	= 168
30g Protein (x 4 cals/gram)	= 120
Total Calories (rounded)	= 520

Calorie Levels for Weight Loss

Start with a calorie-controlled diet that allows a moderate weight loss of ½ - 1 pound per week. Weight loss is usually much greater in the first few weeks due to extra fluid losses.

Note: It is better to increase exercise rather than lessen food calories too drastically.

Suggested Calories for Weight Loss

Women:	Non-active	1000 - 1200
	Active	1200 - 1500
Men:	Non-active	1200 - 1500
	Active	1500 - 1800
Teenagers:		1200 - 1800

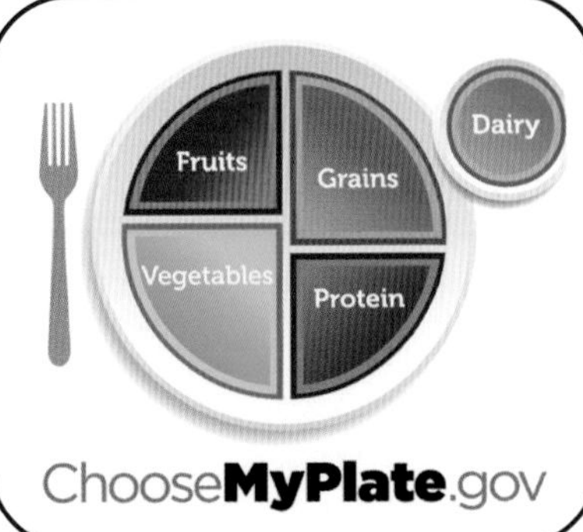

The MyPlate symbol represents the recommended proportion of foods from each food group. It focuses on the importance of making smart food choices in every food group, every day. Daily physical activity is also important. *(More info: www.ChooseMyPlate.gov)*

Examples of Single Serving Sizes

Grains (Eat 3-4 servings per day):

- 1 slice wholegrain bread (1 oz)
- ½ bun, small bagel or English muffin
- 4 small crackers or 1 tortilla
- 1 oz ready-to-eat wholegrain cereal
- ½ cup cooked cereal, rice or pasta

Vegetables (Eat 3-5 servings per day):

- 1 cup raw leafy vegetables
- 1½ cups raw chopped vegetables
- ½ cup cooked vegetables
- ½ - ¾ cup vegetable juice

Fruit (Eat 2-3 servings per day):

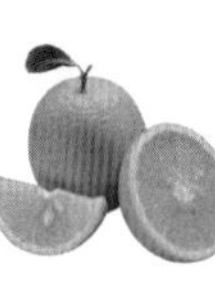

- 1 medium apple, orange, banana
- ½ cup canned fruit (in own juice)
- ¼ cup dried fruit
- ½ cup fruit juice (unsweetened)
- ¼ medium avocado

Protein (2-3 servings per day):

- 2-3 oz (cooked) meat/poultry/fish
- 2 eggs **or** 6 oz tofu **or** ¼ cup nuts
- 1 cup (cooked) dried beans **or** chickpeas

Dairy (2-3 servings per day):

- 1 cup (8 fl.oz) milk/soy (enriched)/yogurt
- 1 ½ oz cheese or ½ cup cottage cheese

Portion Size Counts!

Food portion size is critical to controlling calorie intake for weight control.

Supersized food servings have become more common when eating out and in the home. This can mean a day's worth of calories being consumed in one meal; or a snack being equivalent to a full meal.

For example, some giant size bakery items such as muffins and sweet buns can have more calories, fat and carbs than a large burger – as shown below.

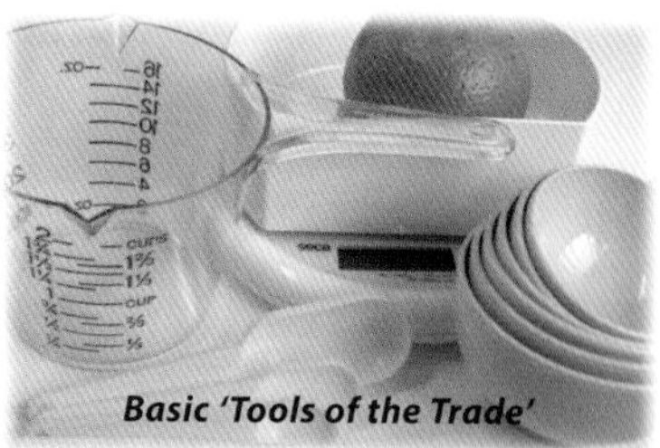

Basic 'Tools of the Trade'

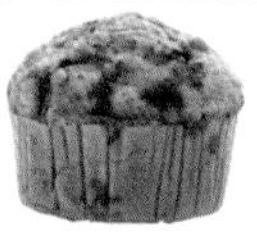

Hostess Double Choc Mega Muffin (5.5 oz):
580 calories, **33g fat, 71g carbs**

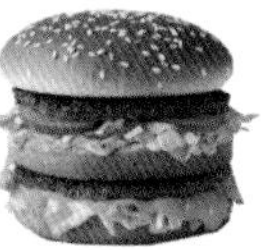

McDonald's Big Mac:
550 calories, 30g fat, 45g carbs

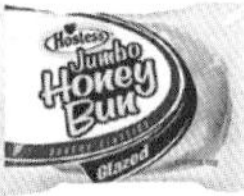

Hostess Jumbo Honey Bun (4.75 oz):
560 calories, 29g fat, 68g carbs

CalorieKing Portion Watch

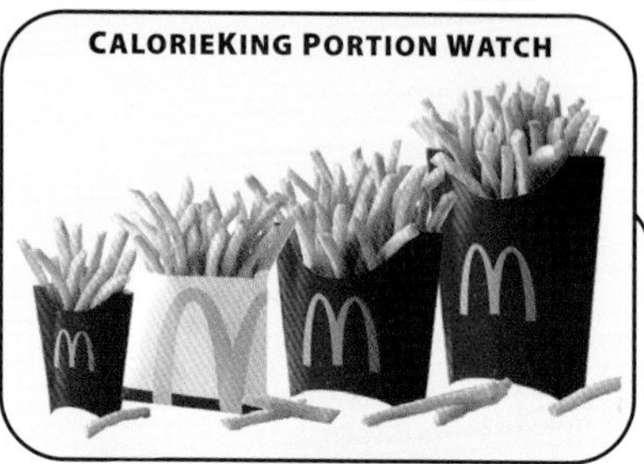

Fries	Cal	Fat	Carb
Kids	110	5	15
Small	220	10	29
Medium	320	15	43
Large	490	23	66

Weigh and Measure Your Portions

It is easy to underestimate portion size of foods and drinks, and unwittingly consume excess calories – even if the fat content is low or even zero!

To more accurately estimate portion size of different foods, weigh and measure your food with food scales, measuring spoons and cups. Better control of calories will result.

Allow for Extra Calories in Packaged Food

The actual weight of packaged foods is usually 5-10% more than the label net weight (the minimum legal weight) – and in some cases up to 50% more (particularly in-store bakery items such as muffins). However, manufacturers calculate the calories based on the net weight. For actual calories, weigh the product and calculate the extra calories.

CalorieKing Portion Watch

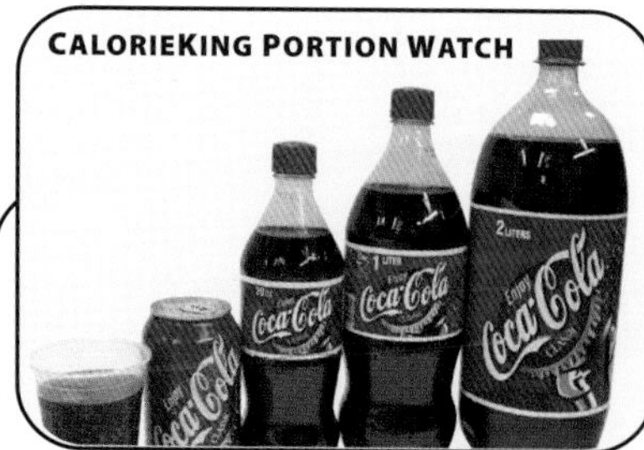

Cola	Cal	Fat	Carb
8 fl.oz Cup	100	0	25
12 fl.oz Can	150	0	37
20 fl.oz Bottle	250	0	63
1 Liter Bottle	400	0	100
2 Liter Bottle	800	0	200

Dietary Fats

► Fats in the diet are essential for good health.

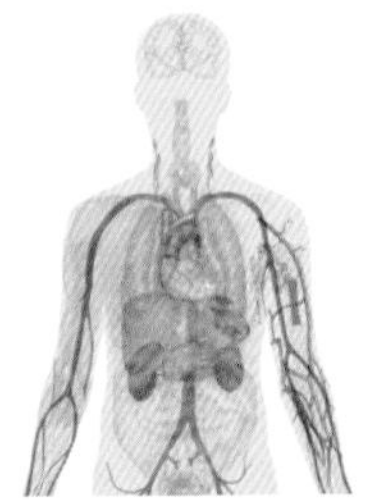

Healthy dietary fats are essential for good health.

Examples of fats' roles in the body include:

- important concentrated fuel source of energy for all cells
- major storage form of energy in the body
- provides structure and functionality to all body cell membranes
- important component of brain tissues
- helps the absorption of nutrients such as fat-soluble vitamins
- satisfies hunger more readily than fat-free foods
- produce important hormones
- protects your organs and keeps the body warm

Dietary fats and oils have over double the calories (9 calories per gram) of carbohydrates or proteins (4 calories per gram).

Low Fat vs Higher Fat Diets:

While low-fat diets have generally been recommended for weight control in past decades, they have not been successful in reducing the incidence of obesity, In fact, obesity rates have been steadily increasing. **Some problems with low-fat diets include:**

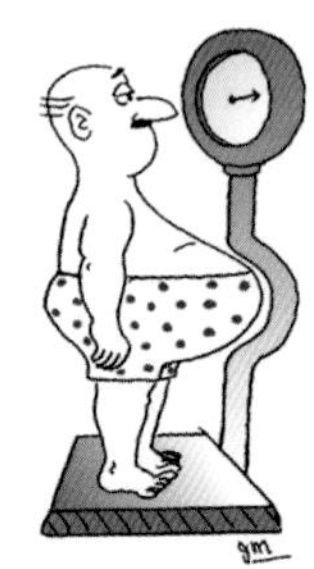

Low-fat diets have not been successful in reducing obesity.

- **Carbohydrates take the place of fats,** so the diet becomes a 'low-fat, high-carbohydrate' diet. This can lead to greater difficulty in losing weight from adipose fatty tissue. When those extra carbohydrates are largely refined ones, this can also result in excessive fat triglycerides in the blood (a risk factor for heart disease), unstable blood sugar levels and a fatty liver leading to insulin resistance and Type 2 diabetes.
- **Low-fat diets do not generally satisfy the hunger** that often results from reduced calories.

Subsequently, research has shown **a diet lower in carbohydrate and higher in fat to be more effective for weight loss**. It is more sustainable and better satisfies hunger. Additionally, there are generally improvements in blood glucose levels, blood triglyceride fats and 'good' HDL-cholesterol levels – which in turn lowers the risk of heart disease and diabetes. This is in the context of sensible portion sizes, and incorporating healthy, high-quality foods.

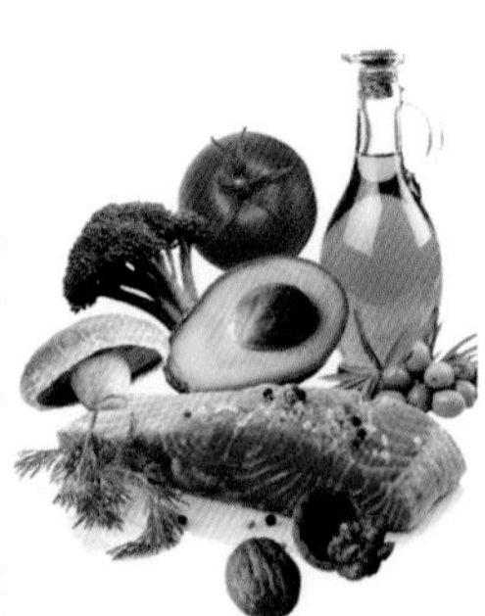

Mediterranean Diet food examples

The Mediterranean Diet is often used as a good example of healthy eating. It includes moderate amounts of meat, regular fish meals, generous lower starch vegetables, fruit, legumes, whole-grains, extra-virgin olive oil, nuts, seeds and herbs. Other important aspects include avoidance of highly processed foods as well as adequate physical activity, clean air, sunshine and sleep.

Of course, there is no one perfect or 'one-size-fits-all' diet that suits all people. Rather, a personalized diet should also consider the person's food philosophy, food allergies / sensitivities, medical condition, medications and genetic predisposition.

Healthy Fats vs Unhealthy Fats

There are three main types of fat in food: saturated fats, monounsaturated fats, and polyunsaturated fats.

Different foods generally have a mixture of all three types with animal fats being rich in saturated fats, and plant foods generally higher in mono- and polyunsaturated fats. *(Extra notes on fats and heart health ~ See page 206)*

When consumed as part of wholefoods (unprocessed), these fats have important functions in maintaining our health. Examples of foods with healthy fats include avocados, olives, nuts, seeds, cheese, milk, fish, meats and eggs.

However, when fats and oils are isolated from their naturally occurring wholefood source, their physico-chemical properties can be altered; and there is the potential for them to affect our health. Ultraprocessing of foods can destroy the accompanying vitamins and antioxidants that would normally protect the fats or oils from oxidation.

Such is the case with so-called 'seed oils' or 'industrial vegetable oils' (such as corn, sunflower, safflower, soy bean and canola oils) which have a high omega-6 fatty acid content. Their polyunsaturated chemical structure is unstable and makes them more prone to oxidation – particularly when used in high-heat cooking

Oxidized fats can damage cellular components, cause inflammation and lead to metabolic dysfunction.

Oxidized fats can also adversely affect all body organs including the pancreas (insulin production), liver, brain, kidneys, eyes, lungs; and can even initiate inflammation of artery linings leading to atherosclerosis (by oxidation of lipoprotein carriers of cholesterol in the blood).

Researchers suggest that the 12-fold increase in consumption of these polyunsaturated seed oils over the last 100 years is largely responsible for the epidemics of obesity, insulin resistance, diabetes, heart disease, fatty liver and even many cancers.

Polyunsaturated omega-3 fats in oily fish, walnuts, hempseed, flaxseed and chia seed have an anti-inflammatory effect which can benefit many health conditions including heart health, insulin resistance, diabetes and brain health. Most Americans are deficient in omega-3 fats. *(Extra notes ~ page 263)*

Monounsaturated oil such as extra-virgin olive oil is more stable and has protective antioxidants.

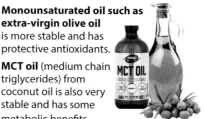

MCT oil (medium chain triglycerides) from coconut oil is also very stable and has some metabolic benefits.

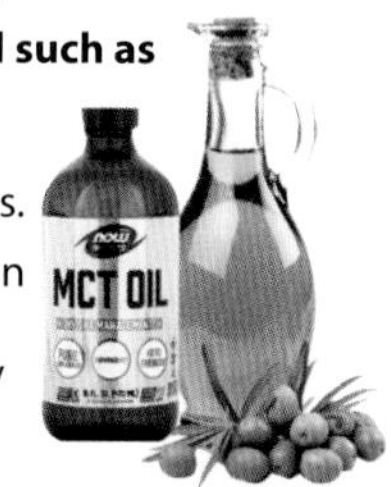

Vegetable seed oils are widely used in processed foods:
Examples:

- spreads, dressings
- sauces, dips
- cakes, cookies, pastries
- fried snacks, snack bars
- vegetarian meat and milk alternatives
- fried foods
- cafe and restaurant foods.

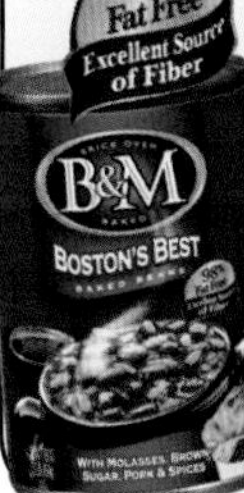

BEWARE OF LOW-FAT & FAT-FREE FOODS

They can be high in sugar!

This brand of baked beans hides 7 teaspoons of sugar (added) per 8 oz serving (½ of 16 oz can).

Carbohydrates ~ Friend or Foe?

Naturally-Friendly Carbs

Carbohydrate foods in their more natural wholefood forms (minimally processed) are essential to good health. They are the main source of fuel for the body, and also provide important vitamins, minerals, antioxidants and fiber.

How Much Do We Need?

Most Americans consume excessive amounts of carbohydrate – particularly as refined white flour and sugar. This greatly increases the risk of obesity, high blood glucose levels, and insulin resistance – which can lead to Type 2 diabetes, fatty liver, heart disease and many other chronic diseases.

As such, many health authorities are now recommending a much lower carbohydrate intake – around 20-25% of total calories. *(See chart below)*

This lower carbohydrate intake still allows for adequate intake of fruit, vegetables and wholegrains in their wholefood forms.

The emphasis is on minimizing refined carbohydrates and sugar.

LOW CARBOHYDRATE DIET ~ DAILY AMOUNTS (Grams) ~

Calories		Carbohydrate
1200 Cals	~	60 - 75g
1600 Cals	~	80 - 100g
2000 Cals	~	100 - 125g
2400 Cals	~	120 - 150g

Note: The carbohydrate range for each calorie level corresponds to 20-25% of total calories.

Ketogenic diets generally contain 20-50 grams of carbohydrate (5-10% total calories). This diet is best planned and supervised by your doctor and dietitian – particularly if on medications to control blood glucose and/or thyroid hormone levels. (Dosage strength of medications may need to be adjusted.)

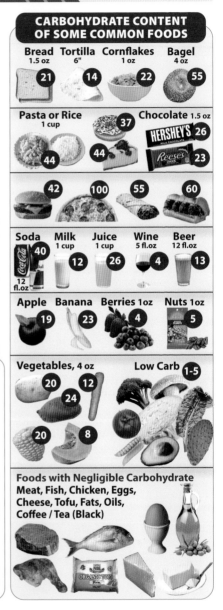

- **Excess Sugar:**

  Many overweight, inactive people consume over 500 calories of refined sugars per day, either self-added or as part of food products. This is equivalent to over 30 level teaspoons. For context, just one 12-ounce can of soda contains 10 teaspoons of added sugar.

  Note: Naturally occurring sugars in fruits, vegetables and milk are fine when consumed in normal recommended amounts. These foods are also rich in other nutrients.

  Refined sugar is referred to as having **'empty calories'**. Sugar supplies calories but negligible nutrients and no fiber.

- **Most sugar in our diet is 'hidden'** in processed foods such as soft drinks, fruit drinks, candy, cookies, cake, jam, sauces, ice cream, desserts, canned foods, and processed breakfast cereals.

  For serious weight control, as well as better control of blood glucose and blood fat levels, severely limit these foods and substitute healthier, higher fiber wholefoods.

- **Be aware that sugar comes in different forms** such as sucrose, glucose, fructose, malt, high-fructose corn syrup, molasses, honey and maple syrup. Check the label.

- **Sugar alcohols** such as sorbitol, mannitol and maltitol are carb-based and have ½ - ¾ the calories of regular sugar. While not counted as sugar on food labels, they do add to the carb count. Excess amounts can cause bloating, gas and diarrhea.

- **Sugar-free sweeteners** make it easy to reduce sugar in drinks and recipes. However, use minimally since research suggests possible ill-effects of some artificial sweeteners on friendly gut microbes. This may increase the risk of glucose intolerance and an increase in appetite.

  Plant-based sweeteners like stevia or monk fruit appear to be better choices.

SUGAR CONTENT OF SOME COMMON FOODS

	Teaspoons of Sugar
Coca Cola or *Pepsi*, 12 fl.oz	10
20 fl.oz size	17
Iced Tea, sweetened, 12 fl.oz	8
Energy Drink *(Red Bull)*, 8.4 fl.oz	7
Chocolate Milk, 12 fl.oz	6
Frappuccino, 16 fl.oz	6
Fruit Drink, sweetened, 8 oz	6
Slurpee, 12 oz	6
Gatorade, 12 fl.oz	5
Shakes, medium, 16 fl.oz	12
Baked Beans *(B&M)*, 8 oz	5
Honey Smacks Cereal, 1 cup, 1 oz	4.5
Popcorn, caramel, 1 cup	3.5
Chocolate Bar, 1.5 oz	5
M&M's, 1.7 oz pkg	7
Baby Ruth, King Size, 3.5 oz	8
Jelly Beans (10 medium), 1 oz	6
Life Saver, 1 roll, 1.2 oz	8
Lollipop, medium, 1 oz	6
Marshmallows, 4 pcs, 1 oz	5
Snickers Bar, 1.9 oz	6
Ice Pop/Popsicle	5
Ice Cream, ½ cup	4
Yogurt, sweetened, 6 oz	4
Muffin, large, 4 oz	6
Honey Bun, jumbo, 4.75 oz	6
Twinkies (2)	8
Choc Chip Cookie, 1 oz	2
Donut, iced	6
Apple Pie, 1 piece	7
Jell-O, snack cup, 3.5 oz	4
Jam, 1 Tbsp, ¾ oz	2.5
Nutella, 1 Tbsp	2.5
Syrup, maple, 1 Tbsp	3

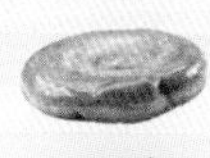

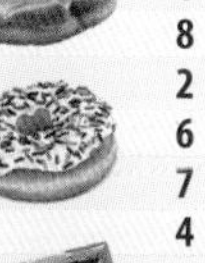

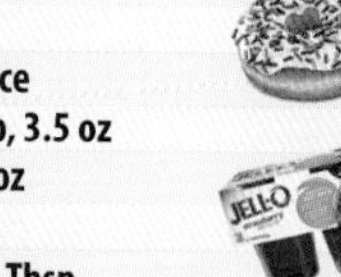

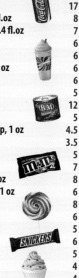

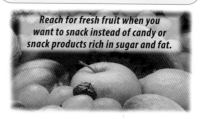

Reach for fresh fruit when you want to snack instead of candy or snack products rich in sugar and fat.

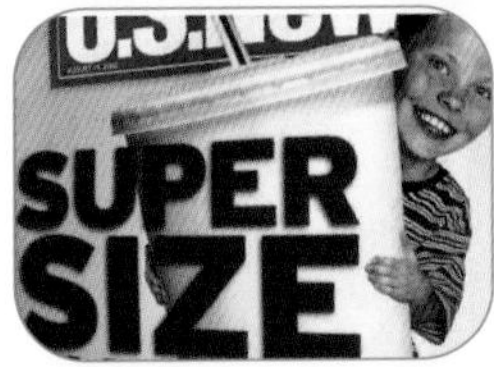

The XL Generation

Some 20% of American kids and adolescents are obese; and childhood obesity has doubled over the last 20 years. Diabetes, high blood pressure and high cholesterol are major problem areas for overweight children and adolescents, as are depression, low self-esteem, sleep apnea and bone joint problems.

To address this problem, cooperation is required between kids, parents, schools and government. Weight control is a family and community affair.

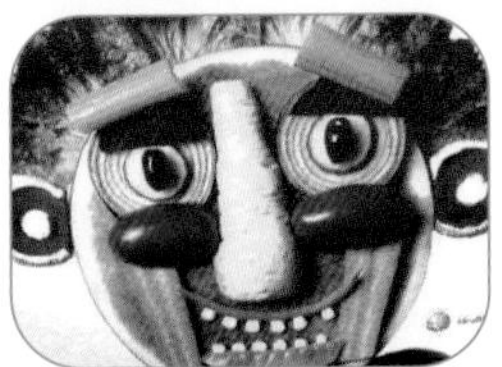

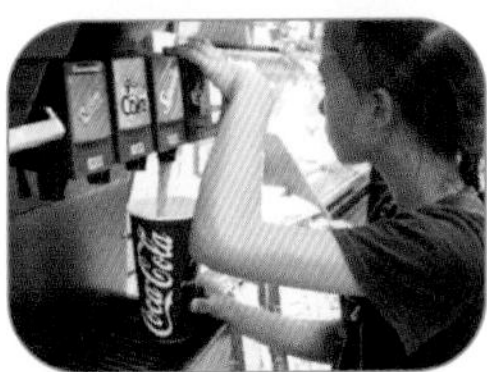

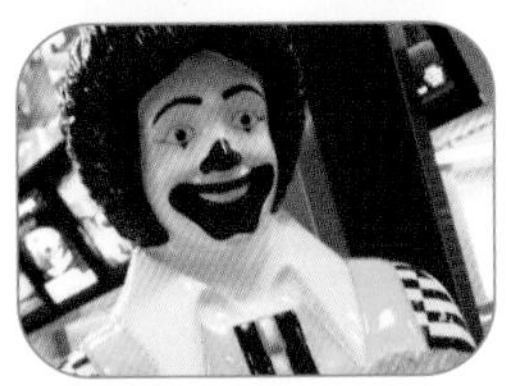

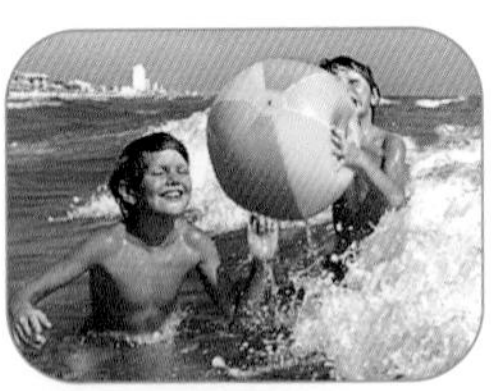

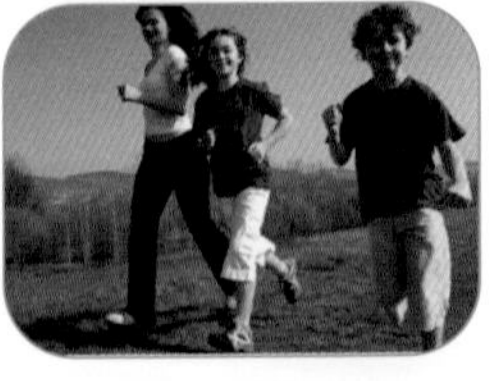

Five Simple Tips To Get Started:

1 Watch Soda Intake

Limit soda and sugary drinks to one serving on the weekends. Soda should not be an everyday beverage – water should be. When at restaurants or using a soda fountain, choose small servings with ice or choose diet soda instead. Schools should provide water and restrict access to soda as should parents when eating out or in the home!

Also limit sports and energy drinks, fruit juice and flavored milks.

2 Cut back on Fast-Foods and Eating Out

Many more calories are consumed when you eat out. Healthy meals prepared at home are best for the whole family.

3 Say "No" to Super-Sizing

When meals are upsized, loads more calories are consumed. Choose sensible portion sizes when eating out and at home. Use smaller plates and choose smaller package sizes.

4 Limit Between-Meal Snacking

Watch out for high-fat and high-calorie snacks – they can have more calories than a meal! Keep your eye on portion sizes and limit salty snack foods and candy to parties and special occasions. Choose fresh fruit, vegetables, nuts and milk instead.

5 Get Moving ~ Watch Less TV

Kids need at least 60 minutes of physical activity every day. It's critical for their fitness, and greatly lessens the risk of obesity.

Encourage kids to be active out of school hours. Wearing a pedometer can be highly motivational for kids to move more – as can playing dance video games such as *Dance Dance Revolution. Dance Central* (XBox360) and *Wii Fit (Nintendo)* are also excellent fitness motivators.

Limit TV and non-active computer games to just one hour per day. Also limit the accompanying snacks! Include exercise in family activities.

Sample Meal Plan ~ 1400 Calories

For Healthy, Overweight Persons ~ Not for Persons With Any Medical Condition ~ Please Check With Your Doctor & Dietitian ~

Breakfast (approx. 300 cal)

	1 Small Fruit or ½ oz Dried Fruit
Plus	*Cereal: 1½ oz Dry (high fiber)*
	or 1 cup cooked Oatmeal/Quinoa *or ½ Avocado*
Plus	*½ oz Almonds/Seeds*
Plus	*Milk (from daily allowance) or Yogurt (low-fat)*

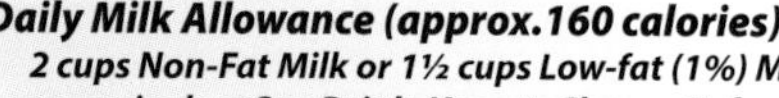

Daily Milk Allowance (approx.160 calories)
2 cups Non-Fat Milk or 1½ cups Low-fat (1%) Milk or equivalent Soy Drink, Yogurt, Cheese, Tofu

Fat Allowance (140 calories; 15g Fat)
4 teasp. Butter/Spread or 3 teasp. Oil or 1½ Tbsp Mayonnaise or ½ medium Avocado or 1½ Tbsp Peanut Butter or 30g Nuts/Seeds

Lunch (approx. 440 calories)

	1 slice Wholegrain Bread (1 oz) *or 2 Crispbreads/Crackers or 6" Pita*
Plus	*3 oz lean Meat, Chicken or Turkey* *or 3-4 oz Tuna (in water) or Salmon* *or 1½ oz Cheese or ¾ cup (6 oz) Cottage Cheese* *or ½ cup (4 oz) Ricotta Cheese* *or ¾ cup (6 oz) Fruit Yogurt (sugar-free)* *or ¾ cup (6 oz) Bean Salad*
Plus	*Large Salad (low-fat dressing)*
Plus	*1 small Fruit or ½ oz Dried Fruit*

Dinner (approx. 360 calories)

	Soup (Vegetable), low-fat
Plus	*3 oz lean Meat (cooked weight)* *or 4 oz Chicken Breast (no skin)* *or 3 oz Chicken Thigh/Leg (no skin)* *or 5 oz Fish (grilled)* *or ¾ cup (6 oz) Beans (Soy, Kidney, Pinto etc)/Lentils*
Plus	*1 small Potato* *or ½ cup Brown Rice/Pasta/Sweet Corn* *or 1 slice Wholegrain Bread*
Plus	*2-3 servings Vegetables (non-starchy)* *or large Salad*
Plus	*1 small fruit* *or ½ oz dark chocolate (over 70% cocoa)*

Brealfast ~ Choice 2

	1 Small Fruit
Plus	*2 Eggs (no added fat)* *or 2 oz Cheese (low-fat)* *or 4 oz Cottage Cheese (low-fat)* *or 2 oz Lean/Canadian Bacon*
Plus	*1 Tomato*
Plus	*1 Slice Wholegrain Toast*

Between Meals

- *Water, Coffee, Tea (sugar-free)*
- *Fruit from main meals; Raw Vegetables*
- *Milk from Daily Allowance*

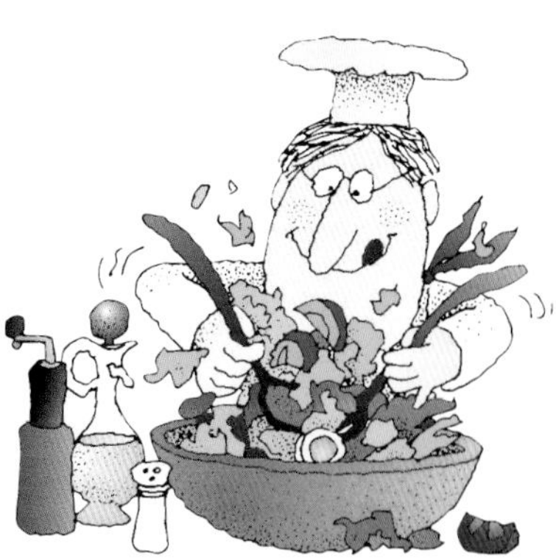

Exercise & Weight Control

- **Persons who exercise regularly lose more weight** and keep it off longer than non-exercisers. Blood glucose control also improves; as do beneficial gut microbes.
- **Exercise also improves general health and well-being.** Mood, confidence and self-esteem are also enhanced.
- **Exercise** is a good way to 'wake up' a sluggish metabolism and burn excess body fat.
- **Aerobic (huff and puff) exercise most days** is great for burning calories and for cardiovascular fitness. But, it is strength training that mainly builds the muscles that burn calories.
- **Strength training is the key to retaining or rebuilding muscles.** As we age, we lose some 6 pounds of muscle per decade. This results in a lower metabolism and fewer calories burnt.

  Muscles are the furnaces that burn calories. The more muscle you have, the more calories burnt – and as a bonus, the more food you can eat.
- **Regular strength training (2-3 times weekly)** can increase our metabolic rate for several days following exercise – with up to an extra 100 calories per day being burnt.

  While 2-3 pounds of muscle may be gained in the first 8-10 weeks, weight from exercised muscles is okay. It is excess fat (particularly abdominal fat) that is a potential health hazard.
- **Body reshaping** is enhanced by gaining muscle and losing fat - even if the scales don't show it.
- **Avoid injury** by beginning with walking, low impact aerobics, or weight-supported exercise (e.g. swimming, cycling). Avoid competitive sports. Allow 2-3 days of recovery between strength training sessions. Get professional advice.
- **How Much?** Start with 10-20 minutes per day and progress to 30-60 minutes per day. Also walk up stairs instead of using elevators. Take a brisk walk at lunch. Use an exercise bike, treadmill or stair machine while watching TV. Walk the dog.
- **How Often?** While aerobic fitness may require only 3-4 sessions weekly, **weight control is a daily event which requires daily exercise to burn calories.** Also add in strength training 2-3 times weekly.

Note: Persons on cholesterol-lowering statin drugs may experience muscle pains and weakness (as well as damage to muscle microfibrils). Supplementing with coenzyme Q10, magnesium, selenium, vitamins D and K2, may be beneficial. Check with your healthcare provider.

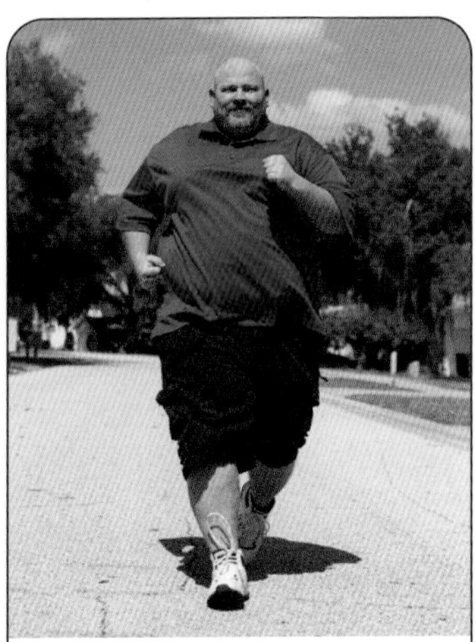

Brisk walking each day is a safe and effective way to burn calories and keep fit. Try it – you'll like it!

Be sure to wear sun-protective clothing.

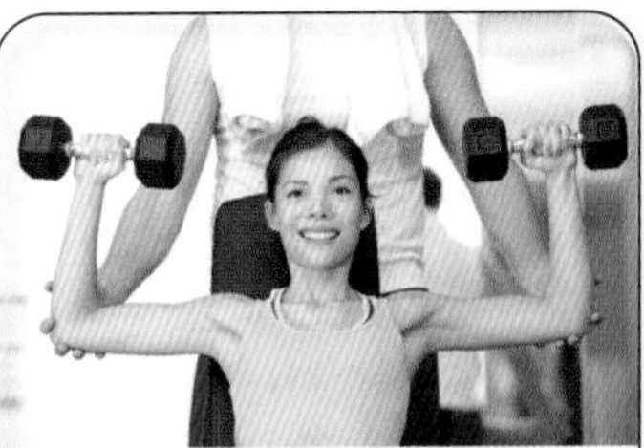

Strength training is the key to retain or rebuild muscles.

Exercized muscles burn extra calories even while you sleep.

For extra guidance and motivation, seek a qualified trainer or join a gym.

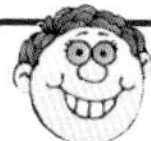

Calories Used in Exercise

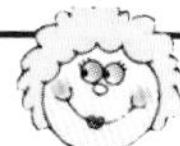

LIGHT	MODERATE	HEAVY
130 lbs ~ 3 Cals/Min	130 lbs ~ 5 Cals/Min	130 lbs ~ 8 Cals/Min
170 lbs ~ 4 Cals/Min	170 lbs ~ 6 Cals/Min	170 lbs ~ 10 Cals/Min
220 lbs ~ 5 Cals/Min	220 lbs ~ 7 Cals/Min	220 lbs ~ 12 Cals/Min
• Walking, slow	• Walking, brisk	• Walking (power), Jogging
• Cycling, light	• Cycling, moderate	• Cycling (vigorous)
• Frisbee playing	• Swimming, crawl	• Swimming, strenuous
• Gardening, light	• Weight-training, light	• Weight-training, heavy
• Golf, social	• Tennis, moderate	• Wrestling/Judo, advanced
• Tennis, doubles	• Racquetball, beginners	• Racquetball, advanced
• Housework, cleaning	• Aerobics, light	• Tae Bo, Kick Boxing
• Calisthenics, light	• Football, touch	• Football, training
• Bowling	• Basketball, Baseball	• Basketball (Pro)
• Ping-pong, social	• Walking Downstairs	• Climbing Stairs
• Ice Skating, light	• Snow Skiing (downhill)	• Skipping Rope
• Aquarobics, light	• Shovelling snow	• Skiing (cross country)
• Skate Boarding	• Dancing (ballroom)	• Aquarobics, advanced
• Line/Square Dancing	• Rowing, moderate	• Dancing (strenuous), Zumba
• Tai Chi, Yoga	• Volleyball, competitive	• Rowing, vigorous
• Volleyball		• Martial Arts

Note: Only those sports or activities that are sustained over a period of time (e.g running) qualify for heavy exercise. Stop-start sports such as tennis are considered 'moderate'.

WALKING PROGRAM

USE DISTANCE, STEPS OR TIME

Weeks	Distance	Steps (Pedometer)	Time
1-2	1 mile	2000	20 mins
3-5	1.5 miles	3000	28 mins
6-8	2 miles	3500	35 mins
9-10	2.5 miles	4500	45 mins
11+	3.5 miles	6000	60 mins

10,000 STEPS PER DAY

A pedometer can motivate you to be more active. It clips to your belt or waist band and registers each step.

Alternatively, use a *Fitbit*, *Garmin* or *Striiv* activity tracker, or your smartphone inbuilt accelerometer.

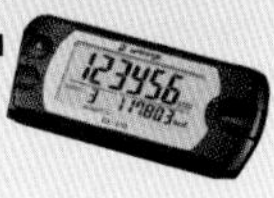

Aim for 8,000 - 10,000 steps per day, insead of an average of only 3,000 - 4,000 steps.

Reshaping Eating Behaviors

- Eating is a behavior that is largely controlled by people with whom we live or socialize, places in which we carry out our lives, and our emotions. Become aware of those situations that commonly lead to extra food being eaten.
- We may also be unaware of 'bad' eating habits that can lead to excess calorie intake; e.g. eating quickly, large mouthfuls, eating when tense or bored, finishing a large serving of food when not hungry.

Tips to help uncover and correct those 'bad' or problem eating habits:

- **Don't eat while engaged in other activities;** for example, watching TV, reading. Eat only at the table, not at the fridge or while standing.
- **Don't eat quickly.** Chewing slowly allows time to register a feeling of fullness. Don't use fingers, only utensils. Cut food into smaller pieces. Don't load your fork until the previous mouthful is finished.
- **Don't purchase problem high calorie foods.** Shop from a set list to prevent impulse buying. Avoid shopping with children.
- **Buy snack foods** in the smallest package. The larger the serving size or package, the more you are likely to eat or drink.
- **Plan meals in advance. Stick to a set menu.**
- **Plan a strategy to avoid uncontrolled eating** and drinking at social events, or when your emotions urge you to binge.

  Rehearse repeatedly in your mind exactly what you will do in such situations. Remind yourself several times each day that you are in charge of your actions and that you can be strong-willed. Seek counseling or coaching on various strategies.
- **Distract yourself** when you feel the urge to snack impulsively. Engage in some activity that will distract you from thinking about food. Examples: go for a walk, brush your teeth, phone a friend.

  If you eat out of boredom, find some new hobby or interest that gets you out of the house. Even enrol in an adult education class.

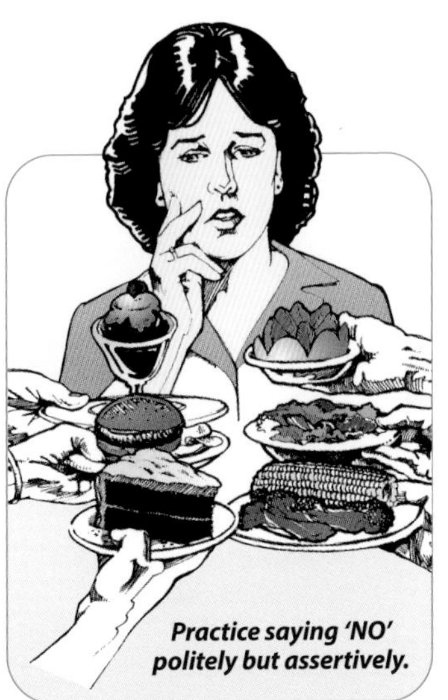

Practice saying 'NO' politely but assertively.

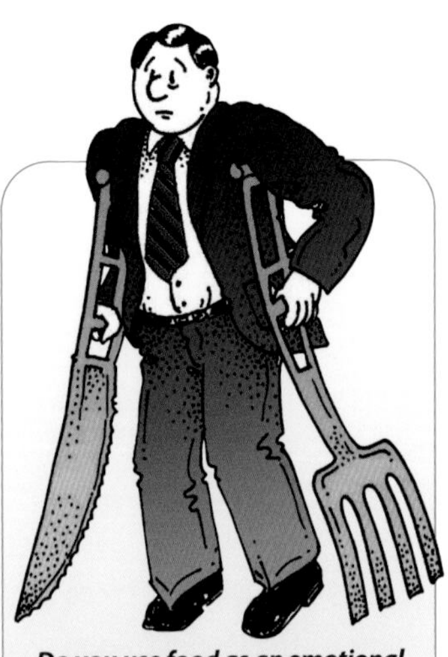

Do you use food as an emotional crutch? If so, professional counseling may be helpful.

The Value of a Food Journal

The food journal is the most powerful proven aid for dieters. Persons who keep a food and exercise journal not only lose more weight, they also keep it off. Here are some of the reasons:

- **Recording your eating and exercise habits** jolts you into realizing just what you do eat and drink each day; and also whether you exercise sufficiently.
- **Helps you identify problem foods** and drinks with excessive calories and fat.
- **Helps identify moods**, situations and events that lead to excessive eating of unwanted calories. You can then plan to overcome or avoid them.
- **Prevents 'calorie amnesia'**, the forgetfulness that leads to rebound weight gain after successful weight loss. Recording puts you back on the right track.
- **Helps you develop greater self-discipline.** You will think twice about overindulging if you have to record it - especially if someone checks your journal regularly. It certainly keeps you honest!
- **Motivates you** to carefully plan your meals and to exercise each day.
- **Serves as a check system** for your doctor, dietitian or counselor to assess your progress and make recommendations.

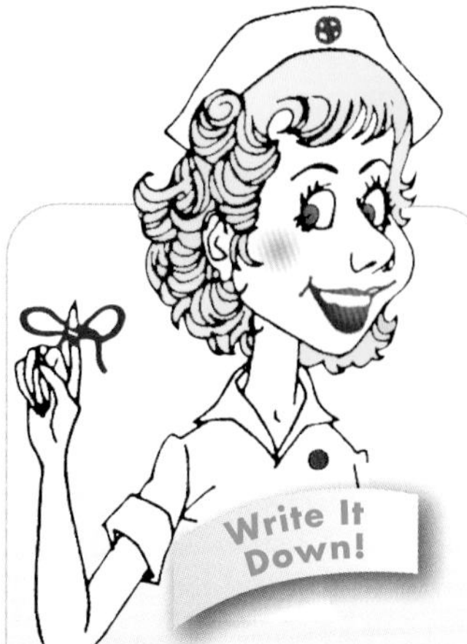

"Keeping a journal gives me feedback on exactly what I eat and drink each day.

It helps prevent 'calorie amnesia' and reminds me to exercise each day.

It's a 'must' for successful weight control!"

3 Easy Ways to Track Your Food & Exercise Calories!

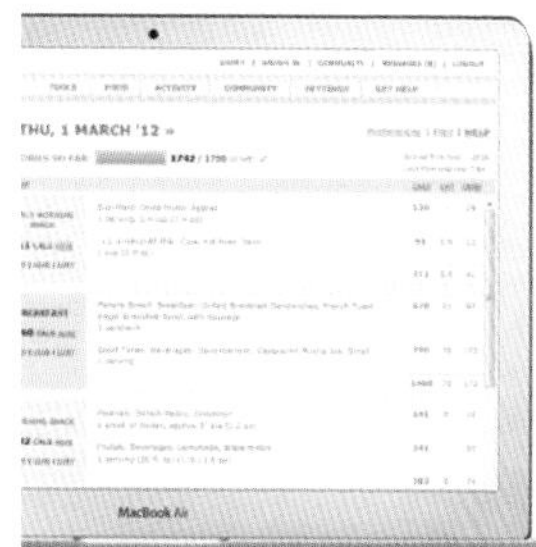

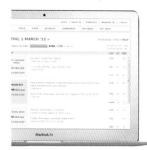

CalorieKing Online

Part of a comprehensive personalized program that includes tools, reports and a supportive community.

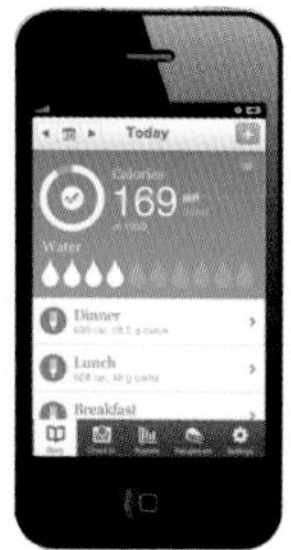

CalorieKing App

ControlMyWeight

Make smart food choices wherever you are!
Easy to use.

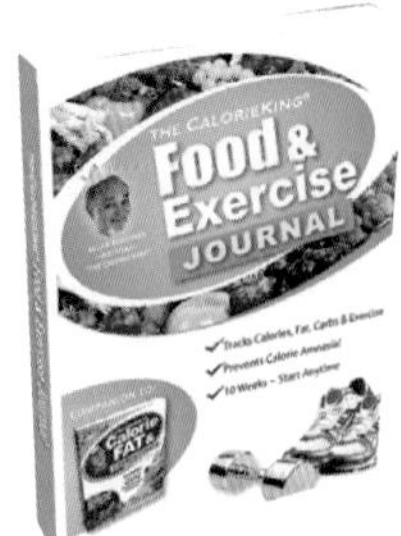

Book

A 10-week journal that fits in your pocket. Includes Weekly Summary page and Progress Checklist.

Extra Information ~ www.CalorieKing.com

Diabetes Guide

What is Diabetes?

Diabetes occurs when the body has difficulty processing glucose sugar in the blood.

- **After digestion**, sugar and starches are changed into **glucose** – the simplest form of sugar vital for body energy and growth.
- **Insulin** is the hormone which acts like a key that opens the door to body cells and allows glucose to enter.
- **Without enough insulin**, glucose builds up in the blood and passes into the urine. High blood glucose levels lead to frequent urination, extreme thirst, and tiredness.
- **Untreated diabetes increases the risk of damage to nerves and blood vessels.** This, in turn, increases the risk of heart disease, stroke, blindness, kidney damage, foot ulcers and gangrene (with amputation), impotence, Alzheimer's Disease and other problems.

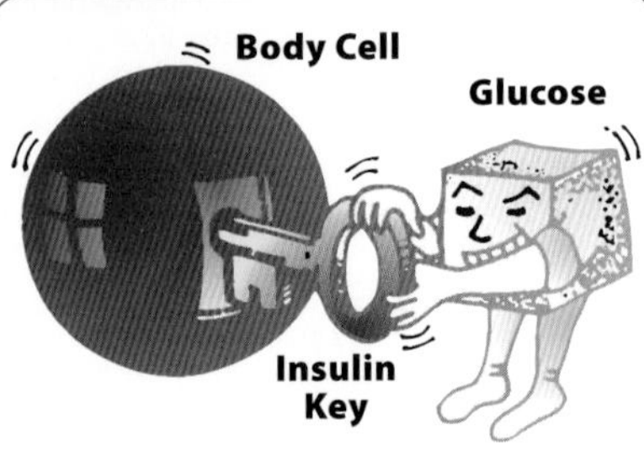

Insulin acts like a key. It opens the door to body cells and allows glucose to enter.

People with type 1 diabetes and some with type 2 have too few or no keys. They require insulin injections.

Others (primarily type 2) make enough insulin but the body doesn't use it as well as it should – particularly if obese and inactive.

SYMPTOMS OF DIABETES

- Frequent urination
- Extreme thirst
- Unusual hunger
- Rapid weight loss
- Extreme fatigue
- Blurred vision
- Skin infections that are slow to heal
- Tingling/numbness in feet

Note: Diabetes can be present even without symptoms.

DON'T IGNORE DIABETES

IT'S A SERIOUS DISEASE!

TYPE 2 DIABETES

- Occurs in 90% of diabetes cases
- Occurs mainly in adults - particularly in overweight and inactive persons
- Insulin is produced but body cells resist its action and glucose cannot enter cells
- Usually treated with meal planning and physical activity. Sometimes requires medication (pills or insulin)

TYPE 1 DIABETES

- Occurs in 10% of diabetes cases
- Usually in children and young adults
- Pancreas produces little or no insulin. Daily insulin injections (or use of an insulin pump) are necessary, as well as:
  - matching pre-meal insulin to the amount of carbohydrate eaten
  - weight control and regular physical activity

GESTATIONAL DIABETES

- Occurs in some women during pregnancy. It usually disappears after the baby's birth but still leaves mothers (1 in 3) at high risk of type 2 diabetes within 5-10 years.
- Check your blood glucose **before** and during pregnancy. High levels can harm the fetus, especially in the first 6 weeks.
- Requires weight control, a healthy lifestyle and regular medical checks.

Are You At Risk for Diabetes?

Prediabetes ~ An Early Warning!

Prediabetes means your blood glucose levels are higher than normal, but not high enough to be called diabetes.

Be aware that **prediabetes is not harmless – and may already be harming your arteries, heart, kidneys and brain.**

The good news is that you can start taking steps to prevent diabetes by making healthy lifestyle changes – such as losing weight if overweight, and being more physically active.

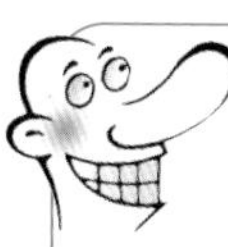

WHAT'S YOUR RISK?

Find out if you're at risk for diabetes by answering the following questions:

- ☐ I have been told I have prediabetes
- ☐ I have a family history of diabetes
- ☐ I am African American, Latino American, Asian American, Native American or a Pacific Islander
- ☐ I have had gestational diabetes (diabetes during pregnancy)
- ☐ I am over age 45
- ☐ I am overweight
- ☐ My waist is larger than: 35 inches (for a woman) or 40 inches (for a man)
- ☐ I get little or no physical activity
- ☐ My blood pressure is higher than 130 over 85
- ☐ My HDL (good cholesterol) is too low
- ☐ My triglycerides (blood fats) are too high

CHECK YOUR RESULT

- **If you've put a check mark in two or more of the boxes, you may be more likely to develop type 2 diabetes.**
- **Talk with your healthcare provider to see if you should have a blood test for diabetes.**

BLOOD GLUCOSE CLASSIFICATION OF DIABETES

Normal:	**Below 100 mg/dl***
Prediabetes:	**100-125 mg/dl***
Diabetes:	**Over 125 mg/dl***

(*Fasting Blood Glucose)

KNOW YOUR BGL

(Blood Glucose Level)

Everyone over the age of 45 should have a blood glucose test every three years.

Importance of Weight Control

- **Type 2 diabetes** is more common in people who are overweight.
- **Being overweight** means that your insulin doesn't work as well to control blood glucose levels.
- **Losing just 10 to 20 pounds** can help you better manage your diabetes and lower your risk for heart disease.

Keys to weight control include:

- Follow a healthy eating plan
- Control food portions.
- Be physically active every day. Track your daily activity.
- Keep food records ~ *See Page 15*
- Get the support of family and friends.
- **Work with a registered dietitian** who can help you reach a weight that's ideal for you.

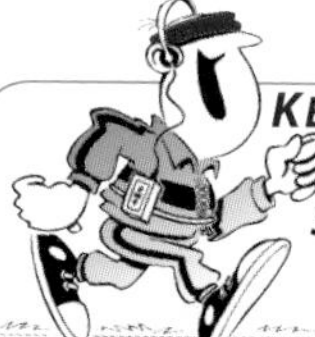

KEEP MOVING!

Every day, do at least 30 minutes of moderate intensity exercise. (even in 5-minute sets)

It's the key to improving insulin action. Add muscle strength training 3-4 times a week to double the benefits.

Managing Diabetes

Don't battle diabetes alone. Establish a partnership with your doctor, dietitian, certified diabetes educator, and pharmacist.

Extra Support:

- *American Association of Diabetes Educators*
- *American Diabetes Association*
- *BeyondType1.org*
- *Joslin Diabetes Center*
- *Juvenile Diabetes Research Foundation*
- *National Diabetes Education Program*

Tips to keep blood glucose within safe limits:

- **Control your food intake.** Know what and when you will eat. Seek referral to a dietitian for expert advice.
- **Exercise daily.** It assists weight control and can improve sensitivity of body cells to insulin. Plan physical activity into your daily routine.
- **Take insulin or oral medication as prescribed.** If on insulin, know what action to take if hypoglycemia (low blood glucose) occurs. Also educate your family and friends.
- **Monitor your blood glucose** at home and work with a blood glucose meter or CGM system. It will help you become familiar with your blood glucose patterns, and the effects of food, activity and medication.
- **Continuous glucose monitoring (CGM) tracks** your glucose levels every few minutes by using a sensor (skin patch or insert) that measures glucose levels in the tissue just below the skin. This allows the user to see a graph of glucose levels – not just single measurements from fingerstick testing. Seeing trends and patterns can help to better manage diabetes. **This results in greater awareness of unnoticed highs and lows** (as illustrated below). CGM can also help to reduce A1C with less risk of hypoglycemia for people on insulin.

Blood glucose meter systems and insulin pumps can greatly improve control of diabetes

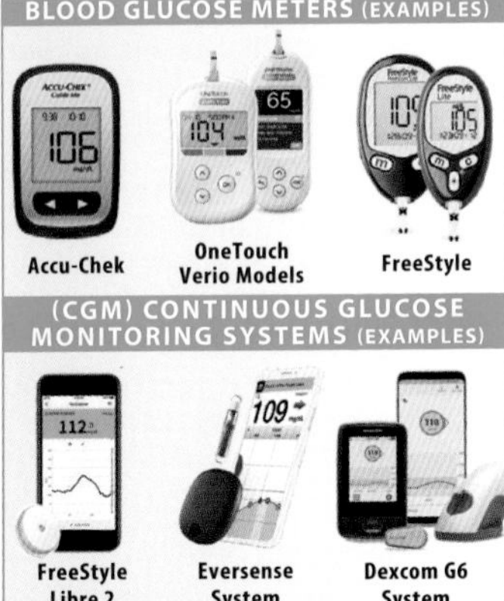

INSULIN PUMPS & SYSTEMS (EXAMPLES)

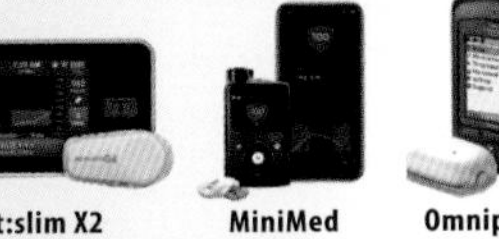

Hemoglobin A1C Target:
The hemoglobin A1C (A-one-C) test reflects your average blood glucose levels over the last 3 months. **Aim for less than 6.5%.**

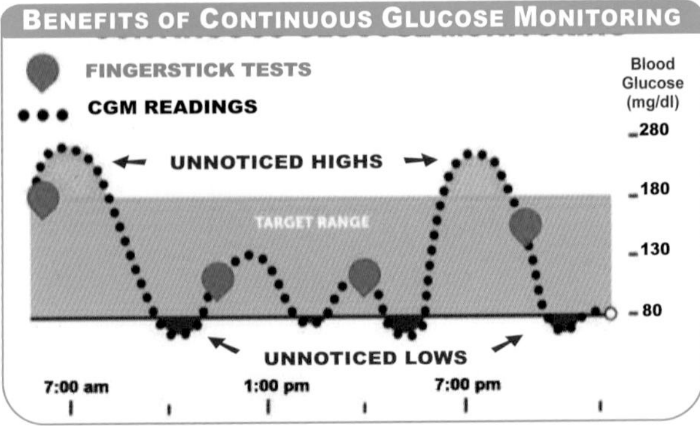

Target Blood Sugar Levels (ADA):

Before Meals:
Between 80 and 130 mg/dL

2 Hours After Meals:
Less than 180 mg/dL

Diabetes Guide ~ Meal Planning Tips

Guidelines for choosing a healthy diet apply equally to people with or without diabetes.

Eat a wide variety of wholefoods that are minimally processed, low in refined grains/flour and added sugar, high in fiber, and moderate in protein.

However, actual food quantities, as well as when you eat, will also influence control of blood glucose. Your dietitian will individualize a meal plan to suit your food preferences, lifestyle and medical status.

Healthy Diet Tips:

- **Maintain a healthy weight.** If overweight, even a modest weight loss plus daily physical activity can help manage blood glucose in type 2 diabetes.
- **Don't skip meals.** If you take insulin or an oral hypoglycemic agent, regular meals are important.

  If on insulin, eat meals at the same time each day. Eat a similar amount of food at each meal. Eating about the same amount of carbohydrate over the day will make best use of insulin and prevent wide variations in blood glucose levels.
- **Know which foods contain carbohydrate;** and learn how to check the *Nutrition Facts Label* on foods. Check the serving size, total fat and total carbohydrate – not just the sugar content. All carbohydrate breaks down to sugars after digestion.
- **Choose wholegrain breads, cereals and pasta.** Eat fresh fruits, vegetables and legumes. These foods contain more fiber and slow the release of glucose into your blood after a meal.
- **Limit sugars and foods high in added sugar** particularly if overweight. *(Extra Notes: Page 9)*
- **Choose foods with healthy fats** such as fatty fish, avocados, olives and nuts, flaxseeds, chia seeds, hemp seeds.Avoid excess use of seed oils. Ideally, use extra virgin olive oil. Avoid fried foods. Frying can oxidize seed oils that can harm our health.

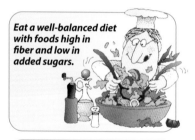

Eat a well-balanced diet with foods high in fiber and low in added sugars.

A fiber-rich diet assists the growth of friendly gut microbes that can benefit our metabolism, weight and blood glucose levels – as well as hunger, mood and our immune system.
(Also see Fiber Guide ~ Page 264)

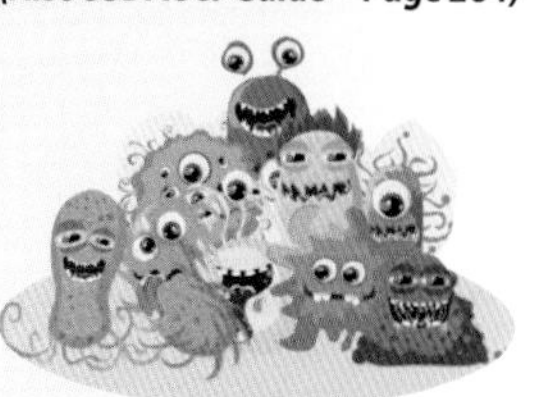

ALCOHOL TIPS

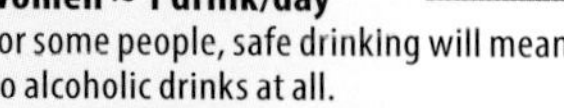

- **If you drink alcohol, have only moderate amounts:**
  Men ~ 1-2 drinks/day
  Women ~ 1 drink/day
  For some people, safe drinking will mean no alcoholic drinks at all.

(Also see Alcohol Guide ~ Page 23)

- **Drink along with your food –** especially if you use insulin or diabetes medication pills.
- **Do not omit any carb food** in exchange for an alcoholic drink. However, non-alcoholic beers (12 fl oz) count as one carb exchange.
- **Alcohol increases the risk of hypoglycemia** (low blood sugar) and drug interactions if you take insulin and certain types of diabetes pills.
- **Check with your doctor and dietitian.**

Notes for Prediabetes & Type 2 Diabetes

(Please discuss with your doctor)

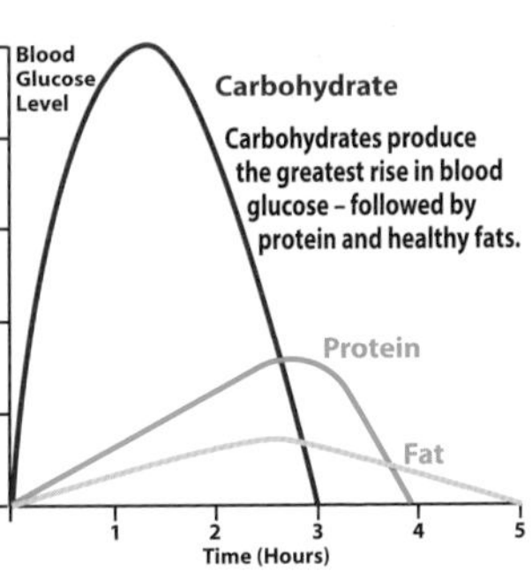

• Benefits of Lower Carb Eating:
Generally, following a lower carbohydrate pattern of eating is associated with more stable blood glucose levels (fewer highs and lows).

A reduction in blood glucose variation (high to low) can greatly reduce the need for diabetes medications (as assessed by your doctor) – as well as the risk of hypoglycemia and diabetic health complications.

Greater improvements are also usually seen with blood triglyceride fat levels and HDL-cholesterol.

• Eat earlier in the day rather than at night. The body's circadian rhythms allow for more efficient processing of foods in the first half of the day - with likely greater tissue sensitivity to insulin resulting in lower blood glucose levels. Eating late at night can lead to higher blood glucose levels and potential greater damage to body tissues – as well as reduced quality of sleep. Ideally make breakfast or lunch the main meal of the day.

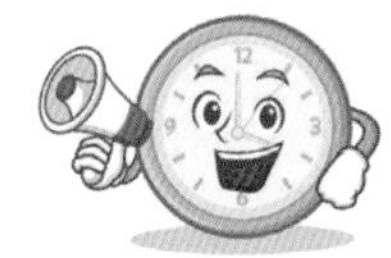

• Consume fats and oils mainly as wholefoods in which they naturally occur such as avocados, olives, cheese, milk, meats, fish, poultry and eggs.

Once vegetable seed oils (such as corn, sunflower, safflower, soy, canola) are isolated from their original food source, their unstable polyunsaturated chemical structure makes them more prone to oxidation particularly when used in high-heat cooking (broiling, frying, baking). The oxidative by-products can be toxic to body tissues and organs, including the pancreas which produces insulin *(Extra Notes ~ See page 6-7)*.

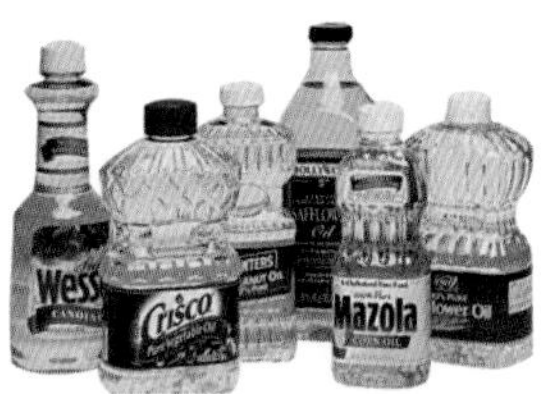

Avoid vegetable seed oils and processed foods that contain them.

• Eat your protein and vegetables before carbohydrate-rich foods such as fruit juice and bread. This greatly improves post-meal blood glucose balance (with fewer spikes), as well as insulin sensitivity. Post-meal insulin levels are also reduced.

• Benefits of Nutrition Supplements:
Persons with Type 2 diabetes are at greater risk of nutritional deficiencies due to the extra inflammatory stresses throughout the body. Further deficiencies can also result from prescribed drugs, such as statin cholesterol-lowering drugs, anti-inflammatory drugs for pain relief, stomach acid-suppressing drugs and antibiotics.

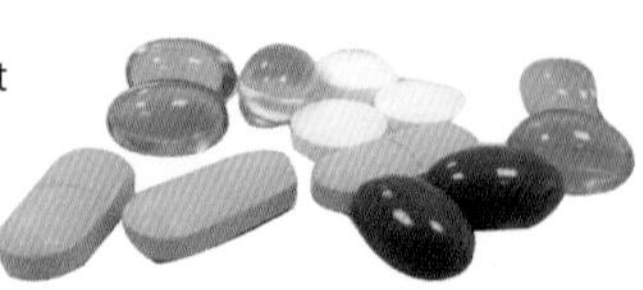

People with diabetes may benefit from nutrition supplements. Check with your doctor.

Check with your doctor about the potential benefits of supplements such as coenzyme Q10, multi-vitamins, vitamins D and K2, magnesium, omega-3 fish or algal oils, astaxanthin, berberine (if statin-intolerant), curcumin – all of which have clinical studies showing potential health benefits.

Carb Type Affects Blood Glucose

The various forms of carbohydrate affect blood glucose levels in different ways. It is difficult to predict the effect of particular foods, sugars, or meals, simply by their carbohydrate content.

Thus the same amount of carbohydrate from different foods may affect blood sugar levels very differently. **Many factors affect the rate of digestion and absorption such as:**

- the type of sugar, starch, and fiber
- the degree of processing and cooking (which increases digestion rate)
- the amount of protein and fat (which slow stomach emptying and digestion).

Additionally, the effect of particular foods on blood glucose can differ markedly between individuals.

Glycemic Index (GI)

The GI is a method of ranking carbohydrate foods on a scale (0-100) according to how they affect blood glucose levels. (See next column).

The higher the GI value, the greater the food's ability to rapidly raise blood glucose levels; and the more insulin that is needed by the body (not desirable).

Eating low-GI foods may lead to better control of blood glucose and insulin levels (which in turn lowers the risk of damage to blood vessels and nerves). The slower digestion of low-GI foods may also help to delay hunger pangs and benefit weight control.

Cautionary Notes on GI

Choosing low-GI foods is not a license to eat unlimited amounts. Calorie restriction and portion control for weight control is of prime importance.

Also remember, **low-GI foods are carbohydrate foods** and must still be counted as part of any dietetic carbohydrate plan.

GI is not meant to be used by itself without regard to portion size, and other dietary recommendations for healthy eating. Foods are not good or bad on the basis of their GI.

LOWER-GLYCEMIC FOODS

Slower-Acting Carbohydrates

These foods are more slowly digested and absorbed. They help maintain more even blood glucose levels, as long as excessive amounts are not eaten. Use these foods regularly but still limit portion size for weight control.

Examples:

- **Dried beans, peas, lentils**
- **Nuts and seeds**
- **Wholegrain breads**
- **Bran cereals, oats**
- **Sweet corn, barley, quinoa buckwheat**
- **Wholegrain pasta, basmati rice**
- **Fresh fruit: apples, avocados, bananas (firm), berries, cherries, grapefruit, grapes, olives, oranges, pears, plums. Fresh juices.**
- **Vegetables: broccoli, yam, nopales, salad greens**
- **Milk, yogurt, soy drinks**
- **Dark chocolate, cacao**
- **Sugar alcohols (sorbitol, maltitol)**

HIGHER-GLYCEMIC FOODS

Quicker-Acting Carbohydrates

These foods more rapidly raise blood glucose levels. Eat only in moderation.

- **White bread, rice cakes, bagels, croissants, doughnuts**
- **Low-fiber cereals: Cornflakes, *Rice Krispies, Froot Loops***
- **White potatoes, white rice**
- **Watermelon, ripe bananas, cantaloupe, pineapple**
- **Soda, sugar-sweetened sports and energy drinks**
- **Sugar, candy, popcorn (plain)**
- **Ice cream (low-fat), frozen yogurt**

High-GI fruits and potatoes can be healthy choices when eaten in moderate amounts.

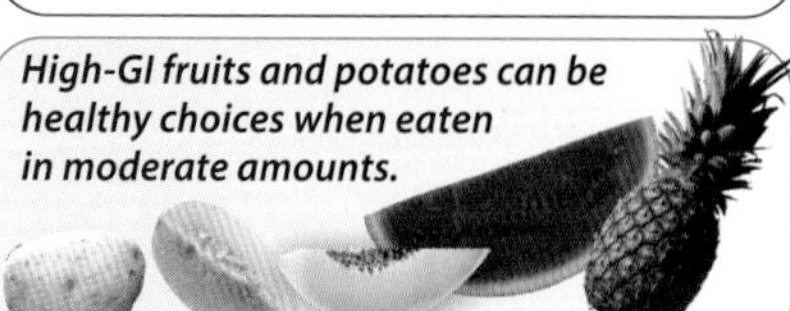

» **Calorie and fat values have been rounded off.**
Calories ~ to the nearest 5 or 10 calories.
Fat ~ to nearest half gram. **Note:** Trace amounts of fat (less than 0.3 grams) have been treated as zero.

» **Carbohydrate figures** in this book are for total carbohydrate, and not **Net Carbs** (which deducts fiber, polydextrose and sugar alcohols from total carbs).

» Because manufacturers' figures on labels are rounded off, figures in this book may differ slightly from the label. Serving sizes may also vary.

IMPORTANT DISCLAIMER

* The authors and publishers of this book are not physicians and are not licensed to give medical advice.This book is not a substitute for professional advice.Users should consult their medical professional before making any health, medical or other decisions based on the material contained herein.

* This book is a compilation of original material from other sources intended for educational purposes only. Because food manufacturers constantly change their products, only they are the authoritative source for food's most current nutritional information.

* Persons using the information herein for any medical purposes, such as matching insulin dosage to carbohydrate intake, should not rely solely on the accuracy of figures herein and should independently check food labels or contact the food manufacturer for the latest data.

Canadian Readers:

Please note that figures in this book are based on U.S. food products and restaurants. Equivalent Canadian foods may vary and should be checked independently.

* WARRANTY DISCLAIMER:

THE AUTHOR AND PUBLISHER DISCLAIM ANY LIABILITY ARISING DIRECTLY OR INDIRECTLY FROM THE USE OF THIS BOOK.THE INFORMATION HEREIN IS PROVIDED "AS IS" AND WITHOUT ANY WARRANTY EXPRESSED OR IMPLIED. ALL DIRECT, INDIRECT, SPECIAL, INCIDENTAL, CONSEQUENTIAL OR PUNITIVE DAMAGES ARISING FROM ANY USE OF THIS INFORMATION IS DISCLAIMED AND EXCLUDED.

This information is also provided subject to Family Health Publications' Terms and Conditions found at the website, www.calorieking.com/terms and incorporated herein.

C ~ Calories

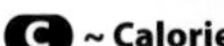

F ~ Fat (grams)

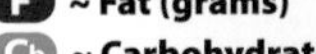

Cb ~ Carbohydrate (grams)

Abbreviations

tsp = teaspoon
Tbsp or T = Tablespoon
oz = ounce(s)
c = cup
fl.oz = fluid ounce(s)
g = gram(s)
avg = average
pkg = package

Volume Measures

(All measures are level)

3 tsp = 1 Tbsp
2 Tbsp = 1 fl.oz
½ cup = 4 fl.oz
1 cup = 8 fl.oz
2 cups = 1 Pint
2 Pints = 1 Quart

Note: 8 oz weight is not the same as 8 fl oz volume (space occupied). Dense foods weigh more per set volume. Examples:

1 cup popcorn weighs ½ oz
1 cup milk weighs 8½ oz
1 cup pudding weighs 10 oz

Metric Conversion

½ oz = 14 grams
1 oz = 28.4 grams
2 oz = 57 grams
3½ oz = 100 grams
1 fl.oz = 30 mls
1 cup (8 fl.oz) = 240 mls
33 fl.oz = 1 liter (volume)

INFORMATION SOURCES

- U.S. Dept. of Agriculture
- U.S. Food Manufacturers
- Food Industry Boards & Councils
- Author extrapolations

FEEDBACK WELCOME!

Please contact the author with your queries and suggestions.
feedback@calorieking.com

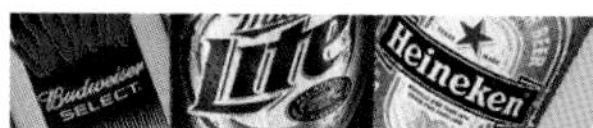

- **Health Hazards: Excessive alcohol intake** contributes to obesity, high blood pressure, stroke, heart and liver disease, some cancers, and even impotence. **Concentration and short-term memory** are reduced as well as athletic performance.

  Other alcohol hazards include: Fetal Alcohol Syndrome, stomach upsets, gut dysbiosis, menstrual and menopausal problems, depression, snoring, sleep problems, work absenteeism, impaired judgement, risky behaviors and social/family problems.
- **Alcohol contributes to obesity** through its high calories and by lessening the body's ability to burn fat. Fat storage is promoted, particularly in the belly – a health danger zone. Alcohol can also stimulate the appetite; and weaken the dieter's resolve!
- **Alcohol is potentially more harmful while dieting:** Blood sugar levels may drop with resultant fatigue and further impairment of concentration, reflexes and driving skills.

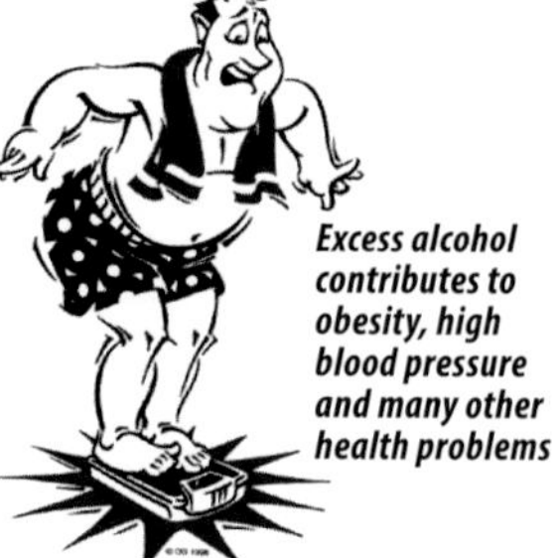

Excess alcohol contributes to obesity, high blood pressure and many other health problems

LOWER RISK ALCOHOL LIMITS

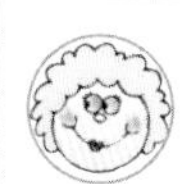

WOMEN:
No more than
1 drink per day

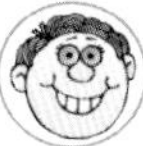

MEN:
No more than
2 drinks per day
(1 drink if over 65 y.o.)

(At least 2 days a week should be alcohol-free)

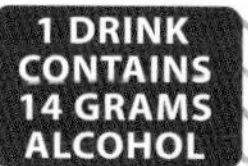

1 DRINK CONTAINS 14 GRAMS ALCOHOL
- **12 fl.oz Regular Beer (5% Alc.)**
- **OR 14 fl.oz Light Beer (4.2% Alc.)**
- **OR 5 fl.oz Wine (12% Alc.)**
- **OR 1½ fl.oz Spirits (80 Proof)**

Note: You cannot save daily drinks for one occasion. Binge drinking is particularly harmful: 4 drinks for males or 3 drinks for females (within 2 hours).

For some people, safe drinking means no alcohol at all. Even one drink may impair driving skills, particularly if tired. For women who drink frequently, breast cancer risk is increased by 9% for each drink after the first drink. In men, just 2 drinks a day doubles the risk of cancers of the mouth and throat.

It is advisable not to drink at all if you are:
- pregnant, trying to conceive or breastfeeding
- taking medication or have liver or heart disease (unless approved by your doctor or pharmacist)
- planning to drive, use machinery or play sports
- studying or needing to concentrate
- a child or adolescent

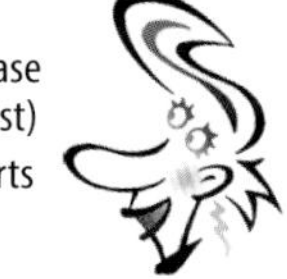

Women and adolescents are more prone to alcohol's ill-effects due to their lower body weight, smaller livers and lesser capacity to metabolize alcohol. As we age, our ability to handle alcohol decreases.

HOW TO CALCULATE ALCOHOL CONTENT

Percent alcohol on label refers to alcohol volume (ml alcohol/100ml). Note: 100ml = 3½ fl.oz

To convert to grams (weight) of alcohol, multiply the alcohol volume by 0.8 – since 1 ml of alcohol weighs only 0.8 grams.

EXAMPLE:
12 fl.oz Can Beer (5% alcohol)

5% alc. volume
= 5% of 12 fl.oz = 0.6 fl.oz
= 18ml alcohol (Note: 1 fl.oz = 30ml)
Weight (18ml x 0.8) = 14.4g alcohol

GOVERNMENT WARNINGS!

(1) According to the Surgeon General, women should not drink alcoholic beverages during pregnancy because of the risk of birth defects.

(2) Consumption of alcoholic beverages impairs your ability to drive a car or operate machinery, and may cause health problems.

EXTRA INFORMATION

Alcohol & Diabetes ~ See Page 19
Alcohol & The Heart ~ See Page 18
Tips to Avoid Harmful Drinking ~ Page 19

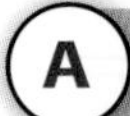

Alcohol ~ Beers ◊ Ales (with Alcohol Counts)

Quick Guide

Alc ~ Alcohol (Grams)
Cb ~ Carbohydrate

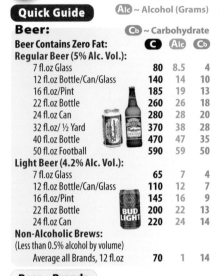

Beer:

Beer Contains Zero Fat:	C	Alc	Cb
Regular Beer (5% Alc. Vol.):			
7 fl.oz Glass	**80**	8.5	4
12 fl.oz Bottle/Can/Glass	**140**	14	10
16 fl.oz/Pint	**185**	19	13
22 fl.oz Bottle	**260**	26	18
24 fl.oz Can	**280**	28	20
32 fl.oz/ ½ Yard	**370**	38	28
40 fl.oz Bottle	**470**	47	35
50 fl.oz Football	**590**	59	50
Light Beer (4.2% Alc. Vol.):			
7 fl.oz Glass	**65**	7	4
12 fl.oz Bottle/Can/Glass	**110**	12	7
16 fl.oz/Pint	**145**	16	9
22 fl.oz Bottle	**200**	22	13
24 fl.oz Can	**220**	24	14
Non-Alcoholic Brews:			
(Less than 0.5% alcohol by volume)			
Average all Brands, 12 fl.oz	**70**	1	14

Beer ~ Brands

Note: Figure shown are for the United States except for the states of Utah, Colorado, Kansas and Oklahoma who have certain restrictions limiting the alcohol content to not more than 4% by volume (3.2% by weight).

Percentage alcohol listed is by volume - not by weight.

Per 12 fl.oz Serving	C	Alc	Cb
Aguila (3.9%)	**125**	12	14
Amstel, Light (3.5%)	**95**	10	5
Anchor: Porter (5.6%)	**210**	16	23
Steam (4.9%)	**160**	14	14
Asahi: Kuronama (5.3%)	**165**	14	14
Select (4.7%)	**140**	13	11
Super Dry (4.9%)	**150**	14	11
Bass, Pale Ale (5.1%)	**155**	14	12
Beck's: Original (5%)	**145**	14	11
Premier Light (2.3%)	**65**	7	4
Sapphire (6%)	**160**	17	9
Big Sky: Original IPA (6.2%)	**195**	18	17
Moose Drool (5.3%)	**175**	15	16
Scape Goat (4.7%)	**155**	14	14
Trout Slayer Ale (4.7%)	**145**	14	12
Blatz: Original (4.6%)	**145**	13	13
Light (3.9%)	**110**	11	8
Blue Moon:			
Belgian White (5.4%)	**170**	15	14
Mango Wheat (5.4%)	**175**	15	16
Bohemia (4.73%)	**140**	14	12
Bud Ice (5.5%)	**125**	16	4

Brands (Cont)

Alc ~ Alcohol (Grams)

Per 12 fl.oz Serving	C	Alc	Cb
Bud Light: Regular (4.2%)	**110**	12	7
Chelado: Clamato (4.2%)	**150**	12	16
Extra Lime; Mangonada (4.2%), av.	**155**	12	17
Lemonade (4.2%)	**150**	12	16
Lime (4.2%)	**115**	12	8
Orange; Grapefruit (4.2%)	**145**	12	14
NEXT (4%)	**80**	11	0
Platinum (6%)	**140**	17	3
Budweiser: Lager (5%)	**145**	14	11
Chelado Clamato (5%)	**185**	14	20
Select (4.3%)	**100**	12	3
Select 55 (2.4%)	**55**	7	2
Supreme (4.6%)	**145**	13	12
Zero (0%)	**50**	0	12
Busch: Beer (4.3%)	**115**	12	7
Ice (5.9%)	**135**	17	4
Light (4.1%)	**95**	12	3
NA (0.4%)	**60**	1	13
Carlsberg, Pilsner (5%)	**135**	14	10
Carta Blanca (4.6%)	**145**	13	11
Cerveza, Aguila (4%)	**125**	11	11
Colorado Native, Amber (5.5%)	**170**	16	15
Colt 45, Malt Liquor (5.6%)	**155**	16	11
Coors: Banquet (5%)	**145**	14	12
Light (4.2%)	**100**	12	5
Non-Alcoholic	**60**	0	12
Corona: Extra (4.6%)	**150**	13	14
Light (4%)	**100**	11	5
Non-Alcoholic	**60**	0	17
Premier (4%)	**90**	11	11
Dos Equis XX: Ambar (4.7%)	**145**	14	12
Lager (4.5%)	**140**	13	11
Extra Gold (5%)	**150**	14	12
Fosters: Lager (5%)	**145**	14	11
Premium Ale (5.5%)	**160**	16	13
Genesee: Beer (4.5%)	**145**	13	13
Light (4%)	**100**	10	4
George Killian's, Irish Red (5.4%)	**170**	16	15
Goose Island, So-Lo (3%)	**100**	8	9
Grolsch, Premium (5%)	**145**	14	10
Guinness: Draught (4%)	**125**	12	10
Extra Stout (6%)	**175**	17	14
Blonde American (5%)	**150**	14	11
Nitro IPA (5.8%), 11.2oz	**155**	19	5
Hamm's, Premium (4.7%)	**145**	13	12
Heineken: Original (5%)	**140**	14	11
Premium Light (3.5%)	**100**	10	7
Silver (4%)	**95**	11	3
0.0 (Alcohol-Free)	**75**	0	12
Hop Valley: Bubble Stash (6.2%)	**195**	17	16
Citrus Mistress (6.5%)	**190**	18	14
Hurricane: Malt Liquor (6%)	**140**	17	4
High Gravity (8.1%)	**185**	23	6
Icehouse, Original (5.5%)	**150**	16	10

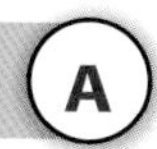

Brands (Cont)

Alc ~ Alcohol (Grams) Cb ~ Carbohydrate

Beer Contains Zero Fat:
Per 12 fl.oz Serving

	C	Alc	Cb
King Cobra (6%)	135	17	4
Kirin: Ichiban (5%)	145	14	11
Light (3.2%)	95	9	8
Kokanee (5%)	145	14	11
Labatt: Blue (5%)	135	14	10
Blue Light (4%)	110	11	8
Laqunitas, Daytime (4%)	100	12	3
Landshark, Lager (4.6%)	150	13	13
Leinenkugel's: Original (4.7%)	150	13	15
Summer Shandy (4.2%)	135	12	13
Lone Star: Pale Lager (4.65%)	135	13	11
Light (3.85%)	110	11	8
Lowenbrau, Original (5%)	140	14	12
Magic Hat, #9 (5.1% alc)	165	15	15
Michelob Ultra:			
Ultra Amber (4%)	100	11	5
Ultra Infusions, Lime (4%)	95	11	5
Ultra Light (4.2%)	95	12	3
Ultra Pure Gold (3.8%)	85	12	3
Mickey's, Malt Liquor (5.6%)	155	16	11
Miller:			
Genuine Draft/High Life (4.6%)	140	13	12
High Life Light (4.1%)	110	12	6
Lite (4.2%)	95	12	3
Miller64 (2.8%)	65	8	3
Milwaukee's Best:			
Light (4.1%)	95	12	4
Premium (4.8%)	145	14	12
Minnesota's Best, Original (4.9%)	140	14	10
Modelo, Especial (4.4%)	145	13	14
Molson Canadian: Ice (5.6%)	170	16	14
Lager (5%)	150	14	12
Canadian 67 (3%)	70	8	3
Moosehead, Lager (5%)	150	14	11
Natural: Ice (5.9%)	130	17	4
Light (4.2%)	95	12	3
Negra Modelo (5.4%)	175	15	16
Newcastle, Brown Ale (4.7%)	130	13	10
O'Douls: Amber (0.4%)	90	1	18
Original (0.4%)	65	1	13
Old Milwaukee: Lager (4.6%)	145	13	13
Light (3.8%)	110	11	8
Non-Alcoholic (0.4%)	60	1	12
Old Style: Lager (4.7%)	145	13	12
Light (4.2%)	115	12	7
Pabst: Blue Ribbon (4.8%)	145	13	12
Low Calorie (3.8%)	110	11	8
Pacifico, Clara (4.4%)	145	12	13

Per 12 fl.oz Serving	C	Alc	Cb
	Unless Indicated		
Palmier, (4.2%), 11.2 fl.oz	90	11	3
Peroni, Nastro Azzurro (5.1%)	150	14	12
Piels, Lager (4.3%)	125	12	9
Pilsner Urquell, Lager (4.4%)	155	12	16
Point: Amber Classic (4.7%)	160	13	14
Special Lager (4.7%)	150	13	12
Presidente (5%)	175	14	5
Redbridge, Lager (4%)	135	10	14
Red Dog, Lager (4.8%)	145	14	12
Red Hook: ESB (5.8%)	185	16	16
India Pale Ale (4.7%)	190	13	19
Red Stripe, Jamaican Lager (4.7%)	150	13	14
Redd's: Apple Ale (5%), 12 fl.oz	165	14	17
Wicked Hard Ale (8%), av. 10 fl.oz	230	19	25
Samuel Adams:			
Boston Lager (4.9%)	175	14	17
Sam Adams, Light Lager (4%)	120	13	8
Sapporo, Prem. Lager (4.9%)	135	14	9
Schaefer: Lager (4.6%)	145	13	12
Light (3.9%)	110	11	8
Schell's: Deer (4.7%)	145	14	13
Light (3.5%)	100	10	7
Schlitz: Pale Lager (4.6%)	145	13	12
Light (3.8%)	110	11	8
Schmidt's: Pale Lager (4.6%)	145	13	13
Light (3.8%)	110	11	8
Sharps, *(Miller)*, N.A., 12 fl.oz	60	0	12
Sheaf, Stout (5.7%)	190	16	19
Shock Top: Belgian White (5.2%)	165	15	15
Lemon Shandy (4.2%)	145	12	15
Sierra Nevada: Bigfoot (9.6%)	330	28	32
Draft Pale Ale (5%)	155	14	13
Pale Ale (5.6%)	175	16	14
Sol: Lager (4.5%)	140	13	12
Chelada (3.5%)	160	10	20
Sparks, Lager (6%)	250	17	34
Steel Reserve:			
High Gravity Malt Liquor (8.1%)	220	23	15
Steel 6.0 (6%)	165	17	11
Stella Artois, (5%), 11.2 fl.oz	140	14	11
Stroh's: Classic (4.5%)	145	13	12
Light (4.1%)	120	12	7
Tecate: Pale Lager (4.6%)	140	13	11
Light (4%)	110	11	8
Third Shift, Amber Lager (5.3%)	185	15	18
Trader Jose: Premium, 11.2 fl.oz	145	14	14
Light (3.8%), 11.2 fl.oz	105	14	8
Victoria Lager (4%)	135	11	14
Wild Blue, Lager (8%)	240	23	20
Yuengling: Light (3.2%)	99	9	9
Traditional Lager (4.5%)	140	13	12
ZeigenBock, Amber (4.9%)	145	14	11

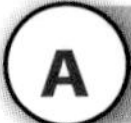

Alcohol ~ Cider ◆ Wine

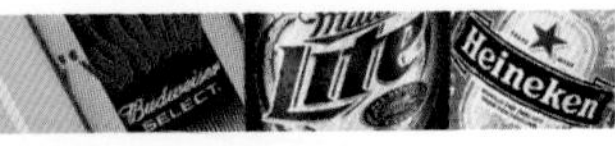

Alc ~ Alcohol (Grams) Cb ~ Carbohydrate

Ciders ~ Alcoholic/Hard

Per 12 fl.oz Unless Indicated	C	Alc	Cb
Ace: Apple (5%), 12 fl.oz	145	14	12
Berry (5%), 12 fl.oz	155	14	14
Joker (6.9%), 12 fl.oz	190	19	13
Perry (5%), 12 fl.oz	170	14	18
Pineapple (5%), 12 fl.oz	175	14	19
Angry Orchard: Crisp Apple (5%)	190	14	25
Green Apple (5.5%), 12 fl.oz	210	14	31
Hard Core (8%), 12 fl.oz	235	22	20
Pear (5%), 12 fl.oz	160	14	17
Rosé (5.5%), 12 fl.oz	170	16	17
Bold Rock: Apple, (4.7%), 12 fl.oz	140	13	12
Carolina Draft (4.7%), 12 fl.oz	145	13	13
IPA (4.7%), 12 fl.oz	140	13	12
Pear (4.7%), 12 fl.oz	140	13	12
Premium Dry (6%), 12 fl.oz	140	17	6
Crispin, Original (5%), 12 fl.oz	160	24	15
Hornsby's: Amber (5.5%)	180	16	19
Crisp (5.5%), 12 fl.oz	190	16	26
Johnny Appleseed, (5.5%)	210	16	26
Magners, (4.5%)	125	13	9
Michelob, Ultra Light Cider (4%)	120	10	10
Schilling: Big Zesty (6.9%)	200	19	17
Excelsior Apple (8.5%)	230	24	16
Grapefruit & Chill (6%)	185	17	16
Local Legend (5.2%)	135	15	7
Moon Berries (5.2%)	150	15	11
Smith & Forge, Hard Apple (6%)	220	17	26
Stella Artois Cidre, (4.5%)	180	13	22
Strongbow: *Per 11.2 fl oz*			
Gold Apple (5%)	170	13	19
Original Dry (5%):			
8.5 fl.oz mini can	105	10	7
16.9 fl.oz can	205	20	14
2 Towns Ciderhouse:			
Brightcider Apple (6%), 12 fl.oz	145	17	7
Ginger Ninja (6%), 12 fl.oz	145	17	7
Made Marion (6%), 12 fl.oz	150	17	8
Outcider (5%), 12 fl.oz	155	14	14
Pacific Pineapple (5%), 12 fl.oz	150	14	12
Woodchuck: Amber (5%)	200	14	21
Granny Smith (5%), 12 fl.oz	160	14	11
Pear (4%), 12 fl.oz	150	12	18
Raspberry (4%), 12 fl.oz	170	12	22
Woodchuck 100, (4.2%), 12 fl.oz	100	12	5
Wyder's: Berry Ginger (5%), 12 fl.oz	170	14	20
Pear (4%), 12 fl.oz	140	11	22
Prickly Pineapple (5%), 12 fl.oz	180	14	22
Raspberry (4%), 12 fl.oz	120	11	17
Reposado (6.9%), 12 fl.oz	250	19	30

Quick Guide ~ Table Wines

Average all Varieties (11.5% Alc.) (Wine Contains Zero Fat)	C	Alc	Cb
4 fl.oz, 1 small wine glass OR ½ large wine glass	100	11	3
6 fl.oz, (¾ large wine glass)	145	16	5
8 fl.oz, (1 large wine glass)	200	21	7
½ Carafe/Bottle, 12 fl.oz	300	32	10
1 Bottle, 750ml, 25.4 fl.oz	620	68	21
Red Wines: *Per 4 fl.oz*			
Burgundy/Cabernet/Merlot, av.	100	11	4
White Wines: *Per 4 fl.oz*			
Dry (Chenin; Fume Blanc; Chardonnay)	95	11	4
Sparkling, 4 fl.oz	95	11	4
Zinfandel Sweet, (Moselle/Sauterne), 4 fl.oz	85	11	2

Other Wines

	C	Alc	Cb
Champagne: *Per 4 fl.oz*			
Average all types, 1 glass	85	11	2
with Orange Jce (3:1 orange)	75	8	4
with Orange Jce (1:1 orange)	65	5	7
Mulled Wine *(Gluhwein)*, 4 fl.oz	180	14	20
Non-Alcoholic Wine: *Less than 0.5% Alcohol*			
Ariel: White varieties, average, 4 fl.oz	35	0.5	8
Red varieties, average, 4 fl.oz	25	0.5	5
Flavored/Reduced Alcohol Wine:			
Average All Brands (6% alcohol): (Arbor Mist, Wild Vines, Boone's Farm):			
1 small wine glass, 4 fl.oz	80	6	10
1 large wine glass, 8 fl.oz	160	11	20
Skinnygirl, Red/White, (8.5%), 5 fl.oz	100	10	5
Sake *(Gekkeikan)*, (16%), 4 fl.oz	120	15	5
Sangria *(Skinnygirl)*, (4%), 5 fl.oz	130	5	23

Dessert Wines

	C	Alc	Cb
Madeira (18%), 2 oz	85	9	5
Marsala (18%), 2 oz	110	9	11
Port, Muscatel (18%), 2 oz	85	9	5
Sherry (15%), 2 oz:			
Dry, 1 Sherry glass	90	7	7
Sweet/Cream, average	90	7	8
Vermouth *(Martini & Rossi)*:			
Extra Dry (18%), 2 oz	65	9	2
Martini Rosso (16%), 2 oz	90	8	8

Cooking Wines

	C	Alc	Cb
Holland House:			
Marsala, (14%), 2 T., 1 fl.oz	45	4	4
Red/White, (10%): 2 T., 1 fl.oz	20	2	1
1 cup, 8 fl.oz	160	18	8
Sherry, (17%), 2 Tbsp, 1 fl.oz	45	5	2

Quick Guide

Alc ~ Alcohol (Grams)

Spirits/Liquors:
Includes Bourbon, Brandy, Gin, Rum, Scotch, Tequila, Vodka, Whiskey.
Note: All spirits with same alcohol proof have similar calories and zero fat.

Average All Brands	C	Alc	Cb
80 Proof (40% Alcohol by Volume):			
1 fl.oz	**65**	9.5	0
1.5 fl.oz (1 shot)	**100**	14	0
3 fl.oz (Double shot)	**195**	28	0
½ Bottle, 350 ml (12 fl.oz)	**770**	113	0
1 Bottle, 700 ml (24 fl.oz)	**1540**	227	0
86 Proof (43% Alc), 1.5 fl.oz shot	**105**	15	0
100 Proof (50% Alc), 1.5 fl.oz	**125**	18	0
Shochu (Soju), av., (25% alc), 2 fl.oz	**65**	12	0

Flavored Spirits

	C	Alc	Cb
Captain Morgan: *Per 1.5 fl.oz*			
Original (35%)	**85**	12	0.5
Black Spiced (47.3%)	**115**	14	1
Parrot Bay (21%), average	**90**	7.5	10
Silver Spiced (35%)	**95**	12	2
Malibu Rum, Orig,/Fruit (21%), 1.5 fl.oz	**80**	8	8
Southern Comfort (35%), 1.5 fl.oz	**100**	13	3

Hard Lemonade, Sodas, Seltzers & Tea

	C	Alc	Cb
Bud Light Seltzers, (5%), 12 fl.oz	**100**	14	2
Corona Seltzers, (4.5%), avg. 12 fl.oz	**100**	12	3
Henry's Hard Soda:			
Grape (4.2%), 12 fl.oz	**225**	12	35
Lemon Lime/Orange (4.2%), 12 fl.oz	**190**	12	28
Labatt Blue Light Seltzer, (5%)	**100**	14	1
Mike's Hard Lemonade:			
Black Cherry (5%), 11.2 fl.oz	**220**	13	33
Lite (5%), 11.2 fl.oz	**150**	13	15
Hard Freeze (5%), avg. 12 fl.oz	**220**	14	33
Lemonade (5%), 11.2 fl.oz	**220**	13	33
Harder (8%), 16 fl.oz	**395**	31	44
Zero Sugar (4.8%(, 12 fl.oz	**100**	13	0
Not Your Father's Root Beer, (5.9%), 12 fl.oz	**195**	17	20
Pabst Hard Coffee, (5%), 11 fl.oz	**250**	13	31
Pura Still, (4.5%), 11.2 fl.oz	**90**	12	1
Redd's Wicked, (8%), av. 10 fl.oz	**230**	19	25
Social Club Seltzer, (7%), 12 fl.oz	**150**	20	2
Sparks, Original (6%), 16 fl.oz	**335**	23	45
Twisted Tea: Original (5%)	**220**	14	31
Half & Half (5%)	**260**	14	34
White Claw, Hard Seltzers (5%), avg.	**100**	14	11
Zumbida Mango, (4.2%), 12 fl.oz	**150**	12	17

Coolers & Premix Cocktails

Ready-To-Drink: *Zero Fat Unless Indicated*	C	Alc	Cb
Bacardi: *Per 4 fl.oz*			
Party Drinks (Ready To Pour):			
Bahama Mama; Mai Tai (10%)	**130**	9	16
Mojito (15%)	**160**	14	16
Rum Island Ice Tea (12.5%)	**150**	12	16
Bacardi Silver: *Per 12 fl.oz*			
Lemonade/Sangria (6%), av.	**270**	17	41
Mojito/Raz/Strawberry (5%)	**240**	14	36
Bartles & Jaymes: *Per 11.2 fl.oz*			
Malt Based Coolers (3.2%):			
Exotic Berry	**195**	9	31
Fuzzy Navel	**215**	9	36
Margarita; Pina Colada, av.	**245**	9	44
Pomegranate Raspberry	**205**	9	35
Sangria	**240**	9	40
Strawberry Daiquiri	**205**	9	34
Cape Lime, Cocktails (4.5%), av. 12 fl.oz	**120**	13	9
Captain Morgan's, Parrot Bay (4.1%), all var. av., 11.2 fl.oz	**210**	10	35
Chi Chi's: Long Is. Iced Tea, 4 fl.oz	**145**	12	17
Mojito, 4 fl.oz	**160**	11	21
Pina Colada, 4 fl.oz (6g fat)	**240**	4	42
White Russian, 4 fl.oz (7g fat)	**245**	2	43
Daily's, Frozen Pouches (5%), average all flavors, 10 fl.oz	**285**	12	47
Jack Daniels, Country Cocktails (4.8%), average all varieties, 10 fl.oz	**200**	9	30
Jose Cuervo:			
Margaritas: Classic Lime (10%), 6 fl.oz	**210**	14	29
Golden (12.7%), 4.7 fl.oz	**170**	14	19
Pabst, Hard Coffee (5%), 11 fl.oz	**250**	13	31
Ritas: Lime-A-Rita (8%), 8 fl.oz	**220**	15	29
Spritz (6%), av., 12 fl.oz	**200**	17	21
Seagram's:			
Escapes Coolers (3.2%):			
Bahama Mama, 11.2 fl.oz	**200**	9	36
Strawb. Daiquiri, 11.2 fl.oz	**225**	9	41
Skinnygirl:			
Vodka with flavors (30%), 1.5 fl.oz	**75**	11	0
Cocktails (10%), av., 3 fl.oz	**70**	8	4
Smirnoff:			
Ice (4.5%): Original, 11.2 fl.oz	**220**	13	33
Mango; Pineapple, av., 11.2 fl.oz	**230**	13	35
Sourced, Fruit Flavors, (4.5%), 11.2 fl.oz	**160**	12	20
Spiked Sparkling Seltzer, (4.5%), all flav., 12 fl.oz can	**90**	13	1
TGI Friday's:			
On The Rocks: *Per 6 fl.oz*			
Long Island Ice Tea (15%)	**250**	21	28
Margarita (7.5%)	**185**	11	29
Mudslide (10%)	**365**	14	31
Blenders (12.5%), Mudslide, 6 fl.oz	**365**	18	31
White Claw, Vodka + Soda (4.5%), avg	**100**	12	21

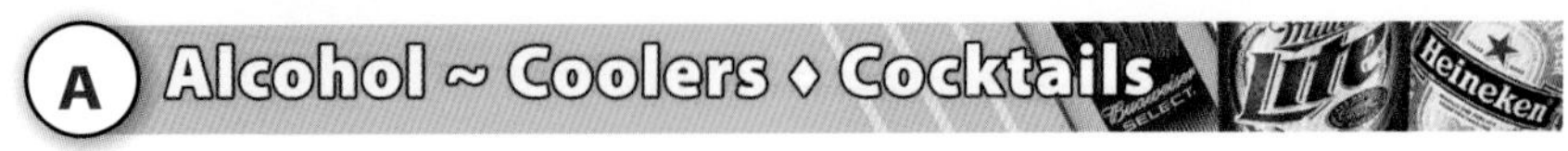

Coolers & Premix Cocktails (Cont)

Ready-To-Drink:

The Club Premix Cocktails: *Per 3.4 oz Serving (½ can)*

	C	Alc	Cb
Censored on Beach; Margarita (7.5%)	**105**	6	17
Gin/Vodka Martini (21%), av.	**155**	17	0.2
Ice Tea (15%)	**145**	12	17
Manhattan (17%)	**115**	13	5
Mudslide/Pina Colada (10%), av.	**200**	8	16
Screwdriver (7.5%)	**95**	6	14
Whiskey Sour (10%)	**95**	8	11

Shooters

Alc ~ Alcohol (Grams)

	C	Alc	Cb
Alabama Slammer	**110**	14	2
Amaretto Sour	**120**	6	19
B52	**145**	14	11
Beam Me Up Scotty	**145**	13	13
Blue Tequila	**160**	18	6
Jager Bomb	**205**	8	30
Jager Bomb, w/ Sugar-Free Red Bull	**155**	8	18
Jell-O Shot: 3 oz, with 1.5 oz Vodka	**180**	14	19
with Diet Jell-O	**110**	14	0
Kamikaze	**75**	8	3
Kool-Aid	**160**	15	14
Orgasm	**100**	12	6
Peppermint Patty	**195**	8	11
Stinger	**170**	18	12
Surfer on Acid	**90**	7	11

Cocktail Mixers ~ Non-Alcoholic

	C	Alc	Cb
Bacardi: *Per 8 fl.oz, Prepared from 2 fl.oz Concentrate*			
Daiquiris; Rum Runner	**120**	0	32
Margarita	**90**	0	25
Mojito	**110**	0	30
Pina Colada	**170**	0	36
Baja Bob's: *Per 4 fl.oz*			
Cranberry Cosmo Martini	**10**	0	2
Pina Colada	**30**	0	4
Jose Cuervo:			
Margaritas: Av. all flav., 4 fl.oz	**85**	0	21
Light (Sugar Free), Lime, 4 fl.oz	**5**	0	1
Mr & Mrs T:			
Bloody Mary: Original, 5 oz	**30**	0	7
Bold & Spicy, 4 oz	**35**	0	7
Mai Tai	**130**	0	32
Margarita	**100**	0	26
Pina Colada	**170**	0	44
Strawberry Daiquiri	**180**	0	46
TGI Friday's:			
Mudslide, 2.3 fl.oz	**110**	0	23
Cosmo; Berrytini, 2 fl.oz	**80**	0	20
Strawb. Daiquiri; Marg., 4 fl.oz	**190**	0	46

Cocktails

Alc ~ Alcohol (Grams)

Made to Standard Recipes (Standard Size):

(Main Reference: The New American Bartender's Guide)

Zero Fat Unless Indicated

	C	Alc	Cb
Adios Mother F.	**260**	23	23
Bacardi & Coke (with 1.5 oz Bacardi)	**160**	14	17
Bellini, 4.5 fl.oz	**95**	11	7
Bloody Mary (with 1.5 oz Vodka)	**125**	10	7
Blushin' Russian (20g fat)	**405**	14	23
Bourbon & Soda (with 2 oz Bourbon)	**130**	19	0
Brandy Alexander (10g fat)	**300**	20	15
Chupa Naranjas (with 1.5 oz Tequila)	**150**	16	8
Cosmopolitan	**215**	24	12
Daiquiri (w/ 2 oz Rum), av. all types	**140**	19	4
Frozen Daiquiri (with 2 oz Rum):			
without fruit	**155**	19	6
with fruit (with 1.5 oz Rum)	**145**	14	11
Grasshopper	**260**	17	28
Harvey Wallbanger (2 oz)	**200**	19	17
Highball (1.5 oz Whiskey)	**100**	14	0
Irish Coffee (10g fat)	**205**	14	2
Kahlua Mudslide: with milk (3g fat)	**145**	11	12
with cream (12g fat)	**230**	11	10
Lemon Drop, 4 fl.oz	**130**	14	10
Long Island Iced Tea (with 3 oz Cola)	**270**	19	32
with 3 oz Diet Cola	**235**	19	22
Mai Tai (with 2 oz Rum)	**290**	24	33
Manhattan	**130**	17	5
Margarita	**160**	18	7
Martini: Dry, with 1.5 oz gin	**100**	14	0
Sour Apple, w/ 2 oz Vodka/1 oz Schnapps	**250**	31	10
Mint Julep (with 2½ oz Bourbon)	**180**	24	4
Mojito (with 2 oz rum)	**170**	19	9
Moscow Mule (with 1.5 oz Vodka)	**180**	14	20
Pina Colada (10g fat), 6 oz	**250**	15	18
Red Bull & Vodka (with 1.5 oz vodka)	**210**	14	28
with Sugar Free Red Bull	**105**	14	3
Rum & Coke (with 1.5 oz Rum)	**160**	14	17
Sake Bomb (1.5 oz Sake & 5 oz Beer)	**105**	12	7
Sangria: with 1 oz Fruit Juice, 5 oz	**120**	12	9
with 0.5 oz Brandy, 5.5 oz	**150**	17	9
Screwdriver	**160**	14	15
Sex On The Beach	**235**	19	25
Spritzer (with 3 oz Wine)	**65**	8	2
Tequila Sunrise	**200**	14	25
Tom Collins (with 2 oz Gin)	**210**	19	18
Vodka Soda (with 1.5 oz Vodka)	**100**	14	0
Vodka Tonic (with 1.5 oz Vodka)	**165**	14	18
Whiskey Sour (w/ 2 oz Whiskey)	**155**	19	7
White Russian (10g fat)	**240**	19	7
Non-Alcoholic:			
Cinderella	**45**	0	11
Shirley Temple (with 6 oz Ginger Ale)	**140**	0	34

Liqueurs/Cordials

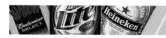

Per 1 fl.oz	C	Alc	Cb
Advocaat (36 Proof; 2g fat)	**85**	4	9
Alizé: Cognac (80 Proof)	**70**	9	2
Gold/Red Passion (32 Proof)	**105**	4	11
Amaretto (56 Proof)	**110**	7	17
Baileys Irish Cream (34 Proof; 4g fat)	**100**	4	8
Benedictine (80 Proof)	**90**	9	5
Chambord (33 Proof)	**105**	4	11
Chartreuse (80 Proof)	**100**	9	9
Cherry Brandy (48 Proof)	**80**	6	9
Coffee Liqueur (53 Proof)	**115**	7	16
Cointreau (80 Proof)	**95**	9	7
Creme de Cacao (54 Proof)	**100**	6	15
Creme de Menthe (72 Proof)	**125**	9	14
Curacao (70 Proof)	**95**	8	6
Drambuie (80 Proof)	**105**	9	9
Frangelico (40 Proof)	**65**	5	12
Galliano (86 Proof)	**100**	10	8
Grand Marnier (80 Proof)	**100**	9	7
(40 Proof)	**85**	5	14
Kirsch (68 Proof)	**80**	8	6
Midori (42 Proof)	**80**	5	11
Ouzo (80 Proof)	**105**	9	11
Pernod (80 Proof)	**75**	9	11
Sambuca (84 Proof)	**100**	10	11
Schnapps (100 Proof)	**115**	12	9
Southern Comfort (70 Proof)	**65**	8	3
Tia Maria (40% Proof)	**90**	7	10

Liqueur Coffee & Hot Drinks

Per Standard Drink	C	Alc	Cb
Liqueur Coffee: Av. all types	**200**	10	10
Irish, 1.5 oz Whiskey & 1 oz whip	**205**	9	4
Hot Toddy, with 1½ oz liquor, av. all	**170**	9	19
Mulled Wine *(Glühwein)*, 4 fl.oz, av	**195**	14	25

"The doctor told him to cut down to just one glass a day."

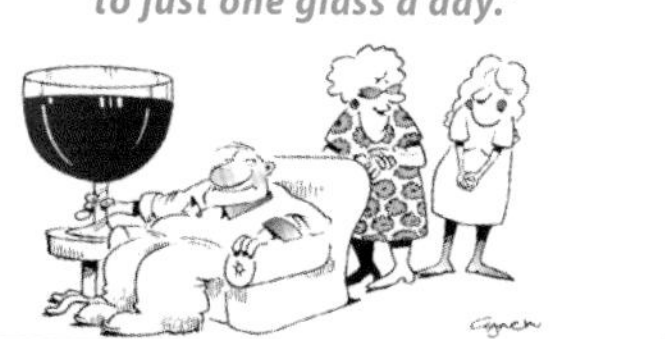

TEN TIPS TO AVOID HARMFUL DRINKING

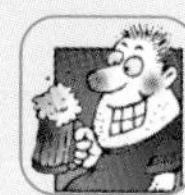

1. **Add up the alcohol** you typically drink each day and on social occasions. How does this compare with 'low risk' amounts? *(See page 23)*
2. **Compare the alcohol content** of different drinks and select the lowest. Request half shots of alcohol in cocktails and mixed drinks. Dilute them and keep topping off with non-alcoholic drinks.
3. **Go easy on 'Light' beers.** At 4% alcohol, on average, they are still high in alcohol compared to regular beer (5% alcohol).
4. **Try low alcohol or non-alcohol** alternatives such as fruit juices and mineral water. Take your own to parties.
5. **Before drinking alcohol,** quench your thirst with water and non-alcoholic drinks – particularly after vigorous exercise or sports.
6. **Slow the rate of drinking.** Chugging or drinking fast is the major cause of illness and death from alcohol poisoning.
7. **Avoid drinking in 'rounds'.**
8. **Have a non-alcoholic 'spacer'** between drinks (e.g. mineral water, orange juice).
9. **Don't drink on an empty stomach.** Food slows the rate of alcohol absorption.
10. **Keep track of the number of drinks** and know when to stop. Stick to a set limit.

Note: Alcohol can be very dangerous when taken with prescription or street drugs, or when you are very tired.

Extra Info: www.CalorieKing.com

Cocktail Mixers & Extracts

	C	Alc	Cb
Angostura Bitters, ¼ tsp	**2**	0	0.5
Grenadine, ½ tsp	**6**	0	2
Lime/Lemon Juice, 2 Tbsp, 1 oz	**10**	0	2
Maraschino Cherry, 1 small	**8**	0	2
Simple Syrup, 1 Tbsp, av.	**50**	0	14
Sweet & Sour Mix, 2 Tbsp, 1 oz	**30**	0	7
Tonic Water, 8 fl.oz	**80**	0	22
Flavor Extracts *(McCormick)*:			
Pure Lemon (83%), 1 tsp	**0**	3.5	0
Pure Vanilla (35%), 1tsp	**0**	1.5	0

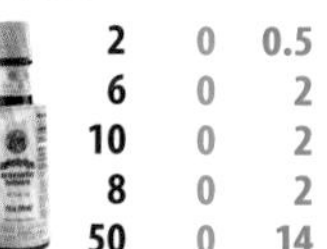
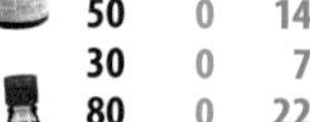
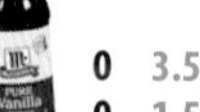
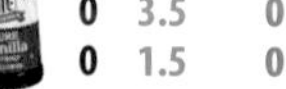

B Baking Ingredients

Baking Ingredients

	C	F	Cb
Almond Flour, ¼ cup, 1 oz	160	10	10
Almond Paste, (Marzipan), 2 Tbsp	170	7	24
Apple Pie Filling, Sweetened, 9.4 oz	290	0	69
(Bean Water), ¼ c., 2 oz	10	0	2
Amaranth Flour *(Bob's Red Mill)*, ¼ cup, 1 oz	110	2	20
Baking Powder: Regular, 1 tsp	5	0	1
Cream of Tartar, 1 tsp	10	0	2
Baking Mix (*Bisquick*): Original, ⅓ cup, 1.5 oz	160	5	26
Batter Mix (*Golden Dipt*), All Purpose, ¼ cup	100	0	20
Butter/Margarine, ½ cup, 4 oz	800	88	1
Stick (*Land O' Lakes*), 0.5 oz	100	11	0
Cacao Butter, 2 Tbsp, 1 oz	240	28	0
Cacao Powder, raw: 1 Tbsp, 0.3 oz	35	2	3
¼ cup, 1 oz	150	9	11
Carob Flour, ½ cup	115	1	46
Cassava Flour, ½ cup, 70g	260	0	62
Chia Seed Protein Powder, 2 T., 0.5 oz	25	0	8
Chocolate Baking Bars: *Average all Brands*			
Sweet (*Baker's*): 1 oz portion	120	7	16
4 oz bar	470	28	64
Semi-sweet, 1 oz	140	9	16
White Baking, 1 oz	160	9	16
Unsweetened: 1 oz	140	14	8
Grated, 1 cup, 4.5 oz	660	69	39
Chocolate Baking Chips: *Average all Brands*			
Milk Choc./Semi Sweet, 1 oz	140	8	18
½ cup, 3 oz	420	24	54
1 cup, 6 oz	840	48	108
Dark, 1 Tbsp, 0.5 oz	70	5	3
Mini Kisses (*Hershey*), 1 piece	5	1	1
Cocoa Powder, unsweetened: 1 Tbsp, 0.2 oz	15	1	3
⅓ cup, 1 oz	60	4	17
Coconut, dried: Sweetened/Flaked: 1 oz	130	8	15
½ cup, 1.3 oz	195	12	22
Tsd (*Baker's*), 1 oz	170	13	13
Unsweetened, 1 oz	190	18	7
Coconut Cream/Milk ~ *See Page 89*			
Coconut Flour, 2 Tbsp, 0.5 oz	60	2	8
Coconut Manna (*Nutiva*), 1 Tbsp	100	9	3
Cornstarch, 1 Tbsp	30	0	7
Eggs: Large (1)	75	5	0
Jumbo (1)	90	6	1
Egg White: 1 Egg White	15	0	0
½ cup (4 egg whites), 4 oz	60	0	1

	C	F	Cb
Flour:			
Whole Wheat, 1 cup, 4.2 oz	400	2	84
White: 1 Tbsp, 0.3 oz	25	0	6
1 cup, 4.2 oz	400	1	88
Flavor Extracts: *Av. all Brands*			
Imitation, 1 tsp	10	0	2
Pure Extract, 1 tsp	10	0	1
Almond; Vanilla, 1 tsp	10	0	1
Fruit Pectin: Swtnd, ¼ tsp	5	0	1
Unsweetened, ¼ tsp	0	0	0
Gelatin, dry, unsweetened, 0.3 oz	20	0	0
Glaze *(Duncan Hines)*: Choc., 2 T.	150	7	21
Vanilla, 2 Tbsp	140	6	22
Hazelnut Meal/Flour, ¼ cup, 1 oz	160	12	8
Hemp Protein Powder, ¼ cup, 1.1 oz	120	3	10
Honey, ½ cup, 6 oz	515	0	145
Lemon/Orange Peel, ¼ cup	25	0	6
Lighter Bake *(Sunsweet)*: (Butter & Oil replacement)			
1 Tbsp, ½ oz	35	0	9
¼ Cup, 2.7 oz	140	0	36
Masa Harina *(Bob's Red Mill)*, ½ cup, 2 oz	220	2	47
Milk: Whole, 1 cup, 8 fl.oz	150	8	12
2%, 1 cup, 8 fl.oz	120	5	12
1%, 1 cup, 8 fl.oz	100	3	12
Fat-Free, 1 cup, 8 fl.oz	90	1	13
Oat Flour *(Bob's Red Mill)*, ⅓ cup, 1.5 oz	120	3	26
Pastry ~ *See Page 134*			
Pie Crusts ~ *See Page 134*			
Pie Fillings, Fruits ~ *See Page 134*			
Lemon Creme, ⅓ cup	130	2	28
Mincemeat, 3.5 oz	190	5	45
Pumpkin, 1 cup, 9.3 oz	270	2	60
Prune Puree, ¼ cup, 3 oz	220	0	55
Quinoa Flour, ¼ cup, 1 oz	110	2	18
Raisins, ½ cup, 2.8 oz	240	1	63
Rennin, 0.4 oz pkt	10	0	2
Rice Flour, ½ cup, 2.8 oz	290	1	63
Soy Milk ~ *See Pages 49-50*			
Soy Flour, *(Bob's Red Mill)*, 100% Whole Ground, ¼ cup, 1 oz	120	6	8
Sprinkles, all types, 1 tsp	20	1	3
Sugar: 1 Tbsp, 0.5 oz	55	0	14
1 oz	110	0	28
1 cup, 7 oz	775	0	195
16 oz (1 lb)	1760	0	454
Sweeteners & Sugar Substitutes ~ *See Page 156*			
Vinegar, average all types, 1 oz	5	0	1
Whey, sweet, dry, 1 oz	100	1	21
Yeast:			
Active, dry, 0.3 oz pkg	25	1	3
Bakers, compressed, 1 oz	30	1	5
Fleischmann's, 0.6 oz pkg	0	0	0

Note: Actual weight of bars is usually 5-10% more than label Net Weight. Weigh bar and allow extra calories.

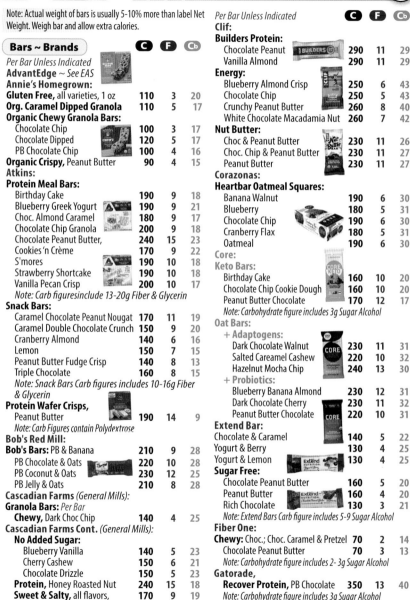

Bars ~ Brands

Per Bar Unless Indicated	C	F	Cb
AdvantEdge ~ *See EAS*			
Annie's Homegrown:			
Gluten Free, all varieties, 1 oz	110	3	20
Org. Caramel Dipped Granola	110	5	17
Organic Chewy Granola Bars:			
Chocolate Chip	100	3	17
Chocolate Dipped	120	5	17
PB Chocolate Chip	100	4	16
Organic Crispy, Peanut Butter	90	4	15
Atkins:			
Protein Meal Bars:			
Birthday Cake	190	9	18
Blueberry Greek Yogurt	190	9	21
Choc. Almond Caramel	180	9	17
Chocolate Chip Granola	200	9	18
Chocolate Peanut Butter,	240	15	23
Cookies 'n Crème	170	9	22
S'mores	190	10	18
Strawberry Shortcake	190	10	18
Vanilla Pecan Crisp	200	10	17
Note: Carb figuresinclude 13-20g Fiber & Glycerin			
Snack Bars:			
Caramel Chocolate Peanut Nougat	170	11	19
Caramel Double Chocolate Crunch	150	9	20
Cranberry Almond	140	6	16
Lemon	150	7	15
Peanut Butter Fudge Crisp	140	8	13
Triple Chocolate	160	8	15
Note: Snack Bars Carb figures includes 10-16g Fiber & Glycerin			
Protein Wafer Crisps,			
Peanut Butter	190	14	9
Note: Carb Figures contain Polydextrose			
Bob's Red Mill:			
Bob's Bars: PB & Banana	210	9	28
PB Chocolate & Oats	220	10	28
PB Coconut & Oats	230	12	25
PB Jelly & Oats	210	8	28
Cascadian Farms *(General Mills):*			
Granola Bars: *Per Bar*			
Chewy, Dark Choc Chip	140	4	25
Cascadian Farms Cont. *(General Mills):*			
No Added Sugar:			
Blueberry Vanilla	140	5	23
Cherry Cashew	150	6	21
Chocolate Drizzle	150	5	23
Protein, Honey Roasted Nut	240	15	18
Sweet & Salty, all flavors,	170	9	19

Per Bar Unless Indicated	C	F	Cb
Clif:			
Builders Protein:			
Chocolate Peanut	290	11	29
Vanilla Almond	290	11	29
Energy:			
Blueberry Almond Crisp	250	6	43
Chocolate Chip	250	5	43
Crunchy Peanut Butter	260	8	40
White Chocolate Macadamia Nut	260	7	42
Nut Butter:			
Choc & Peanut Butter	230	11	26
Choc. Chip & Peanut Butter	230	11	27
Peanut Butter	230	11	27
Corazonas:			
Heartbar Oatmeal Squares:			
Banana Walnut	190	6	30
Blueberry	180	5	31
Chocolate Chip	190	6	30
Cranberry Flax	180	5	31
Oatmeal	190	6	30
Core:			
Keto Bars:			
Birthday Cake	160	10	20
Chocolate Chip Cookie Dough	160	10	20
Peanut Butter Chocolate	170	12	17
Note: Carbohydrate figure includes 3g Sugar Alcohol			
Oat Bars:			
+ Adaptogens:			
Dark Chocolate Walnut	230	11	31
Salted Careamel Cashew	220	10	32
Hazelnut Mocha Chip	240	13	30
+ Probiotics:			
Blueberry Banana Almond	230	12	31
Dark Chocolate Cherry	230	11	32
Peanut Butter Chocolate	220	10	31
Extend Bar:			
Chocolate & Caramel	140	5	22
Yogurt & Berry	130	4	25
Yogurt & Lemon	130	4	25
Sugar Free:			
Chocolate Peanut Butter	160	5	20
Peanut Butter	160	4	20
Rich Chocolate	130	3	21
Note: Extend Bars Carb figure includes 5-9 Sugar Alcohol			
Fiber One:			
Chewy: Choc.; Choc. Caramel & Pretzel	70	2	14
Chocolate Peanut Butter	70	3	13
Note: Carbohydrate figure includes 2- 3g Sugar Alcohol			
Gatorade,			
Recover Protein, PB Chocolate	350	13	40
Note: Carbohydrate figure includes 3g Sugar Alcohol			

Bars ~ Brands (Cont)

Per Bar Unless Indicated	C	F	Cb
General Mills:			
Milk 'n Cereal Bar,			
Honey Nut Cheerios	160	4	28
Glucerna:			
Snack Bars,			
Crispy Oats & Nuts	160	6	18
Note: Carbohydrate figure includes 4g Sugar Alcohol			
Mini Snack Bar, average	80	4	11
Note: Carbohydrate figure includes 2g-7g Sugar Alcohol			
Great Value *(Walmart):*			
Fruit & Grain Cereal Bars,			
Apple Cinn; Mixed Berry; Strawberry	130	3	24
Chewy Granola:			
Chocolate Chip Dipped	150	6	22
S'Mores,	90	2	19
Sweet & Salty, Cashew	160	6	23
Crunchy Granola,			
Oats & Honey, 2 bars	190	7	29
Grenade:			
Choc Chip Cookie Dough	210	8	24
Chocolate	220	8	20
Peanut Nutter	220	9	15
Note: Carbohydrate figure includes 6- 14g Sugar Alcohol			
Health Valley,			
Multigrain, Cobbler Cereal Bars, all flavors	130	3	26
HMR, Benefit Bars, average	160	5	22
Note: Carbohydrate figure includes 6- 9g Sugar Alcohol			
Init:			
Dark Chocolate Cherry & Cashew	180	10	22
Mixed Nut & Sweet Berries	180	9	24
Roasted Nuts & Honey Chipotle	190	13	18
Kates Real Food:			
Almond Bars:			
Dark Chocolate Cherry Almond	260	9	40
Lemon Coconut	300	20	30
Oatmeal Cranberry & Almond	260	12	36
Peanut Bars: Dark Chocolate	260	12	34
Hemp & Flax	240	12	36
Milk Chocolate	260	12	36
Kellogg's:			
Nutrigrain ~ *See page 33*			
Special K ~ *See page 34*			
Kind Bars:			
Breakfast Bars:			
Blueberry Almond (2)	210	8	23
Honey Oat (2)	210	7	33
Peanut Butter (2)	220	10	29

Per Bar Unless Indicated	C	F	Cb
Kind Bars (cont):			
Breakfast Bars (Cont):			
Protein Breakfast:			
Almond Butter (2)	220	9	28
Dark Chocolate Cocoa (2)	210	8	28
PB Banana Dark Chocolate (2)	220	10	27
Caramel Almond & Seasalt	170	15	16
Dark Chocolate:			
Cherry Cashew	170	10	22
Nuts & Seasalt	180	15	16
Drizzled: *Per Bar*			
Dark Chocolate P'nut Butter	140	6	22
Milk Chocolate Chunk	140	5	23
Healthy Grains:			
Dark Chocolate Chunk	150	5	23
Oats & Honey with Toasted Coconut	150	5	23
Peanut Butter Dark Chocolate	150	6	23
Thins,			
P'nut Butter Dark Chocolate	100	7	10
Kuli Kuli:			
Moringa Energy Bars:			
Black Cherry	170	4	29
Dark Chocolate	210	11	22
Larabar:			
Original:			
Almond Butter Chocolate Chip	210	12	23
Almond Cookie	230	14	20
Banana Choc. Chip	190	9	26
Cashew Cookie	220	12	25
Cherry Pie	200	8	28
Chocolate Peanut Caramel Truffle	210	9	27
Cocoa Coconut Chew	210	11	23
Peanut Butter & Jelly	210	10	25
Minis, Mint Chocolate Chip	100	5	13
Luna Bars:			
Gluten Free: Blueberry Bliss	190	6	29
Chocolate Cupcake	190	6	29
Chocolate Peppermint Stick	200	6	28
Minis, 0.81 oz	90	3	14
LemonZest	190	6	28
Nutz Over Chocolate	210	10	24
White Chocolate Macadamia	200	7	27
Mash-Ups, Lemon Zest Blueberry	190	6	29

Bars ~ Brands (Cont)

Per Bar Unless Indicated	C	F	Cb
Mars, Hi Protein Bar, 2.3 oz	230	5	26
Made Good:			
Granola Bars:			
Chocolate Banana	100	3	17
Chocolate Chip	100	4	17
Chocolate Drizzled: B'Day Cake	110	4	17
Cookie Crumble	110	4	16
Vanilla Flavor	110	4	17
Cookies & Cream	100	3	17
Mixed Berry	100	3	18
Met-Rx: *Per Bar*			
Big 100:			
Birthday Cake	420	13	47
Chocolat Chip Cookie Dough	410	12	45
Crispy Apple Pie	400	10	48
P'nut Buttter Pretzel	410	12	47
Super Cookie Crunch	410	14	42
Protein Plus:			
Chocolate Chocolate Chunk, 3 oz	310	10	29
Peanut Butter Cup	300	10	34
Mojo Bars ~ *See Clif*			
Muscle Milk *(Cytosport):*			
15G Protein Bars: Cookies & Cream	180	5	23
Peanut Butter Cookie	190	6	22
20G Protein Bar, Choc P'nut Butter	250	9	27
Note: Protein Bars Carb figures include 6-14g Sugar Alcohol			
Nature's Path:			
Crunch, 2 bars, average all varieties	195	8	27
Sunrise Chewy B'fast, average	140	4	25
Nature Valley: *Per Bar*			
Chewy, XL Prot., Salted Caramel Dk Choc.	290	17	23
Crunchy, 2 bars, average all flavors	200	8	28
Fruit & Nut, Trail Mix, all flavors	150	5	25
Savory Nut Crunch, White Cheddar	130	8	11
Soft Baked Muffin, average all flav.	150	6	23
Sweet & Salty:			
Granola, av. all flavors	160	8	20
Nut, average all flavors	160	7	21
Wafer Bars, average all flavors	200	12	18

Per Bar Unless Indicated	C	F	Cb
NuGo:			
Dark, average all varieties	200	6	25
Fiber d'Lish: Chocolate Brownie	150	5	30
Peanut Chocolate Chip	160	6	29
Gluten Free, average all flavos	175	5	27
Organic, all flavors	200	7	25
Slim: Espresso	170	6	18
Average other flavors	175	6	18
Smarte Carb: Choc. Black Berry, 1.76 oz	150	3	22
Peanut Butter Crunch	160	5	19
Note: Carbohyrate figures include 12-14 g Sugar Alcohol			
Stronger: Peanut Cluster	330	14	36
Average other flavors	320	11	38
Nutri-Grain *(Kellogg's):*			
Bites, all varieties	140	4	27
Soft Baked B'fast Cereal Bars, all varieties	130	4	25
NutriSystem: *Per Bar*			
Breakfast, Apple Streudel Bar	160	3	28
Lunch:			
Chewy Trail Mix Bar	200	8	24
Chocolate Peanut Butter Bar	200	8	25
Chocolaty Fudge Graham Bar	200	7	24
Double Chocolate Caramel Bar	180	6	28
One: *Per Bar*			
Almond Bliss	240	9	22
Birthday Cake	220	8	23
Blueberry Cobbler	230	8	23
Chocolate Chip Cookie Dough	230	8	23
Cookies & Cream	220	8	23
Lemon Cake	220	8	23
Maple Glazed Doughnut	230	8	23
Note: Carbohydrate figure includes 5-6g Sugar Alcohol			
Optifast, Chocolate Bar	160	5	17
PowerBar:			
Protein Plus, average	210	6	27
Power Crunch *(BNRG): Per Bar*			
Power Crunch, average all flavors	215	12	11
Pro, Peanut Butter Fudge	300	21	15

Note: Actual weight of bars is usually 5-10% more than label Net Weight. Weigh bar and allow extra calories.

Bars ~ Brands (Cont)

Per Bar Unless Indicated	C	F	Cb
Promax: *Per Bar*			
Original 20G Protein, Nutty Butter	300	9	38
Average other varieties	285	6	37
Proti Bars *(Bariatrix):*			
Caramel Nut	160	6	15
Choc A Lot Chip	160	6	19
Note: Carbohydrate figure include 2g Sugar Alcohol			
VLC, Chocolate Crisp, 1.6 oz	160	7	17
PureFit, Protein, av. all flavors	210	8	21
Pure Protein:			
20G Protein, average all flavors	195	6	18
Note: Carbohydrate figures include 3- 9g Sugar Alcohol			
Nut Bars: Caramel Almond Sea Salt	180	14	19
PB Dark Chocolate	200	14	18
Note: Carbohydrate figures include 1g Sugar Alcohol			
Quaker:			
Chewy Granola Bars:			
25% Less Sugar, average	95	4	17
Big, average all varieties	175	6	30
Note: Big Bar Carbohydrate figure include 2g Sugar Alcohol			
Classic, averge	95	3	18
Dipps, average	140	6	21
Yogurt, Strawberry	140	5	25
Note: Yogurt Carbohydrate figure include 2g Sugar Alcohol			
Quest Bar:			
Hero: Chocolate Peanut Butter	200	11	19
Cookies & Cream	200	11	19
Note: Carbohydrate figure includes 5g Sugar Alcohol			
Protein, Chocolate Peanut Butter	200	9	22
Note: Carbohydrate figures includes 6g Sugar Alcohol			
RX Bar:			
Plant Based, average all varieties	210	9	25
Protein: Blueberry	230	9	29
Average other varieties	215	9	24
Skratch Bars,			
Anytime Energy,			
Peanut Butter & Chocolate	270	14	30

Per Bar Unless Indicated	C	F	Cb
Slim-Fast:			
Intermittent Fasting,			
average all flavors	185	9	19
Note: Carb includes 5g Sugar Alcohol			
Meal Replacement Delights,			
Whippped Peanut Butter Chocolate	190	14	15
Note: Carb includes 3g Sugar Alcohol			
Snickers, 20G Protein Bar	240	10	19
Solo, Gi, average all varieties	195	7	26
Special K:			
12G Protein,			
Chocolate Peanut Butter	190	9	19
thinkThin: *Per Bar*			
High Protein, Brownie Crunch	240	10	23
Note: Carbohydrate figure includes 10g Sugar Alcohol			
Keto, Choc. Peanut Butter Pie	180	14	14
Note: Carbohydrate figure includes 7g Sugar Alcohol			
Protein + 150 Calorie, average	150	5	20
Vegan High Protein:			
Chocolate Mint	200	7	25
PB Chocolate Chip	190	6	23
Sea Salt Almond Chocolate	220	9	25
Note: Carbohydrate figure includes 7-8g Sugar Alcohol			
Trader Joe's:			
ABC Bar	160	8	19
Five Seed Almond Bar	100	4	16
Protein, Chewy Chocolate & PB	190	11	15
U Can:			
Energy Bars: Cherry Berry Almond	160	7	26
Choc. Almond Butter; PB Fudge, av.	160	8	23
Chocolate Fudge	150	6	24
Zone Perfect:			
Classic:			
Choc. Chip Cookie Dough	180	5	24
Chocolate Mint	220	6	30
Chocolate Peanut Butter	220	8	24
Fudge Graham	220	7	25
Strawberry Yogurt	210	6	25
Gluten Free,			
Oatmeal Choc Chunk	180	8	18
Macros, average	205	8	23
Note: Carbohydrate figure includes 4-8g Sugar Alcohol			

Cocoa & Hot Chocolate

	C	F	Cb
Cocoa:			
Small (8 fl.oz):			
with Whole Milk	205	9	22
with Nonfat Milk	145	1	23
Tall (12 fl.oz): with Whole Milk	280	12	26
with Nonfat Milk	185	1	28
Hot Chocolate:			
Small (8 fl.oz): with Whole Milk	180	7	26
with Nonfat Milk	140	2	27
Tall (12 fl.oz): with Whole Milk	260	10	36
with Nonfat Milk	190	2	37
Cinnabon, Mochalatta Chill, 16 oz	420	17	63

Cocoa - Chocolate Mixes

Add extra cals/fat/carbohydrate for milk

	C	F	Cb
Caffé D'Vita: *Per Singe Serve Envelope*			
Hot Cocoa, 1 oz	110	2	24
Hot Cocoa, Sugar Free	70	5	7
Carnation Breakfast Drinks ~ *See Page 38*			
Carnation: *Per 3 Tbsp*			
Malted Milk: Original	90	2	15
Chocolate	90	1	18
Ghirardelli:			
Premium Hot Cocoa:			
with Chocolate Chips, 1 oz	110	2	23
Double Chocolate, 2 Tbsp	90	1	20
Hershey's, Cocoa, Natural, unsweetened, 1 Tbsp, 0.2 oz	10	1	3
Land O Lakes:			
Arctic White Coccoa, 1.3 oz	160	6	26
Other varieties, 1.3 oz	140	4	26
Nestle: *Per Per Single Serve Envelope*			
Rich Milk Chocolate:			
Regular	80	2	15
Fat Free	25	0	4
with Mini Marshmallows	80	2	15
Nesquik Powder: *Per 2 Tbsp*			
Chocolate	50	0	12
No Added Sugar	40	1	8
Strawberry	45	0	12
Ovaltine, av. all flav., 2 Tbsp	40	0	10
Swiss Miss: *Per Single Serve Envelope*			
Cafe Blends, Mocha	150	3	28
Classics: Marshmallow Lovers	190	3	39
Milk Chocolate	160	3	34
Indulgent Collection:			
Caramel Delight	160	3	34
Dark Chocolate Sensation	150	4	28
Sensibly Sweet, Milk Choc. Flavor, No Sugar Added	80	2	14
Simply Cocoa, Milk Chocolate	100	0	22

Instant Coffee

	C	F	Cb
Powder/Granules: *Regular or Decaffeinated,*			
1 level tsp	2	0	1
1 rounded tsp	4	0	1
Ground, 3 tsp	7	0	2
Brewed/Percolated, 1 cup, 8 fl.oz	4	0	1
Coffee with Milk/Cream/Creamers: *Per 8 oz Cup*			
Black:	4	0	1
with Whole Milk: Dash, 1 Tbsp	15	1	2
2 Tbsp, 1 fl.oz	25	1	3
with 2% Milk, 2 Tbsp	20	1	3
with 1% Milk, 2 Tbsp	20	1	3
with Fat Free Milk, 2 Tbsp	15	0	3
with Soy Milk: 1 Tbsp	10	0	2
2 Tbsp, 1 oz	15	1	2
with Half & Half: 2 Tbsp	50	3	3
1/4 cup, 2 fl.oz	90	6	4
with Cream (light coffee), 2 Tbsp	65	6	2
with Coffee Mate: Liquid, reg., 1 T.	20	1	3
Liquid Fat Free, 1 Tbsp	25	0	2
Powder, 1 heaping tsp	15	1	2
Sugar ~ Add Extra: 1 heaping tsp	25	0	6
Single portion, 1 package, 4g	15	0	4
Sweeteners, *(Equal/Splenda/Sweet N Low),*			
Powder, 1 package	0	0	0

Flavored Coffee Mixes

	C	F	Cb
Chicory:			
Instant Coffee, 1 tsp	5	0	1
Coffee Essence, 1 tsp	15	0	4
Caffé D'Vita:			
Cappuccino: Caramel, 3 tsp	60	2	10
English Toffee, 3 tsp	70	3	11
French Vanilla, 3 tsp	70	3	10
Mocha; Peppermint Mocha, av., 3 tsp	60	3	11
Iced, Caramel Latte, 3 tbsp	180	6	32
Sugar Free Cappuccino, Mocha, 2 tsp	40	3	4
General Foods International:			
Cappuccino: Hazelnut Belgian,1.3 oz	160	4	29
Suisse Mocha, 1.3 oz	150	5	28
White Chocolate Caramel, 1.3 oz	150	3	30
Hills Bros: *Per 3 Tbsp, 1 oz*			
Cappuccino: French Vanilla	110	4	19
Sugar Free	50	2	8
Double Mocha, Sugar Free	50	2	8
English Toffee	110	3	19
White Chocolate Caramel	120	5	19
Nescafe, Memento, 1 stick, average all varieties	100	3	19

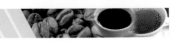

Coffee Shops/Restaurants

Per 8 fl.oz Cup (Unless Indicated)	C	F	Cb
Coffee, Regular/Percolated/Filtered	5	0	0
Americano Drip Coffee, 1 cup	8	0	2
Cafe Au Lait: 1 cup, 8 fl.oz	60	4	5
Nonfat Milk, 1 cup, 8 fl.oz	35	0	5
Caffe Latté:			
8 fl.oz cup: with Whole Milk	110	6	9
with 2% Milk	100	4	9
with Nonfat Milk	70	0	10
12 fl.oz: with Whole Milk	180	9	14
with Nonfat Milk	100	0	15
16 fl.oz: with Whole Milk	220	11	18
with Nonfat Milk	130	0	19
Cafe Mocha (Mochaccino): 8 fl.oz	150	6	20
12 fl.oz	230	9	31
16 fl.oz	290	12	41
Cappuccino:			
8 fl.oz cup: with Whole Milk	90	4	7
with 2% Milk	80	3	8
with Nonfat Milk	50	0	8
12 fl.oz: with Whole Milk	110	6	9
with 2% Milk	90	4	9
with Nonfat Milk	60	0	9
16 fl.oz: with Whole Milk	140	7	11
with 2% Milk	120	4	11
with Nonfat Milk	80	0	12
Mocha: *With Cream*			
8 fl.oz: with Whole Milk	200	11	22
with Nonfat Milk	160	6	22
12 fl.oz: Whole Milk	290	15	33
with Nonfat Milk	230	8	34
Iced Mocha: *Without Cream*			
12 fl.oz: with Whole Milk	170	6	26
with Nonfat Milk	130	2	27
Espresso: Single (Solo), 1 fl.oz	5	0	1
Double (Doppio), 2 fl.oz	10	0	2
Espresso con Panna,			
(w/ dollop wh. cream), solo, 1 fl.oz	30	3	2
Espresso Macchiato, solo, 1 fl.oz	5	0	1
Frappuccino: Tall, 12 fl.oz	180	3	37
Grande, 16 fl.oz	240	3	48
Frappuccino Mocha:			
(with Cream): Tall, 12 fl.oz	280	11	43
Grande, 16 fl.oz	380	15	57

Iced Latte, Similar to Caffe Latte

McCafe (McDonald's) ~ *See Fast Food, Page 216*
Starbucks ~ *See Fast-Foods Section , Page 243*

Coffee Substitute Mixes

	C	F	Cb
Roasted Cereal Beverages ~ *(No Caffeine)*			
Cafix, Instant Beverage, 1 tsp	5	0	1
Kaffree Roma, Instant Beverage, 1 tsp	10	0	2
Teeccino, Herbal Coffees, 1 tsp	10	0	2

Irish & Liqueur Coffees

	C	F	Cb
Irish Coffee, without sugar	175	10	0
Liqueur Coffee, with cream,			
all varieties, av., 1 fl.oz	100	5	7

Coffee Extras

	C	F	Cb
Chocolate (Cocoa) Topping, ½ tsp	5	0	1
Flavored Syrups: Regular, 2 Tbsp	80	0	20
Sugar-free, 2 Tbsp	0	0	0
Half & Half Cream: 2 Tbsp	40	4	1
Single serve pkg, 3/8 fl.oz	15	2	1
Light whipped cream, 2 Tbsp	15	2	1
Marshmallows, miniature (2)	5	0	1
Sugar:			
1 single portion, pkg, 4g	15	0	4
1 level tsp, 4g	15	0	4
1 heaping tsp, 6g	25	0	6
Equal/Splenda/Sweet 'N Low	0	0	0

Coffee Shop ~ Cakes, Cookies

	C	F	Cb
Cookies:			
Biscotti, 1 oz	140	7	18
Chocolate Chip, 3 oz	350	15	54
Oatmeal Raisin, 3 oz	350	12	56
Peanut Butter, 3 oz	410	25	39
White Choc. Macadamia, 3.33 oz	420	20	55
Cakes/Pastries:			
Almond Croissant, 5 oz	620	35	67
Apple Danish, 5 oz	450	18	67
Banana Walnut, 4.5 oz	410	17	60
Brownie, 3 oz	390	24	42
Bundt, Chocolate, 4 oz	440	21	61
Carrot Cake, 4 oz	400	22	45
Chocolate Cake, 5 oz	530	28	65
Crumble Coffee Cake, 4.5 oz	500	25	65
Cupcake, 3 oz	330	16	43
Pound Cake, av., 3 oz	330	17	40
Cinnamon Roll, 6 oz	500	15	83
Donuts:			
Sugared, 1.8 oz	220	11	27
Glazed, 2 oz	250	12	34
Pretzel, large, 4 oz	290	5	52

Starbucks Bakery Items ~ *See Page 244*

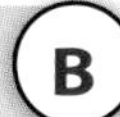

Ready To Drink Coffee

	C	F	Cb
Bottled & Chilled:			
Califia Farms: *With Almond Milk*			
Cold Brew Coffee:			
Almond Milk Mocha Latte, 12 fl.oz	**120**	5	20
Oatmilk Caramel Latte, 12 fl.oz	**130**	5	23
Dunkin:			
Brownie Batter Donut, 11 fl.oz	**200**	6	32
Coffee Cake Muffin, 11 fl.oz	**200**	6	32
Mocha, 13.7 fl.oz	**270**	8	43
International Delight: *Per 12 fl.oz*			
Iced: Caramel Macchiato	**180**	4	32
Connamon Churro	**180**	4	31
Mocha	**180**	4	32
Vanilla	**180**	5	33
Light varieties, 12 fl.oz	**120**	4	18
Kahlua, Cappuccino Shake, 10.5 fl.oz	**130**	2	24
Private Selection *(Kroger): Per 12 fl.oz*			
Cold Brew: Espresso	**15**	0	4
Medium Roast, Slightly Sweetened	**60**	0	15
Vanilla	**60**	0	15
Rise:			
Nitro Cold Brew: Original Black	**10**	0	2
Oat Milk: Latte, 7 fl.oz	**110**	4	18
Mocha, 7 fl.oz	**150**	5	23
Salted Caramel, 7 fl.oz	**120**	6	16
Vanilla Latte, 7 fl.oz	**120**	4	21
Starbucks:			
Cold Brew: *Per 11 fl.oz Unless Indicated*			
Black, sweet	**50**	0	12
Black, unsweetened	**15**	0	3
Cocoa & Honey, with Cream	**150**	4	23
Nitro, 9.6 fl.oz	**80**	2	13
Vanilla Sweet Cream, 12 fl.oz	**90**	2	17
Frappuccino Coffee Drink:			
AlmondMilk Mocha	**120**	4	21
Mocha, 13.7 fl.oz	**260**	5	47
Vanilla, 13.7 fl.oz	**290**	5	53
Macchiato Latte, Caramel, 14 fl.oz	**220**	5	36

Starbucks Refreshers ~ *See Page 40*

Tips to Reduce the Calories in Your Coffee Drinks:

- Request non-fat milk in place of whole or 2% milk
- Downsize to 8 fl.oz or 12 fl.oz
- Avoid cream on frappuccinos
- Replace sugar with *Equal, Splenda, Stevia* or *Sweet 'N Low*
- Avoid syrup add-ons

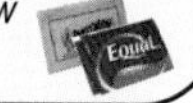

Caffeine Counter

Moderate caffeine intake is not harmful to healthy adults. However, frequent large amounts (over 400 mg/day) may cause dependency ('caffeinism') and adversely affect health. **To be safe, limit caffeine to 200mg/day.** Avoid if pregnant, breastfeeding, a child under 8, have sleep problems, an overactive bladder or heart arrhythmia.

	Caffeine (mg)
Coffee: Instant: Weak, 1 level teaspoon	30
Medium, 1 rounded teaspoon	60
Strong, 1 heaping teaspoon	100
Decaffeinated, 1 rounded teaspoon	2
Bags (Folgers), 1 bag (6-8 fl.oz)	115
Ground, 1 Tbsp, 0.2 oz	60
Bottled (Ready-To-Drink), 9.5 fl.oz	70
Coffee Shop: Brewed, 8 fl.oz	110 -150
Cappuccino/Latte: 1 cup, 8 fl.oz	75
Tall, 12 fl.oz	110
Large, 16 fl.oz	150
Decappuccino, decaffeinated	5
Espresso: Regular/Single/Solo	75
Double/Doppio	150
Iced Coffee w/o Milk, 12 fl.oz	140
Latte, 1 cup, 8 fl.oz	75
Mocha, 1 cup, 8 fl.oz	90
Hot Chocolate, 8 fl.oz	15
Black Tea: Weak, 1 cup	20
Medium Strength, 1 cup	40
Strong, 1 cup	70
Decaffeinated Tea, 1 cup	0-5
Herbal Tea, 1 cup	0
Green Tea, 1 cup	20
Iced Tea, tall glass/can, 12 fl.oz	20-30
Soft Drinks: *Per 12 fl.oz Can*	
Coca-Cola; Pepsi (Regular/Diet)	35
Diet Coke; TAB; RC Cola (Regular)	45
Dr. Pepper; Sunkist Orange	40
Pepsi One; Mountain Dew; Mellow Yellow; Surge	55
Pepsi Max (Regular/Diet) Sun Drop (Reg/Diet)	70
7-Up, Fanta, Sprite, Fresca, Diet Rite Cola	0
Energy Drinks (with added caffeine): *(AMP, Adrenaline Rush, Full Throttle Monster, No Fear, Red Bull, Rockstar)*	
Average all brands: 8 fl.oz	80
16 fl.oz	160
NOS Energy, 16 fl.oz	260
Chocolate Bars: Milk Chocolate, 2 oz	20
Dark Chocolate, 2 oz	30
Choc Chip Cookies, 2 medium, 2 oz	6
Chocolate Syrup, 2 Tbsp, 1.4 oz	5
Guarana, *GNC*, 1 tablet	90
Medicinals: *Excedrin Extra*/Migraine, 1 tab.	65
Jet Alert/NoDoz, 1 tablet	200
Stay Awake (Walgreens), *Vivarin*, 1 tab.	200

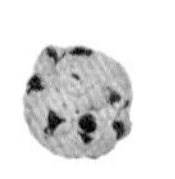

Energy/Protein Drinks	C	F	Cb
5-hour Energy, 1.93fl.oz	4	0	1
AllSport:			
Powder Drink Mix:			
Body Quencher, 2 Tbsp	100	0	25
Zero, 3 grams	5	0	2
AMP ~ *See Mountain Dew*			
Arbonne:			
Essential Meal Protein Shakes,			
all flavors, 2 scoops, 1.4 oz	200	7	11
Feel Fit Pea Protein Shake:			
Chocolate, 1.48 oz	160	4	13
Coffee; Vanilla, 1.2 oz	130	5	5
TrueSport Workout Fuel,			
Orange Pineapple Flavor, 1 stick	50	0	9
Arizona:			
Caution Extreme Performance:			
Classic, 11 fl.oz	160	0	40
Fruit Punch, 11.5 fl.oz	130	0	33
Low Carb Performance, 11 fl.oz	30	0	7
Atkins: *Per 11 fl.oz*			
Plus 30G Prot. Shakes, Choc./Van., av.	190	5	9
Shakes, average all flavors	165	9	7
Bariatrix:			
Proti-Max, Ready to Drink,			
Chocolate/Vanilla, av., 8.45 fl.oz	100	3	7
VHP Shakes, av. all flav., powder,2.36 oz	250	4	19
Bawls Guarana, all flavors, 10 fl.oz	120	0	29
BodyArmor:			
Sports Drinks: Original, 12 fl.oz	90	0	21
Lyte, 12 fl.oz	15	0	14
Bolthouse: *Per 15.2 fl.oz*			
Parfait, Mixed Berry	350	5	65
Protein Plus: Nut Butter , av.	400	15	39
Banana Honey	400	10	50
Coffee	400	7	55
Oatmilk, Chocolate Salted Caramel	270	4	41
Strawberry	340	6	42
Vanilla Bean	340	6	45
Boost *(Nestle):*			
Original, all flavors, 8 fl.oz	240	6	37
High Protein, all flav, 8 fl.oz	250	6	28
Glucose Control, 8 fl.oz	190	7	16
Plus, all flavors, 8 fl.oz	360	14	45
Very High Calorie, all flavors, 8 fl.oz	530	26	52

Carnation:	C	F	Cb
B'Fast Essentials, Powder: *Unprepared*			
Original,av. all flav., 1.3 oz envelope	135	0	27
Light Start, Rich Milk Chocolate. , 0.7 oz	65	1	11
Ready To Drink: Orig., all flav., 8 fl.oz	240	4	41
High Protein, average, 8 fl.oz	220	6	27
CeraSport:			
Powders: Endurance, Vanilla, 1 pkt	150	0	30
Hydration, Berry Flavorm 3 tbsp	80	0	20
Plus Hydration, Strawb., 1 pkt	120	0	30
Champion Performance:			
Heavyweight High Density Mass Gainer,			
av. all flavors, 4 scps, 5.4 oz	580	7	97
Pure Whey Protein Stack,			
average, 1 scoop, 1.2 oz	140	3	4
Clif: Hydration Mix, 0.4 oz pkt	40	0	10
Shot, 1.2 oz packet, Chocolate	110	2	23
Cocaine, Energy, 12 fl.oz can	90	0	23
Core Power *(fairlife):*			
26g, av. all flavors, 14 fl.oz	170	5	7
Elite, 42g, av. all flav., 14 fl.oz	230	4	8
Curves, Protein Drink,			
Choc.; Vanilla, 2 scoops, 1 oz	120	1	12
Ensure:			
Powder, all flavors, prepared, 3.4 fl.oz	100	3	14
Plus, all flavors,3.4 fl.oz	150	5	20
Plus Strength, all flavors, 3.4 fl.oz	150	5	17
TwoCal HN, all flavors, 3.4 fl.oz	200	9	21
Enterex, Diabetic, all flavors, 8 fl.oz	220	8	25
Enu, Nutritional Shakes, 8.5 fl.oz	400	16	45
Evolve (Vegan):			
Plant Based Protein Shake,			
Chocolate, 11 fl.oz	140	2	16
FRS, Protein RTD, Blackberry Acai, 12 fl.oz	150	1	14
Full Throttle: *Per 16 fl.oz*			
Energy, Citrus; True Blue	230	0	57
Gatorade G Series:			
Energy: Gel, 1.3 oz pouch	80	0	20
Fast Twitch, Strawb W'melon, 12 fl.oz	10	0	2
Hydration: Gatorde Fit, 16.9 fl.oz	15	0	3
Thirst Quencher Powder, 1.23 oz	130	0	34
Zero Powder, Fruit Punch, 3 g	5	0	2
Protein:			
G Essntl Whey Protein Isolate,			
Vanilla, ⅓ cup, 0.85 oz	90	0	1
Super Shake, 30G Protein,			
Chocolate, 11.16 fl.oz	180	1	11
Glaceau,			
Vitaminwater,			
average all varieties, 20 fl.oz	100	0	27

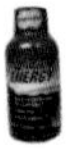

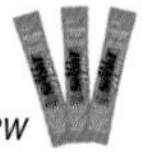

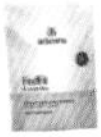

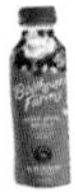

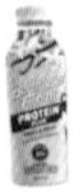

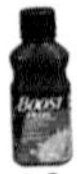

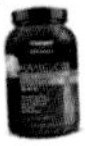

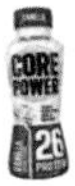

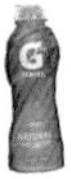

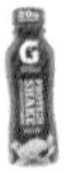

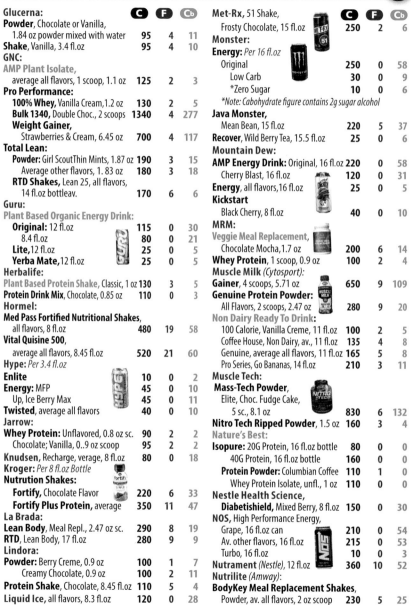

	C	F	Cb
Glucerna:			
Powder, Chocolate or Vanilla,			
1.84 oz powder mixed with water	95	4	11
Shake, Vanilla, 3.4 fl.oz	95	4	10
GNC:			
AMP Plant Isolate,			
average all flavors, 1 scoop, 1.1 oz	125	2	3
Pro Performance:			
100% Whey, Vanilla Cream,1.2 oz	130	2	5
Bulk 1340, Double Choc., 2 scoops	1340	4	277
Weight Gainer,			
Strawberries & Cream, 6.45 oz	700	4	117
Total Lean:			
Powder: Girl ScoutThin Mints, 1.87 oz	190	3	15
Average other flavors, 1. 83 oz	180	3	18
RTD Shakes, Lean 25, all flavors,			
14 fl.oz bottleav.	170	6	6
Guru:			
Plant Based Organic Energy Drink:			
Original: 12 fl.oz	115	0	30
8.4 fl.oz	80	0	21
Lite,12 fl.oz	25	0	5
Yerba Mate,12 fl.oz	25	0	5
Herbalife:			
Plant Based Protein Shake, Classic, 1 oz	130	3	5
Protein Drink Mix, Chocolate, 0.85 oz	110	0	3
Hormel:			
Med Pass Fortified Nutritional Shakes,			
all flavors, 8 fl.oz	480	19	58
Vital Quisine 500,			
average all flavors, 8.45 fl.oz	520	21	60
Hype: *Per 3.4 fl.oz*			
Enlite	10	0	2
Energy: MFP	45	0	10
Up, Ice Berry Max	45	0	11
Twisted, average all flavors	40	0	10
Jarrow:			
Whey Protein: Unflavored, 0.8 oz sc.	90	2	2
Chocolate; Vanilla, 0..9 oz scoop	95	2	2
Knudsen, Recharge, verage, 8 fl.oz	80	0	18
Kroger: *Per 8 fl.oz Bottle*			
Nutrution Shakes:			
Fortify, Chocolate Flavor	220	6	33
Fortify Plus Protein, average	350	11	47
La Brada:			
Lean Body, Meal Repl., 2.47 oz sc.	290	8	19
RTD, Lean Body, 17 fl.oz	280	9	9
Lindora:			
Powder: Berry Creme, 0.9 oz	100	1	7
Creamy Chocolate, 0.9 oz	100	2	11
Protein Shake, Chocolate, 8.45 fl.oz	110	5	4
Liquid Ice, all flavors, 8.3 fl.oz	120	0	28

	C	F	Cb
Met-Rx, 51 Shake,			
Frosty Chocolate, 15 fl.oz	250	2	6
Monster:			
Energy: *Per 16 fl.oz*			
Original	250	0	58
Low Carb	30	0	9
*Zero Sugar	10	0	6
**Note: Cabohydrate figure contains 2g sugar alcohol*			
Java Monster,			
Mean Bean, 15 fl.oz	220	5	37
Recover, Wild Berry Tea, 15.5 fl.oz	25	0	6
Mountain Dew:			
AMP Energy Drink: Original, 16 fl.oz	220	0	58
Cherry Blast, 16 fl.oz	120	0	31
Energy, all flavors,16 fl.oz	25	0	5
Kickstart			
Black Cherry, 8 fl.oz	40	0	10
MRM:			
Veggie Meal Replacement,			
Chocolate Mocha,1.7 oz	200	6	14
Whey Protein, 1 scoop, 0.9 oz	100	2	4
Muscle Milk *(Cytosport):*			
Gainer, 4 scoops, 5.71 oz	650	9	109
Genuine Protein Powder:			
All Flavors, 2 scoops, 2.47 oz	280	9	20
Non Dairy Ready To Drink:			
100 Calorie, Vanilla Creme, 11 fl.oz	100	2	5
Coffee House, Non Dairy, av., 11 fl.oz	135	4	8
Genuine, average all flavors, 11 fl.oz	165	5	8
Pro Series, Go Bananas, 14 fl.oz	210	3	11
Muscle Tech:			
Mass-Tech Powder,			
Elite, Choc. Fudge Cake,			
5 sc., 8.1 oz	830	6	132
Nitro Tech Ripped Powder, 1.5 oz	160	3	4
Nature's Best:			
Isopure: 20G Protein, 16 fl.oz bottle	80	0	0
40G Protein, 16 fl.oz bottle	160	0	0
Protein Powder: Columbian Coffee	110	1	0
Whey Protein Isolate, unfl., 1 oz	110	0	0
Nestle Health Science,			
Diabetishield, Mixed Berry, 8 fl.oz	150	0	30
NOS, High Performance Energy,			
Grape, 16 fl.oz can	210	0	54
Av. other flavors, 16 fl.oz	215	0	53
Turbo, 16 fl.oz	10	0	3
Nutrament *(Nestle)*, 12 fl.oz	360	10	52
Nutrilite *(Amway)*:			
BodyKey Meal Replacement Shakes,			
Powder, av. all flavors, 2 oz scoop	230	5	25

Energy/Protein Drinks (Cont)

	C	F	Cb
Optifast: *(Nestle):*			
HP Shake Mix, 1 pkg	200	6	11
Ready To Drink Shakes, 8 fl.oz	200	6	12
Shake Mix, 1 pkg	160	4	18
Optimum Nutrition: *Powder*			
Amino Energy, average, 12 fl.oz	5	0	1
Gold Standard: 12 fl.oz			
100% Plant, 1 scoop, 1.3 oz	150	4	5
100% Whey, av. all flav., 1 oz scp	120	2	4
Optisource *(Nestle)*,			
Very High Prot. Drink, Strawb., 8 fl.oz	200	6	12
OrGain:			
Organic Nutritional Shakes: *Per 11 fl.oz*			
Milk Based, all flavors	250	7	32
Plant Based, average	235	7	29
Clean Protein, avg., 11 fl.oz	130	2	10
Protein Shakes:			
Milk Based, average, 14 fl.oz	160	4	15
Plant Based, Creamy Choc., 11 fl.oz	140	5	8
Powerade, average all flav., 20 fl.oz	135	0	35
PowerBar, Power Gel Smoothie,			
Mango Apple	145	0	35
Premier Protein *(Premier Nutrition):*			
Clear, Peach; Tropical Punch, 16.9 fl.oz	90	0	1
Protein Shakes, average, 11.5 fl.oz	160	3	4
Protein2O: *Per 16.9 fl.oz*			
Protein Water, Peach Mango	70	0	7
Protein Water Plus, Orange Mango	90	0	7
Pure Protein: *P er 11 fl.oz Bottle or Can*			
30 Gram Shakes, average	140	1	6
Whey Powder, Vanilla, 1.4 oz scoop	160	3	9
Red Bull:			
Energy Drink:			
Regular: 8.4 fl.oz	110	0	29
12 fl.oz can	160	0	40
Sugar-Free, 8.4 fl.oz	10	0	2
Zero Calories, 8.4 fl.oz	0	0	0
Rhino, Rush Drink, all flav., 2 fl.oz	6	0	2
Rip It, Energy Fuel, Citrus X, 16 fl.oz	200	0	52
Rockstar: *Per 16 fl.oz Can*			
Energy Drink: Original	270	0	63
Sugar Free	25	0	1
Rumble: *Per 12 fl.oz*			
Milk Based Supershake, Dutch Choc.	250	10	23
Plant Based, Latte	220	12	12
Rush: *Per 8.4 5fl.oz*			
Energy Drink: Original	120	0	32
with Maca	130	0	30

Shakeology:	C	F	Cb
Plant Based, Vanilla, 1.34 oz	160	3	15
Whey Proein, Chocolate, 1.48 oz	160	3	18
Skratch Labs:			
Hydration Drink Mix,			
Lemon Lime, 0.9 oz	80	0	21
Recovery Sports Mix, Strawb., 1.76 oz	210	4	36
Super High-Carb,			
Lemon + Lime Mix, 1.9 oz	200	0	50
Slim-Fast:			
Original: Protein Shakes,			
average all flavors, 11 fl.oz	180	5	25
Powder, average, 0.9 oz scoop	110	3	18
Advanced: High Protein, 11 fl.oz	180	9	7
Smoothie Mix, 1 scoop, 0.9 oz	100	3	7
Keto Meal Shake, 11 fl.oz bottle	180	14	7
SoBe,			
Citrus Energy Fruit Drink, 20 fl.oz	250	0	64
Spiru-Tein *(Natures Plus):*			
High Protein Energy Meal,			
Cappuccino, 1.13 oz	100	0	13
Chocolate PB Swirl, 1.1 oz	110	1	13
Protein Powder Meal:			
Banana, 1.3 oz scoop	120	0	16
Gold: Chocolate, 1.3 oz scoop	90	0	21
Vanilla,1.3 oz scoop	100	0	20
Note: Gold Products Contains 12-15 grams Xylitol			
Sport, Vanilla, 2.26oz	260	7	27
Whey, Chocolate, 1.13 oz	110	2	10
Starbucks ~ Doubleshot Energy ~ See page 37			
Steaz: *Per 16 fl.oz*			
Antioxidant Brew Green Tea:			
Regular, all flavors	90	0	21
Zero, all flavors	0	0	0
Twin Lab, Sports Pre Workout, 0.4 oz	30	0	7
Vega, Real Food Smoothie,			
Chocolate Peanut Butter Blast, 1.3 oz	150	4	9
Venom, av all flavors, 16 fl.oz	160	0	40
Vital: Organic Greens, 0,17 oz	20	0.2	2.3
Pea & Hemp Protein, 0.9 oz	100	2	5
XS *(Amway)*, Energy Drinks, 12 fl.oz	15	0	1
ZOA, Energy Drinks: 12 fl.oz	10	0	2
Zola,			
Flavored Coconut Water, av., 8 fl.oz	60	0	14

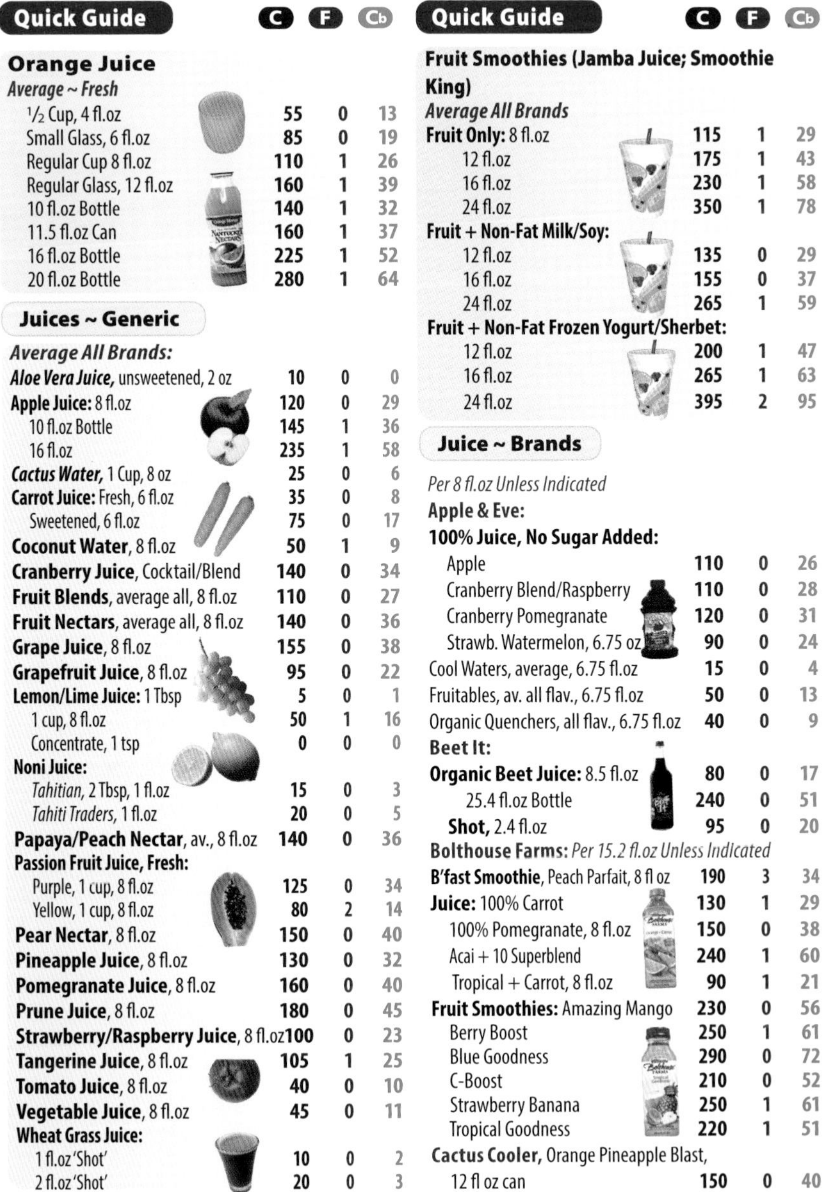

Quick Guide

Orange Juice

Average ~ Fresh

	C	F	Cb
½ Cup, 4 fl.oz	55	0	13
Small Glass, 6 fl.oz	85	0	19
Regular Cup 8 fl.oz	110	1	26
Regular Glass, 12 fl.oz	160	1	39
10 fl.oz Bottle	140	1	32
11.5 fl.oz Can	160	1	37
16 fl.oz Bottle	225	1	52
20 fl.oz Bottle	280	1	64

Juices ~ Generic

Average All Brands:

	C	F	Cb
Aloe Vera Juice, unsweetened, 2 oz	10	0	0
Apple Juice: 8 fl.oz	120	0	29
10 fl.oz Bottle	145	1	36
16 fl.oz	235	1	58
Cactus Water, 1 Cup, 8 oz	25	0	6
Carrot Juice: Fresh, 6 fl.oz	35	0	8
Sweetened, 6 fl.oz	75	0	17
Coconut Water, 8 fl.oz	50	1	9
Cranberry Juice, Cocktail/Blend	140	0	34
Fruit Blends, average all, 8 fl.oz	110	0	27
Fruit Nectars, average all, 8 fl.oz	140	0	36
Grape Juice, 8 fl.oz	155	0	38
Grapefruit Juice, 8 fl.oz	95	0	22
Lemon/Lime Juice: 1 Tbsp	5	0	1
1 cup, 8 fl.oz	50	1	16
Concentrate, 1 tsp	0	0	0
Noni Juice:			
Tahitian, 2 Tbsp, 1 fl.oz	15	0	3
Tahiti Traders, 1 fl.oz	20	0	5
Papaya/Peach Nectar, av., 8 fl.oz	140	0	36
Passion Fruit Juice, Fresh:			
Purple, 1 cup, 8 fl.oz	125	0	34
Yellow, 1 cup, 8 fl.oz	80	2	14
Pear Nectar, 8 fl.oz	150	0	40
Pineapple Juice, 8 fl.oz	130	0	32
Pomegranate Juice, 8 fl.oz	160	0	40
Prune Juice, 8 fl.oz	180	0	45
Strawberry/Raspberry Juice, 8 fl.oz	100	0	23
Tangerine Juice, 8 fl.oz	105	1	25
Tomato Juice, 8 fl.oz	40	0	10
Vegetable Juice, 8 fl.oz	45	0	11
Wheat Grass Juice:			
1 fl.oz 'Shot'	10	0	2
2 fl.oz 'Shot'	20	0	3

Quick Guide

Fruit Smoothies (Jamba Juice; Smoothie King)

Average All Brands

	C	F	Cb
Fruit Only: 8 fl.oz	115	1	29
12 fl.oz	175	1	43
16 fl.oz	230	1	58
24 fl.oz	350	1	78
Fruit + Non-Fat Milk/Soy:			
12 fl.oz	135	0	29
16 fl.oz	155	0	37
24 fl.oz	265	1	59
Fruit + Non-Fat Frozen Yogurt/Sherbet:			
12 fl.oz	200	1	47
16 fl.oz	265	1	63
24 fl.oz	395	2	95

Juice ~ Brands

Per 8 fl.oz Unless Indicated

	C	F	Cb
Apple & Eve:			
100% Juice, No Sugar Added:			
Apple	110	0	26
Cranberry Blend/Raspberry	110	0	28
Cranberry Pomegranate	120	0	31
Strawb. Watermelon, 6.75 oz	90	0	24
Cool Waters, average, 6.75 fl.oz	15	0	4
Fruitables, av. all flav., 6.75 fl.oz	50	0	13
Organic Quenchers, all flav., 6.75 fl.oz	40	0	9
Beet It:			
Organic Beet Juice: 8.5 fl.oz	80	0	17
25.4 fl.oz Bottle	240	0	51
Shot, 2.4 fl.oz	95	0	20
Bolthouse Farms: *Per 15.2 fl.oz Unless Indicated*			
B'fast Smoothie, Peach Parfait, 8 fl oz	190	3	34
Juice: 100% Carrot	130	1	29
100% Pomegranate, 8 fl.oz	150	0	38
Acai + 10 Superblend	240	1	60
Tropical + Carrot, 8 fl.oz	90	1	21
Fruit Smoothies: Amazing Mango	230	0	56
Berry Boost	250	1	61
Blue Goodness	290	0	72
C-Boost	210	0	52
Strawberry Banana	250	1	61
Tropical Goodness	220	1	51
Cactus Cooler, Orange Pineapple Blast, 12 fl oz can	150	0	40

Juice Brands (Cont)

Per 8 fl.oz Unless Indicated	C	F	Cb
Campbell's:			
Tomato Juice: 11.5 fl.oz can	70	0	14
8 fl.oz	50	0	10
Califia Farms: *Per 8 fl.oz Unless Indicated*			
Ginger Limeade	80	0	21
Meyer Lemonade	80	0	21
Orange Juice, 10. 5 fl.oz	140	1	32
Tangerine	110	0	25
Tart Cherry Lemonade	110	0	27
Capri Sun: *Per 6 fl.oz*			
100% Juice, average,	85	0	21
Juice Drinks,			
(25% Less Sugar), all flavors	50	0	14
Refreshers, average, 6 fl.oz	45	0	11
Roarin' Waters, all flav., 6 fl.oz	30	0	8
Sport, average, 6 fl.oz	30	0	8
Sun Adventures, av., 6 fl.oz	50	0	13
Clamato: *Per 8 fl.oz*			
Original Tomato Cocktail	60	0	12
Picante	60	0	13
Coco Joy:			
Natural Coconut Water, 8.4 fl.oz	60	0	15
Sparkling Coconut Water, all, 11 fl.oz	80	2	20
Coco Libre, Flav. Coconut Water, 11 fl.oz	75	0	18
CocoZia, Coconut Water:			
100% Organic, 11.1 fl.oz pkg	70	0	16
Original, 8 fl.oz	40	0	10
Chocolate, 8 fl.oz	60	1	13
Dole: *Per 8 fl.oz*			
Canned: 100% Juice, 6 fl.oz	100	0	25
Jaya Juice, av. all flavors, 8 fl.oz	145	0	36
Florida's Natural: *Per 8 fl.oz*			
Apple Juice	120	0	29
Lemonades, all flavors	110	0	28
Orange, No Pulp	110	0	26
Light Orange Juice	50	0	12
Ruby Red Grapefruit	90	0	22
Fuze: *Per 12 fl.oz*			
Blueberry Lemonade	80	0	21
Pineapple + Mango	80	0	21
Goya: *Per 9.6 fl.oz Can*			
Cocktail, Passion Fruit	130	0	34
Juice, Pineapple	110	0	27
Nectar: Mango	180	0	47
Peach	140	0	36
Pear & Passion Fruit	140	0	36
Soursop	130	0	35

Per 8 fl.oz Unless Indicated	C	F	Cb
Great Value *(Walmart):*			
100% Juice: *Per 8 fl.oz*			
Apple	110	0	28
Cranberry Blend	120	0	30
Grape	150	0	38
Orange	110	0	27
White Grape	140	0	38
Hansen's:			
Junior Juice,			
100% Juice, av. of flavors,			
4.23 oz box	60	0	16
Natural, (64 fl.oz Bottles): *Per 8 fl.oz*			
Apple	120	0	28
Apple Strawberry	110	0	27
Cranberry Apple	110	0	27
Cranberry Grape	140	0	35
Grape	120	0	33
Orange Pineapple	110	0	27
White Grape	140	0	36
Hawaii's Own, Frozen Concentrate,			
100% Juice, average all flavors,			
8 fl.oz prepared	105	0	27
Hi-C Juice Drinks: *Per 6.75 fl.oz Box*			
Flashin' Fruit Punch	90	0	25
Orange Lavaburst	90	0	25
Poppin' Lemonade	100	0	27
Hood: *Per 8 fl.oz*			
Lemonade	110	0	29
Orange	120	0	30
Jamba Juice ~ *See Fast-Foods Section*			
Juicy Juice *(Nestle):*			
Juicy Waters, 6.75 fl.oz	0	0	0
Organic Juice : *Per 8 fl.oz Unless Indicated*			
100%, Apple Juice; Fruit Punch	120	0	28
Fruitfuls, all flavors	70	0	16
6.75 fl.oz box	50	0	13
Plus Protein, all flavors, 6 fl.oz	90	0	17
Splashers, all f lavors, 1 pouch	40	0	9
Kerns:			
Nectars: *Per 11.5 fl.oz Can*			
Apricot	210	0	52
Guava; Strawberry, av.	180	0	45
Pear; Strawb. Banana, av.	195	0	46
Pineapple Coconut	230	6	43
L & A: *Per 8 fl.oz*			
All Cherry	180	0	45
All Cranberry	60	0	14
Papaya Delight	130	0	32
Pineapple Coconut	140	3	28

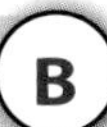

Juice Brands (Cont)

Per 8 fl.oz Unless Indicated	C	F	Cb
Lakewood Organic: *Per 8 fl.oz*			
Organic Blends:			
Black Cherry	130	0	32
Blueberry Blend	120	0	29
Pineapple Coconut	190	8	29
Pom Blue	120	0	29
Kale	80	0	19
Papaya	110	0	27
Tart Cherry	130	0	31
Veggie	80	0	17
Organic Pure: Beet	100	0	23
Blueberry	110	0	26
Carrot	90	0	20
Cranberry	80	0	19
Noni	5	0	1
Orange	120	0	28
Pineapple	130	0	31
Pink Grapefruit	110	0	26
Prune	180	0	43
Langers: *Per 8 fl.oz*			
100% Juice:			
Apple Juice	120	0	28
Red/White Grape Juice	160	0	40
Juice Cocktails (27% Juice):			
Blueberry Cranberry	135	0	34
Cranberry	140	0	35
Cranberry Grape	165	0	41
Cranberry Raspberry	140	0	35
20% Juice, all flavors	120	0	30
Martinellli's:			
Juice, 100% Apple, all varieties, 8 fl.oz	140	0	35
Sparkling: Apple Juice, 10 fl.oz	180	0	43
Apple Grape, 8.4 fl.oz	130	0	33
Apple-Pear Cider, 8 fl.oz	120	0	29
Apple Pomegranate, 8fl.oiz	120	0	30
Blush, 10 fl.oz	160	0	40
Cider, 8 fl.oz	140	0	35
Pear Cider, 8.4 fl.oz	130	0	31
Rose, 10 fl.oz	160	0	40
Minute Maid:			
12 fl.oz Bottles: *Per Bottle*			
Apple Juice	170	0	41
Cranb. Apple Raspberry	180	0	48
Cranberry Grape	190	0	50
Pineapple Orange	180	0	43

Per 8 fl.oz Unless Indicated	C	F	Cb
Minute Maid (Cont):			
Orange Juice,			
Original, 8 fl.oz	110	0	27
Just 15 Calories, Lemonade, 8 fl.oz	15	0	4
Kid's Juice Boxes, 100% Juice,			
Apple White Grape, 6.75 fl.oz	90	0	22
Light Juice, Cherry Limeade, 8 fl.oz	4	0	1
Soft Frozen Concentrate,			
Limeade, 8 fl.oz prepared	90	0	25
Mott's:			
100% Juice:			
Original Apple, 8 fl.oz	120	0	29
Apple Mango, 8 fl.oz	120	0	29
Apple White Grape, 6.75 fl.oz	130	0	31
Fruit Punch, 4.23 fl.oz	60	0	15
Juice Drink, Light Apple, 8 fl.oz	50	0	12
Mott's For Tots (47-54% Juice):			
40% Less Sugar: Fruit Punch, 8 fl.oz	70	0	16
Other flavors, 8 fl.oz	60	0	16
Sensibles, all flavors, 8 fl.oz	90	0	21
Naked Juice: *Per 15.2 fl.oz Unless Indicated*			
Core: Berry Blast	220	1	55
Mighty Mango	290	0	68
Orange Mango	230	0	59
Pina Colada	290	3	65
Strawberry Banana	270	0	52
Tropical Guava	260	0	62
Craveworthy: Chocolate Protein	410	6	61
Key Lime, 12 fl.oz	220	6	36
Orange Vanilla Creme, 12 fl.oz	260	6	45
Vanilla	370	6	48
Functional: Double Berry Protein	370	2	55
Mighty Berry	290	0	69
Orange Carrot Mango Immune	220	0	55
Tropical Protein	390	2	62
Machines: Blue	320	0	76
Green	270	0	63
Power-C	220	0	55
Rainbow	260	0	61
Red	320	9	59
Suerfood	270	3	58

Juice Brands (Cont)

Per 8 fl.oz Unless Indicated	C	F	Cb
Nantucket Nectars:			
Juice: *Per 16 fl.oz*			
Orange Mango	220	0	59
Peach Orange	260	0	63
Pineapple Orange Banana	290	0	69
Pineapple Orange Guava	210	0	52
Pomegranate Cherry	230	0	57
Pomegranate Pear	230	0	57
Premium Orange Juice	220	0	51
Pressed Apple	240	1	59
Red Plum	220	0	55
Watermelon Strawberry	220	0	55
Juice Cocktail, Cranberry	240	0	59
Lemonade, Squeezed	180	0	47
Newman's Own: *Per 8 fl.oz*			
Lemonade, Regular; Pink	110	0	27
Limeade	140	0	34
Fruit Juice Cocktail:			
Grape	110	0	29
Orange Mango Tango	130	0	33
Northland: *Per 8 fl.oz*			
100% Juice:			
Blueberry Blackberry Acaí	110	0	27
Cranb. Blackberry/Raspberry, av.	110	0	27
Cranberry Cherry	120	0	30
Cranberry Grape	110	0	28
Cranberry Mango	120	0	29
Ocean Spray: *Per 8 fl.oz*			
Juice Cocktails:			
Cranberry	110	0	28
100% Juice Blends:			
Cranberry Concord Grape	130	0	36
Cranberry Mango	120	0	31
Cranberry Pineapple	110	0	31
Cranberry Raspberry	120	0	32
Juice Drinks:			
Cran-Apple	100	0	27
Cran-Grape	100	0	28
Cran-Tangerine	100	0	28
Diet Juice Drinks, all flavors	5	0	2
Growing Goodness, av., 6.75 fl.oz	45	0	12
Light Juice Drinks, av. all flavors	50	0	13
Sparkling, av. all flavors, 8.4 fl.oz	70	0	20

Per 8 fl.oz Unless Indicated	C	F	Cb
Orange Julius:			
Originals:			
Medium: Mango Pineapple	320	0.2	78
Orange	260	1	63
Strawberry	300	0.2	75
Large: Mango Pineapple	470	0.5	117
Orange	400	1	98
Strawberry	450	0.5	113
Smoothies ~ *See Fast-Foods Section*			
Orangina, 10 fl.oz bottle	130	0	32
Pom Wonderful,			
100% Juice (8 fl.oz Bottle),			
Pom Blueberry/Cherry/Pomegranate	155	0	38
R.W. Knudsen: *Per 8 fl.oz*			
Organic, 100% Juice: Apple	110	0	28
Acai Berry	110	0	26
Concord Grape	160	0	39
Cranberry Blueberry	110	0	27
Mango Nectar	120	0	29
Orange Carrot	110	0	27
Tomato	45	0	10
Natural, 100% Juice:			
Mango Peach	120	0	30
Papaya Nectar	130	0	32
Razzleberry	110	0	28
Rio Red Grapefruit	140	0	34
Just Juice:			
Just Blueberry	90	0	23
Just Black Cherry	190	0	45
Just Black Currant	110	0	24
Simply Nutritious:			
Lemon Ginger Echinacea	110	0	27
Average other flavors	115	0	28
Shots: Apple Cider Vinegar, 2.5 fl.oz	10	0	2
Beet , 2.5 fl.oz	25	0	5
Carrot, Black Pepper & Turmeric, 2.5 fl.oz	25	0	5
Pineapple Ginger, 2.5 fl.oz	30	0	9
Sparkling: Caramel Apple	110	0	28
Cranberry	110	0	27
Cherry; Pomegranate	130	0	32
Organic Pear	120	0	30

Juice Brands (Cont)

Per 8 fl.oz Unless Indicated

	C	F	Cb
R.W. Knudsen (Cont):			
Organic Veggie Blends:			
Beet, Carrot Orange	90	0	22
Carrot Ginger Turmeric	70	0	16
Celery Apple Cucumber	50	0	11
Sweet Potato	100	0	24
Very Veggie; Low Sodium	50	0	10
Spicy	45	0	10
ReaLemon – ReaLime:			
Lemon/Lime Juice (from concentrate):			
1 teaspoon	0	0	0
2 Tbsp, 1 fl.oz	10	0	3
Santa Cruz: *Per 8 fl.oz*			
Organic, 100% Juice:			
Apple; Apricot Mango, average	115	0	29
Concord/White Grape	160	0	39
Orange Mango; Red Tart Cherry	120	0	29
Pear Nectar	140	0	34
Lemonade:			
Regular; Peach	90	0	22
Blueberry; Raspberry; Strawberry, av.	90	0	23
Cherry	100	0	25
Peach	80	0	21
Simply Orange Juice Company:			
Lemonade; Limeade, average	120	0	31
Lemonade, with Raspberry	110	0	28
Mixed Berry; Tropical	100	0	26
Orange Juice, with or without pulp	110	0	26
Snap•E•Tom, Tomato & Chili Cocktail, 11.5 fl.oz can	70	0	15
Snapple: *Per 16 fl.oz Bottle*			
Juice: Go Bananas.	230	0	55
Grapeade; Orangeade	190	0	46
Fruit Punch	200	0	48
Kiwi Strawberry	190	0	46
Mango Madness	190	0	45
Watermelon Lemonade	150	0	35
Diet, Cranberry Raspberry	20	0	5
Ssips, Juice Boxes, av. all flavors, 6 fl.oz box	80	0	21

Per 8 fl.oz Unless Indicated

	C	F	Cb
SunnyD: *Per 8 fl.oz*			
Blue Raspberry	60	0	15
Fruit Punch	60	0	16
Lemonade	60	0	15
Orange Mango/Strawberry	60	0	16
Orange Peach	60	0	17
Orange Pineapple	60	0	16
Orange Strawberry	60	0	16
Smooth Orange	50	0	14
Tangy Original	60	0	16
Sunsweet: *Per 8 fl.oz*			
Plum Smart: Original	160	0	36
Light	60	0	15
Prune Juice: Original	180	0	42
Light	100	0	26
Trader Joe's:			
All Natural Pasteurized, 32/64 fl.oz Bottle: *Per 8 fl.oz*			
100% Cranberry	70	0	16
Blueberry Pomegranate	140	0	34
Just Blueberry	100	0	24
Just Pomegranate	150	0	37
Mango PassionFruit	130	0	32
Omega Orange Carrot	110	0	26
Organic, 32/64 fl.oz Bottle: *Per 8 fl.oz*			
Apple Juice	120	0	30
Concord Grape Juice	160	0	39
Cranberry	70	0	18
Grapefruit Sunset	120	0	30
jalapeno Limeade	100	0	25
Mango Nectar	130	0	32
Pink Lemonade	130	0	32
Strawberry Lemonade	120	0	29
White Grape Juice	160	0	40
Cold Presssed, 12 fl.oz:			
Coconut Carrot	70	0	16
Spiced Fuji Apple Cider	200	0	48
Spiced Cider	130	0	31
Winter Wassail	100	0	26
Joe's Kids: *Per 6.75 oz Box*			
From Concentrate: Apple	90	0	23
Apple Grape	100	0	24
White Grape	120	0	30
10% Juice, Lemonade	90	0	22
Sparkling Juices, 25.4 fl.oz Bottle: *Per 8 fl.oz*			
Blueberry	120	0	30
Cranberry	140	0	35
Pomegranate	130	0	31

Juice Brands (Cont)

Per 8 fl.oz Unless Indicated	C	F	Cb
Tree Top:			
100% Juice, 64 fl.oz Bottle: *Per 8 fl.oz*			
Apple Berry/Grape, average	125	0	31
Mango Cherry	120	0	29
Orange Passionfruit ; P'apple Orange	120	0	30
5.5 fl.oz can, apple	80	0	19
6.75 fl.oz Box, Apple; Pear	100	0	24
Fruit & Water: Tropical, 6 fl.oz	45	0	11
All other Flavors, 6 fl.oz	50	0	12
Tropicana: *Per 8 fl.oz*			
Essentials Fiber,			
Strawberry Banana	140	0	35
Premium Drinks:			
Island Punch	90	0	21
Lemonade: Peach	110	0	27
Raspberry; Tangerine, average	100	0	25
Strawberry Peach	100	0	24
Pure Premium Orange Juice:			
Grovestand, Lots of Pulp	110	0	26
No Pulp	110	0	26
Trop 50: Pomegranate Blueberry	50	0	14
Orange Mango/Peach, av.	50	0	12
Tru Nopal:			
Cactus Water: 1 Cup, 8 fl.oz	25	0	6
16.9 fl.oz carton	50	0	12
Turkey Hill: *Per 12 fl.oz*			
All Natural Lemonade: Original	170	0	41
Blackberry; Watermelon	160	0	39
Pink	150	0	37
Watermelon	160	0	39
Fruit Punch	150	0	39
V8 Juices & Drinks *(Campbell's):*			
Original/Spicy 100% Vegetable Juice:			
5.5 fl.oz can	35	0	7
8 fl.oz cup	45	0	9
11.5 fl.oz can	70	0	14
12 fl.oz bottle	75	0	15
Blends: Peach Mango, 8 fl.oz	110	0	27
Healthy Greens; Carrot Mango, 8 fl.oz	60	0	14
Red Radiance, 8 fl.oz	70	0	17
Sparkling V8-Energy:			
Orange Pineapple, 11.5 fl.oz	140	5	20
Strawberry Kiwi, 11.5 fl.oz	50	0	12
Veryfine:			
100%: Apple, 8 fl.oz	120	0	29
Apple Strawb., Krazy Kiwi, 11.5 fl.oz	170	0	43
Orange, 8 fl.oz	120	0	30

Per 8 fl.oz Unless Indicated	C	F	Cb
Vita Coco: *Per 8 fl.oz*			
Coconut Water: Regular	45	0	11
with Peach & Mango	90	3	16
with Pineapple	60	0	14
Walnut Acres: *Per 8 fl.oz*			
Organic: Apple	110	0	29
Apricot; Raspberry	130	0	32
Cherry	140	0	34
Concord Grape	120	0	31
Incredible Vegetable	50	0	12
Orange Carrot	110	0	27
Welch's: *Per 8 fl.oz Unless Indicated*			
100% Juice: Concord Grape	140	0	38
Red Sangria	140	0	34
White Grape	140	0	38
White Grape Peach	140	0	34
Juice Drink, Fruit Punch, 10 fl.oz	120	0	31
Refrigerated Cocktails: CherryBurst	100	0	23
Mango Twist	120	0	28
Peach Medley	100	0	25
Sparkling Juice Cocktail:			
Red/White Grape, av.	150	0	40
Rose; Mimosa, average	75	0	18
Zola:			
Acai: *Per 12 fl.oz Bottle*			
Original	185	3	38
with Blueberry/Pomegranate	180	3	38
Coconut Water, 17.5 oz Can:			
Original,	50	0	13
Chocolate, 8 fl.oz	50	0	12
Espresso, 8 fl.oz	60	0	13

CalorieKing Portion Watch

ORANGE JUICE	C	Cb
8 fl.oz	110	26
16 fl.oz	220	52
24 fl.oz	330	78
32 fl.oz	440	104

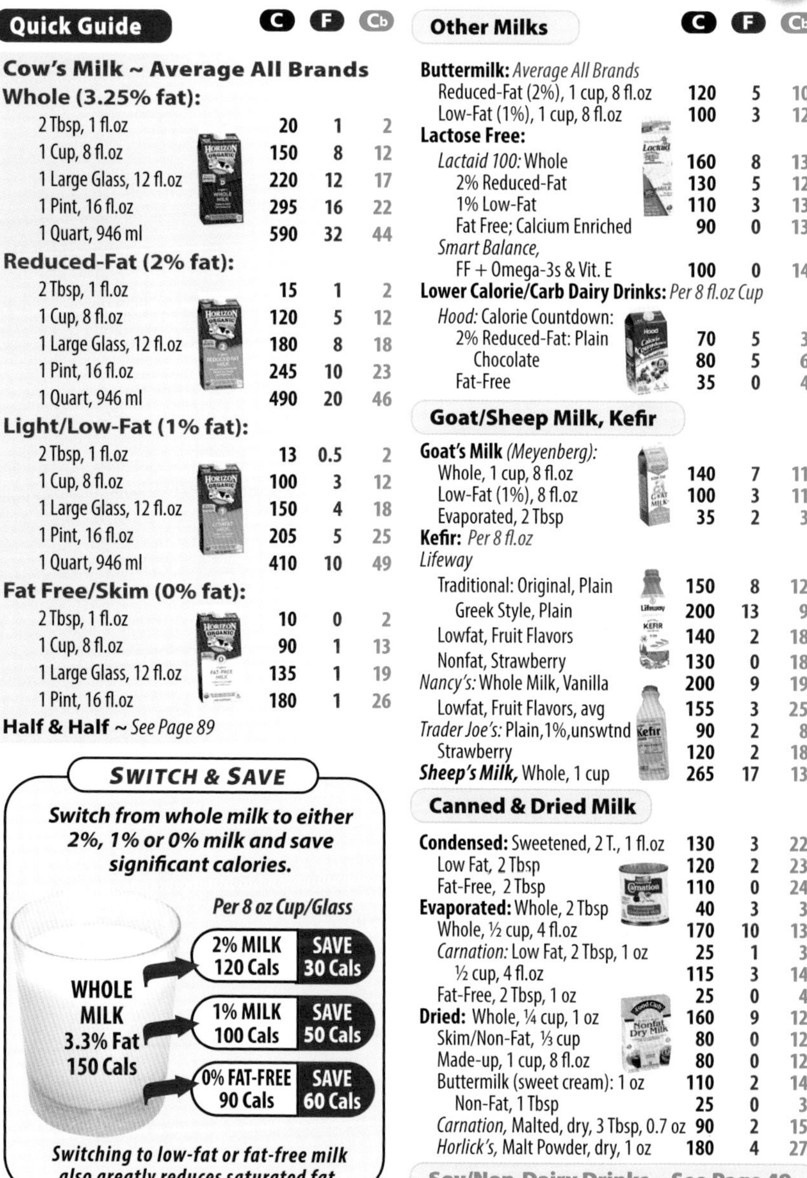

Quick Guide

Cow's Milk ~ Average All Brands

	C	F	Cb
Whole (3.25% fat):			
2 Tbsp, 1 fl.oz	20	1	2
1 Cup, 8 fl.oz	150	8	12
1 Large Glass, 12 fl.oz	220	12	17
1 Pint, 16 fl.oz	295	16	22
1 Quart, 946 ml	590	32	44
Reduced-Fat (2% fat):			
2 Tbsp, 1 fl.oz	15	1	2
1 Cup, 8 fl.oz	120	5	12
1 Large Glass, 12 fl.oz	180	8	18
1 Pint, 16 fl.oz	245	10	23
1 Quart, 946 ml	490	20	46
Light/Low-Fat (1% fat):			
2 Tbsp, 1 fl.oz	13	0.5	2
1 Cup, 8 fl.oz	100	3	12
1 Large Glass, 12 fl.oz	150	4	18
1 Pint, 16 fl.oz	205	5	25
1 Quart, 946 ml	410	10	49
Fat Free/Skim (0% fat):			
2 Tbsp, 1 fl.oz	10	0	2
1 Cup, 8 fl.oz	90	1	13
1 Large Glass, 12 fl.oz	135	1	19
1 Pint, 16 fl.oz	180	1	26

Half & Half ~ *See Page 89*

SWITCH & SAVE

Switch from whole milk to either 2%, 1% or 0% milk and save significant calories.

Per 8 oz Cup/Glass

WHOLE MILK 3.3% Fat 150 Cals

2% MILK 120 Cals	SAVE 30 Cals
1% MILK 100 Cals	SAVE 50 Cals
0% FAT-FREE 90 Cals	SAVE 60 Cals

Switching to low-fat or fat-free milk also greatly reduces saturated fat.

Other Milks

	C	F	Cb
Buttermilk: *Average All Brands*			
Reduced-Fat (2%), 1 cup, 8 fl.oz	120	5	10
Low-Fat (1%), 1 cup, 8 fl.oz	100	3	12
Lactose Free:			
Lactaid 100: Whole	160	8	13
2% Reduced-Fat	130	5	12
1% Low-Fat	110	3	13
Fat Free; Calcium Enriched	90	0	13
Smart Balance,			
FF + Omega-3s & Vit. E	100	0	14
Lower Calorie/Carb Dairy Drinks: *Per 8 fl.oz Cup*			
Hood: Calorie Countdown:			
2% Reduced-Fat: Plain	70	5	3
Chocolate	80	5	6
Fat-Free	35	0	4

Goat/Sheep Milk, Kefir

	C	F	Cb
Goat's Milk *(Meyenberg):*			
Whole, 1 cup, 8 fl.oz	140	7	11
Low-Fat (1%), 8 fl.oz	100	3	11
Evaporated, 2 Tbsp	35	2	3
Kefir: *Per 8 fl.oz*			
Lifeway			
Traditional: Original, Plain	150	8	12
Greek Style, Plain	200	13	9
Lowfat, Fruit Flavors	140	2	18
Nonfat, Strawberry	130	0	18
Nancy's: Whole Milk, Vanilla	200	9	19
Lowfat, Fruit Flavors, avg	155	3	25
Trader Joe's: Plain,1%,unswtnd	90	2	8
Strawberry	120	2	18
Sheep's Milk, Whole, 1 cup	265	17	13

Canned & Dried Milk

	C	F	Cb
Condensed: Sweetened, 2 T., 1 fl.oz	130	3	22
Low Fat, 2 Tbsp	120	2	23
Fat-Free, 2 Tbsp	110	0	24
Evaporated: Whole, 2 Tbsp	40	3	3
Whole, ½ cup, 4 fl.oz	170	10	13
Carnation: Low Fat, 2 Tbsp, 1 oz	25	1	3
½ cup, 4 fl.oz	115	3	14
Fat-Free, 2 Tbsp, 1 oz	25	0	4
Dried: Whole, ¼ cup, 1 oz	160	9	12
Skim/Non-Fat, ⅓ cup	80	0	12
Made-up, 1 cup, 8 fl.oz	80	0	12
Buttermilk (sweet cream): 1 oz	110	2	14
Non-Fat, 1 Tbsp	25	0	3
Carnation, Malted, dry, 3 Tbsp, 0.7 oz	90	2	15
Horlick's, Malt Powder, dry, 1 oz	180	4	27

Soy/Non-Dairy Drinks ~ **See Page 49**

Quick Guide

Chocolate Milk:	C	F	Cb
Average All Brands:			
Whole Milk, (3.3%):			
8 fl.oz cup	220	8	29
1 Pint, 16 fl.oz	440	16	58
Reduced-Fat, (2%):			
8 fl.oz cup	190	5	30
1 Pint, 16 fl.oz	380	10	60
Low-Fat, (1%):			
8 fl.oz cup	160	3	26
1 Pint, 16 fl.oz	315	5	52

Flavored Milk ~ Brands

	C	F	Cb
Ready-To-Drink: *Per 8 fl.oz Unless Indicated*			
fairlife, Chocolate , reduced fat	140	5	13
Great Value *(Walmart)*, Chocolate, low fat	140	3	21
Hood:			
Chocolate: Premium, 8 fl.oz	230	8	30
Lowfat, 8 fl.oz	160	3	28
Lowfat (1%), 14 fl.oz bottle	300	5	50
Whole Milk, 14 fl.oz bottle	220	8	30
Coffee, lowfat, 14 fl.oz bottle	290	5	48
Horizon Organic: *Per 8 fl.oz*			
Lowfat: Chocolate	150	3	23
Strawberry	150	3	24
Vanilla	140	3	22
Kroger: *Per 8 fl.oz*			
Chocolate: CARBmaster, Non Fat	80	0	7
1% Lowfat	170	3	29
Simple Truth Organic:			
Chocolate: Lowfat	130	3	20
Whole Milk, regular	210	8	28
Muscle Milk ~ *See Energy Protein Drinks*			
Nesquik: *Per 14 fl.oz*			
Low Fat, Choc.; Strawberry	250	4	41
TruMoo: *Per 8 fl.oz*			
Whole Milk: Chocolate	200	8	24
Strawberry	210	8	27
1% Low-Fat, Chocolate	130	3	19
High Protein 1% (25g), Lowfat, all flavors	360	5	55
Yoo-Hoo:			
Chocolate: 6.5 fl.oz box	220	2	51
12 fl.oz bottle	170	2	39
15.5 fl.oz bottle	220	2	51
Cookies & Cream, 6.5 fl.oz	100	1	23
Strawb./Vanilla, av. 6.5 fl.oz	100	1	22

Bottled Coffee Drinks ~ *See Page 37*

Shakes

	C	F	Cb
Arby's Shakes: *Per Regular with Drizzle & Whipped Cream*			
Chocolate	540	17	86
Jamocha	540	16	74
Vanilla	480	17	70
Burger King Shakes: *Per 16 fl.oz Without Toppings*			
Chocolate	590	14	103
Chocolate Oreo	670	17	116
Classic Oreo	640	17	109
Strawberry	610	14	110
Vanilla	560	14	96
Carl's Jr Shakes: *Per Medium, With Whipped Topping*			
Hand Scooped Ice Cream Shakes:			
Chocolate	690	36	84
Strawberry	690	35	83
Vanilla	700	35	86
Denny's Shakes: *With Whipped Cream*			
Chocolate, 16 oz	870	43	111
Oreo, 17 oz	1050	56	125
Strawberry, 17 oz	780	34	114
Vanilla, 16 oz	800	43	97
Hardees Shakes: *Per Medium, with Whipped Topping*			
Hand Scooped Ice Cream Shakes:			
Vanilla, 4 oz	700	35	86
Chocolate;Strawberry, average	690	35	84
McDonald's Shakes: *With Whipped Light Cream*			
Chocolate: Small	520	14	85
Medium	650	17	107
Large	790	20	134
Strawberry/Vanilla: *Average*			
Small	475	13	79
Medium	585	16	99
Strawberry, Large	850	21	143

Other Restaurants ~ *See Fast-Foods Section*

Smoothies

	C	F	Cb
Made Up Ready-To-Drink:			
8 fl. oz Milk/Soy + Fruit: *Per 12 fl.oz*			
Average all flavors:			
with Whole Milk	300	8	50
+ Ice Cream, 1 scoop	400	13	62
with Non-Fat Milk	240	0	50

Freshens; Jamba Juice; TCBY ~ *See Fast Foods*

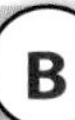

Nut, Pea, Rice & Cereal Drinks

Per 8 fl.oz Cup Unless Indicated	C	F	Cb
Almond Breeze *(Blue Diamond):*			
Almondmilk: Original	60	3	8
Chocolate	100	3	21
Hint of Honey	60	3	9
Vanilla	80	3	14
Extra Creamy, regular	80	7	4
Reduced Sugar, Vanilla	60	3	8
Unsweetened, Original; Vanilla	30	3	1
Blends:			
Almond Coconut, Unsweetened Original	40	4	1
Blended with Bananas	80	2	14
Almond Dream ~ *See Dream*			
Better Than Milk			
Organic: Almond	80	4	9
Oat	130	5	22
Rice Hazelnut	170	4	32
Cacique,			
Orig; Strawb. Horchata, 12 fl.oz	230	5	46
Califia Farms: *Per 8 fl.oz Cup*			
Almond Milk:			
Organic Unsweetened	60	5	1
Unsweetened	60	5	1
Barista Blend:			
Almond, 8 fl.oz	70	5	6
Unsweetened, 8 fl.oz	40	3	1
Oat, 8 fl.oz	130	7	13
Organic Oatmilk, Original	80	1	14
Don Jose: *Per 8 fl.oz Cup*			
Horchata Rice Drink	140	4	25
Dream: *Per 8 fl.oz Cup*			
Almond Dream, unsweetened	35	3	2
Coconut Dream ~ *See page 50*			
Horchata, Traditional, 8 fl.oz	170	3	35
Ricemilk: 2% Fat, 8 fl.oz	150	5	25
Classic: Original, 8 fl.oz	120	3	24
Vanilla, 8 fl.oz	130	3	28
Whole, 8 fl.oz	170	8	25
Milkadamia: *Per 8 fl.oz Cup*			
Macadamia Milk: Creamy	60	4	7
Unsweetened	40	4	1
Barista, unsweetened	45	4	1
Soy Dream ~ *See page 50*			

Note: Rice/Oat/Nut Drinks are very low in protein. Unless enriched with protein (and calcium), they are not suitable for infants as a substitute for milk or calcium-enriched soy drinks.

Nut, Pea, Rice & Cereal Drinks

Per 8 fl.oz Cup Unless Indicated	C	F	Cb
Pacific Foods: *Per 8 fl.oz Cup*			
Organic:			
Almond: Original, unsweetened	40	3	2
Vanilla, unsweetened	40	3	2
Cashew, Original, unsweetened	50	4	2
Hemp: Original	140	6	19
Unsweetened, Original or Vanilla	60	5	0
Vanilla	170	6	23
Oat: Original	130	2	25
Vanilla	130	2	25
Ripple:			
Pea Protein: Original	100	5	6
Unsweetened	80	5	1
Chocolate	140	5	17
Vanilla	140	5	16
Unsweetened	80	5	1
Silk: *Per 8 fl.oz Cup*			
Almond: Original	60	3	8
Unsweetened	30	3	1
Dark Chocolate	100	2	19
Vanilla: Regular	80	3	14
Less Sugar	45	2	7
Unsweetened	30	3	1
Cashew, Unsweetned Original; Vanilla	25	2	1
Oat: Creamy Lowfat	45	3	5
Nextmilk: Whole Fat	110	8	7
Reduced Fat, 2%	90	5	7
Protein, Chocolate	150	5	8
Trader Joe's,			
Oat Beverage, 8 fl.oz	90	5	9

Soy Milk ~ Ready-To-Drink

	C	F	Cb
365 Organic *(Whole Foods): Per 8 fl.oz Cup*			
Original, unsweetened	70	4	3
Chocolate, unsweetened	40	3	1
8th Continent: *Per 8 fl.oz*			
Original	80	3	7
Vanilla	100	3	11
Dream: *Per 8 fl.oz*			
Original, with Calcium & Vit D	120	5	9
Edensoy: *Per 8 fl.oz Cup*			
Organic: Original	130	5	11
Unsweetened	120	6	4
Carob; Vanilla	150	4	23
Cocoa	200	5	32
Extra: Original	130	5	12
Vanilla	150	3	23
Great Value *(Walmart)*, Orig. Soy	100	4	9

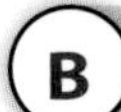

Beverages ~ Soy ◊ Coconut

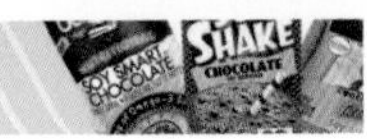

Soy Milk ~ Ready-To-Drink (Cont)

Per 8 fl.oz Unless Indicated	C	F	Cb
O Organics *(Albertsons): Per 8 fl.oz*			
Original Soy, unsweetened	80	5	4
Pacific: *Per 8 fl.oz*			
Soy, Organic, Orig., unswtnd	90	4	5
Ultra Soy, Original	140	5	13
Pearl *(Kikkoman): Per 8 fl.oz*			
Organic: Original; Creamy Vanilla	130	5	13
Unsweetened	90	5	4
Organic Smart: Original	130	5	13
Unsweetened	90	5	4
Chocolate	150	5	18
Creamy Vanilla	140	5	17
Silk *(Whitewave): Per 8 fl.oz*			
Organic: Original; Vanilla, av.	105	4	10
Unsweetened Orig.; Vanilla	80	4	3
Chocolate	150	5	19
Very Vanilla	130	4	18
Slim-Fast *~ See Page 40*			
Soy Dream *(Dream): Per 8 fl.oz*			
Enriched, Original	100	5	6
Soylent:			
Ready To Drink Bottles: *Per 14 fl.oz*			
Original; Banana	400	24	37
Cacao; Strawberry	400	21	37
Cafe Chai or Mocha	400	24	38
Creamy Chocolate; Vanilla	400	24	36
Mint Chocolate	400	24	36
Complete Protein,			
Chocolate, 11.15 fl.oz	250	13	10
Soy Slender *(Westsoy): Per 8 fl.oz*			
Chocolate Soy Milk	70	3	5
Organic Soy Milk: Original Plain	130	5	15
Unsweetened, Plain or Vanilla	100	5	4
Organic Plus: Plain	110	5	9
Vanilla	120	5	11
WestSoy:			
Organic Soy Milk:			
Original	130	5	15
Unsweetened: Plain	100	5	4
Vanilla	100	5	4
Organic Plus: Plain	110	5	9
Vanilla	120	5	11

Soy Powder Mix

1 oz (¼ cup) mix makes 8 fl.oz Cup	C	F	Cb
Soy Protein Isolate, dry, 1 oz	95	1	2
Better Than Milk:			
Original, 2 Tbsp	90	2	18
Vanilla, 2 Tbsp	90	2	18
Now:			
Soy Protein Isolate:			
Plain, ⅓ cup, 0.8 fl.oz	90	1	0
Creamy Chocolate, 1 scoop, 1.6 oz	160	2	9
Creamy Vanilla, 1 scoop, 1.6 oz	180	3	13
Soylent:			
Meal Replacement Powders:			
Original, ⅔ cup, 3.2 oz	400	19	42
Cacao, 2 rounded scoops, 3.2 oz	400	20	41
Total Soy *(Natureade): Per 2 Scoops*			
Meal Replacement:			
Bavarian Chocoate, 1.4 oz	150	2	20
French Vanilla, 1.4 oz	150	2	21
Strawberry Delight, 1.4 oz	150	2	21
Weight Loss:			
Chocolate, 1.27oz	140	3	17
Horchata, 1.27 oz	140	3	17
Vanilla, 1.27 oz	130	3	17

Coconut Milk Drinks

	C	F	Cb
Califia Farms: *Per 8 fl.oz Cup*			
Blend, Coconut Almond, Chocolate	50	4	1
Go Coconuts, Coconut Water Blend	45	4	1
Coconut Dream *(Dream): Per 8 fl.oz Cup*			
Enriched: Unsweetened	60	5	1
Vanilla	90	5	9
Great Value *(Walmart),*			
Original Unsweetened	50	5	1
Pacific:			
Organic: Original	60	4	5
Unsweetened: Original	45	4	1
Vanilla	50	4	2
Silk: Original	70	5	6
Unsweetened	40	4	2
So Delicious: *Per 8 fl.oz cup*			
Organic: Original	70	5	8
Unsweetened	45	4	2
Vanilla	80	5	9
Unsweetened	50	5	2
Organic Vegan: Unsweetened	45	5	1
Vanilla Unsweetened	45	5	1
Trader Joes: *Per 8 fl.oz cup*			
Unsweetened	60	5	1
Vanilla	90	5	9

(Enriched with calcium + vitamins D & B12)

Quick Guide

	C	F	Cb
Cola:			
Drinks: *Average all Brands*			
8 fl.oz Cup/Can	100	0	26
12 fl.oz Can	150	0	39
16 fl.oz Bottle	200	0	52
20 fl.oz Bottle	250	0	65
24 fl.oz (Pepsi)	300	0	84
1-Liter Bottle (34 fl.oz)	400	0	100
2-Liter Bottle (68 fl.oz)	800	0	200
Other Soda Drinks: *Per 12 fl.oz, average all brands*			
Club Soda	0	0	0
Cream Soda	190	0	48
Ginger Ale	125	0	31
Lemonade, Regular/Pink	180	0	45
Orange	180	0	45
Root Beer	150	0	39
Tonic Water	125	0	32
Mineral Water: Plain	0	0	0
Sweetened/flavored	150	0	37
with Fruit Juice	120	0	30
Soda Water/Seltzer: Plain/Diet	0	0	0
Sweetened/flavored	155	0	39
with Fruit Juice	160	0	40

Fountain, Movie Theater & Take-Out

Average All Flavors	C	F	Cb
Small Cup, 12 fl.oz: No Ice	160	0	40
with ⅓ Ice	120	0	30
Regular, 16 fl.oz: No Ice	215	0	53
with ⅓ Ice	160	0	40
Medium, 22 fl.oz: No Ice	295	0	73
with ⅓ Ice	220	0	55
Large, 32 fl.oz: No Ice	430	0	105
with ⅓ Ice	320	0	80

Note: ⅓ Cup of Ice = ¼ Cup Liquid

Soft Drink ~ Brands

Per 12 fl.oz Unless Indicated	C	F	Cb
A&W: Root Beer, 20 fl.oz	290	0	78
Cream Soda, 20 fl.oz	170	0	46
Albertson's:			
Signature Select: Cola	160	0	44
Diet Cola	0	0	0
Barq's: Root Beer	160	0	44
Creme Soda: Fr. Vanilla	160	0	45
Red	170	0	45
Big Red, Red Soda, 20 fl.oz	250	0	63
Blue Sky, Root Beer	130	0	32

Soft Drink Brands (Cont)

Per 12 fl.oz Unless Indicated	C	F	Cb
Bubble Up,			
Lemon-Lime Soda	140	0	42
Cactus Cooler	150	0	40
Canada Dry:			
Club Soda; Diet Ginger Ale	0	0	0
Ginger Ale; Tonic Water, av.	140	0	36
Cheerwine	150	0	42
Coca-Cola:			
Classic; Orange/Cherry Vanilla	140	0	39
Vanilla	150	0	42
Diet Coke; Zero	0	0	0
Energy: Regular	140	0	39
Cherry	140	0	39
Zero Sugar	0	0	0
Life	140	0	39
Crush: *Per 20 fl.oz*			
Cherry; Strawberry	290	0	77
Grape; Orange	270	0	72
Peach; Pineapple, average	315	0	84
Dad's: Cream Soda, 12 fl.oz	200	0	51
Root Beer, 12 fl.oz	180	0	45
Diet Rite, Pure Zero	0	0	0
Dr Pepper: *Per 12 fl.oz Can*			
Regular	150	0	40
Cherry	160	0	43
Ten	10	0	3
Fanta: Orange	160	0	44
Zero, all flavors	0	0	0
Fresca, all flavors	0	0	0
Great Value *(Walmart)*, Cream Soda	180	0	49
GuS, Cola; Dry Ginger Ale, average	95	0	23
Hansen's: *Per 12 fl.oz*			
Natural Cane Sugar:			
Original Cola; Root Beer	160	0	41
Pomegranate	140	0	35
Diet, all flavors	0	0	0
Hawaiian Punch, all flavors	60	0	15
Henry Weinhard's: Root Beer	170	0	43
Orange/Vanilla Cream, av.	180	0	44
Hires, Root Beer	170	0	45
IBC: Cream Soda; Black Cherry	175	0	44
Root Beer; Cherry Limeade, av.	165	0	40
Icee: Cola; Orange; Lemon Lime, 6 fl.oz	80	0	20
Average other flavors	80	0	21
Jarritos, av. all flavors, 8 fl.oz	110	0	28
Jelly Belly, all flavors	180	0	42
Jolt, Cola, 16 fl.oz	190	0	50

Soft Drink Brands (Cont)

Per 12 fl.oz Unless Indicated	C	F	Cb
Jones Soda:			
Regular, all flavors, 12 fl.oz	160	0	36
Stripped, all flavors, 12 fl.oz	30	0	8
Zilch, sugar free, 12 fl.oz	0	0	0
Kool Aid, Bursts, av., 6.75 fl.oz	20	0	5
Mello Yello: Regular, 12 fl.oz can	170	0	47
Cherry; Peach, 20 fl.oz	290	0	78
Mountain Dew: All flavors, can	170	0	46
Diet, 20 fl.oz	10	0	1
Dewshine, 12 fl.oz can	160	0	42
Kickstart, all flavors, 16 fl.oz	80	0	20
Mug, Root Beer	160	0	43
Natural Brew: Draft Root Beer	170	0	43
Outrageous Ginger Ale	180	0	44
Vanilla Cream Soda	160	0	39
Nehi, Peach	190	0	51
Pepsi: *Per 12 fl.oz*			
Regular; Mango Flavor	150	0	41
7.5 fl.oz, Regular	100	0	26
Black Currant; Citrus Flav.	150	0	39
Zero	0	0	0
Perrier, Carbonated Water	0	0	0
Pibb: Xtra	140	0	38
Zero	0	0	0
RC Cola: Regular, 12.fl.oz	160	0	43
Cherry, 12.fl.oz	160	0	45
Reed's: Ginger Beer, all var.	145	0	35
Ginger Ale	140	0	35
Refreshe *(Signature Select): Per 12 fl.oz*			
Dr Dynamite	150	0	45
Strawberry	180	0	44
7•UP: Lemon Lime; Cherry	140	0	39
Diet flavors	0	0	0
Signature Select,			
Ginger Ale, 12 fl.oz	140	0	37
Schweppes: Ginger Ale	120	0	33
Tonic Water	130	0	33
Shasta: Cream Soda	190	0	47
Cola	130	0	33
Club Soda; Diet, all flavors	0	0	0
Dr. Shasta	150	0	38
Ginger Ale; Orange	130	0	33
Lemon Lime	120	0	29
Tiki Punch	150	0	39
Average other flavors	170	0	41
Sierra Mist, Lemon Lime	120	0	30
Sprite: Original, 12 fl.oz	140	0	37
Zero, all flavors	0	0	0

Per 12 fl.oz Unless Indicated	C	F	Cb
Squirt, Ruby Red	170	0	45
Stewarts: Cherries 'n Cream	190	0	46
Grape; Orange 'n Cream	180	0	45
Root Beer	150	0	38
Average Other Flavors	180	0	44
Sun Drop: Citrus Soda, 20 fl.oz	290	0	76
Diet Citrus Soda	10	0	1
Sunkist: Orange; Grape, av., 12 fl.oz	165	0	45
Pineapple, 12 fl.oz	190	0	51
Surge, Original 16 fl.oz	230	0	62
Tab, Original	0	0	0
Tampico: *Per 8 fl.oz*			
Lemonade, with Lime	50	0	14
Punch: Blue Raspberry	60	0	14
Pineapple Coconut	70	0	17
Average other flavors	55	0	14
Thomas Kemper: *Per 12 fl.oz*			
Black Cherry	170	0	44
Ginger Ale; Vanilla Cream	150	0	36
Root Beer	160	0	41
Trader Joe's:			
Sparkling:			
French Berry Lemonade:			
1 cup, 8 fl.oz	130	0	31
1 bottle, 33.8 fl.oz	520	0	124
Lime Ade: 1 cup, 8 fl.oz	110	0	28
1 bottle, 33.8 fl.oz	440	0	108
Pink Lemonade: 1 cup, 8 fl.oz	130	0	31
1 Bottle, 33.8 fl.oz	520	0	124
Vernors, Ginger Soda, 20 fl.oz	240	0	65
Virgil's, Root Beer	160	0	42
Walgreens: *Per 12fl.oz*			
Nice: Cherry Cola	170	0	45
Diet Cola	0	0	0
Root Beer	160	0	45
Zevia, all flavors,	0	0	0

Powdered Soft Drink Mixes

Per 8 fl.oz Prepared, Unless Indicated	C	F	Cb
Country Time: *Per 12 fl.oz*			
Lemonade; Pink Lemonade	100	0	26
Strawberry Lemonade	130	0	33
Crystal Light *(Kraft):*			
Fruit Drinks, all flav., ½ tsp	5	0	0
On The Go, 1 pkt, 3 grams	10	0	3
Flavor Aid, ⅛ package	0	0	0
Kool-Aid, sweetened, 0.6 oz	60	0	16
Tang, Regular, 1 cap, 0.9 oz	90	0	22

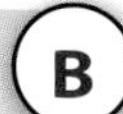

Quick Guide

	C	F	Cb
Teas			
Regular: Bag, Loose or Instant			
Brewed, 1 cup, 8 fl.oz (Add extra for sugar/milk)	2	0	1
Herbal, av. all flav., 1 cup	2	0	1
Bubble Milk Tea, w/ Pearls, 8 fl.oz	175	0	41
Chai Tea Latte Mix, 1 oz	110	1	24
Kombucha Tea, *Average all Brands:*			
Low Sugar, 1 cup, 8 fl.oz	30	0	7
Higher Sugar, 1 cup, 8 fl.oz	50	0	12
Iced Tea			
Average All Brands			
Sweetened: 8 fl.oz cup	90	0	22
12 fl.oz glass/can	140	0	35
16 fl.oz bottle	180	0	45
20 fl.oz bottle	225	0	55
Unsweetened, 8 fl.oz	0	0	0

Iced Tea Mixes

Per 8 fl.oz Made-Up Unless Indicated

	C	F	Cb
4C Iced Tea: *Per 12 fl.oz*			
Average all flavors, 0.9 oz	100	0	25
Light, all flavors, 1 Tbsp	25	0	6
Crystal Light, sugar free	5	0	0
Lipton:			
Sweetened: Lemon	70	0	18
Mango; Peach	80	0	19
Unsweetened	0	0	0
Diet, all varieties	5	0	1

Bottled & Canned Teas

	C	F	Cb
Arizona: *Per 8 fl.oz*			
Brewed Tea, Southern Style, Sweet	130	0	33
Green Tea, with Ginseng & Honey	70	0	18
Half & Half, Mango	50	0	14
Iced Tea, Lemon Flavor	100	0	25
White Tea, Blueberry	70	0	19
Fuze: *Per 12 fl.oz*			
Lemon + Sweet Black Tea	80	0	22
Strawberry + Peach Green Tea	80	0	21
Watermelon + Lime Green Tea	80	0	21
Gold Peak, Lemon, 18.5 fl.oz	180	0	45
Health-Ade: *Per 8 fl.oz*			
Original Kombucha	30	0	7
Blood Orange Carrot Ginger	35	0	7
Ginger Lemonade	35	0	7
Pink Lady Apple; Bubbly Rose	40	0	9

Bottled & Canned Teas (Cont)

	C	F	Cb
Honest Tea:			
Honey Green Tea, 16.9 fl.oz	70	0	19
Mango White Tea, 16 fl.oz	70	0	19
Peach Oolong, 16.9 fl.oz	70	0	19
Lipton:			
Green Tea, Citrus Flav. & Juice, 20 fl.oz	100	0	25
Half & Half	90	0	24
Flavored Iced Tea:			
Lemon Flavor, 12 fl.oz	70	0	19
Mango Flavor, 20 fl.oz	120	0	30
Peach Flavor, 12 fl.oz	70	0	18
Pear & Peach, 20 fl.oz	100	0	26
Tropical, 16.9 fl.oz	90	0	22
Sweet Tea, Black, 12 fl.oz	70	0	17
Nestea:			
Classics, all flavors, 8 fl.oz	50	0	13
Flash Brewed, all flavors, 17.6 fl.oz	100	0	25
POM:			
Antioxidant Super Tea: *Per 12 fl.oz*			
Pomegranate:			
Honey Green Tea	130	0	35
Lemonade Tea	140	0	35
Peach Passion White Tea	130	0	32
Sweet Tea	120	0	30
Snapple: *Per 16 fl.oz*			
Green Tea	120	0	31
Diet Green Tea	0	0	0
Half & Half	210	0	51
Lemon Tea; Raspberry Tea	150	0	37
Zero Sugar Tea, Lemon	5	0	0
Straight Up Tea: *Per 18.5 fl.oz Bottle*			
Sorta Sweet	90	0	22
Sweet	180	0	45
SoBe, Elixir, Green Tea, 20 fl.oz	200	0	52
Ssips, Lemon Iced Tea, 8 fl.oz	100	0	24
Steaz, Iced Green Tea, lightly sweetened, av., 16 fl.oz	80	0	20
Tampico, Iced Tea, Peach, Lemon, 8 fl.oz	40	0	10
Tazo, Giant Peach, 13.8 fl.oz	150	0	37
TeaZazz, NaturalZ,all flav., 12.8 fl.oz	70	0	20
Trader Joe's:			
Hibiscus Tea & Lemonade, 16 fl.oz	40	0	9
Organic Tea & Lemonade, 8 fl.oz	100	0	25
Turkey Hill: Iced Tea, 12 fl.oz	120	0	31
Orange Tea, 12 fl.oz	150	0	38
Peach Tea, 12 fl.oz	140	0	34
365 Organic *(Whole Foods)*:			
Unsweetened: Black Tea	0	0	0
Green Tea	0	0	0

B Bread & Bread Products

Note: Most breads have similar calories on a weight basis. However, volume may vary.

For example, 1 oz of bread may equal 1 slice regular bread or 2 slices of a lighter bread. It is best to weigh bread used and calculate using: 1 oz bread = 70 calories, 14g carb.

Quick Guide

	C	F	Cb
Bread			
White or Wheat: *Average Per Slice*			
Thin or Light, 0.85 oz	65	1	12
Regular slice, 1 oz	75	1	14
Thick or Large, 1.5 oz	115	2	21
Thick, 2 oz	150	2	28
Extra Thick, 3 oz	225	3	42
Whole Loaf, 16 oz	1200	16	224
Multi Grain/Whole Wheat: *Per Slice*			
Regular Slice, 1.3 oz	90	1	16
Thick Slice, 1.5 oz	110	2	19
Toast: *Based on same counts as White/Wheat as above*			
1 Thick Slice (1.5 oz untoasted):			
with 1 tsp butter/margarine	150	6	21
with 1 tsp "light" butter/marg.	135	4	21
with 2 tsp butter/margarine	185	10	21
with 2 tsp "light" butter/marg.	155	7	21

Breads

Per Slice Unless Indicated	C	F	Cb
12-Grain, 1.5 oz	110	2	22
Bran style/Dark, 1 oz	70	1	14
Buttermilk, average, 1.5 oz	110	1	22
Challah, 0.75 oz	85	2	17
Chapati, 1 oz	110	3	18
Ciabatta, 2 oz	130	1	26
Cornbread, average, 3 oz	220	6	37
Cracked Wheat Sourdough, 1.5 oz	130	1	27
Croissants ~ *See Page 134*			
Crustless Bread, regular, slice, 0.75 oz	40	1	9
Crusts Only, regular slice, 0.25 oz	30	0	7
English Toasting, 2 oz	140	2	27
Flax & Grain, 1.5 oz	120	3	19
Foccacia: Plain, 2 oz serve	150	3	28
Cheese & Garlic; Pesto, 2 oz serve	160	6	21
Tomato & Olive, 2 oz serve	150	5	21

Breads (Cont)

Per Slice Unless Indicated	C	F	Cb
French Stick/Baguette, 1 oz	70	1	15
French Toast: Slice, 1.5oz	140	2	26
Aunt Jemima, Sticks, av., 2 oz	110	2	18
Garlic Bread/Toast:			
Small slice + 1 tsp spread, 0.75 oz	80	5	7
Medium slice + 2 tsp spread, 1.5 oz	160	10	14
Thick slice + 3 tsp spread, 1.8 oz	220	14	20
Pepperidge Farm, Texas, 1 sl., 1.4 oz	150	8	15
Hawaiian Sweet Bread, 1.5 oz	110	2	19
Hemp Bread, 1.2 oz	95	2	12
Italian Bread, 2 oz	140	1	28
Lower Carb, (higher protein/fiber), average all brands, 1 oz	50	2	9
MultiGrain, 1.5 oz	100	2	21
Naan Flatbread, 2 oz	160	4	29
Nut/Health Nut, 1.35 oz	90	2	18
Oatmeal/Oatbran Bread, 1.5 oz	90	1	19
Pita, average all types:			
Small (4" diam), 1 oz	90	0	18
Large (6½" diam), 2 oz	140	2	27
Extra Large (9" diam), 4 oz	300	2	60
Popovers, (1), without butter	130	2	18
Pumpernickel:			
Cocktail/Party size	30	1	6
Large slice, 1.35 oz	80	0	15
Raisin Bread, 1 oz	80	1	15
Rye: 1 thin slice, av., 1 oz	80	1	14
1 thick slice, 2 oz	150	2	25
Cocktail size, 0.4 oz	25	1	4
Sandwich Pockets, 2 oz	140	2	27
Sourdough: Regular, 1.5oz	120	1	25
French Style,1 oz	75	0	14
Spelt, 1.6 oz	130	1	26
Sprouted 7-Grain, 1.5 oz	110	1	18
Squaw, 1.1 oz	85	1	13
Tacos/Tortillas ~ *See Page 172*			
Turkish/Middle Eastern, 1 oz	80	2	16
Wheat-Free Breads: Spelt, 1.6 oz	130	1	26
Rice, with Fruit Juice, 1.5 oz	110	2	21
Healthseed Rye, 1.6 oz	90	1	20
Millet, 1.5 oz	100	1	20

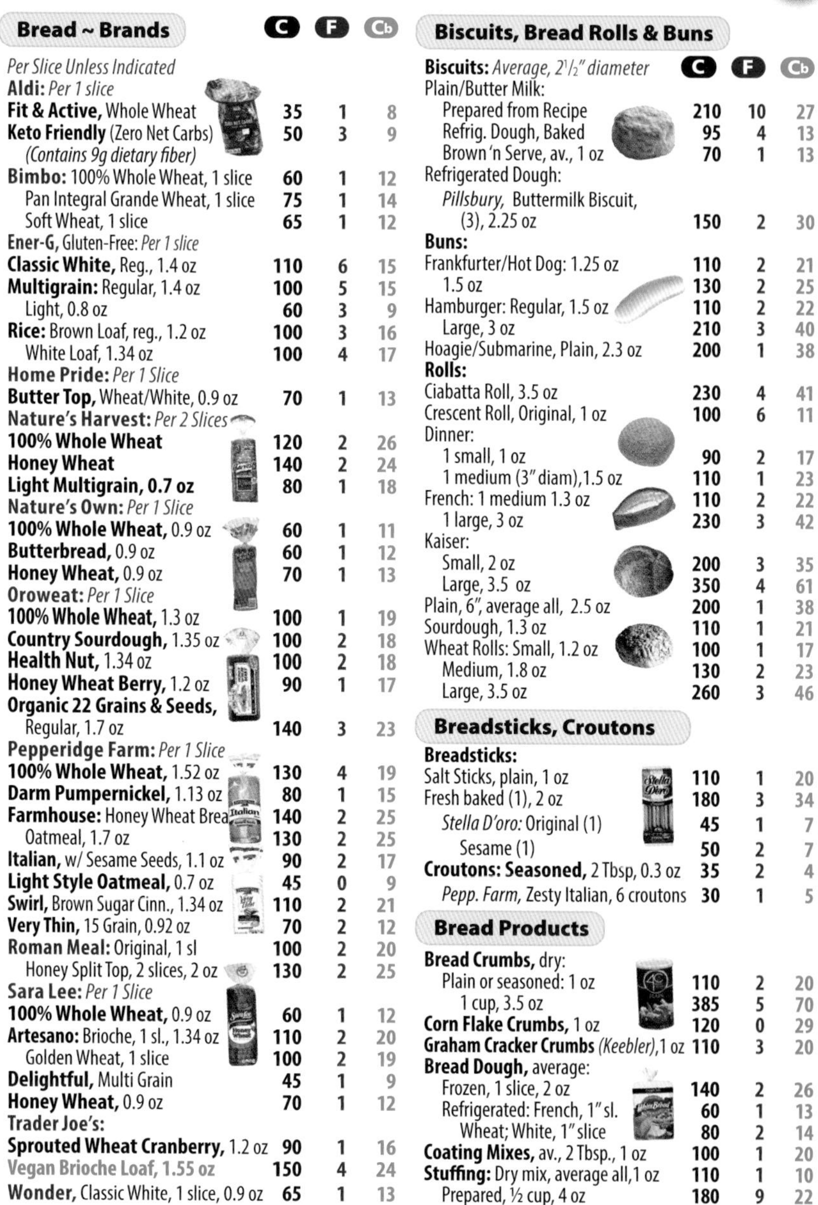

Bread ~ Brands

Per Slice Unless Indicated

	C	F	Cb
Aldi: *Per 1 slice*			
Fit & Active, Whole Wheat	35	1	8
Keto Friendly (Zero Net Carbs)	50	3	9
(Contains 9g dietary fiber)			
Bimbo: 100% Whole Wheat, 1 slice	60	1	12
Pan Integral Grande Wheat, 1 slice	75	1	14
Soft Wheat, 1 slice	65	1	12
Ener-G, Gluten-Free: *Per 1 slice*			
Classic White, Reg., 1.4 oz	110	6	15
Multigrain: Regular, 1.4 oz	100	5	15
Light, 0.8 oz	60	3	9
Rice: Brown Loaf, reg., 1.2 oz	100	3	16
White Loaf, 1.34 oz	100	4	17
Home Pride: *Per 1 Slice*			
Butter Top, Wheat/White, 0.9 oz	70	1	13
Nature's Harvest: *Per 2 Slices*			
100% Whole Wheat	120	2	26
Honey Wheat	140	2	24
Light Multigrain, 0.7 oz	80	1	18
Nature's Own: *Per 1 Slice*			
100% Whole Wheat, 0.9 oz	60	1	11
Butterbread, 0.9 oz	60	1	12
Honey Wheat, 0.9 oz	70	1	13
Oroweat: *Per 1 Slice*			
100% Whole Wheat, 1.3 oz	100	1	19
Country Sourdough, 1.35 oz	100	2	18
Health Nut, 1.34 oz	100	2	18
Honey Wheat Berry, 1.2 oz	90	1	17
Organic 22 Grains & Seeds,			
Regular, 1.7 oz	140	3	23
Pepperidge Farm: *Per 1 Slice*			
100% Whole Wheat, 1.52 oz	130	4	19
Darm Pumpernickel, 1.13 oz	80	1	15
Farmhouse: Honey Wheat Brea	140	2	25
Oatmeal, 1.7 oz	130	2	25
Italian, w/ Sesame Seeds, 1.1 oz	90	2	17
Light Style Oatmeal, 0.7 oz	45	0	9
Swirl, Brown Sugar Cinn., 1.34 oz	110	2	21
Very Thin, 15 Grain, 0.92 oz	70	2	12
Roman Meal: Original, 1 sl	100	2	20
Honey Split Top, 2 slices, 2 oz	130	2	25
Sara Lee: *Per 1 Slice*			
100% Whole Wheat, 0.9 oz	60	1	12
Artesano: Brioche, 1 sl., 1.34 oz	110	2	20
Golden Wheat, 1 slice	100	2	19
Delightful, Multi Grain	45	1	9
Honey Wheat, 0.9 oz	70	1	12
Trader Joe's:			
Sprouted Wheat Cranberry, 1.2 oz	90	1	16
Vegan Brioche Loaf, 1.55 oz	150	4	24
Wonder, Classic White, 1 slice, 0.9 oz	65	1	13

Biscuits, Bread Rolls & Buns

Biscuits: *Average, 2½″ diameter*	C	F	Cb
Plain/Butter Milk:			
Prepared from Recipe	210	10	27
Refrig. Dough, Baked	95	4	13
Brown 'n Serve, av., 1 oz	70	1	13
Refrigerated Dough:			
Pillsbury, Buttermilk Biscuit,			
(3), 2.25 oz	150	2	30
Buns:			
Frankfurter/Hot Dog: 1.25 oz	110	2	21
1.5 oz	130	2	25
Hamburger: Regular, 1.5 oz	110	2	22
Large, 3 oz	210	3	40
Hoagie/Submarine, Plain, 2.3 oz	200	1	38
Rolls:			
Ciabatta Roll, 3.5 oz	230	4	41
Crescent Roll, Original, 1 oz	100	6	11
Dinner:			
1 small, 1 oz	90	2	17
1 medium (3″ diam),1.5 oz	110	1	23
French: 1 medium 1.3 oz	110	2	22
1 large, 3 oz	230	3	42
Kaiser:			
Small, 2 oz	200	3	35
Large, 3.5 oz	350	4	61
Plain, 6″, average all, 2.5 oz	200	1	38
Sourdough, 1.3 oz	110	1	21
Wheat Rolls: Small, 1.2 oz	100	1	17
Medium, 1.8 oz	130	2	23
Large, 3.5 oz	260	3	46

Breadsticks, Croutons

	C	F	Cb
Breadsticks:			
Salt Sticks, plain, 1 oz	110	1	20
Fresh baked (1), 2 oz	180	3	34
Stella D'oro: Original (1)	45	1	7
Sesame (1)	50	2	7
Croutons: Seasoned, 2 Tbsp, 0.3 oz	35	2	4
Pepp. Farm, Zesty Italian, 6 croutons	30	1	5

Bread Products

	C	F	Cb
Bread Crumbs, dry:			
Plain or seasoned: 1 oz	110	2	20
1 cup, 3.5 oz	385	5	70
Corn Flake Crumbs, 1 oz	120	0	29
Graham Cracker Crumbs *(Keebler)*,1 oz	110	3	20
Bread Dough, average:			
Frozen, 1 slice, 2 oz	140	2	26
Refrigerated: French, 1″ sl.	60	1	13
Wheat; White, 1″ slice	80	2	14
Coating Mixes, av., 2 Tbsp., 1 oz	100	1	20
Stuffing: Dry mix, average all,1 oz	110	1	10
Prepared, ½ cup, 4 oz	180	9	22

Quick Guide

	C	F	Cb
Bagels			
Average All Brands			
Plain/Onion:			
1 mini/bagelette, 1 oz	65	1	13
1 small bagel, 2 oz	145	1	29
1 medium bagel, 3 oz	220	2	43
1 large bagel, 4 oz	290	2	57
Bagel Chips, 1 oz	130	5	19
Pizza Bagel Bites (Bagel Bites), average all varieties., 4 pieces, 3 oz	190	6	27
Bagel Crisps *(New York Style)*, average all varieties, 6 crisps, 1 oz	130	5	17
Bagel Thins *(Thomas')*, 1, 1.5 oz	110	1	25

Bagel ~ Brands

	C	F	Cb
Per Bagel			
Bubba's: Plain	220	2	45
Blueberry	230	2	49
Cinnamon Raisin	230	2	48
Costco Bakery: Plain	330	2	70
Cinnamon Raisin	340	2	73
Whole Grain	300	5	56
Lender's, Refrigerated:			
Blueberry, 2.85 oz	230	2	45
Cinnamon, 3.3 oz	240	2	46
Egg, 2.85 oz	220	2	45
French Toast, 2.86 oz	230	2	46
Panera Bread: Plain, 3 oz	230	1	47
Cinnamon Swirl & Raisin, 3 oz	230	2	47
Everything, 3 oz	240	2	47
Sara Lee:			
Delux: Plain, 3.35 oz	260	2	52
Blueberry, 3.35 oz	260	2	51
Cinnamon Raisin, 3.35 oz	260	2	52
Everything, 3.35 oz	280	4	50
Onion, 3.35 oz	270	2	52
Western, The Alternatives, av., 2 oz	120	1	29

Bagel Spreads

	C	F	Cb
Cream Cheese:			
Plain: 2 Tbsp, 1 oz	100	9	1
2 oz mini-tub	200	18	2
Reduced Fat: 2 Tbsp, 1 oz	60	5	2
2 oz mini-tub	120	10	4
Flavors: Lox, 1 oz	90	8	2
Honey Nut, 1 oz	80	7	4
Strawberry, 1 oz	90	7	5
Sundried Tomato, 1 oz	80	7	2
Vegetable, 1 oz	90	8	2

English Muffins

	C	F	Cb
Average All Brands			
Plain/Whole Wheat: Regular, 2 oz	135	2	26
Heavier, 2.5 oz	155	2	31
Super Size, 3.2 oz	190	2	38
Raisin-Cinnamon, 2.2 oz	150	1	30

Note: Actual weight of packaged muffins can be 10-15% heavier than stated net weight.

Rice Cakes

	C	F	Cb
Lundberg, (Organic):			
Minis, av. all flavors, 13 pieces	140	5	23
Thin Stackers, av. all flavors, (4)	105	1	23
Quaker: Apple Cinnamon (1)	50	0	11
Chocolate, (1)	60	1	12
Tomato & Basil (1)	50	2	9
White Cheddar (1)	45	1	8
Signature Select, White Cheddar (1))	45	1	9

Tortillas & Shells

	C	F	Cb
Tortillas: *Per Tortilla*			
Corn Flour, White/Yellow: 6", 1 oz	55	1	11
7", 1.2 oz	75	1	14
Wheat Flour:			
6", 1.2 oz	100	3	16
8", 1.4 oz	130	4	20
10", 2.3 oz	200	6	31
Shells: *Per Shell, without Fillings*			
Corn Taco Shells: Mini, 3", 0.2 oz	25	1	3
Medium, 5", 0.5 oz	60	3	8
Large, 6½", 0.7 oz	100	5	13
Salad Shell, 10"	310	17	34
Tostada Shells, fried:			
White Corn, 5½" diam., 0.4 oz	55	3	8
Yellow Corn, 5½" diam., 0.5 oz	80	4	11
Sopes, 1 shell, 4" 2 oz	110	2	23
La Tortilla Factory:			
Non GMO:			
Gluten Free, Casava Flour, 1.4 oz	90	3	20
Hand Made, Wh. Corn & Wheat, 1.45 oz	90	1	15
Low Carb, Quinoa & Flax, 1.45 oz	60	2	15
Protein, Whole Wheat, 1.76 oz	120	4	12
Traditional, Flour, Burrito Size, 2 oz	170	4	28
Mission Foods:			
Corn, Yellow, Super Soft:			
Low Fat, 2 Tortillas, 1.65 oz	100	2	20
Flour, Super Soft,			
Burrito Size (1), 2.47 oz	210	4	37
Ortego:			
Cauli & Corn, Taco Shell (3)	170	9	20
Cauli & Flour, Tortilla (1)	120	2	22

Quick Guide

	C	F	Cb
Cooked Cereal			
Barley, pearled, cooked, 1 cup	195	1	44
Buckwheat Groats, roasted:			
Dry, ½ cup, 3 oz	285	2	61
Cooked, 1 cup, 6 oz	155	1	34
Bulgur: Dry, ½ cup, 2.5 oz	240	1	53
Cooked, 1 cup, 6.5 oz	150	1	34
Corn/Hominy Grits:			
Dry: Regular, ¼ cup, 1.4 oz	140	1	32
Instant: 0.8 fl.oz packet	75	0	18
w/ Imitation Bacon Bits, 1 oz	100	1	22
Cooked, ¾ cup, 6.5 oz	110	1	23
Cream of Rice, cooked, ¾ cup, 6.5 oz	95	0	21
Cream of Wheat:			
Cooked: Regular, ¾ cup, 6.5 oz	95	1	20
Instant, ¾cup, 6.5 oz	105	1	21
Quick, ¾ cup, 6.5 oz	100	1	22
Farina, cooked, ¾ cup, 6 oz	95	1	19
Millet, dry, ½ cup, 1.8 oz	190	2	36
Oat Bran: Raw, ⅓ cup, 1 oz	70	2	19
Cooked, ½ cup, 3.8 fl.oz	45	1	13
Oatmeal:			
Dry: Regular, ⅓ cup, 1 oz	100	2	18
Instant: Regular, average, 1 oz	105	2	18
Flavored, average, 1.5 oz	165	2	34
Cooked: Regular, ¾ cup, 6 oz	125	3	21
1 cup, 8 fl.oz	165	4	28
Whole Wheat, cooked, ¾ cup, 6.5 oz	115	1	25

Brans, Wheat Germ, Add-Ons

	C	F	Cb
Bee Pollen Granules, 1 Tbsp, 0.3 oz	25	1	2
Bran:			
Oat Bran: Raw, 1 Tbsp, 0.2 oz	20	1	3
⅓ cup, 1 oz	100	2	17
Rice Bran: Raw, 1 Tbsp, 0.2 oz	15	1	3
¼ cup, 1 oz	95	6	15
Fruit: Dried, average, 1 oz	70	0	18
Banana, ½ medium	55	0	14
Prunes in Syrup (5), 3 oz	90	0	23
Honey, 1 Tbsp, 0.75 oz	65	0	17
Lecithin Granules, 1 Tbsp, 0.4 oz	55	4	1
Nuts, Almonds (6), 0.3 oz	40	4	2
Psyllium Husks, 1 Tbsp, 0.2 oz	10	0	4
Wheat, unprocessed, 1 Tbsp	5	0	2
Wheat Germ: Raw, 1 Tbsp, 0.3 oz	25	1	4
¼ cup, 1 oz	105	3	15

Hot/Cooked Cereals ~ Brands

Per Serving, Dry Mix only	C	F	Cb
Albers,			
Quick Grits, ¼ cup, 1.4 oz	140	1	31
B&G:			
Cream of Wheat Instant:			
Original, 1 oz	120	0	25
Banana & Cream, 1.23 oz	130	0	29
Maple Brown Sugar, 1.3 oz	130	0	28
Bob's Red Mill:			
7 Grain Hot Cereal, 1.4 oz	150	1	30
Brown Sugar & Maple,			
Instant Oatmeal, 1.23 oz	140	3	25
Creamy Wheat, 1.4 oz	140	0	30
Great Value *(Walmart):*			
Instant Oatmeal:			
Apples & Cinn.,1.23 oz	130	2	27
Original, 1 oz packet	110	2	19
McCann's:			
Instant Irish Oatmeal:			
Original, 1 oz pkt	100	1	20
Apples & Cinnamon, 1.3 oz	130	1	29
Maple & Brown Sugar, 1.5 oz	160	1	35
Microwaveable,			
Vanilla Honey, 1.94 oz Cup	200	1	44
Quick Cooking, Original, 1.4 oz	140	1	30
Malt-O-Meal: Orig.; Creamy, 1.23 oz	130	0	27
Maple Brown Sugar, 1.6 oz	170	0	38
Natures Path, Flax Plus, 1,76 oz pkt	210	3	38
NutriSystem,			
Oatmeal, Maple Brown Sugar, 1 pkg	150	2	29
Quaker:			
Gluten Free, Maple Br. Sugar, 1.5 oz	160	3	32
Instant Grits, Butter, 1.45 oz	150	2	32
Quick Grits, Old Fash., ¼ cup, 1.4 oz	140	1	32
Instant Oatmeal::			
High Fiber:			
Cinnamon Swirl, 1.6 oz	150	2	34
Maple & Brown Sug.,1.5 oz	150	2	35
Protein: Banana Nut, 2.15 oz	230	5	40
Cranberry Almond, 2.2 o	230	5	41
Wegmans: *Per Packet*			
Instant Oatmeal:			
Maple Brown Sugar, 1.51 oz	160	2	32
Peaches & Cream, 1.23 oz pkt	130	2	27

B Breakfast Cereals

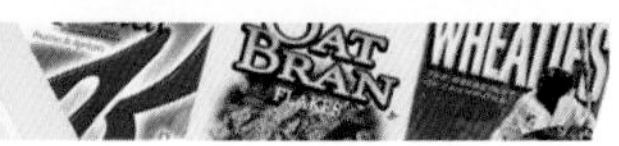

Quick Guide

Cold Cereals

Average All Brands	C	F	Cb
Bran Flakes, ¾ cup, 1 oz	95	1	24
Corn Flakes, 1 cup, 1 oz	100	0	22
Frosted Flakes, ¾ cup, 1 oz	110	0	27
Granola, 100% Nat., ½ cup, 1.7 oz	205	6	35
Oat Bran Cereal, ½ cup, 1.5 oz	145	3	25
Puffed Rice, 1 cup. 0.5 oz	55	0	13
Puffed Wheat, 1 cup, 0.5 oz	45	0	10
Raisin Bran, ½ cup, 1 oz	90	1	22
Rice Crisps, 1 cup, 1 oz	105	1	24
Shredded Wheat, 1 biscuit, 1 oz	85	1	20
Wheat Flakes, ¾ cup, 1 oz	105	1	24

Breakfast/Cereal Bars ~ *See Page 31*

Ready-To-Eat Cereal ~ Brands

Dry Cereal Only

	C	F	Cb
Arrowhead Mills:			
Organic: Bulgar Wheat, 1.55 oz	160	1	32
Flakes: Amaranth, 2.1 oz	210	3	42
Maple Buckwheat, 2 oz	190	2	43
Oat Bran, 1.94 oz	170	3	37
Spelt, 2 oz	190	1	41
Puffed: Corn, 0.5 oz	60	1	11
Kamut, 0.5 oz	60	0	11
Millet, 0.5 oz	50	1	11
Rice, 0.5 oz	50	0	12
Back to Nature (Plant Based):			
Gluten Free Granola: *Per ½ Cup*			
Chocolate Delight, 1.76 oz	210	5	37
Classic, 1.76 oz	200	3	40
Van. Almond Agave, 1.76 oz	210	6	36
Grain Free Granola: *Per ⅓ Cup*			
Cinnamon Apple Crunch, 1.1oz	170	13	8
Vanilla Almond Crunch, 1.1 oz	160	12	8
Granola Clusters,			
Peanut Butter, 1.8 oz	230	9	29
Lower Sugar Granola: *Per ½ Cup*			
Cinnamon Pecan, 1.1 oz	160	14	10
Dark Chocolate, 1.1 oz	150	13	10

Barbara's Bakery:	C	F	Cb
Morning Oat Crunch, 2.1 oz	210	3	45
Organic, Corn Flakes, 1.4 oz	150	0	34
Shredded Wheat, 2 biscuits, 1.8 oz	170	1	41
Spoonfuls, Multigrain, 1.4 oz	140	2	31
Bear Naked: *Per ½ Cup*			
Granola: Banana Nut, 1.9 oz	250	13	33
Cacao & Cashew, 1.9 oz	250	11	34
Fruit & Nut, 2.1 oz	270	12	39
Maple Pecan, 2.1 oz	260	9	43
Peanut Butter, 2 oz	260	12	35
Triple Berry Crunch, 1.83 oz	210	6	38
Vanilla Almond Crisp, 1.83 oz	220	9	34
Bob's Red Mill:			
Granola: Coconut Spice, 1oz	150	8	17
Cranberry Almond, 1 oz	140	6	19
Lemon Blueberry, 1 oz	140	6	19
Maple Sea Salt, 1 oz	150	8	17
Peanut Butter, 1 oz	140	7	18
Vanilla Shake, 1 oz	150	7	19
Muesli: Fruit & Seed,1.1oz	130	4	21
Gluten Free, European Style, 1 oz	120	4	19
Paleo Style, Grain Free, 0.85 oz	140	10	9
Cascadian Farm:			
Berry Vanilla Puffs, 1.5 oz	170	2	37
Buzz Crunch, Honey Almond, 1.9 oz	210	3	44
Cinnamon Crunch, 1.3 oz	140	3	29
Graham Crunch, 1.3 oz	150	3	30
Granola:			
Cinnamon Raisin, 2.1 oz	250	7	43
Dark Chocolate Almond, 2.2 oz	260	8	45
French Vanilla Alm., 2 oz	240	7	42
Fruit & Nut, 2.2 oz	270	9	44
No Sugar Added,			
BlueberryVanilla, 1.83 oz	250	11	33
Honey Nut O's, 1.5 oz	160	2	35
Multi Grain Squares,			
1¼ cups, 2 oz	260	2	54
Raisin Bran, 2.2 oz	210	2	50
EnviroKidz (Vegan): *Per 1.4 oz*			
Amazon Frosted Flakes	160	0	36
Gorilla Munch	150	1	35
Leapin' Lemurs	160	2	33
Panda Puffs	170	5	31

Ready-To-Eat Cereal (Cont)

Dry Cereal Only

Ezekiel 4.9 (Vegan):	C	F	Cb
Sprouted Grain, Low Sodium, 2 oz	190	1	38
Sprouted Whole Grain Cereal:			
Original, 2 oz	180	1	35
Almond, 2 oz	200	3	34
Golden Flax, 2 oz	190	3	65
Sprouted Flakes:			
Almond, ¾ cup, 1.94 oz	200	3	40
Flax & Chia, ¾ cup, 1.94 oz	200	2	41
Original, ¾ cup, 1.94 oz	210	1	42
Raisin, 1.94 oz	190	1	42
General Mills:			
Cheerios: *Per Cup Unless Indicated*			
Original, 1.4 oz	140	3	29
Apple Cinnamon, 1.3 oz	140	2	30
Chocolate, 1.3 oz	140	2	29
Chocolate PB, 1.27 oz	150	4	26
Cinnamon, 1.3 oz	140	2	29
Frosted, 1.3 oz	140	2	30
Multi Grain, 1.4oz	150	2	32
Oat Crunch, Cinnamon. 1.9 oz	220	5	42
Very Berry, 1.3 oz	140	2	29
Chex: Blueberry, 1.4 oz	170	4	33
Chocolate, 1.5 oz	180	4	35
Cinnamon, 1.4 oz	170	4	33
Corn, 1.4 oz	150	1	33
Honey Nut,1.4 oz	160	2	37
Rice,1.4 oz	160	1	35
Wheat, 2 oz	210	1	51
Cinnamon Toast Crunch:			
Original, 1.45 oz	170	4	33
Chocolate, 1.4 oz	170	5	31
Churros, 1.45 oz	160	5	32
Fiber One: Original, ⅔ cup, 1.4 oz	90	1	34
Honey Clusters, 1.8 oz	170	2	45
Kix: Original, 1½ cups,1.4 oz	160	1	34
Berry Berry; Honey, av., 1½ cups, 1.4 oz	160	2	34
Lucky Charms:			
Original, 1 cup, 1.27 oz	140	2	30
Chocolate, 1.27 oz	140	2	31
Puffs: Cocoa, 0.95 oz	100	2	23
Reese's 1 oz	120	3	22
Raisin Nut Bran, 1.73 oz	180	3	40
Total, Whole Grain, 1.4 oz	140	1	33
Wheaties, 1.4 oz	130	1	30

Great Value *(Walmart)*:	C	F	Cb
Almond Crunchy Honey Oats, 1.4 oz	160	2	33
Berry Crunch, 1.9 oz	150	2	33
Cinnamon Crunch, 1.48 oz	180	5	32
Cinn. Oat Crunch, 1.48 oz	160	2	34
Crunchy Honey Oats, 1.4 oz	150	2	33
Frosted Flakes, 1.45 oz	160	0	37
Fruit Spins, 1.48 oz	170	2	36
Honey Graham Crunch, 1.48 oz	170	5	32
Honey Nut O's, 1.1 oz	160	2	33
Magic Treasures, 1.45 oz	160	2	35
P'nut Butter Chocolate Puffs, 1.4 oz	170	5	31
Rice Crisps, 1.45 oz	160	1	36
Shredded Frosted Wheat, 21 biscuits	210	1	50
Strawberry Awake, 1..4 oz	140	1	34
Kashi *(Organic)*:			
Clusters, Blueberry, 1.9 oz	200	2	44
Go: Original, 2.2 oz	200	2	43
Crisp: Cinnamon, 2.2 oz	220	5	40
Toasted Berry,1.87 oz	200	5	37
Crunch: Original, 2 oz	190	3	38
Chocolate, 1.83 oz	200	7	32
Honey Almond Flax, 1.83 oz	200	5	35
Peanut Butter, 1.84 oz	220	9	31
Kellogg's:			
All-Bran: Original, 1.4 oz	120	2	32
Bran Buds, 1.6 oz	120	2	36
Complete Wheat Flakes, 1.3 oz	120	1	30
Apple Jacks, 1.4 oz	150	2	34
Cocoa Krispies, 1.4 oz	160	1	35
Corn Flakes: Original, 1.4 oz	150	0	36
Honey Flavor, 1.4 oz	150	0	35
Corn Pops, 1.4 oz	150	0	36
Cracklin' Oat Bran, ¾ cup, 2 oz	230	8	41
Crispix, Original, 1.4 oz	150	0	34
Despicable Me, Brown Sugar 1 cup, 1.13 oz	120	1	27
Froot Loops:			
Original, 1.4 oz	150	2	34
Marshmallows, 1.4 oz	140	1	34

continued next page...

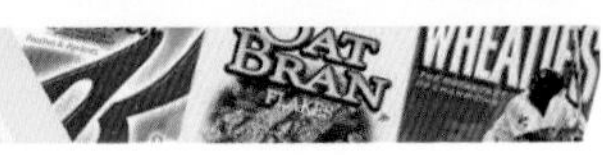

Ready-To-Eat Cereal (Cont)

Dry Cereal Only

Kellogg's (Cont):	C	F	Cb
Frosted Flakes: *Per Cup*			
Chocolate, 1.4 oz	150	1	33
Cinn. French Toast, 1.3 oz	140	1	32
Original Flakes, 1.3 oz	130	0	33
Strawberry Milkshake, 1.3 oz	140	0	33
Frosted Mini-Wheats:			
Original (25), 2 oz	210	2	51
Blueberry (25), 2 oz	210	1	51
Cinnamon Roll (25), 2 oz	210	1	50
Strawberry (25), 2 oz	210	1	51
Little Bites: Original, 2 oz	190	1	47
Chocolate, 2 oz	190	2	45
Honey Smacks, 1.3 oz	130	1	32
Krave, Chocolate, 1.45 oz	170	5	32
Krispies:			
Cinnamon Sugar, 1.48 oz	160	0	38
Cocoa, 1.48 oz	160	1	35
Frosted, 1.35 oz	150	0	35
Rainbow, 1.4 oz	220	2	43
Rice, 1.4 oz	150	0	36
Mueslix, 2.36 oz	250	4	50
Raisin Bran: Original, 2 oz	190	1	47
with Cranberries, 2 oz	200	1	50
Crunch, Original, 1.94 oz	190	1	46
Smart Start,			
Orig. Antioxidants, 2.25 oz	240	1	56
Special K: Original, 2 oz	150	1	29
Blueberry,1.45 oz	150	1	36
Choc. Dipped w/ Almonds, 2.2 oz	250	5	50
Cinnamon & Pecan,1.45 oz	160	3	33
Red Berries, 1.4 oz	140	1	34
Protein,			
Honey Almond Ancient Grain, 2.1 oz	220	3	38
Kind: *Per 2.3 oz Unless Indicated*			
Granola: Cinnamon Oat with Flax	240	7	42
Maple Quinoa with Chia	240	6	42
Ot & Honey	250	5	45
Raspberry with Chia Seeds	230	4	45
Vanilla Blueberry with Flax	240	6	43
Soft Baked: Dark Choc. Chunk, 2 oz	230	7	34
Dark Choc. Peanut Butter, 2 oz	230	10	33
Clusters:			
Almond Butter, 2.3 oz	250	5	41
Dark Chocolate, 2.3 oz	240	6	38
Peanut Butter, 2.3 oz	260	8	37

Malt-O-Meal:	C	F	Cb
Apple Zings, 1.4 oz	150	1	34
Cocoa Roos, 1.5 oz	170	2	38
Frosted Flakes, 1.4 oz	160	0	37
Frosted Mini Spooners,			
21 biscuits	210	1	50
Golden Puffs, 1.35 oz	150	1	34
Honey Nut Scooters, 1.4 oz	160	2	33
Marshmallow Mateys, 1.4 oz	160	2	35
Peanut Butter Cups, 1.4 oz	170	5	31
Raisin Bran, 2.1 oz	190	1	48
S'Mores, 1 cup, 1.4 oz	160	4	33
Tootie Fruities, 1.48 oz	170	2	36
Waffle Crunch, 1.4 oz	160	2	34
Nature's Path:			
Flax Plus:			
Cinnamon Flakes, 1.4 oz	160	2	32
Maple Pecan Crunch, 2.1 oz	230	7	39
Multibran Flakes, 1.4 oz	150	2	31
Pumpkin Raisin Crunch, 2 oz	210	5	39
Raisin Bran, 2 oz	210	3	45
Red Berry Crunch, 2 oz	210	5	41
Heritage: Flakes, 1.4 oz	160	2	31
O's, 2 oz	220	2	42
Granola:			
Love Crunch Granola:			
Apple Chia, 1 oz	140	4	22
Dark Chocolate:			
& Coconut, 1 oz	150	6	20
& Hazelnut Butter, 1 oz	120	6	16
& PB, 1 oz	150	5	18
& Red Berries, 1 oz	130	5	20
Double chocolate Chunk, 1 oz	140	5	21
Espresso Vanilla Cream,.1 oz	130	5	21
Keto, Dark Chocolate Flavor, 1.4 oz	110	3	20
Mesa Sunrise, 1.4 oz	160	2	32
Qi'a Superfood Superflakes,			
Buckwheat & Hemp, 1 oz	140	7	13
Sunrise:			
Crunchy Honey, 1.4 oz	150	2	35
Crunchy Maple, 1.4 oz	150	2	34
New England Natural Bakers:			
Organic Granola:			
Blueberry Harvest, 2 oz	270	7	41
Salted Caramel Apple, 2 oz	260	7	43
Toasted Coconut, 2 oz	270	10	42
Unsweetened, Berry Coconut, 2 oz	290	13	37
Organic Granola Clusters	240	9	36
NutriSystem,			
NutriFlakes, 1 pkt	90	1	22

Ready-To-Eat Cereal ~ Brands (Cont)

Dry Cereal Only

	C	F	Cb
Post:			
Better Oats,			
Maple & Br. Sugar, 1 oz	100	2	18
Bran Flakes, 1.3 oz	110	1	29
Grape-Nuts: Original, 2 oz	200	1	47
Flakes, 1.45 oz	150	2	34
Great Grains:			
Banana Nut Crunch, 2 oz	230	5	45
Cranberry Almond Crunch, 2 oz	210	3	44
Crunchy Pecan, 1.95 oz	210	6	39
Honey Bunches of Oats:			
Cinnamon Bunches, 1.45 oz	160	2	34
French Vanilla Almond, 2.22 oz	270	9	45
Maple & Pecans, 1.45 oz	170	4	32
With: Almonds, 1.42 oz	170	3	34
Strawberries, 1.45 oz	160	2	34
Vanilla, 1.45 oz	160	2	34
Granola, French Vanilla, ⅔ cup, 2.22 oz	270	9	45
Honey-Comb, Original, 1.4 oz	160	1	35
Honey Maid, S'mores, 1.4 oz	160	4	33
Malt O Meal ~ *see Page 60*			
Oreo O's, 1.4 oz	160	3	34
Pebbles: Crunch'd varieties	140	2	31
Fruity, 1.27 oz	140	2	31
Premier Protein, all flavors, 1.48 oz	180	5	14
Raisin Bran, 2.15 oz	190	1	48
Shredded Wheat, Spoon Size:			
Original, 2 oz	210	2	49
Wheat 'N Bran, 2 oz	210	2	49
Big Biscuit, Original (2)	170	1	41
Waffle Crisp, 1.4 oz	160	2	34
Quaker:			
Chewy Granola:			
Crispy Clusters: Chocolate, 1.87 oz	220	6	38
Strawberry, 1.94 oz	230	6	40
Life, all flavors, 1.48 oz	160	2	33
Oatmeal Squares, all flavors, 2 oz	210	3	44
Quisps, 1.52 oz	170	3	37
Sweet Home Farm:			
Granola:			
French Vanilla with Almond, 2 oz	250	8	41
Honey Nut with Almonds, 1.87 oz	240	10	36
Maple Pecan with Syrup, 2 oz	260	9	42

Trader Joe's:	C	F	Cb
Almond Butter Puffs, 1.4 oz	200	10	20
Flakes & Strawberries, 1.4 oz	140	1	33
Honey O's, 1.45 oz	160	2	34
Joe's O's, 1.45 oz	160	3	31
Just The Clusters,			
Maple Pecan Granola, 2.25 oz	290	11	45
Maple Pecan Clusters, 1.87 oz	230	7	39
Peanut Butter Protein Granola, ¾ cup, 2 oz	260	12	29
Tiny Fruity Cuties, 1.4 oz	150	2	33
Udi's: *Per ½ Cup*			
Granola ~ Gluten Free:			
Original, 2 oz	280	12	42
Almond Butter, 2 oz	280	12	36
Au Naturel, 2 oz	240	8	38
Chocolate Coconut, 2 oz	280	12	40
Cranberry, 2 oz	260	10	42
Vanilla, 2 oz	280	12	42
Uncle Sam,			
Original Wheat Berry Flakes, ¾ cup, 2 oz	220	6	43
Weetabix,			
3 biscuits, 1.84 oz	180	1	43
Wegmans:			
Apple Snaps, 1.4 oz	150	1	34
Cinnamon Squares, 1.48 oz	180	5	32
Crispy Rice, 1.45 oz	160	1	36
Frosted Fruit O's, 1.48 oz	170	2	36
Marshmallow Treasures, 1.49 oz	160	2	35
P'nut Butter & Cocoa Corn Crunch, 1.4 oz	170	5	30
Rice Squares, 1.45 oz	150	0	35
Shredded Wheat:			
Frosted Bite Size: Original, 2.1 oz	210	1	50
Blueberry, 2.1 oz	210	1	49
Toasted Oats, Honey & Nut, 1.45 oz	160	2	33
Whole Foods 365:			
Bran Flakes, 1.4 oz	130	1	32
Corn Flakes, 1.4 oz	150	0	34
Cocoa Rice Crisps, 1.4 oz	140	1	31
Hazelnut Cocoa Pillows, 1.3 oz	140	3	27
Morning O's, 1.4 oz	150	3	30
Raisin Granola, 2 oz	250	8	41
Wheat Waffles, 1.4 oz	140	1	33

Ready-to-Eat

Per Piece/Slice	C	F	Cb
Angel Food, Plain: without oil, 2 oz	145	0	33
with oil, 2 oz	145	1	27
with Cream Frosting	255	7	45
Almond Croissant, 5 oz	620	35	67
Apple Danish, 5 oz	450	18	67
Apple Pie ~ *See Pies/Tarts Page 134*			
Baklava, 1½" square, 1.75 oz	200	10	27
Banana Cake, with Butter Cream, 2 oz	230	9	37
Banana Walnut Cake, 3 oz	270	11	40
Bear Claw, 4.5 oz	540	24	71
Black Forest, 3 oz	345	11	59
Brownie: Small, 2" Square, 1 oz	130	8	14
Large, 3 oz	390	24	42
Bundt Cakes, av. all types:			
3 oz slice	300	13	42
Mini-Bundt, 5 oz	500	22	70
Cannoli's: Mini, 1 oz	85	3	11
Regular, 2.5 oz	215	8	28
Carrot Cake: Plain, 3 oz	300	16	37
with Cream Cheese Frosting	400	22	48
Cheesecake:			
Small serving, 3 oz	240	13	26
Large serving, 5 oz	400	21	44
with Low-Fat Cheese/Fruit, 3 oz	170	4	28
Denny's, NY Style, 5oz	510	34	43
Chocolate Cake:			
with Choc. Frosting, 4 oz	415	18	62
without Frosting, 1/12 of 9", 3.5 oz	340	14	51
Chocolate Croissant, 4.25 oz	470	26	54
Chocolate Eclair, w/ custard, 3.5 oz	260	16	24
Chocolate Fudge Cake, 3 oz	270	12	40
Chocolate Meringue, 2.5 oz	320	13	48
Churros, 1 stick, 1.5 oz	165	8	21
Cinnamon Crumb Cake, 2.5 oz	260	9	40
Cinnamon Rolls: Small, 2 oz	220	8	34
Regular, 4 oz	440	16	68
Large, 6 oz	660	24	102
Brands ~ *See Page 67*			
Coffee Cake, 2 oz	180	6	30
Concha: Small, (3") 2.5 oz	250	8	38
Large (5" diam.), 5.5 oz	550	18	84
Cream Puff, custard filled, 4.6 oz	335	20	30
Cream Horn, 3 oz	210	5	36
Crumble Coffee Cake, 4.5 oz	500	25	65
Danish Pastries:			
Small, 2.5 oz	250	14	25
Large, 5 oz	500	28	50
Donuts ~ *See Page 66*			
Eclair, Chocolate, custard filled, 3.5 oz	260	16	24
Fig Bars, average	160	3	31

Ready-to-Eat (Cont)

Per Piece/Slice	C	F	Cb
Fruit Cake, Dark/Light, 2 oz	185	5	34
Fudge Nut Brownie, 3.5 oz	380	18	54
Gingerbread, from mix, 3" square	210	4	41
Honey Bun, glazed, large, 4.75 oz	560	29	68
Jelly Roll, 1/12 roll, 1.8 oz	150	2	32
Key Lime Pie, 4.3 oz	400	25	41
Kringles: Almond; Pecan, average	205	12	24
Blueberry: Cherry; Raspberry, av.	165	8	24
Lady Finger, 3 oz	310	5	59
Lemon Cake, 4 oz	440	24	49
Marble Cake, 4 oz	430	23	50
Mississippi Mud Pie, 4 oz	480	22	67
Mud Cake, 4.5 oz	380	20	44
Muffins ~ *See Page 67*			
Palmier Cookie, large, 4.5 oz	490	25	62
Pineapple Upside Down Cake,			
2.5 oz	230	9	36
Peach Melba, 3.5 oz	300	8	52
Pecan Sticky Roll, 6.5 oz	690	22	91
Pecan Twirls, 1.3 oz	170	7	26
Pies & Tarts ~ *See Page 134*			
Pound Cakes: Iced Lemon, 3.5 oz	360	17	50
Marble, 3.75 oz	350	13	53
Raspberry Rugulah,			
1.2 oz	110	9	7
Scone, fruit, 2 oz	200	9	30
Sponge Cake: Plain, 2.5 oz	220	10	33
with Chocolate Frosting	290	12	45
with Cream & Strawberry Jam	390	12	69
Starbucks Cakes ~ *Page 244*			
Strawberry Cream Cake, 4.7 oz	400	27	33
Strudel Bites, 0.75 oz	60	3	9
Strudel, fruit, av., 4.5 oz	300	17	32
Swiss Rolls, 1 oz	135	6	19
Tiramisu, 4.5 oz	440	22	34
Turnovers, fruit, average, 3 oz	290	15	35

Cupcakes

Average all Varieties	C	F	Cb
Regular:			
Cake only, 1.5 oz	140	6	20
Cake + Icing, 2.5 oz	260	13	34
Large, (Muffin Size):			
Cake only, 2.5 oz	235	9	34
Cake + Icing, 5 oz	520	27	67
Mini, (2-Bite):			
Cake only, 0.4 oz	40	2	6
Cake + Icing, 1 oz	110	6	13
Icing Only: Per 1 oz	115	7	13
Thick/Tall amount, 2.5 oz	290	17	32

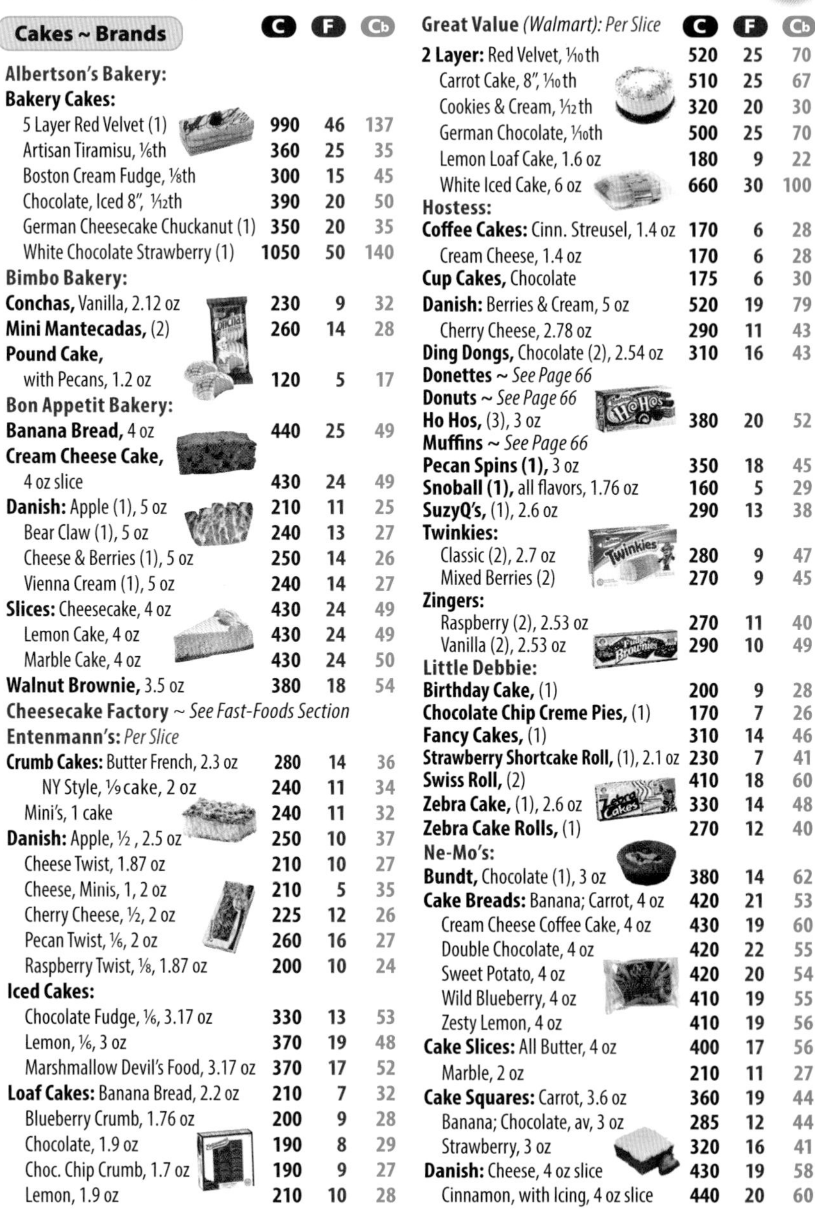

Cakes ~ Brands

	C	F	Cb
Albertson's Bakery:			
Bakery Cakes:			
5 Layer Red Velvet (1)	990	46	137
Artisan Tiramisu, ⅙th	360	25	35
Boston Cream Fudge, ⅛th	300	15	45
Chocolate, Iced 8", 1/12th	390	20	50
German Cheesecake Chuckanut (1)	350	20	35
White Chocolate Strawberry (1)	1050	50	140
Bimbo Bakery:			
Conchas, Vanilla, 2.12 oz	230	9	32
Mini Mantecadas, (2)	260	14	28
Pound Cake, with Pecans, 1.2 oz	120	5	17
Bon Appetit Bakery:			
Banana Bread, 4 oz	440	25	49
Cream Cheese Cake, 4 oz slice	430	24	49
Danish: Apple (1), 5 oz	210	11	25
Bear Claw (1), 5 oz	240	13	27
Cheese & Berries (1), 5 oz	250	14	26
Vienna Cream (1), 5 oz	240	14	27
Slices: Cheesecake, 4 oz	430	24	49
Lemon Cake, 4 oz	430	24	49
Marble Cake, 4 oz	430	24	50
Walnut Brownie, 3.5 oz	380	18	54
Cheesecake Factory ~ *See Fast-Foods Section*			
Entenmann's: *Per Slice*			
Crumb Cakes: Butter French, 2.3 oz	280	14	36
NY Style, 1/9 cake, 2 oz	240	11	34
Mini's, 1 cake	240	11	32
Danish: Apple, ½ , 2.5 oz	250	10	37
Cheese Twist, 1.87 oz	210	10	27
Cheese, Minis, 1, 2 oz	210	5	35
Cherry Cheese, ½, 2 oz	225	12	26
Pecan Twist, ⅙, 2 oz	260	16	27
Raspberry Twist, ⅛, 1.87 oz	200	10	24
Iced Cakes:			
Chocolate Fudge, ⅙, 3.17 oz	330	13	53
Lemon, ⅙, 3 oz	370	19	48
Marshmallow Devil's Food, 3.17 oz	370	17	52
Loaf Cakes: Banana Bread, 2.2 oz	210	7	32
Blueberry Crumb, 1.76 oz	200	9	28
Chocolate, 1.9 oz	190	8	29
Choc. Chip Crumb, 1.7 oz	190	9	27
Lemon, 1.9 oz	210	10	28

Great Value *(Walmart): Per Slice*	C	F	Cb
2 Layer: Red Velvet, 1/10th	520	25	70
Carrot Cake, 8", 1/10th	510	25	67
Cookies & Cream, 1/12th	320	20	30
German Chocolate, 1/10th	500	25	70
Lemon Loaf Cake, 1.6 oz	180	9	22
White Iced Cake, 6 oz	660	30	100
Hostess:			
Coffee Cakes: Cinn. Streusel, 1.4 oz	170	6	28
Cream Cheese, 1.4 oz	170	6	28
Cup Cakes, Chocolate	175	6	30
Danish: Berries & Cream, 5 oz	520	19	79
Cherry Cheese, 2.78 oz	290	11	43
Ding Dongs, Chocolate (2), 2.54 oz	310	16	43
Donettes ~ *See Page 66*			
Donuts ~ *See Page 66*			
Ho Hos, (3), 3 oz	380	20	52
Muffins ~ *See Page 66*			
Pecan Spins (1), 3 oz	350	18	45
Snoball (1), all flavors, 1.76 oz	160	5	29
SuzyQ's, (1), 2.6 oz	290	13	38
Twinkies:			
Classic (2), 2.7 oz	280	9	47
Mixed Berries (2)	270	9	45
Zingers:			
Raspberry (2), 2.53 oz	270	11	40
Vanilla (2), 2.53 oz	290	10	49
Little Debbie:			
Birthday Cake, (1)	200	9	28
Chocolate Chip Creme Pies, (1)	170	7	26
Fancy Cakes, (1)	310	14	46
Strawberry Shortcake Roll, (1), 2.1 oz	230	7	41
Swiss Roll, (2)	410	18	60
Zebra Cake, (1), 2.6 oz	330	14	48
Zebra Cake Rolls, (1)	270	12	40
Ne-Mo's:			
Bundt, Chocolate (1), 3 oz	380	14	62
Cake Breads: Banana; Carrot, 4 oz	420	21	53
Cream Cheese Coffee Cake, 4 oz	430	19	60
Double Chocolate, 4 oz	420	22	55
Sweet Potato, 4 oz	420	20	54
Wild Blueberry, 4 oz	410	19	55
Zesty Lemon, 4 oz	410	19	56
Cake Slices: All Butter, 4 oz	400	17	56
Marble, 2 oz	210	11	27
Cake Squares: Carrot, 3.6 oz	360	19	44
Banana; Chocolate, av, 3 oz	285	12	44
Strawberry, 3 oz	320	16	41
Danish: Cheese, 4 oz slice	430	19	58
Cinnamon, with Icing, 4 oz slice	440	20	60

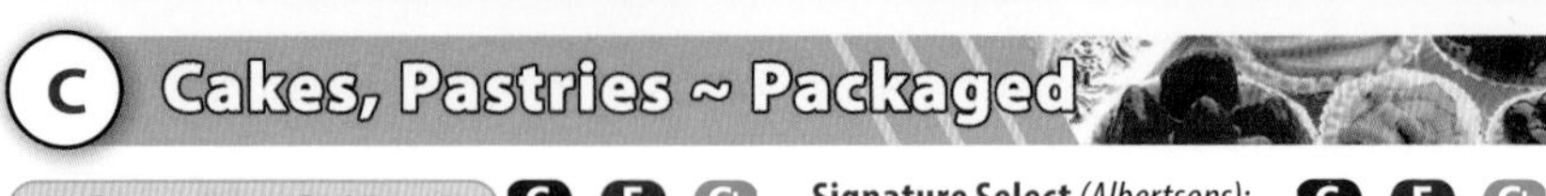

Cakes ~ Brands (Cont)

	C	F	Cb
Pepperidge Farm:			
Layer Cakes (Frozen): *Per ⅛ Cake, 2.43 oz*			
Chocolate Fudge	240	13	32
Chocolate Fudge Stripe	250	13	32
Classic Coconut	250	12	34
Golden	240	13	31
German Chocolate	240	12	31
Lemon; Tangy Key Lime; Vanilla	240	12	34
Red Velvet	240	13	30
Pop-Tarts *(Kellogg's): Per 2 Pop Tarts*			
Brown Sugar Cinnamon	400	13	68
Frosted: Apple Jacks	370	9	70
Banana Bread	360	8	71
Brown Sugar	400	13	68
Cherry	370	9	70
Chocolate Chip	380	11	67
S'Mores	370	9	67
Unfrosted: Blueberry; Strawberry	380	10	69
Brown Sugar	410	15	66
Prairie City:			
Ooey Gooey: Butter Cake (1)	220	9	33
Lemon (1)	210	9	32
Fudge Molten Lava (1)	400	21	48
Peanut Butter Molten Lava (1)	410	24	47
Salted Caramel Molten Lava (1)	380	20	50
Sara Lee:			
Frozen			
Butter Streusel Coffee Cake, 1.91 oz	190	9	26
Classic Cheesecakes:			
Original, 4.27 oz	320	16	38
Cherry, 4.76 oz	320	12	55
Strawberry, 4.76 oz	300	12	45
French Style Cheesecakes:			
Classic, 4.7 oz	290	20	24
Strawberry, 4.34 oz	230	14	25
NY Style, 5 oz	480	27	52
Pecan Coffee Cake, ⅙ Cake, 1.9 oz	190	9	25
Rich Caramel Truffle Cheesecake, 1 cheesecake, 3 oz	290	18	27
Pound Cakes: *Per ¼ Cake*			
All Butter, 2.66 oz	300	16	35
Classic Pound, 2.68 oz	310	19	31
Lemon, 2.68 oz	240	8	39

Signature Select *(Albertsons):*	C	F	Cb
7 Layer Square, ½ square, 1.76 oz	230	14	27
Artisan Fruit Topped Mousse Cake, 2.5 oz slice	140	8	15
Bakery: Black and White Cake, 4 oz	500	30	60
Triple Chocolate Cake, 4 oz	490	25	60
Cheesecake: 9" Platter, 1 slice	330	20	33
Four Variety Cheesecake, 2 slice	420	25	45
NY Choc. Cheesecake Platter,1 slice	330	20	32
Cheesecake Bars: *Per 5 oz*			
Cookies 'n Cream	540	27	63
Lemon Mascarpone	560	31	62
Strawberry Crumble	500	24	60
Wild Blueberry	520	28	58
Chocolate Lava Cake (1)	390	23	43
Colossal Unicorn Cake, 5 oz slice	600	30	90
Decadent Chocolate Cake, 2.68 oz	270	17	27
Lemon Squares, ½ square, 1.76 oz	180	7	26
Pumpkin Cake Roll, 3 oz slice	340	14	49
Strawb. White Choc. Shortcake, 2.78 oz slice	220	11	28
Tuxedo Truffle Cake, 7.2oz	740	50	80
Special K, Pastry Crisps, all varieties, 1 pouch, 0.9 oz	100	2	20
Tastykake:			
Creme Filled Cupcakes:			
Chocolate (2), 2.4 oz	270	10	42
Koffee Cake (2), 2.1 oz	240	9	38
Swirly Choc. (1), 2 oz	200	6	35
Kandy Kake: Coconut (2)	180	9	23
Peanut Butter (3)	280	16	31
Krimpets: Butterscotch (2)	220	6	39
Creme Filled (2)	280	11	44
Jelly (2)	190	4	37
Lemon Flavored (2)	220	6	40
Toaster Strudel *(Pillsbury): Per 2 Pastries*			
Cinnamon Roll	340	12	54
Cream Cheese & Stawberry	350	13	53
Fruit Flavors	340	12	54
Trader Joe's:			
Banana Bread with Walnuts, 2 oz	210	9	30
Cinnamon Coffee Cake, 2 oz	240	12	31
Frozen:			
Chocolate Lava Cake (1)	370	22	42

Cakes ~ Mixes

	C	F	Cb
Betty Crocker: *Dry Mix Only*			
Brownie Mix:			
Fudge, 1 oz	120	1	26
Milk Chocolate, 1 oz	120	1	26
Reese's, 1 oz	130	3	24
Salted Caramel, 1.15 oz	120	2	26
Supreme: Original, 1 oz	110	2	24
Chocolate Chunk, 1 oz	130	2	27
Fudge, 1.2 oz	130	2	27
Triple Chunk, 1 oz	130	2	27
Walnut, 1 oz	120	3	23
Cake Mix: Angel Food, 1.34 oz	140	0	32
Angel Food Confetti, 1.4 oz	150	0	33
Gingerbread, 1.8 oz	220	6	40
Pound Cake, 2 oz	230	3	48
Dessert Bars: *Dry Mix Only*			
PB Cookie Brownie Bars, 1.1 oz	130	3	25
Reese's Premium Bar Mix,	130	2	27
Supreme Lemon Bar Mix, 1.1 oz	130	4	24
Super Moist Delights Cake Mix: *Per 1.5 oz Dry Mix*			
Butter Pecan	160	1	37
Carrot	160	1	37
Cherry Chip	160	1	37
Dark Chocolate; Devils Food	160	2	36
French Vanilla	160	1	37
German Chocolate	160	1	36
Lemon	160	1	37
Party Rainbow Chip	160	1	37
Red Velvet	160	1	36
Strawberry	160	1	37
Triple Chocolate Fudge	160	2	36
White Cake, 1.58 oz	180	2	40
Duncan Hines: *Dry Mix Only*			
Brownie Mix: Chewy Fudge, 0.9 oz	110	2	22
Dark Chocolate Fudge, 1 oz	120	2	24
Classic Perfectly Moist:			
Butter Golden, 1.5 oz	170	2	36
Classic White, 1.5 oz	170	2	35
Dark Choc. Fudge, 1.5 oz	170	2	34
Keto, Chewy Fudge, 0.85 oz	140	7	17
Signature Perfectly Moist: *Per 1.52 oz Dry Mix*			
Carrot	170	3	34
French Vanilla	170	2	36
German Chocolate	170	4	35
Strawberry Supreme, 1.52 oz	170	2	36
Swiss Chocolate	170	2	35

	C	F	Cb
Jell-O: *Dry Mix Only*			
No Bake: Candy Cane, 1.76 oz	210	6	40
Classic Cheesecake, 1.83 oz	220	5	42
Double Chocolate, 1.55 oz	180	5	33
Strawberry, 2.43 oz	210	4	44
Krusteaz: *Dry Mix Only*			
Bars: Meyer Lemon, 1.1 oz	130	3	26
Pumpkin Pie, 0.9 oz	110	1	24
Cakes: Cinnamon Swirl, 1.52 oz	180	3	36
Vanilla Pound, 2 oz	180	1	42
Gluten Free: Chocolate., 1.24 oz	130	1	29
Yellow Cake, 1.52 oz	170	1	37
Quick Bread: Banana, 1.23 oz	130	1	30
Cinnamon Swirl, 1.23 oz	140	1	32
Cranberry Orange, 1.23 oz	140	2	29
Pillsbury: *Per 1 oz Dry Mix Only*			
Classic Brownie Mix: Choc Fudge	110	1	25
Dark Chocolate	110	1	25
Milk Chocolate	110	1	25
Funfetti Brownie Mix:			
With Candy Bits, 0.9 oz	110	1	24
With Oreo Cookie Pieces, 1 oz	120	2	25
Premium Brownie Mix:			
Cheesecake Swirl, 1 oz	120	2	25
Funfetti Cake Mix, all flavors, 1.5 oz	160	2	35
Moist Supreme Cake Mix:			
Devil's Food, 1.5 oz	160	2	34
White/Yellow, 1.5 oz	160	2	35
Traditional Cake Mix:			
Vanilla Flavored, 1.5 oz	130	2	29
Other Flavors, 1.5 oz	160	2	35

Cake Frostings

	C	F	Cb
Betty Crocker: *Per 2 Tbsp*			
Rich & Creamy: Coconut Pecan, 1.23 oz	140	8	18
Average other flavors, 1.23 oz	135	5	23
Whipped, av. all flavors., 0.9 oz	100	5	15
Cool Whip, Original, 2 Tbsp, 0.3 oz	25	2	3
Duncan Hines: *Per 2 Tbsp*			
Creamy, average all flavors, 1.23 oz	140	6	23
Whipped, average all flavors, 0.9 oz	100	5	15
Pillsbury: *Per 2 Tbsp*			
Creamy Supreme:			
Chocolate, 1.16 oz	130	6	20
Strawberry, 1.16 oz	140	5	22
Funfetti: Choc. Fudge, 1.2oz	140	6	21
Fluffy S'mores, 0.88 oz	110	5	16
Hot Pink Vanilla1.2 oz	140	5	23
Vanilla, 1.2 oz	140	5	23

Quick Guide

	C	F	Cb
Donuts			
Average All Brands			
Cake: Plain, 1.8 oz	205	12	23
Chocolate Iced, 2 oz	255	14	29
Sugared, 0.8 oz	205	10	29
Non-Cake, Glazed, 2 oz	225	11	29
Croissant-Donuts			
(Includes Cronuts/Frissants)			
Average all Brands			
Cream-filled, 3.5 oz	430	26	45
Custard-filled, 3.5 oz	360	19	45

Extra Listings ~ *See CalorieKing.com*

(Cronut is a trademark of Dominique Ansel Bakery, New York)

Donuts ~ Brands

	C	F	Cb
Albertson's:			
Donut Holes:			
Glazed Old Fashioned (4)	240	12	31
Powdered Sugar (4)	210	12	24
Gem Donuts: Plain Cake (3)	190	12	20
Cinnamon Sugar (3)	240	15	23
Glazed (1)	140	6	21
Bon Appetit:			
Mini Donuts:			
Chocolate (4)	270	16	29
Crumb (4)	240	12	32
Powdered (4)	250	12	34
Dunkin':			
Apple Crumb	290	11	44
Apple N' Spice	230	10	31
Barvarian Kreme	240	11	31
Boston Kreme	270	11	39
Chocolate Frosted	260	11	34
Chocolate Headlight	310	14	41
Coconut	410	21	50
Glazed Chocolate	370	23	41
Jelly Filled	250	10	36
Lemon	230	10	31
Powdered	330	20	34
Strawberry Frosted	260	11	35
Sugared	210	11	24
Vanilla Creme	300	15	37

Extra Listings ~ *See Fast Food Section*

Donuts ~ Brands (Cont)

	C	F	Cb
Entenmann's:			
8 Pack: *Per Donut*			
Apple Cider, 2 oz	240	11	34
Crumb Topped, 1.94 oz	240	11	33
Frosted: Devil's Food, 2.1 oz	290	17	33
Rich Frosted, 2 oz	290	18	30
Pop'ems Donut Holes: Glazed (4)	240	13	28
Party Sprinkled Devil's Food (4)	230	12	31
Rich Frosted (4)	330	26	24
Popettes, Riuch Frosted, 3 pieces	310	22	28
Softees Variety Pack: Plain (1)	180	11	19
Cinnamon; Powdered (1)	210	12	24
Hostess: *15 count Box, Per 3 Donuts*			
Jumbo Donette, Glazed Blueb. (1)	230	9	35
Mini Donettes: Caramel Crunch	250	12	34
Caramel Chocolate	210	10	28
Double Chocolate	280	17	31
Strawberry Cheesecake	240	12	33
Krispy Kreme: *Each*			
Apple Fritter	350	19	42
Chocolate: Iced Cake	340	19	40
Iced Custard Filled	300	15	37
Iced Glazed Cruller	290	15	37
Iced Glazed	240	11	33
Iced Kreme Filled	350	19	41
Iced Glazed with Sprinkles	260	11	36
Cinnamon Twist	210	11	26
Glazed Cruller	240	15	25
Glazed Doughnut Holes: *Each*			
Original	45	3	5
Blueb.; Cake; Choc. Cake	45	2	7
Glazed Kreme Filled	350	19	40
Maple Iced Glazed	240	11	34
New York Cheesecake	350	19	40
Original Glazed	190	11	22
Powdered Cake	310	19	32
Traditional Cake	290	18	29
Little Debbie:			
Glazed Donut Sticks: 1.7 oz	220	13	25
1.9 oz	260	15	29
Tastykake: *10 oz Bags*			
Mini:			
Crunch (6), 3.4 oz package	370	14	57
Frosted (6), 3 oz package	360	16	49
Lemon (4), 2 oz	260	14	30
Powdered (4), 1.9 oz	230	10	31
Salted Caramel Flavored (4), 2 oz	260	10	39

Quick Guide

	C	F	Cb
Muffins: Ready-To-Eat			
Average All Brands			
Small, 1 oz	90	4	14
Medium, 2 oz	185	7	28
Large, 3 oz	275	10	42
Extra Large, 4 oz	365	13	57
Giant, 6 oz	550	20	84
Super Size, 8 oz	730	27	112

Muffins Ready-To-Eat ~ Brands

	C	F	Cb
Albertsons: *Per Muffin*			
Banana Nut, 3.75 oz	410	25	40
Strawberry, 3.5 oz	360	20	45
Entenmann's: *Per Muffin*			
Litttle Bites: Blueberry, 1.38 oz	100	1	19
Chocolate Chip, 1.34 oz	110	2	19
Garden Lites: *Per 2 oz Muffin*			
Banana Chocolate Chip	120	3	22
Blueberry Oat	110	2	21
Carrot Berry	100	2	19
Double Chocolate	110	3	19
Great Value *(Walmart):*			
Banana Nut Filled (4), 4 oz	410	19	56
Blueberry; Choc Chip (4), av.,4 oz	425	19	58
Hostess:			
Mega Muffin: Banana/Blueb., av., 5.5 oz	550	27	71
Double Choc, 5.5 oz	580	33	73
Mini Muffins: Blueberry (4)	210	10	29
Chocolate Chip (4)	220	11	30
Kroger: *Per 3.74 oz Muffin*			
Banana Nut; Blueberry, average	455	23	59
Little Debbie:			
Mini Muffins: Blueberry (1), 1.9 oz	170	6	28
Chocolate Chip (1), 1.9 oz	190	8	27
My Favorite Muffin: *Per Large*			
Banana Nut	650	38	71
Blueberry	590	28	78
Boston Cream Pie	740	33	105
Chocolate Cheesecake	650	38	70
Lemon Poppyseed	670	32	90
Otis Spunkmeyer:			
Banana, 2 oz	220	10	30
Blueberry, 2 oz	210	9	29
Minis, Blueberry (3)	240	10	33
Starbucks ~ *See Fast-Foods Section*			
Trader Joe's: *Per 3.5 oz Muffin*			
Blueberry	360	13	56
Cinnamon Coffee Cake	440	23	56
Vitalicious:			
VitaTops: Banana Choc. Chip, 2 oz	100	0	23
Chocolate Chip, 2 oz	100	2	27
Deep Chocolate, 2 oz	110	2	27

Muffin Mixes

	C	F	Cb
Dry Mix Only			
Betty Crocker: *Makes 2 Muffins*			
Boxed: Banana Nut, 2 oz	230	5	45
Cinnamon Streusel, 2.3 oz	270	6	52
Wild Blueberry, 2.82 oz	230	3	48
Pouch Mix:			
Banana Nut, 2.1 oz	240	5	47
Blueberry, 2.1 oz	240	5	48
Chocolate Chip, 2.1 oz	250	5	48
Krusteaz: *Dry Mix Only*			
Almond Poppy Seed, 1.4 oz	150	2	35
Choc Chunk, 1.5 oz	180	4	35
Cranb. Orange, 1.23 oz	140	0	33

Sweet Rolls & Buns

Note: It is best to weigh for accuracy as actual weight can be 10-50% higher than label weight.

	C	F	Cb
Per Sweet Roll or Bun Unless Indicated			
Bon Appetit, Super Cinn. Roll, 5 oz	480	16	72
Cinnabon: Classic	880	37	129
Caramel Pecanbon	1090	51	149
Minibon	350	15	52
Cloverhill Bakery,			
Big Texas Cinnamon Roll, 4 oz	420	16	63
Entenmann's, Jumbo Glazed Bun	460	22	58
Hostess, Jumbo Honey Bun, 4 oz	480	24	61
Little Debbie:			
Honey Bun: 1.5 oz	230	13	25
Individual, 3 oz Bun	360	20	41
Pecan Spinwheels: Single, 1 oz	110	4	18
2 Pack, 2.1 oz	220	7	37
O&H Danish: *Per 1.95 oz*			
Kringles: Apple; Wisconsin, average	185	10	26
Almond; Turtle, average	225	13	29
Cinn. Roll; Cream Cheese, average	220	14	25
Pillsbury: *Per Roll UnlessIndicated*			
Sweet Rolls, Refrigerated:			
Orig; Cinnamon, w/ Crm Cheese Icing	140	5	24
Cinn., Flaky w/ Butter Cream Icing	160	7	23
Orange, with Orange Icing	160	5	26
Grands, Refrigerated: *Per Roll*			
Cinnabon: Cinnamon Roll, with Cream Cheese Icing	320	10	53
w/ Extra Rich Butter Icing, 3.5 oz	320	10	53
Flaky Cinnamon Roll, with Original Icing, 3.5 oz	360	16	49

Quick Guide

	C	F	Cb
Chocolate:			
Average All Brands			
Milk Chocolate, regular:			
Plain/Nuts/Fruit, average, 1 oz	150	9	17
1.5oz Bar	230	13	25
2 oz Bar	305	17	34
4 oz Block	610	34	68
8 oz Block	1220	68	136
1 Pound, 16 oz	2440	136	272
Dark/White Chocolate: 1 oz	155	9	17
Hershey's, Sugar Free, 5 pieces	110	13	24
Milk Chocolate-Coated:			
Almonds, 5-6, 1 oz	150	10	15
Cherry Cordial Centers, 2 pcs, 1 oz	145	6	21
Clusters, Nut, 3 pieces, 1.2 oz	210	14	20
Coffee Beans, 1.4 oz	220	13	22
Macadamias, 10 pieces, 1.4 oz	220	16	21
Mints, 1 medium, 0.5 oz	55	1	11
Nougat & Caramel, 1 oz	150	9	15
Peanuts, 12 medium, 1 oz	145	10	14
Raisins, 28 medium, 1 oz	110	4	19
Baking Chocolate:			
Baker's: Bittersweet, 1 oz	140	12	14
Semi-sweet, 1 oz	140	9	16
Nestle, Chips: Dark, 1 Tbsp. 0.5 oz	70	5	3
Semi-Sweet, 1 Tbsp. 0.5oz	70	4	9
Unsweetened, 1 oz	140	14	8
Carob, Plain, 1 oz	155	9	16

Candy ~ Brands & Generic

Per Piece/Serving	C	F	Cb
3 Musketeers: Orig., 1 bar, 1.9 oz	240	7	42
2 To Go, 1.7 oz Bar	200	6	36
Fun Size, 3 bars, 1.6 oz	190	6	34
Minis, 7 pieces, 1.4 oz	170	5	32
100 Grand: 1.5 oz bar	190	8	30
Snack Size (1), 0.8 oz	95	4	15
Super Size, 2.8 oz	360	14	58
Abba Zabba, 2 oz bar	250	5	48
After Dinner Mints, 1 small	25	2	3
After Eight Mint, each	35	2	4
Airhead, 1 bar, 0.5 oz	60	1	14
Almond Joy: 2 bars, 1.6 oz	220	13	26
King Size, 4 bars, 3.2 oz	440	26	53
Miniatures, 2 pieces, 1 oz	130	7	15
Snack Size, 2 pieces, 1.2 oz	160	9	20

Per Piece/Serving	C	F	Cb
Almond Roca, 3 pieces, 1.3 oz	200	15	17
Almonds: Sugar-coated (15), 1.4 oz	190	7	27
Jordan, 15 pieces, 1.4 oz	180	8	28
Almond Clusters:			
True North, 5 pieces, 1 oz	170	12	9
Trader Joe's, 2 pieces, 1.2 oz	190	14	13
Almond Pecan Crunch:			
True North, 5 pieces, 1.2 oz	150	11	10
Altoids: Original, 3 mints	10	0	2
Artic, 3 mints	5	0	2
Andes, Thins (8), av. all var., 1.4 oz	205	13	22
Anthon Berg:			
Creamy Mint (4), 1.4 oz	180	6	31
Marzipan with Plum, in Madeira	120	6	14
Atomic Fireball, 1 piece, 0.3 oz	35	0	9
Baby Ruth: King Size, 3.5 oz bar	500	24	66
2 oz bar	280	14	39
Fun size, 2 bars	170	8	24
Minis, 4 bars	210	11	28
Baci *(Perugina),* 1 piece, 0.5 oz	75	6	7
Bark Thins, Snacking Chocolate, Dark Choc. Mint/Pretzel, av., 1 oz	140	6	20
Baskin-Robbins: Sugar Candy, 3 pcs	60	1	12
Sugar Free, 4 pieces, average, 0.6 oz	40	1	16
Note: Carb figure includes 16g sugar alcohol			
Big Hunk, 2 oz Bar	230	3	47
Bit-O-Honey:			
1.7 oz bar	180	4	39
Chews, 6 pcs, 1.4 oz	150	3	32
Blow Pops, each, 0.6 oz	60	0	17
Bon Bons, 3 pieces	65	0	15
Boston Baked Beans, (11)	70	2	11
Brach's: Almond Supremes (10)	200	14	20
Bridge Mix (15)	190	10	26
Double Dippers (15)	210	14	22
Gummi Bears (14)	130	0	30
Lemon Drops, Sugar Free, 4 pieces	35	0	17
Note: Carb figures include 17g Sugar Alcohol			
Mandarin/Orange Slices (3), 1.6 oz	150	0	37
Maple Nut Goodies (8)	190	9	27
Milk Maid Crmls (4)	150	4	25
Peanut Cluster (3)	210	15	20
Breath Savers, (1),all var.	5	0	2
Bubble Gum ~ *See Page 75*			
Bulls Eyes, 3 pieces, 1.2 oz	130	3	23
Buncha Crunch: 1.4 oz	180	9	25
Movie Box, 3.2 oz	450	20	65
Burnt Peanuts, 1.4 oz	170	6	29

Candy ~ Brands & Generic (Cont)

Per Piece/Serving	C	F	Cb
Butterfinger:			
Bars: 1.9 oz bar	250	10	36
Crisp Bar, 1 pkg, 2 oz	300	17	35
Fun Size Bars (2), 1.3 oz	170	7	25
Minis, 1.1 oz	140	6	20
Bites, 6 pieces, 1.1 oz	140	6	20
Dessert Toppers, 2 Tbsp, 1.3 oz	180	7	25
Butter Mints, 7 pieces, 0.5 oz	50	0	12
Butterscotch: 3 pieces	60	0	15
Discs (*Walgreens*), 3 pieces, 0.6 oz	70	0	17
Cadbury *(Hershey's)*:			
Caramello Bar 1.6 oz	220	10	29
Caramel Egg, 1.2 oz	170	8	22
Dairy Milk Bar, 7 pcs, 1.4 oz	200	11	23
Mini Eggs (Candy), 12 pcs, 1.4 oz	190	8	28
Blocks: Caramello, 6 pieces	180	8	24
Fruit & Nut, 5 pieces	140	7	17
Milk Chocolate, 7 pieces	200	11	23
Roasted Almond, 5 pieces	150	8	16
Candy Apple, medium, 6.5 oz	280	0	60
Candy Cane, medium, 5", 0.5 oz	40	0	14
Candy Corn, 20 pieces, 1.4 oz	150	0	38
Candy Jar Mix *(Jewel)*, 3 pcs, 0.6 oz	60	0	14
Candy Necklace *(Smarties)*, (1), 0.8 oz	90	1	20
Caramels: Each, 0.4 oz	40	1	8
Chocolate, each, 0.3 oz	25	1	6
Creams (3), 1.3 oz	130	3	23
Caramel Popcorn, $^{2}/_{3}$ cup	150	6	23
Cella's,			
Milk Choc. Cherries, 3 pcs, 1.5 oz	160	6	27
Certs, Breath Mints, 1 piece	5	0	2
Charleston Chew:			
Chocolate Bar (1), 1.4 oz	160	5	30
Mini Bars, 13 pieces	190	6	34
Charms: Blow Pop	60	0	17
Flat Pop, 0.5 oz	50	0	14
Chew-ets, Peanut Chews,			
Original (4), 1.6 oz	230	12	29
Chewz, 1 roll, 1 oz	120	1	28
Chick O Stick, 2 oz	240	9	42
Chunky Bar *(Nestlé)*,			
King Size, 2.5 oz	340	19	44
Chupa Chups, 1 Pop	50	0	12
Cinn. Buttons *(Walgreens)*, 3 pieces	60	0	16
Cinnamon Disks *(Walmart)*, 3 pieces	70	0	18
Circus Peanuts *(Spangler)*,			
6 pieces, 1.3 oz	165	0	41

Per Piece/Serving	C	F	Cb
CocoaVia, Orig., 0.8 oz	100	6	12
Coconut Stacks, (8)	320	16	46
Coffee Go, Candy, (4)	60	1	12
Conversation Hearts *(Necco)*:			
Small (40), 1.4 oz	160	0	39
1 large	10	0	3
Cookie Dough Bites, 1.4 oz	200	10	27
Cote d'Or: Dark 86% Coca, 4 pcs	270	22	14
Dark, 70%, Orange, 3.5 oz	575	46	34
Dark, Raspberry, 3.5 oz	580	46	34
Milk, Intense, 3.5 oz	575	40	45
Cotton Candy, 1 oz	110	0	28
Cough Drops ~ *See Page 75*			
Cracker Jack, $^{1}/_{2}$ cup, 1 oz	120	2	23
Creme Savers:			
3 pieces, 0.5 oz	60	1	11
Sugar-Free, 3 pieces	30	1	8
Crisped Rice, Choc Chip, 1 bar, 1 oz	115	4	20
Crows, 11 pieces, 1.4 oz	130	0	33
Crunch Bar ~ *See Nestle*			
Dots, 11 dots, 1.4 oz	130	0	33
Double Dip Stick, 1 stick	15	1	3
Dove:			
Milk Choc: Singles Bar, ⅓, 1.05 oz	170	10	19
Large Tablet Bar, 9 pcs, 1.5 oz	230	13	25
Choc. Cov. Almonds, 13 pcs, 1.4 oz	220	15	19
Promises: Milk Choc., 1 pce, 0.3 oz	45	3	5
w/ Caramel, 1 piece, 0.3 oz	40	2	5
w/ Peanut Butter, 1 pce, 0.3 oz	45	3	4
Swirls, all var., 9 pieces 1.5 oz	230	14	25
Dark Choc: Singles Bar, 1.3 oz	220	13	24
Large Tablet Bar, 9 pcs, 1.5 oz	220	14	25
Chocolate Cov. Almds, 13 pcs	210	15	19
Promises, Almond, 1 piece, 0.3 oz	40	3	4
Swirls, Raspberry, 9 pcs, 1.4 oz	220	14	24
Dum Dum Pops *(Spangler)*, 1 pop	25	0	7
Drops *(Hershey's)*:			
Cookies 'n' Creme, 14 pieces, 1.5 oz	210	11	26
Milk Chocolate, 15 pieces, 1.4 oz	200	12	25
Endangered Species (Vegan):			
80% Cocoa 3 oz Dark Choc. Bars,			
Strong Velvety, 1. oz	180	13	11
75% Cocoa 3 oz Dark Choc. Bars,			
Oat Milk Coconut & Almonds, 1 oz	180	13	12
72% Cocoa 3 oz Dark Choc. Bars: *Per 1 oz*			
Almond & Sea Salt Dark Chocolate	170	11	14
Bold & Silky Dark Choolate	170	11	14
Vibrant Cherries & Dark Chocolate	160	10	15
60% Cocoa 3 oz Bar: *Per 1 oz*			
Caramel Sea Salt & Dark Choc.	150	9	16
48% Cocoa 30 oz Bar: *Per 1. oz*			
Fudgey PB Milk Chocolate	170	12	13
Rich Caramel Milk Chocolate	160	10	14

Candy ~ Brands & Generic (Cont)

Per Piece/Serving	C	F	Cb
English Toffee, 1 piece, 0.4 oz	70	4	6
5th Avenue:			
Bars: 2 oz	260	12	38
King Size, 3 pieces, 3.4 oz	450	21	66
Fannie May:			
Buttercreams,			
Milk Chocolate, Vanilla (1), 0.7oz	90	3	16
Mint Meltaway, 3 pcs	150	10	15
Pixie (1), 0.8 oz	110	7	13
Fast Break *(Reese's):*			
Bars: 1.8 oz bar	230	11	32
King Size, 3 pieces, 3.4 oz	450	21	63
Ferrero Rocher:			
Bars: Milk Chocolate, 5 pcs, 1.06 oz	180	13	14
Aero			
Pieces:1 piece	75	5	5
3 pieces, 1.3 oz	230	16	18
Fluffy Stuff *(Charms),*			
Cotton Candy, 2.5 oz	270	0	71
Fondant: Choc-coated, 1.2 oz	125	3	27
Mint, 1 oz	105	0	25
Fran's:			
Gold Bar, Macadamia (1)	230	15	23
GoldBite, Almond (1)	140	8	16
Park Bar (1), 1.5 oz	230	13	22
Fruit Drops, (1), ¼ oz	20	0	4
Fruit Gems *(Sunkist)*, (4), 1.4 oz	130	0	34
Fruit Leathers, average, 0.5 oz	50	1	12
Fruit Pastilles *(Rowntree),* 1 roll	185	0	45
Fruit Roll-Ups *(Betty Crocker/Sunkist),*			
1 roll, 0.5 oz	50	1	12
Fruit Flavored Snacks *(Betty Crocker),*			
all varieties, 0.8 oz	80	1	17
Fudge:			
Chocolate; Mint, 1 oz	130	8	14
P'nut Butter & Choc., 1 oz	130	8	13
Brevin's: Cashew, 1 oz	195	9	28
Triple Decker, 1 oz	165	7	25
Fun Dip*(Ferrero)*, 1 package	45	0	11
Ghirardelli:			
Intense Dark Chocolate Bars:			
60% Cocao, 2 squares	140	10	16
72% Cocao, 2 squares	130	11	11
86% Cocao, 2.5 squares	190	19	11
92% Cocao, 3 squares	190	20	10

Per Piece/Serving	C	F	Cb
Gobstoppers/Jawbreakers,			
9 pieces	60	0	14
Godiva:			
Milk Choc. Bar, 31% Cacao, 4 blocks	210	12	23
Signature Dark Chocolte Mini Bars:			
72% Cacao, 1.2 oz	200	15	10
Roasted Almond,1.2oz	190	14	11
GoLightly:			
Assorted Toffee, 5 pieces, 1 oz	85	2	24
Fruit Chews, 5 pieces, 1 oz	95	2	26
Hard Candy, Assorted (4), 0.5 oz	45	0	15
Note: Carb figures include 15-25g sugar alcohol			
Goobers Peanuts, 3Tbsp., 1.1 oz	180	11	17
Good & Plenty *(Hershey's)*, (33), 1.8 oz	180	0	46
GooGoo Clusters, 1 piece, 1.76 oz	180	12	20
Gum ~ *See Page 75*			
Gum Drops: 1 small, 0.1 oz	15	0	3
5 pieces, 0.5 oz	75	0	15
Gummi *(Shur Fine):*			
Bears (15), 1.4 oz	130	0	29
Chewy Sweet Tarts (4)	160	0	36
Worms (9), 1.5 oz	140	0	31
Guylian:			
Bars: Dark Chocolate (3), 1 oz	150	12	11
Milk Choc. w/ Hazelnuts (3),1 oz	170	11	15
No Sugar Added Bars:			
Milk Chocolate, 3 squares	150	11	16
54% Cocoa, Dark Choc., 3 sqrs.	140	11	16
Seashells:			
Bar, 1.4 oz	210	13	21
Boxed, Originals (1), 0.4 oz	60	4	6
Truffles, (1), 0.4 oz	70	6	5
Heath: Original (1), 1.4 oz	210	13	24
King Size, 2.8 oz	420	26	49
Miniatures, 4 pieces, 1 oz	150	9	17
Hershey's:			
Candy-Coated Eggs,			
Milk Chocolate Center, (5)	140	9	17
Cookies 'n' Creme: 1.55 oz Bar	220	11	29
Crunchers, 1.8 oz pkg	250	11	35
Fangs, 2 pieces	130	7	17
Polka Dot Eggs (6)	150	8	19
Milk Chocolate:			
Harry Potter Bar, 1.52 oz	220	13	26
Nuggets: 3 pieces	150	9	19
w/ Almonds, 3 pcs	150	9	15
Truffles, 3 pieces	150	9	17
Plant Based Oat Choc., 1.55 oz Bar	230	16	24
Kisses ~ See Page 71			

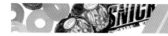

Candy ~ Brands & Generic (Cont)

Per Piece/Serving	C	F	Cb
Hershey's, (Cont):			
Special Dark Chocolate:			
Golden Almond Bar, ⅓ pack	130	9	13
Nuggets with almonds, 3 pieces	140	10	16
Truffles, 3 pieces	150	10	18
Honeycomb: Plain, 1 oz	115	0	27
Choc-coated, 2 pieces	180	7	31
Hot Tamales, 16 pieces, 1.4 oz	110	0	27
Hugs ~ *See Kisses*			
Jawbreakers/Gobstoppers *(Ferrara),* 9 pieces	60	0	14
Jells *(Joyva),* Raspb., 3 rings, 1.34 oz	150	3	32
Jelly Beans, average all brands:			
Small Size: 1 bean	5	0	1
12 beans, 0.5 oz	50	0	13
Regular Size: 1 bean	10	0	2
10 beans, 1 oz	105	0	26
Large Size: 1 bean	15	0	38
10 beans, 1.5 oz	150	0	38
Sugar Free, av. all brands, (27), 1 oz	80	0	29
Note: Carb figure include 26g sugar alcohol			
Jelly Belly: 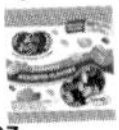			
27 beans, 1.06 oz	110	0	28
Sugar Free, 27 beans, 1.06 oz	80	0	29
Note: Carb figure include 26g sugar alcohol			
Chocolate Dips, all flavors:			
1 bean	4	0	1
27 beans	110	3	18
2.8 oz bag	295	8	48
Jolly Rancher:			
Bites: Filled, 11 pieces	140	0	32
Sours, 16 pieces	130	0	34
Candy Canes, 1 piece	45	0	12
Chews, 7 pieces	120	2	27
Gummies, 7 pieces	100	0	24
Hard Candy, 3 pieces	70	0	17
Jelly Beans, 1.1oz	100	0	26
Lollipops (1), 0.46 oz	45	0	12
Twizzlers, Chery; Watermelon, 2 pcs	90	1	19
Jujyfruits, 15 pieces	130	0	33
Junior Caramels, 9 pieces, 1.5 oz	130	4	23
Junior Mint: 12 pieces	130	3	26
Minis, 42pieces	130	4	26

Per Piece/Serving	C	F	Cb
Justin's:			
Peanut Butter Cups: Dark Choc (2)	220	14	20
Milk Chocolate (2)	230	15	20
White Chocolate (2)	230	16	19
Kinder, Joy, 1 egg, 0.7 oz	110	6	12
Kisses *(Hershey's):*			
Candy Cane Mint (6)	140	8	18
Milk Chocolate: 1 Kiss	20	1	3
7 Kisses	160	9	19
With Almonds (7) 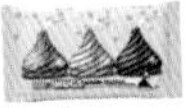	160	10	16
Hugs (7)	160	9	19
Special Dark Chocolate: 7 pieces	150	9	20
Mint Truffles (7)	160	10	20
Kit Kat *(Hershey's):*			
Dark Chocolate: 1.5 oz pkg	200	12	27
King Size , 3 fingers, 3 oz	150	9	20
Milk Chocolate: 4 piece bar, 1.5 oz	210	11	28
Miniatures (4), 1.2 oz	170	9	22
Snack Size (2), 1 oz	140	7	19
Halloween:			
Milk Choc., 2 pieces	140	7	19
Witches Brew White Choc., 2 pcs	140	8	18
Thins, 5 pieces	150	8	20
White Creme Candy Bar, 1.5 oz pkg	220	12	27
Lemon Drops: (4), 0.6 oz	60	0	16
Walgreens, Sugar Free (3), 0.6 oz	50	0	17
Laffy Taffy *(Ferrerro):*			
Bites, all flavors, 10 pieces	120	1	29
Ropes, all flavors, 1 pce	80	2	16
Stretchy & Tangy, all flavors, 1 bar	180	2	35
Lemonhead, (10), 1.4 oz	50	0	12
Licorice:			
Average all varieties, 1oz	100	0	25
Chews *(Panda),* (1) 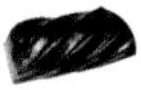	10	0	3
Tid Bits (1)	10	0	2
Twists: Black/Red, av., 1 pc	35	0	8
Sugar Free, 1 piece	15	0	3
Note: Carb figure includes 3g sugar alcohol			
American Licorice Co.:			
Made Simple, Black Licorice Twists (3)	100	0	24
Red Ropes, Snack Size, 2 ropes	100	0	25
Red Vines:			
Black, 3 pieces	100	0	24
Grape; Red, 3 pieces	100	0	25
Sugar Free, Strawberry, 4 pieces	100	0	25
Note: Carb figure includes 11g sugar alcohol			
Super Strings, 3 pieces	100	0	25
Lifesavers: *Per 4 Pieces Unless Indicated*			
Butter Rum	60	0	14
Five flavor Pack; Fruit Variety	60	0	15
Wild Cherry	60	0	15
Gummies, Neons, 7 pieces	90	0	22
Orange Mints, 1 piece	15	0	3

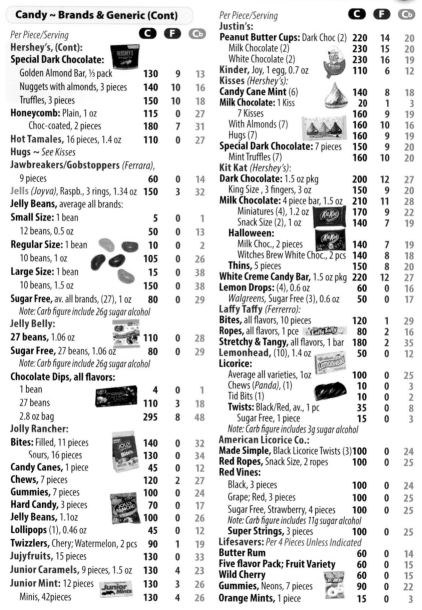

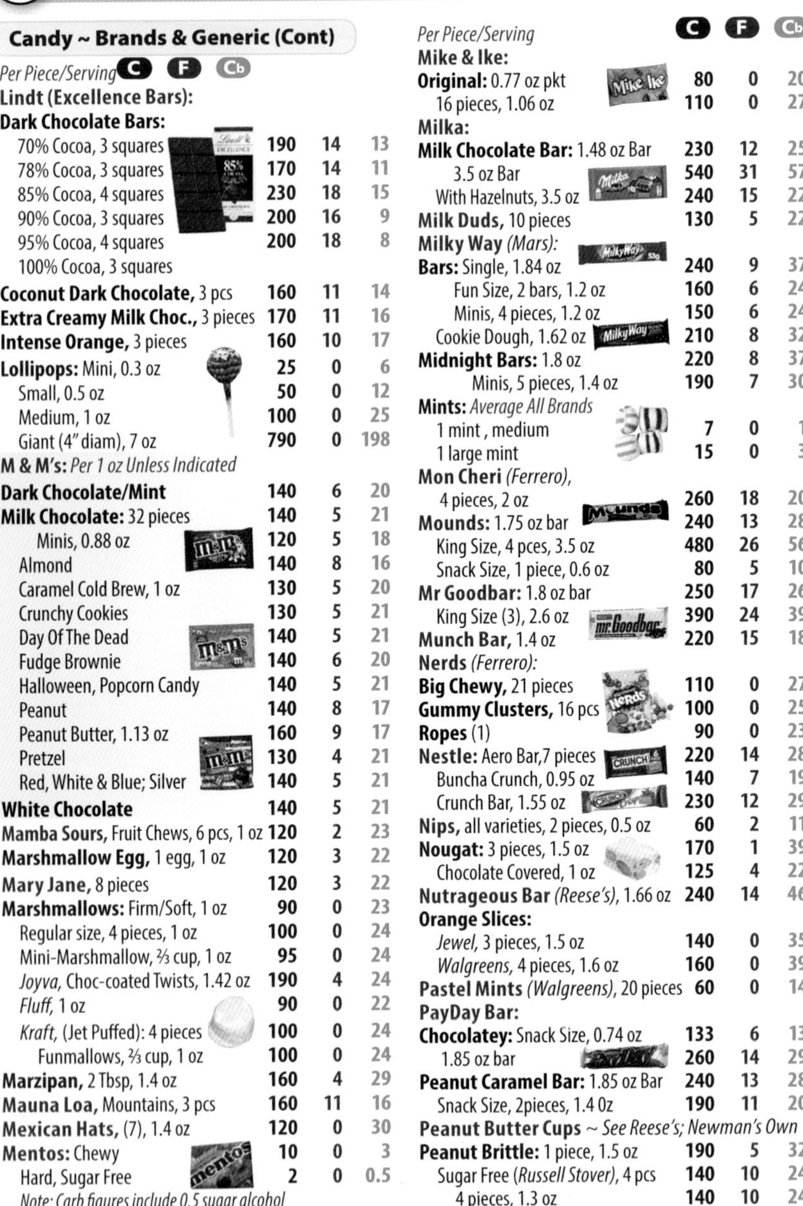

Candy ~ Brands & Generic (Cont)

Per Piece/Serving	C	F	Cb
Lindt (Excellence Bars):			
Dark Chocolate Bars:			
70% Cocoa, 3 squares	190	14	13
78% Cocoa, 3 squares	170	14	11
85% Cocoa, 4 squares	230	18	15
90% Cocoa, 3 squares	200	16	9
95% Cocoa, 4 squares	200	18	8
100% Cocoa, 3 squares			
Coconut Dark Chocolate, 3 pcs	160	11	14
Extra Creamy Milk Choc., 3 pieces	170	11	16
Intense Orange, 3 pieces	160	10	17
Lollipops: Mini, 0.3 oz	25	0	6
Small, 0.5 oz	50	0	12
Medium, 1 oz	100	0	25
Giant (4" diam), 7 oz	790	0	198
M & M's: *Per 1 oz Unless Indicated*			
Dark Chocolate/Mint	140	6	20
Milk Chocolate: 32 pieces	140	5	21
Minis, 0.88 oz	120	5	18
Almond	140	8	16
Caramel Cold Brew, 1 oz	130	5	20
Crunchy Cookies	130	5	21
Day Of The Dead	140	5	21
Fudge Brownie	140	6	20
Halloween, Popcorn Candy	140	5	21
Peanut	140	8	17
Peanut Butter, 1.13 oz	160	9	17
Pretzel	130	4	21
Red, White & Blue; Silver	140	5	21
White Chocolate	140	5	21
Mamba Sours, Fruit Chews, 6 pcs, 1 oz	120	2	23
Marshmallow Egg, 1 egg, 1 oz	120	3	22
Mary Jane, 8 pieces	120	3	22
Marshmallows: Firm/Soft, 1 oz	90	0	23
Regular size, 4 pieces, 1 oz	100	0	24
Mini-Marshmallow, ⅔ cup, 1 oz	95	0	24
Joyva, Choc-coated Twists, 1.42 oz	190	4	24
Fluff, 1 oz	90	0	22
Kraft, (Jet Puffed): 4 pieces	100	0	24
Funmallows, ⅔ cup, 1 oz	100	0	24
Marzipan, 2 Tbsp, 1.4 oz	160	4	29
Mauna Loa, Mountains, 3 pcs	160	11	16
Mexican Hats, (7), 1.4 oz	120	0	30
Mentos: Chewy	10	0	3
Hard, Sugar Free	2	0	0.5

Note: Carb figures include 0.5 sugar alcohol

Per Piece/Serving	C	F	Cb
Mike & Ike:			
Original: 0.77 oz pkt	80	0	20
16 pieces, 1.06 oz	110	0	27
Milka:			
Milk Chocolate Bar: 1.48 oz Bar	230	12	25
3.5 oz Bar	540	31	57
With Hazelnuts, 3.5 oz	240	15	22
Milk Duds, 10 pieces	130	5	22
Milky Way *(Mars):*			
Bars: Single, 1.84 oz	240	9	37
Fun Size, 2 bars, 1.2 oz	160	6	24
Minis, 4 pieces, 1.2 oz	150	6	24
Cookie Dough, 1.62 oz	210	8	32
Midnight Bars: 1.8 oz	220	8	37
Minis, 5 pieces, 1.4 oz	190	7	30
Mints: *Average All Brands*			
1 mint , medium	7	0	1
1 large mint	15	0	3
Mon Cheri (Ferrero),			
4 pieces, 2 oz	260	18	20
Mounds: 1.75 oz bar	240	13	28
King Size, 4 pces, 3.5 oz	480	26	56
Snack Size, 1 piece, 0.6 oz	80	5	10
Mr Goodbar: 1.8 oz bar	250	17	26
King Size (3), 2.6 oz	390	24	39
Munch Bar, 1.4 oz	220	15	18
Nerds *(Ferrero):*			
Big Chewy, 21 pieces	110	0	27
Gummy Clusters, 16 pcs	100	0	25
Ropes (1)	90	0	23
Nestle: Aero Bar,7 pieces	220	14	28
Buncha Crunch, 0.95 oz	140	7	19
Crunch Bar, 1.55 oz	230	12	29
Nips, all varieties, 2 pieces, 0.5 oz	60	2	11
Nougat: 3 pieces, 1.5 oz	170	1	39
Chocolate Covered, 1 oz	125	4	22
Nutrageous Bar *(Reese's)*, 1.66 oz	240	14	46
Orange Slices:			
Jewel, 3 pieces, 1.5 oz	140	0	35
Walgreens, 4 pieces, 1.6 oz	160	0	39
Pastel Mints *(Walgreens)*, 20 pieces	60	0	14
PayDay Bar:			
Chocolatey: Snack Size, 0.74 oz	133	6	13
1.85 oz bar	260	14	29
Peanut Caramel Bar: 1.85 oz Bar	240	13	28
Snack Size, 2pieces, 1.4 Oz	190	11	20
Peanut Butter Cups ~ *See Reese's; Newman's Own*			
Peanut Brittle: 1 piece, 1.5 oz	190	5	32
Sugar Free *(Russell Stover)*, 4 pcs	140	10	24
4 pieces, 1.3 oz	140	10	24

Candy ~ Brands & Generic (Cont)

Per Piece/Serving	C	F	Cb
Peanuts, choc-covered, 14 pieces	230	14	23
Pearson's:			
Mint Patties (2), 1 oz	110	2	23
Salted Nut Roll Bar, ⅓ bar	150	9	14
Peppermints:			
7 small, 0.5 oz	60	0	15
Brach's, Star Brites (3)	60	0	15
Pez, 1 roll	35	0	9
Pretzels: Choc-covered, Mini (6)	200	9	25
White Chocolate Bites (23), 1.4 oz	200	9	25
Raisinets:			
Milk Choc, 1.58 oz pkg	190	8	32
Dark Chocolate, 0.85 oz	110	5	17
Reese's:			
Milk Chocolate:			
Peanut Butter Cups: 1.5 oz	210	12	24
Big Cup, King Size, 2.8 oz	400	24	44
King Size (2), 1.4 oz	200	12	22
Minis, Unwrapped, 9 pieces	160	9	19
Snack Size (1), 0.8 oz	110	6	12
Thins (3), 1.25 oz	170	10	20
Pieces: 38 pieces	150	7	19
2 pkgs, 1.4 oz	210	12	25
Sticks:			
1.5 oz Package	220	13	24
King Size (1)	110	6	12
Take Five ~ *See Page 74*			
Rice Krispies Treats *(Kellogg's),*			
1 bar, average all varieties, 0.78 oz	95	3	17
Riesen, Chocolate Chew (3)	120	5	19
Rocky Road,			
Milk Choc.; Dark Choc. Mint, 1.83 oz	220	10	28
Roca Thins:			
Milk Chocolate (3)	220	15	22
Dark Chocolate (3)	190	13	20
Rolo:			
Creamy Caramels (8)	215	9	32
Dark Salted Caramel (5)	140	7	20
Russell Stover Candy:			
Dark Chocolate Assorted (2)	150	7	19
Milk Chocolate:			
Assorted: Regular (2)	150	8	19
Cremes (2)	130	5	21
Caramels (2)	160	7	23
Chocolate Covered Nuts (2)	160	11	13
Sugar Free: Assorted (2)	130	9	18
Fine Chocolate, Assorted (2)	120	8	18
Peanut Butter (2)	150	12	18

Note: Carbohydrate figure includes 15g-18 sugar alcohol

Per Piece/Serving	C	F	Cb
Russell Stover Candy (Cont):			
Sugar Free: Ass'td Hard Candies (2)	130	10	17
Note: Carbohydrate figures includes 15 g sugar alcohol			
Bags: Cinnamon (3)	40	0	17
Fruit Flavors (3)	40	0	17
Lemon	40	0	17
Note: Carbohydrate figures includes 15 g sugar alcohol			
Salt Water Taffy *(Brach's),* (5)	170	3	36
Seashells *(Guylian),*			
Boxed Originals (1), 0.4 oz	60	4	6
See's Candies (Sugar Free):			
Dark Chocolate Bar: 1.48 oz	200	15	24
Dark Almond Clusters, 2 pieces	170	13	16
Dark Walnut Clusters, 2 pieces	180	15	15
Lollypops: Butterscotch (1)	50	3	13
Butterschotch Little Pops, 4 pieces	35	2	9
Chocolate (1)	60	0	12
Milk Chocoalte Bar, 1.48 oz	190	14	23
Peanut Brittle, 1 oz	120	10	15
Peanut Brittle Bar (1)	130	10	14
Note: Carbohydrate figures include 12-18 g sugar alcohol			
Shari, Root Beer Barrels (2)	50	0	14
Skittles:			
Chewy: Brightside, 2 oz pkt	230	6	52
Original, 2.17 oz	250	3	56
Sour, 1 oz	110	1	26
Wild Berry, 1 oz	110	1	26
Gummies: Original (14)	90	0	23
WildBerry (14)	90	0	23
Skor,			
Toffee Bar (1), 1.4 oz	210	12	25
Smarties:			
Candy Rolls (1)	25	0	6
Giant, 5 tablets	25	0	7
Snickers:			
Dark Choc. Bar, Alm. Brownie, 2 sq.	180	9	23
Milk Chocolate Bars:			
Original, 1.86 oz bar	250	12	32
Fun Size, 2 bars, 1.2 oz	160	8	20
Almond Bar, 1.76 oz	230	10	33
Almond Brownie, 2 squares	180	9	23
Peanut Brownie, 2 squares	180	8	21
Peanut Butter Bar	130	7	15
White Chocolate Bar, 1.4 oz	200	10	23

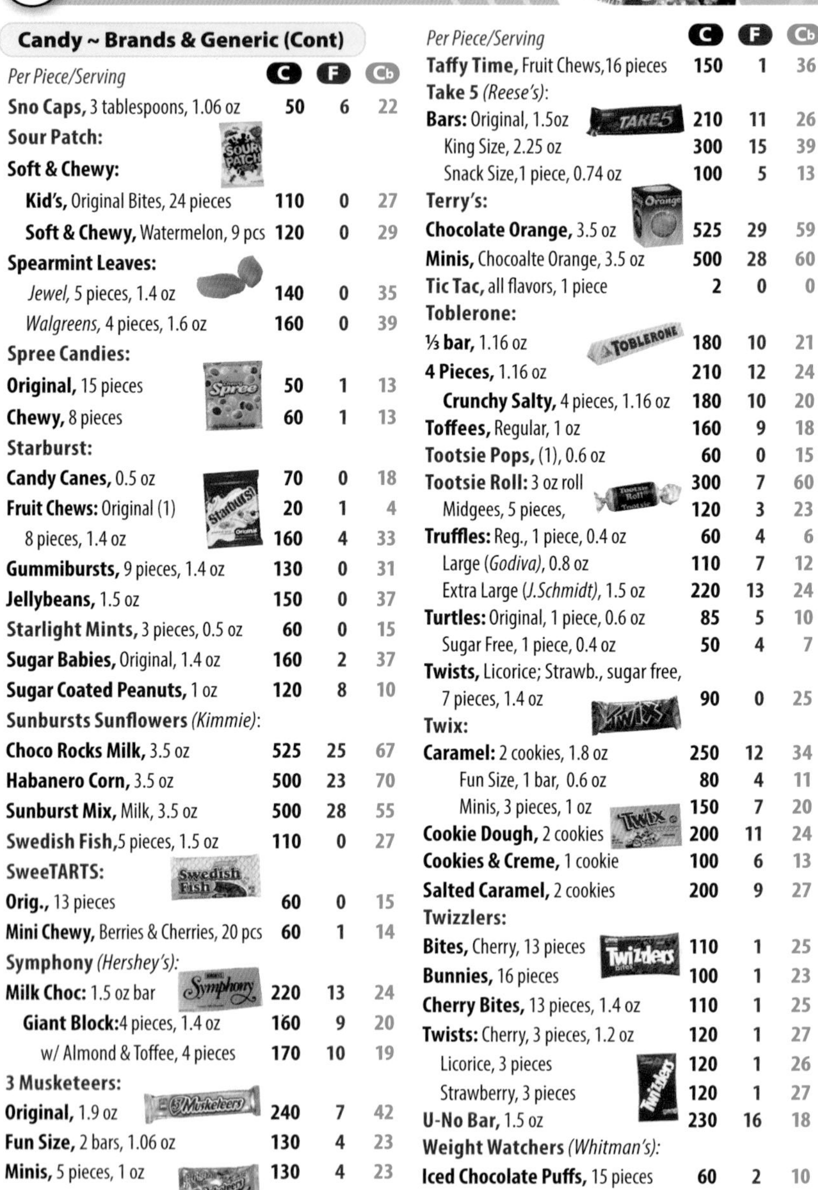

Candy ~ Brands & Generic (Cont)

Per Piece/Serving	C	F	Cb
Sno Caps, 3 tablespoons, 1.06 oz	50	6	22
Sour Patch:			
Soft & Chewy:			
Kid's, Original Bites, 24 pieces	110	0	27
Soft & Chewy, Watermelon, 9 pcs	120	0	29
Spearmint Leaves:			
Jewel, 5 pieces, 1.4 oz	140	0	35
Walgreens, 4 pieces, 1.6 oz	160	0	39
Spree Candies:			
Original, 15 pieces	50	1	13
Chewy, 8 pieces	60	1	13
Starburst:			
Candy Canes, 0.5 oz	70	0	18
Fruit Chews: Original (1)	20	1	4
8 pieces, 1.4 oz	160	4	33
Gummibursts, 9 pieces, 1.4 oz	130	0	31
Jellybeans, 1.5 oz	150	0	37
Starlight Mints, 3 pieces, 0.5 oz	60	0	15
Sugar Babies, Original, 1.4 oz	160	2	37
Sugar Coated Peanuts, 1 oz	120	8	10
Sunbursts Sunflowers *(Kimmie)*:			
Choco Rocks Milk, 3.5 oz	525	25	67
Habanero Corn, 3.5 oz	500	23	70
Sunburst Mix, Milk, 3.5 oz	500	28	55
Swedish Fish,5 pieces, 1.5 oz	110	0	27
SweeTARTS:			
Orig., 13 pieces	60	0	15
Mini Chewy, Berries & Cherries, 20 pcs	60	1	14
Symphony *(Hershey's):*			
Milk Choc: 1.5 oz bar	220	13	24
Giant Block:4 pieces, 1.4 oz	160	9	20
w/ Almond & Toffee, 4 pieces	170	10	19
3 Musketeers:			
Original, 1.9 oz	240	7	42
Fun Size, 2 bars, 1.06 oz	130	4	23
Minis, 5 pieces, 1 oz	130	4	23
Share Size, 1.66 oz	210	6	37

Per Piece/Serving	C	F	Cb
Taffy Time, Fruit Chews,16 pieces	150	1	36
Take 5 *(Reese's)*:			
Bars: Original, 1.5oz	210	11	26
King Size, 2.25 oz	300	15	39
Snack Size,1 piece, 0.74 oz	100	5	13
Terry's:			
Chocolate Orange, 3.5 oz	525	29	59
Minis, Chocoalte Orange, 3.5 oz	500	28	60
Tic Tac, all flavors, 1 piece	2	0	0
Toblerone:			
⅓ bar, 1.16 oz	180	10	21
4 Pieces, 1.16 oz	210	12	24
Crunchy Salty, 4 pieces, 1.16 oz	180	10	20
Toffees, Regular, 1 oz	160	9	18
Tootsie Pops, (1), 0.6 oz	60	0	15
Tootsie Roll: 3 oz roll	300	7	60
Midgees, 5 pieces,	120	3	23
Truffles: Reg., 1 piece, 0.4 oz	60	4	6
Large *(Godiva)*, 0.8 oz	110	7	12
Extra Large *(J.Schmidt)*, 1.5 oz	220	13	24
Turtles: Original, 1 piece, 0.6 oz	85	5	10
Sugar Free, 1 piece, 0.4 oz	50	4	7
Twists, Licorice; Strawb., sugar free, 7 pieces, 1.4 oz	90	0	25
Twix:			
Caramel: 2 cookies, 1.8 oz	250	12	34
Fun Size, 1 bar, 0.6 oz	80	4	11
Minis, 3 pieces, 1 oz	150	7	20
Cookie Dough, 2 cookies	200	11	24
Cookies & Creme, 1 cookie	100	6	13
Salted Caramel, 2 cookies	200	9	27
Twizzlers:			
Bites, Cherry, 13 pieces	110	1	25
Bunnies, 16 pieces	100	1	23
Cherry Bites, 13 pieces, 1.4 oz	110	1	25
Twists: Cherry, 3 pieces, 1.2 oz	120	1	27
Licorice, 3 pieces	120	1	26
Strawberry, 3 pieces	120	1	27
U-No Bar, 1.5 oz	230	16	18
Weight Watchers *(Whitman's):*			
Iced Chocolate Puffs, 15 pieces	60	2	10
Nut Butter Bites (2)	140	5	21

Candy ~ Brands & Generic (Cont)

Per Piece/Serving	C	F	Cb
Werther's:			
Hard Candy: Caramel Coffee (4)	70	1	15
Sugar-Free Original (5)	45	2	14
Note: Carb figure includes 14g sugar alcohol			
Soft, Chocolate Covered (2)	120	5	19
Whatchamacallit: 1.6 oz Bar	230	12	28
King Size Bar, 2.6 oz	370	20	46
Whitman's,			
Boxed Chocolates, Sampler (2)	120	5	17
Whoppers, av. all varieties, 18 pcs	190	7	31
Yogurt Candy, Coated Raisins,1.4 oz	180	8	28
York:			
Peppermint Pattie: 1.4 oz pkg	150	3	32
Share Package, 2 pieces, 0.95 oz	100	2	22
Snack Size, 2 pieces, 1.2 oz	120	3	27
Zagnut, 1.75 oz bar	220	9	35
Zero Bar: 1.85 oz bar	230	8	37
King Size, 3.5 oz	420	15	69

Gum

Per Piece	C	F	Cb
Bazooka	15	0	4
Beechies	6	0	2
Big League Chews	10	0	2
Bubble Yum: Original	25	0	6
Sugarless	10	0	3
Candilicious	30	0	2
Carefree, Sugarless/Regular	5	0	2
Chiclet	5	0	1
Dentyne	5	0	1
Double Bubble Ball	20	0	5
Estee, Bubble/Regular	5	0	2
Extra *(Wrigley's)*, Sugar-Free	5	0	2
Freshen-Up	10	0	3
Hubba Bubba: Regular	25	0	6
Sugar-free, average	14	0	1
Ice Breakers	5	0	2
Jolt Gum	5	0	2
Super Bubble	15	0	4
Trident, Orig.; White	5	0	1
Wrigley's, all flavors	10	0	2

Carob Candy

Per Piece/Serving	C	F	Cb
Carob, Plain/Natural, 1 oz	155	9	15
Carob Coated: Raisins, 1 oz	130	8	15
Almonds/Peanuts, 1 oz	150	10	14
Caramels, 1 oz	110	4	18
Dates, 1 oz	125	5	20
Malt Balls, 1 oz	135	8	15
Soybeans	145	9	16
Trail/Party Mix, 1 oz	150	9	15

Cough Drops

Per Drop/Piece	C	F	Cb
Beech Nut, 1 drop	10	0	2
CVS, Honey Lemon Cough Drops	15	0	4
Diabetic Tussin	0	0	0
Halls, Defense Vitamin C:			
Regular	15	0	4
Sugar Free	5	0	3
Fruit Breezers	15	0	4
Menthol Drops: Regular	15	0	4
Sugar Free	5	0	4
Plus	20	0	5
Listerine *(Amer. Chicle)*, Lozenge	10	0	2
Luden's, Throat Drops: Reg., all var.	10	0	2
Sugar Free	0	0	0
Pine Bros, Cough Drops	10	0	2
Ricola:			
Cough Drops:			
Natural Herbs	10	0	3
Sugar-Free Lemon Mint	0	0	1
Rolaids, Sodium Free	5	0	1
Sathers, Peppermint Lozenges	15	0	3
Sucrets *(Beecham)*, Lozenges	10	0	3
Wintergreen, Lozenges	15	0	3

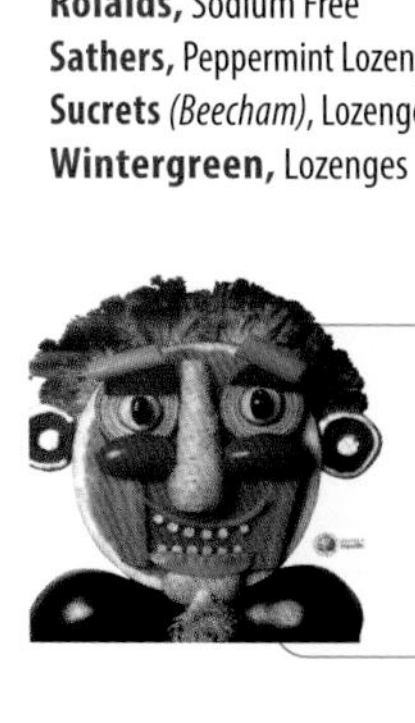

Eat at least 5 servings of fruit and vegetables every day . . . and Enjoy Better Health!

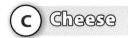

Quick Guide

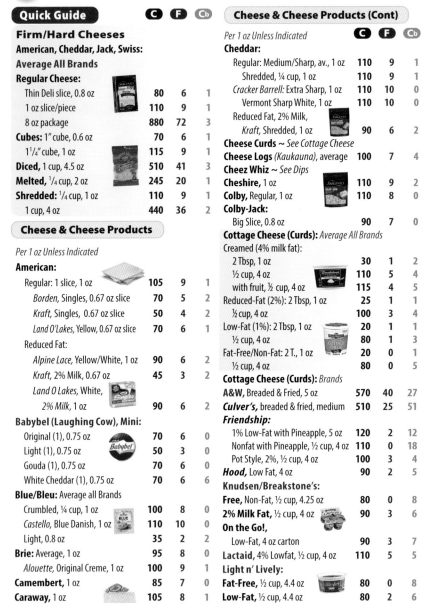

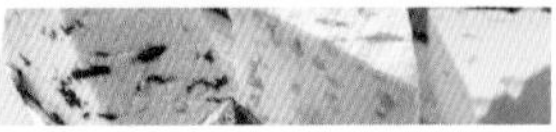

	C	F	Cb
Firm/Hard Cheeses			
American, Cheddar, Jack, Swiss:			
Average All Brands			
Regular Cheese:			
Thin Deli slice, 0.8 oz	80	6	1
1 oz slice/piece	110	9	1
8 oz package	880	72	3
Cubes: 1" cube, 0.6 oz	70	6	1
1¼" cube, 1 oz	115	9	1
Diced, 1 cup, 4.5 oz	510	41	3
Melted, ¼ cup, 2 oz	245	20	1
Shredded: ¼ cup, 1 oz	110	9	1
1 cup, 4 oz	440	36	2

Cheese & Cheese Products

Per 1 oz Unless Indicated	C	F	Cb
American:			
Regular: 1 slice, 1 oz	105	9	1
Borden, Singles, 0.67 oz slice	70	5	2
Kraft, Singles, 0.67 oz slice	50	4	2
Land O'Lakes, Yellow, 0.67 oz slice	70	6	1
Reduced Fat:			
Alpine Lace, Yellow/White, 1 oz	90	6	2
Kraft, 2% Milk, 0.67 oz	45	3	2
Land O Lakes, White, *2% Milk,* 1 oz	90	6	2
Babybel (Laughing Cow), Mini:			
Original (1), 0.75 oz	70	6	0
Light (1), 0.75 oz	50	3	0
Gouda (1), 0.75 oz	70	6	0
White Cheddar (1), 0.75 oz	70	6	6
Blue/Bleu: Average all Brands			
Crumbled, ¼ cup, 1 oz	100	8	0
Castello, Blue Danish, 1 oz	110	10	0
Light, 0.8 oz	35	2	2
Brie: Average, 1 oz	95	8	0
Alouette, Original Creme, 1 oz	100	9	1
Camembert, 1 oz	85	7	0
Caraway, 1 oz	105	8	1

Cheese & Cheese Products (Cont)

Per 1 oz Unless Indicated	C	F	Cb
Cheddar:			
Regular: Medium/Sharp, av., 1 oz	110	9	1
Shredded, ¼ cup, 1 oz	110	9	1
Cracker Barrell: Extra Sharp, 1 oz	110	10	0
Vermont Sharp White, 1 oz	110	10	0
Reduced Fat, 2% Milk, *Kraft,* Shredded, 1 oz	90	6	2
Cheese Curds ~ *See Cottage Cheese*			
Cheese Logs *(Kaukauna),* average	100	7	4
Cheez Whiz ~ *See Dips*			
Cheshire, 1 oz	110	9	2
Colby, Regular, 1 oz	110	8	0
Colby-Jack:			
Big Slice, 0.8 oz	90	7	0
Cottage Cheese (Curds): *Average All Brands*			
Creamed (4% milk fat):			
2 Tbsp, 1 oz	30	1	2
½ cup, 4 oz	110	5	4
with fruit, ½ cup, 4 oz	115	4	5
Reduced-Fat (2%): 2 Tbsp, 1 oz	25	1	1
½ cup, 4 oz	100	3	4
Low-Fat (1%): 2 Tbsp, 1 oz	20	1	1
½ cup, 4 oz	80	1	3
Fat-Free/Non-Fat: 2 T., 1 oz	20	0	1
½ cup, 4 oz	80	0	5
Cottage Cheese (Curds): *Brands*			
A&W, Breaded & Fried, 5 oz	570	40	27
Culver's, breaded & fried, medium	510	25	51
Friendship:			
1% Low-Fat with Pineapple, 5 oz	120	2	12
Nonfat with Pineapple, ½ cup, 4 oz	110	0	18
Pot Style, 2%, ½ cup, 4 oz	100	3	4
Hood, Low Fat, 4 oz	90	2	5
Knudsen/Breakstone's:			
Free, Non-Fat, ½ cup, 4.25 oz	80	0	8
2% Milk Fat, ½ cup, 4 oz	90	3	6
On the Go!,			
Low-Fat, 4 oz carton	90	3	7
Lactaid, 4% Lowfat, ½ cup, 4 oz	110	5	5
Light n' Lively:			
Fat-Free, ½ cup, 4.4 oz	80	0	8
Low-Fat, ½ cup, 4.4 oz	80	2	6

Cheese & Cheese Products (Cont)

Per 1 oz Unless Indicated	C	F	Cb
Cream Cheese: *Average All Brands*			
Regular/Soft:			
2 Tbsp, 1 oz	95	10	1
3 oz package	290	29	4
8 oz package	780	78	9
Light, Plain, 1 oz	60	5	3
Fat-Free, Plain, 1 oz	30	0	2
Better Than Cream Cheese (Tofutti),			
all varieties, 1 oz	85	5	9
Easy Cheese *(Kraft),*			
American, 2 Tbsp, 1.2 oz	80	6	2
Edam, 1 oz	100	8	1
Farmer, Low-Fat, 1 oz	40	3	0
Feta: Regular, 1 oz	75	6	1
Crumbled, ½ cup, 2.5 oz	190	15	3
Athenos, Reduced-Fat,			
1 oz	50	3	1
Fontina, 2 Tbsp, 1 oz	110	9	1
Goat's Milk Cheese:			
Chevre: Original, 2 Tbsp	80	7	0
Semi-Soft, 1 oz	100	9	1
Hard, 1 oz	130	10	1
Chavrie, Logs:			
Original, 2 Tbsp, 1 oz	80	7	0
Honey, 1 oz	80	5	6
Sundried Tomato & Garlic, 1 oz	80	6	2
Gjetost, fresh, 1 oz	130	8	12
Myzithra, grated, 1 oz	80	4	2
Gorgonzola, 1 oz	100	8	1
Galbani, Dolcelatte, 1 oz	95	8	1
Gouda, 1 oz slice	100	8	1
Gruyere, 1 oz	115	9	1
Havarti *(Sargento),* 0.7 oz	80	6	0
Jarlsberg: Average, 1 oz	100	8	0
Reduced Fat, shredded, 1 oz	70	4	0
Labneh, (Lebanese Cream Cheese), 1.8 oz	70	4	4
Laughing Cow:			
Creamy Wedges: Asiago (1)	30	2	1
Original (1)	50	4	1
Light (1)	30	2	1
Lifetime,			
Fat Free, all varieties, 1 Slice, 1 oz	40	0	1

Cheese & Cheese Products (Cont)

Per 1 oz Unless Indicated	C	F	Cb
Limburger, 1 oz	95	8	0
Mascarpone, av., 1 oz	125	13	1
Mexican:			
Cacique: Asadero, sliced	70	5	1
Cotija	90	7	0
Enchilado; Manchego	90	7	0
Panela	80	6	0
Queso Fresco	80	6	0
Queso Quesadilla	90	7	1
Shredded	100	7	1
Ranchero	80	6	0
Chi-Chi's, Salsa Con Quéso, Mild	45	3	4
El Mexicano: Cotija, 1 oz	90	6	0
Oaxaca, 1 oz	90	7	1
Kraft, Mexican Four Cheese; Taco,			
Shredded,	100	8	1
Sargento, 4 Cheese Mexican, Shredded	110	9	2
Supremo, Quéso Chihuahua, 1 oz	100	8	0
Verole, Quéso Oaxaca, 1 oz	70	8	1
Monterey Jack:			
Regular, shredded, 1 oz	100	8	1
Land O Lakes, Co-Jack, 1 oz	90	7	1
Kraft, 1" cube, 1 oz	100	8	0
Mozzarella:			
Whole Milk: Average 1 oz	85	7	1
Land O'Lakes, String, 1 oz	80	6	2
Polly-O, Slice, average, 1 oz	80	6	1
Fat-Free,			
Kraft, Shredded, 1 oz	45	0	2
Reduced Fat,			
Kraft, 2% Milk Fat, Shredded, 1 oz	80	4	2
Part Skim:			
Borden, Shredded, 1 oz	90	6	2
Kraft, Shredded, 1 oz	80	5	2
Kraft, String, 1 oz	80	5	1
Polly-O, Shredded, 1 oz	80	5	0
Muenster:			
Land O Lakes, 1 oz slice	100	9	0
Wisconsin, 1 oz slice	100	8	0
Parmesan:			
Fresh/Block, Dry, 1 oz	110	8	1
Grated (Packaged):,2 tsp	20	2	0
Kraft: Shaker Bottle, 1 oz	110	8	1
Reduced-Fat Topping, 1 Tbsp	20	1	2

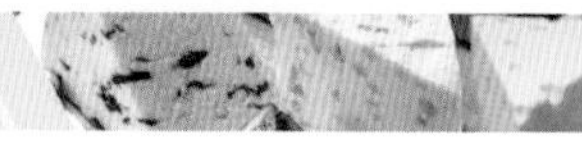

Cheese & Cheese Products (Cont)

Per 1 oz Unless Indicated	C	F	Cb
Philadelphia:			
Cheesecake:			
Crumbles: Chocolate, 3.3 oz	320	17	37
Chocolate Hazelnut, 3.3 oz	320	17	37
Cup, Cherry, 3.25 oz	200	13	18
Cream Cheese Brick:			
Original: 1 oz	100	10	1
8 oz package	800	80	4
⅓ Less Fat, 1 oz	70	6	1
Cream Cheese Tubs:			
Original, 1.1 oz	80	7	2
⅓ Less Fat, 1.1 oz	60	5	2
Smoked Salmon, 1.1 oz	60	5	2
Strawberry, 1.1 oz	70	5	5
Low-Fat, 95%, 1 oz	20	1	1
Whipped: Original, 0.77 oz	50	4	2
Garlic & Herb, 0.77 oz	50	4	2
Port Wine (Kaukauna/WisPride):			
10 oz Ball, 1 oz	100	7	5
Provolone: Regular, 1 oz	100	8	1
Alpine Lace, Reduced-Fat, 1 oz	80	6	1
Sargento, 1 slice, 0.67 oz	70	5	0
Pub *(President)*, average all varieties	75	7	1
Quark: 40% fat	45	3	1
20% fat	30	2	1
Skim/Non-Fat	20	0	2
Ricotta Cheese:			
Whole Milk, 1 oz	50	4	1
Part Skim, 1 oz	40	2	2
Light/Low-Fat, 1 oz	25	1	2
Fat-Free, ½ cup, 4.5 oz	100	0	10
Baked Ricotta, 2 oz	130	9	3
Romano: Block/Loaf	110	8	1
Grated, 1 oz	120	9	1
Roquefort, 1 oz	105	9	1
Sheep's Milk, (Manchego),			
Trader Joes/Wegman's, 1 oz	120	10	0
Smoked Cheddar, average, 1 oz	110	10	0
Stilton, average, 1 oz	110	10	0
String:			
Regular, average all brands	80	6	1
Kraft: Twists/Strings,			
Mozzarella & Cheddar (1), 0.75 oz	60	4	0
Frigo, 1 oz	80	6	1
Light/Lite:			
Polly-O, String,			
2% Red-Fat, 1 oz	70	5	0

Cheese & Cheese Products (Cont)

Per 1 oz Unless Indicated	C	F	Cb
Swiss: Regular, 1 oz	110	8	2
Alpine Lace, Reduced-Fat, 1 oz	90	6	1
Tilsit, 1 oz	100	8	1
Tybo, 1 oz	100	7	1
Velveeta *(Kraft): Per Slice*			
Orig.; 3 Cheese Blend; Jalap., 0.74 oz	40	2	3
Queso Blanco, Mild, 0.74	40	2	3

Plant Based

	C	F	Cb
Daiya:			
Shreds, all varieties,1.05 oz	80	5	8
Slices, all varieties, 0.77 oz	60	5	4
Field Roast:			
Chao: Block/Shreds, 1 oz	80	6	6
Slices, all flavors, 0.7 oz	60	5	4
Follow Your Heart:			
Coconut Oil: Shreds/Feta, av.	85	7	5
Slices, 0.7 oz, all flavors	60	5	4
Palm Fruit, Shreds, av.	80	7	7
Soy Cheese Varieties, av.	85	7	5
Kite Hill:			
Almond Milk Cream Cheese:			
Plain, 2 Tbsp	70	6	2
Chive, 2 Tbsp	60	6	2
Almond Milk Ricotta, ¼ cup, 2 oz	140	12	5
Lisanatti:			
Almond Milk, Chunks/Shreds, 1 oz	70	4	3
Rice Milk, Chunks, average, 1 oz	60	3	2
Miyoko's Creamery:			
Organic Cashew Milk: *Per 1 oz*			
Aged Sharp English Farmhouse	110	8	7
Cream Cheese, Everything	90	8	5
Double Cream Chive	120	11	4
Italian Style Mozzarella	60	5	1
Smoked Mozzarella	60	5	2
Tofutti, Better Than Cheese,			
all flavors, 2 Tbsp	60	5	2
Trader Joes, Soy Cheese, Mozz. Style	70	4	3
Treeline: *Per 1 oz Unless indicated*			
Aged Artisinal Wheel, all flavors	140	11	5
Cream Cheese, average all flavors	90	7	4
Goat Cheese, all flavors	90	6	5
Shreds, all flavors	90	6	7
Slices, all flavors, 0.9 oz	80	5	6
Soft French Style:			
Chipotle-Serrano Pepper	100	8	3
Average other flavors	95	7	3
Vitalite:			
Shreds, average all flavors	90	7	7
Slices, all flavors	60	5	4
Spread, Original Creamy	70	7	1

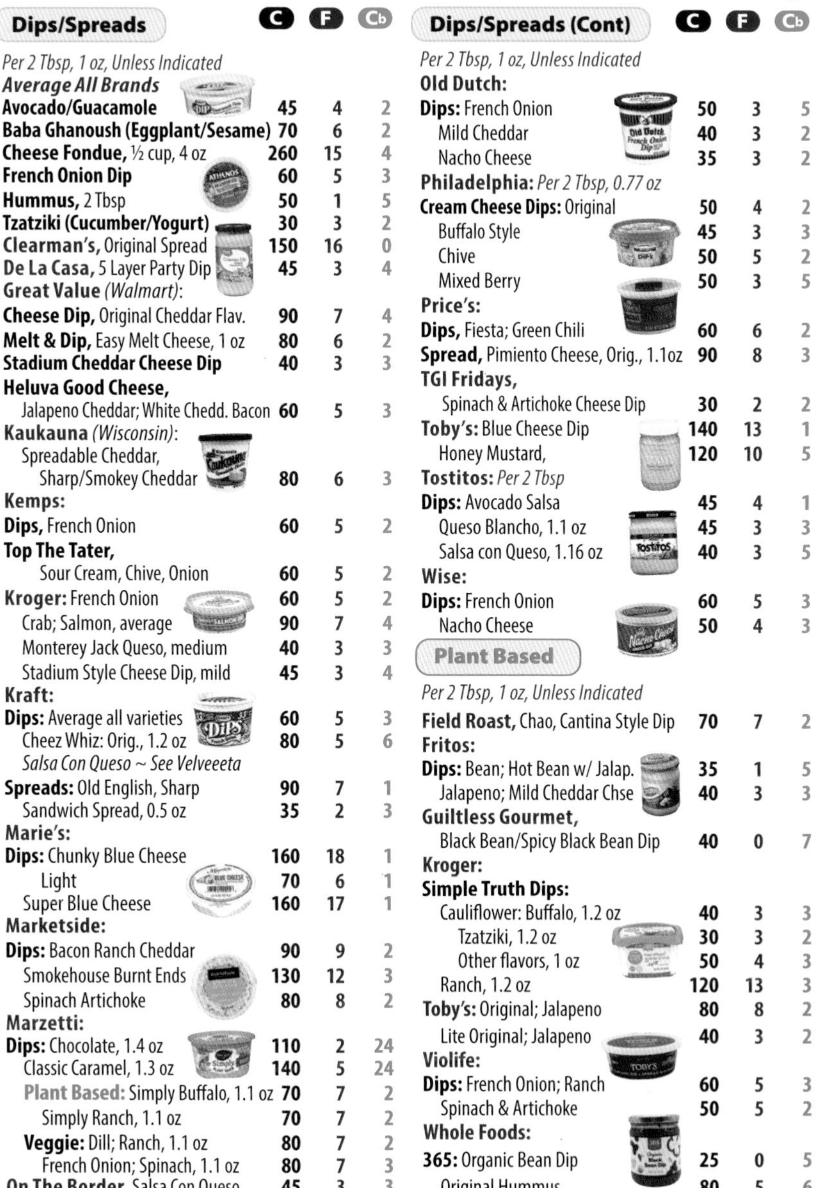

Dips/Spreads

Per 2 Tbsp, 1 oz, Unless Indicated	C	F	Cb
Average All Brands			
Avocado/Guacamole	45	4	2
Baba Ghanoush (Eggplant/Sesame)	70	6	2
Cheese Fondue, ½ cup, 4 oz	260	15	4
French Onion Dip	60	5	3
Hummus, 2 Tbsp	50	1	5
Tzatziki (Cucumber/Yogurt)	30	3	2
Clearman's, Original Spread	150	16	0
De La Casa, 5 Layer Party Dip	45	3	4
Great Value *(Walmart)*:			
Cheese Dip, Original Cheddar Flav.	90	7	4
Melt & Dip, Easy Melt Cheese, 1 oz	80	6	2
Stadium Cheddar Cheese Dip	40	3	3
Heluva Good Cheese,			
Jalapeno Cheddar; White Chedd. Bacon	60	5	3
Kaukauna *(Wisconsin)*:			
Spreadable Cheddar,			
Sharp/Smokey Cheddar	80	6	3
Kemps:			
Dips, French Onion	60	5	2
Top The Tater,			
Sour Cream, Chive, Onion	60	5	2
Kroger: French Onion	60	5	2
Crab; Salmon, average	90	7	4
Monterey Jack Queso, medium	40	3	3
Stadium Style Cheese Dip, mild	45	3	4
Kraft:			
Dips: Average all varieties	60	5	3
Cheez Whiz: Orig., 1.2 oz	80	5	6
Salsa Con Queso ~ See Velveeeta			
Spreads: Old English, Sharp	90	7	1
Sandwich Spread, 0.5 oz	35	2	3
Marie's:			
Dips: Chunky Blue Cheese	160	18	1
Light	70	6	1
Super Blue Cheese	160	17	1
Marketside:			
Dips: Bacon Ranch Cheddar	90	9	2
Smokehouse Burnt Ends	130	12	3
Spinach Artichoke	80	8	2
Marzetti:			
Dips: Chocolate, 1.4 oz	110	2	24
Classic Caramel, 1.3 oz	140	5	24
Plant Based: Simply Buffalo, 1.1 oz	70	7	2
Simply Ranch, 1.1 oz	70	7	2
Veggie: Dill; Ranch, 1.1 oz	80	7	2
French Onion; Spinach, 1.1 oz	80	7	3
On The Border, Salsa Con Queso	45	3	3

Dips/Spreads (Cont)

Per 2 Tbsp, 1 oz, Unless Indicated	C	F	Cb
Old Dutch:			
Dips: French Onion	50	3	5
Mild Cheddar	40	3	2
Nacho Cheese	35	3	2
Philadelphia: *Per 2 Tbsp, 0.77 oz*			
Cream Cheese Dips: Original	50	4	2
Buffalo Style	45	3	3
Chive	50	5	2
Mixed Berry	50	3	5
Price's:			
Dips, Fiesta; Green Chili	60	6	2
Spread, Pimiento Cheese, Orig., 1.1oz	90	8	3
TGI Fridays,			
Spinach & Artichoke Cheese Dip	30	2	2
Toby's: Blue Cheese Dip	140	13	1
Honey Mustard,	120	10	5
Tostitos: *Per 2 Tbsp*			
Dips: Avocado Salsa	45	4	1
Queso Blancho, 1.1 oz	45	3	3
Salsa con Queso, 1.16 oz	40	3	5
Wise:			
Dips: French Onion	60	5	3
Nacho Cheese	50	4	3

Plant Based

Per 2 Tbsp, 1 oz, Unless Indicated	C	F	Cb
Field Roast, Chao, Cantina Style Dip	70	7	2
Fritos:			
Dips: Bean; Hot Bean w/ Jalap.	35	1	5
Jalapeno; Mild Cheddar Chse	40	3	3
Guiltless Gourmet,			
Black Bean/Spicy Black Bean Dip	40	0	7
Kroger:			
Simple Truth Dips:			
Cauliflower: Buffalo, 1.2 oz	40	3	3
Tzatziki, 1.2 oz	30	3	2
Other flavors, 1 oz	50	4	3
Ranch, 1.2 oz	120	13	3
Toby's: Original; Jalapeno	80	8	2
Lite Original; Jalapeno	40	3	2
Violife:			
Dips: French Onion; Ranch	60	5	3
Spinach & Artichoke	50	5	2
Whole Foods:			
365: Organic Bean Dip	25	0	5
Original Hummus	80	5	6

Condiments, Sauces

Average of Brands & Homemade	C	F	Cb
Apple Sauce:			
Sweetened, ¼ cup, 2.5 oz	55	0	13
Unsweetened, ¼ cup, 2 oz	25	0	7
Barbecue Sauce:			
Regular, av. all flavors, 2 Tbsp, 1 oz	40	0	10
Bull's Eye, Original, 1 oz	60	0	14
Bearnaise Sauce, ¼ cup, 2.5 oz	190	19	5
Buffalo Wing Sce: Hon. Mustard, 1 T.	40	3	3
Average other varieties, 1 Tbsp	25	2	2
Cheese, h/made, ¼ cup, 2.5 oz	150	10	12
Chef-Mate, Hot Dog, ¼ cup	70	3	9
Chili Sauce *(Heinz)*, 1 Tbsp	20	0	5
Cocktail Sauce: ¼ cup	110	0	15
Walden Farms, Fat-Free, 1 Tbsp	0	0	0
Cranberry Sauce, av. all varieties: 2 T.	45	0	11
¼ cup, 2.5 oz	110	0	27
Demi Glaze Gold, 2 tsp	30	1	3
Honey Mustard *(French's)*, 2 Tbsp	60	1	12
Horseradish: 1 tsp	2	0	0
Kraft, 1 tsp	15	2	1
Ketchup: Regular, 1 Tbsp	15	0	4
Heinz: Reduced Sugar, 1 Tbsp	5	0	1
Simply Heinz, 1 Tbsp	15	0	4
Mole:			
Dona Maria, av. all varieties., 2 T.	150	10	10
Rogelio Bueno, 2 Tbsp, 1 oz	160	11	12
Mushroom Sce, ½ cup, 2 oz	50	2	5
Mustard, average, 1 tsp	5	0	1
Pesto Sauce, ¼ cup, 2 oz	270	28	2
Pizza Sauce, ¼ cup, 2 oz	30	0	6
Seafood Cocktail Sce, ¼ cup	60	0	15
Soy Sauce: Average all, 1 Tbsp	10	0	1
Kikkoman, Lite Soy, 1 Tbsp	10	0	1
Spaghetti Sce, ½ cup, 4.5 oz	135	6	19
Steak Sauce:			
Kraft, A1, 1 Tbsp, 0.5 oz	15	0	3
Lea & Perrins, 1 Tbsp, 0.5 oz	20	0	5
Strawb. Puree Sauce, Unsweet., 2 T.	10	0	2
Sweet & Sour Sauce:			
Contadina, 1.2 oz	40	1	8
Kraft, 1 Tbsp	60	0	13
Tabasco Sauce, 1 tsp	2	0	0
Taco Sauce, average all, 2 Tbsp, 1 oz	10	0	1
Tartar Sauce: *(Heinz)*, 2 Tbsp, 1 oz	120	11	4
Hellmann's, Regular, 2 Tbsp, 1 oz	80	7	4
McCormick, Fat-Free, 2 Tbsp, 1 oz	30	0	7
Teriyaki Sauce *(Kikkoman)*, 1 T., 0.5 oz	15	0	2
Vinegar, White or Wine, 2 T.	4	0	1
White Sauce, ½ cup, 5 oz	130	7	10
Worcestershire Sauce, 1 tsp	5	0	1

Pickles & Relish

Average All Brands	C	F	Cb
Bread & Butter Pickles, 4 sl.,1 oz	25	0	6
Chutney, 2 Tbsp, 1.25 oz	50	1	11
Dill Pickles:			
Slices, 4 slices, 1 oz	4	0	1
1 large, (3¾"x 1¼" diam.), 2.25 oz	12	0	3
Extra large (4"x 1¾" diam.), 5 oz	30	0	6
Halves: Small, 1 oz	3	0	1
Large, 2.5 oz	8	0	2
Gherkins, sweet, 1 medium, 1 oz	30	0	7
Green Chiles, chopped, 2 Tbsp	5	0	1
Horseradish, 1 Tbsp	10	0	2
Jalapenos, pickled (2), 2 oz	10	1	2
Jalapeno Relish, 1 Tbsp, 0.5 oz	5	0	1
Mustard, av. all brands, 1 tsp	5	0	1
Peppers, Hot/Mild (1), 1.5 oz	20	0	4
Pickled: Beets, ½ cup, 4 oz	75	0	19
Cocktail Onion, 1 onion	2	0	0
Red Cabbage, ½ cup, 3 oz	65	0	15
Pickles: Sweet, 2 Tbsp, 1 oz	35	0	8
Large (3" x ¾ diam.),1.25 oz	40	0	10
Pickle in a Pouch, 1 large	12	0	3
Relishes:			
Cranberry-Orange, 1 Tbsp	30	0	7
Hot Dog *(Heinz)*, 1 T., 0.5 oz	17	0	3
S'wich Spread, 1 tsp	20	1	5
Sweet Pickle, 1 Tbsp, 0.5 oz	20	0	5
Sweet Cauliflower, 1 oz	35	0	8
Sugar Free Relish, 1 tsp	5	0	1
Sweet Gherkins (2), 1 oz	5	0	1
Sauerkraut,			
Drained, 1 cup, 5 oz	25	0	6

Salsa

Average all Types:	C	F	Cb
Regular, w/out oil, 2 T., 1 oz	15	0	4
Made with oil, 2 Tbsp, 1 oz	40	3	8
La Victoria, 2 Tbsp, 1 oz	10	0	2
Old El Paso, 1 Tbsp, 1 oz	10	0	3
TGI Friday's, 1.2 oz	15	0	4

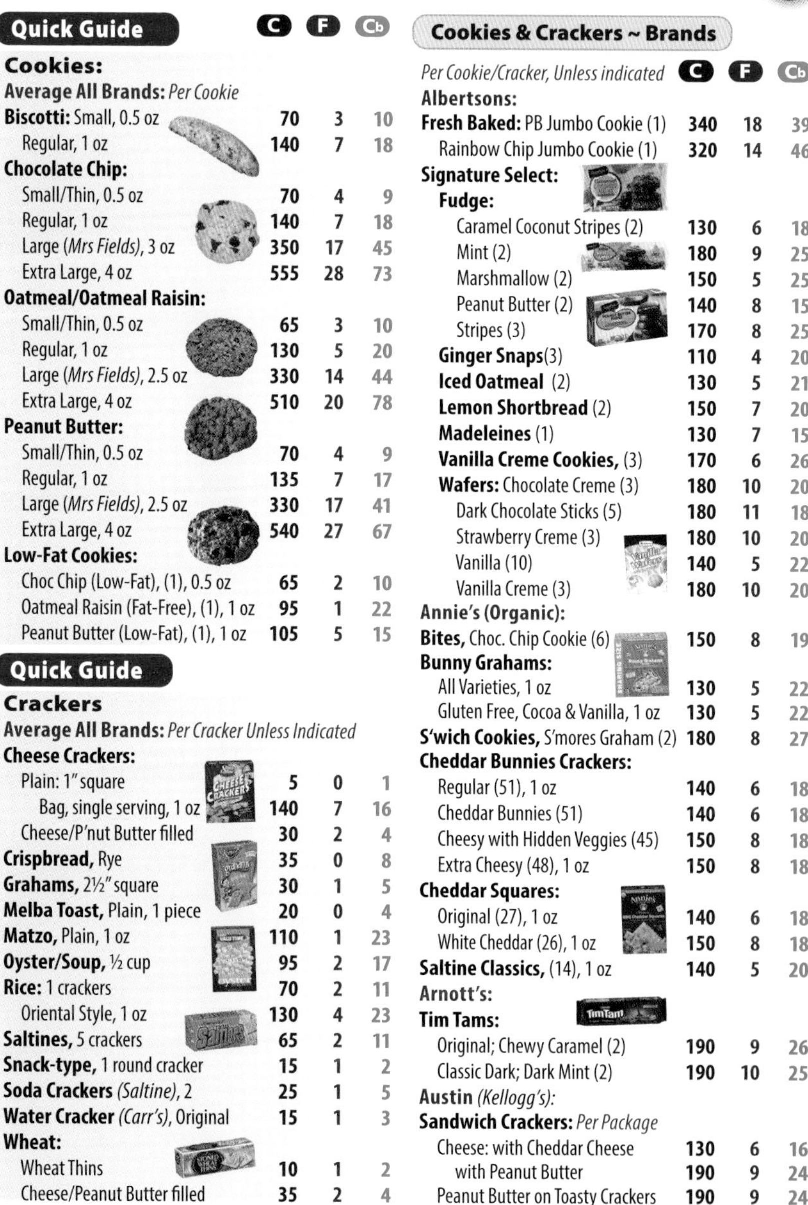

Quick Guide

Cookies:	C	F	Cb
Average All Brands: *Per Cookie*			
Biscotti: Small, 0.5 oz	70	3	10
Regular, 1 oz	140	7	18
Chocolate Chip:			
Small/Thin, 0.5 oz	70	4	9
Regular, 1 oz	140	7	18
Large (*Mrs Fields*), 3 oz	350	17	45
Extra Large, 4 oz	555	28	73
Oatmeal/Oatmeal Raisin:			
Small/Thin, 0.5 oz	65	3	10
Regular, 1 oz	130	5	20
Large (*Mrs Fields*), 2.5 oz	330	14	44
Extra Large, 4 oz	510	20	78
Peanut Butter:			
Small/Thin, 0.5 oz	70	4	9
Regular, 1 oz	135	7	17
Large (*Mrs Fields*), 2.5 oz	330	17	41
Extra Large, 4 oz	540	27	67
Low-Fat Cookies:			
Choc Chip (Low-Fat), (1), 0.5 oz	65	2	10
Oatmeal Raisin (Fat-Free), (1), 1 oz	95	1	22
Peanut Butter (Low-Fat), (1), 1 oz	105	5	15

Quick Guide

Crackers	C	F	Cb
Average All Brands: *Per Cracker Unless Indicated*			
Cheese Crackers:			
Plain: 1" square	5	0	1
Bag, single serving, 1 oz	140	7	16
Cheese/P'nut Butter filled	30	2	4
Crispbread, Rye	35	0	8
Grahams, 2½" square	30	1	5
Melba Toast, Plain, 1 piece	20	0	4
Matzo, Plain, 1 oz	110	1	23
Oyster/Soup, ½ cup	95	2	17
Rice: 1 crackers	70	2	11
Oriental Style, 1 oz	130	4	23
Saltines, 5 crackers	65	2	11
Snack-type, 1 round cracker	15	1	2
Soda Crackers (*Saltine*), 2	25	1	5
Water Cracker (*Carr's*), Original	15	1	3
Wheat:			
Wheat Thins	10	1	2
Cheese/Peanut Butter filled	35	2	4

Cookies & Crackers ~ Brands

Per Cookie/Cracker, Unless indicated	C	F	Cb
Albertsons:			
Fresh Baked: PB Jumbo Cookie (1)	340	18	39
Rainbow Chip Jumbo Cookie (1)	320	14	46
Signature Select:			
Fudge:			
Caramel Coconut Stripes (2)	130	6	18
Mint (2)	180	9	25
Marshmallow (2)	150	5	25
Peanut Butter (2)	140	8	15
Stripes (3)	170	8	25
Ginger Snaps(3)	110	4	20
Iced Oatmeal (2)	130	5	21
Lemon Shortbread (2)	150	7	20
Madeleines (1)	130	7	15
Vanilla Creme Cookies, (3)	170	6	26
Wafers: Chocolate Creme (3)	180	10	20
Dark Chocolate Sticks (5)	180	11	18
Strawberry Creme (3)	180	10	20
Vanilla (10)	140	5	22
Vanilla Creme (3)	180	10	20
Annie's (Organic):			
Bites, Choc. Chip Cookie (6)	150	8	19
Bunny Grahams:			
All Varieties, 1 oz	130	5	22
Gluten Free, Cocoa & Vanilla, 1 oz	130	5	22
S'wich Cookies, S'mores Graham (2)	180	8	27
Cheddar Bunnies Crackers:			
Regular (51), 1 oz	140	6	18
Cheddar Bunnies (51)	140	6	18
Cheesy with Hidden Veggies (45)	150	8	18
Extra Cheesy (48), 1 oz	150	8	18
Cheddar Squares:			
Original (27), 1 oz	140	6	18
White Cheddar (26), 1 oz	150	8	18
Saltine Classics, (14), 1 oz	140	5	20
Arnott's:			
Tim Tams:			
Original; Chewy Caramel (2)	190	9	26
Classic Dark; Dark Mint (2)	190	10	25
Austin (*Kellogg's*):			
Sandwich Crackers: *Per Package*			
Cheese: with Cheddar Cheese	130	6	16
with Peanut Butter	190	9	24
Peanut Butter on Toasty Crackers	190	9	24

Cookies & Crackers ~ Brands (Cont)

Per Cookie/Cracker, Unless Indicated	C	F	Cb
BelVita *(Nabisco):*			
Breakfast Biscuits:			
Crunchy, 1 pack (4 biscuits), average	230	8	35
Sandwich, Peanut Butter, 1.76 oz	230	9	35
Soft Baked, 1.76 oz	200	8	32
Bites, (46), average, 1.8 oz	230	8	37
Blue Diamond:			
Nut Thins:			
Cheddar Cheese (19)	130	4	22
Hint of Sea Salt (19), 1 oz	130	3	24
Average other varieties (19), 1 oz	130	3	24
Carr's:			
Cookies, Ginger Lemon (2)	150	7	20
Crackers: Rosemary (4)	80	4	10
Toasted Sesame (4)	60	2	10
All other Varieties (4)	50	1	10
Cheez•It ~ *See Sunshine, Page 87*			
Chips Ahoy! ~ *See Nabisco, Page 85*			
Ener-G Foods: (Gluten Free):			
Cinnamon Crackers, (7)	110	5	19
Flax Crackers, (9)	90	5	11
Erin Baker's:			
Original Breakfast: *Per 3 oz Cookie*			
Banana Walnut	310	8	55
Caramel Apple	300	6	58
Double Chocolate	300	7	55
Gingerbread	320	8	58
Oatmeal Raisin	300	6	59
Peanut Butter	320	11	51
Peanut Butter Chocolate	330	11	52
Minis: *Per 1 oz Cookie*			
Double Chocolate	100	3	19
Oatmeal Raisin	100	2	19
Grain Free Better Cookie:			
Almond Butter (2)	140	9	16
Salted Chocolate Cashew (2)	130	9	14
Famous Amos: *Per 4 Cookies*			
Bite Size: Belgian Chocolate	280	14	37
British Salted Caramel	140	7	19
Mediterranean Hazelnut	150	9	17
Philippine Coconut	150	9	17
fifty50:			
Chocolate Chip (4)	170	9	22
Hearty Oatmeal (4)	160	7	24

Per Cookie/Cracker, Unless Indicated	C	F	Cb
Fig Newtons ~ *See Nabisco, Page 85*			
Gamesa:			
Arcoiris Marshmallow, 1.8 oz pkg	210	4	41
Chokis, Chocolate Chip (3)	130	6	19
Classics: Barras de Coco (5)	120	3	22
Florentinas (2)	120	4	21
Maravillas (6)	120	4	21
Ricanelas (2)	140	5	24
Emperador: Chocolate (3)	160	6	24
Lime Flavor (3)	140	5	23
Pecan (3)	160	6	25
Mamut, 1 cookie, 1 oz	130	5	21
Marias, 8 cookies, 1 oz	120	2	23
Crackers:			
Sabrosas (5)	70	3	9
Girl Scouts Cookies:			
Adventurefuls (2)	130	6	7
Caramel Chocolate Chip (3)	160	7	21
Caramel deLites (2), av.	140	6	19
Girl Scout S'Mores (2)	150	7	21
Lemonades (2)	150	7	20
Peanut Butter S'wich, (3)	170	8	22
Thin Mints (4)	160	7	22
Trefoils (4)	120	5	19
Goldfish Crackers ~ *See Pepperidge Farm, Page 86*			
Goya:			
Lady Fingers, (4),1 oz	130	1	25
Marias, (5), 1 oz	130	3	23
Chocolate (5), 1 oz	130	4	23
Strawberry Wafers, (5), 1.15 oz	170	8	22
Grandma's *(Fritolay): Per Cookie*			
Chocolate Brownie	190	8	27
Chocolate Chip	200	10	25
Minis, 1 pkg	210	8	31
Oatmeal Raisin	180	7	27
Peanut Butter	190	10	22
Sandwich Cremes:			
Peanut Butter (4)	170	8	22
Vanilla (4)	170	7	23
Great American Cookies: *Per Cookie*			
Chewy Choc. Supreme	180	7	27
Chewy Pecan Supreme	200	10	25
Double Fudge with Reese's	210	10	31
Original with M&M's	220	10	30
Peanut Butter with M&M's	240	13	27
White Chunk Macadamia	240	13	30

Cookies & Crackers ~ Brands (Cont)

Per Cookie/Cracker, Unless Indicated	C	F	Cb
Great American Cookies (Cont): *Per Cookie*			
Double Doozies:			
Original, 5.28 oz	650	32	90
M&M's Big Bite, 1.9 oz	250	12	35
Cookie Cakes:			
16", 3.5 oz	350	16	51
16" M&M, 4 oz	360	17	52
Heart Shaped, 3.5 oz	350	15	61
Great Value *(Walmart):*			
Bars: Peanut Butter Wafer (1)	150	8	16
Strawberry (2)	120	2	24
Caramel Coconut & Fudge, (2)	130	6	18
Chippers: Chewy, (2)	150	6	21
Chunky, (2)	160	8	21
Classic (3)	170	8	22
Fudge: Grahams, (1)	110	5	16
Covered Peanut Butter Filled (2)	160	9	16
Marshmallow (1)	130	5	20
Mint (4)	150	7	20
Iced Oatmeal, (2)	140	5	23
Mini: Chocolate Grahams, 1 oz pack	130	5	22
Chocolate Chip Chippers, 1 oz pack	140	7	19
Oatmeal, (2)	150	5	23
Pecan Shortbread, (2)	170	10	19
Sandwich:	160	6	25
Cremes:			
Duplex Chocolate (3)	160	6	25
Lemon Cremes (3)	160	6	26
Vanilla (3)	170	6	26
Peanut Butter (2)	110	5	17
Twist & Shout: Chocolate (2)	110	5	17
Chocolate Double Filled (2)	140	6	20
Golden (3)	170	7	25
Wafers: Strawberry Creme (4)	160	8	23
Vanilla Creme, (4)	160	7	24
Crackers:			
Buttery Smooth (4), 0.5 oz	70	3	9
Cheddar Cheese (28), 1 oz	150	8	18
Cinnamon Graham, 2 sheets	130	4	24
Multi-Grain (4)	70	3	10

Per Cookie/Cracker, Unless Indicated	C	F	Cb
Keebler:			
Chips Deluxe: Coconut (2)	160	9	19
Dipped Duos (2)	190	11	22
Double Choc. Chip, with M&M's (2)	160	8	19
Fudgy (2)	160	9	19
Soft Batch (2)	150	7	21
With M&M's (2)	160	8	20
Coconut Dreams, (2)	140	8	17
Deluxe Grahams, Original (3)	140	7	18
E.L. Fudge: Original (2)	180	9	24
Double Stuffed (2)	180	9	24
Fudge:			
Caramel Nut Dreams, (2)	190	11	20
Coconut Dreams Fudge Covered (2)	170	9	20
Deluxe Grahams (2)	140	7	18
El Fudge: Original Elfwich (2)	170	7	25
Double Stuffed (2)	180	9	24
Fudge Sticks:			
Original (3)	150	8	20
Fudge Stripes:			
Original (2)	140	7	19
Minis, S'mores, 1.42 oz pouch	190	8	28
Whoopsy!, (2)	170	8	23
Grasshopper, Mint & Fudge (4)	150	7	20
Sandies Shortbread Cookies:			
Classic (2)	160	9	20
Cranberry Almond (2)	170	9	19
Pecan(2)	170	10	19
Sugar Wafers:			
Chocolate (4)	140	7	20
Strawberry (4)	150	6	23
Vanilla Filled (4)	150	7	20
Vienna Fingers,			
Vanilla Fudge Creme (2)	150	6	23
Crackers:			
Town House: Original (5)	80	5	9
Dippers, Game Day Originals (4)	80	4	10
Dipping Thins: Black Pepper (7)	80	4	11
Sea Salt (7)	80	4	11
Flatbread Crisps, all flavors (8)	70	2	11
Flip Side, Original (5)	70	4	10
Pita:			
Everything (6)	70	3	11
Mediterranean Herb (6)	70	3	11

Cookies & Crackers ~ Brands (Cont)

Per Cookie/Cracker, Unless Indicated	C	F	Cb
Kroger:			
Chip Mates: Original Choc. Chip (3)	130	6	17
Candy (2)	140	7	18
Chewy Chocolate Chip (2)	150	7	20
Chunky Chocolate Chip (2)	140	7	18
Peanut Butter (2)	130	7	15
White Chip Chocolate Chunk (2)	140	7	18
Coconut & Caramel Fudge (2)	130	6	18
Fudged Striped Shortbreads (3)	170	7	25
Ginger Snaps (3)	110	4	20
Olde Southern Pecan Shortbread (2)	150	9	16
Peanut Butter Fudge Enrobed (2)	150	8	17
Sandwich Cookies:			
Kaleido:			
Orig. Chocolate (3)	160	6	25
Double Filled (2)	140	6	21
Golden, Dble Filled (2)	140	6	21
Maple Creme (2)	140	5	22
Peanut Butter (2)	110	5	17
Supreme, Choc Chip Van. Creme (2)	170	8	24
Vanilla Wafers (8)	130	4	23
Crackers:			
Grahams, Orig.; Honey, (4)	130	3	24
Saltines, Original (5), 0.5oz	70	2	12
Lance:			
Nekot Sandwich Cookies:			
Fudge, 1.72 oz	230	9	35
Lemon Creme; P'nut Butter, 1.75 oz	240	11	34
Vanilla Creme, 1.59 oz	220	9	33
Crackers:			
Captain's Wafers: *Per Pkg*			
Cream Cheese & Chives	200	10	24
Grilled Cheese	200	10	24
PB & Honey; White Cheddar	190	9	23
Malt, with Peanut Butter Filling	180	10	21
Toastchee,			
Peanut Butter	220	10	25
Toasty, Peanut Butter	180	9	21
Wholegrain: Cheddar Cheese	200	10	19
Peanut Butter	200	9	19
Little Debbie:			
Choc. Chip Cream Pie, (1), 1.34 oz	170	7	26
Fudge Rounds, (1)	150	6	23
Nutty Buddy, (1)	120	7	12

Little Debbie (Cont):	C	F	Cb
Oatmeal Creme Pie (1)	170	7	26
Big Size (1), 2.65 oz	330	12	52
Peanut Butter Cream Pies, (1)	170	7	25
Big Size (1), 3.1 oz	410	19	54
Raisin Creme Pies (1)	150	5	25
Star Crunch (1)	150	6	22
Lu:			
Petit Ecolier:			
Dark Chocolate, (2)	130	7	15
Petit Ecolier, Milk Chocolate (2)	130	6	17
Pim's, Orange (2), 0.9 oz	100	3	17
Manischewitz:			
Almond Cookies, 1.1 oz	140	6	21
Crackers:			
Matzos:			
Everything (1)	80	0	16
Thin Salted (1)	90	0	20
Unsalted (1)	110	0	24
Whole Wheat (1)	120	1	25
Tam Tams, Everything; Original (1)	130	5	20
Mary's Gone Crackers:			
Chocolate Kookies; Honey, av. (6)	150	6	21
Cinnamon (12)	150	6	17
Crackers:			
Average All Flavors, (13)	140	5	21
Gone Cheezee: Cheddar (19)	140	6	19
Plant Based, Cheese & Herb (19)	140	6	19
Super Seed: Rosemary (12)	140	6	17
Avg. Other Varieties (12)	150	7	16
Miss Meringue:			
Meringue Classiques:			
Cappuccino (4), 1 oz	110	0	26
Mint Choc. Chip; Triple Choc. (4), 1 oz	120	2	25
Vanilla Rainbow/Van. (4), 1 oz	110	0	27
Meringue Minis, Low Fat:			
Mini: Chocolate Chip (12), 1 oz	130	2	27
Mint Chocolate Chip (12), 1 oz	120	2	26
Meringue Minis, Fat Free:			
Peppermint Crush (9), 1 oz	110	0	25
Rainbow Vanilla; Vanilla (13), 1 oz	110	0	27
Meringue Petites: Cafe au Lait (7)	100	0	25
Toasted Coconut (6)	120	3	23
Mother's:			
Circus Animal (7)	140	6	20
Sparkling Mythical Creatures (10)	150	7	20

Mrs Fields Cookies ~ *See Page 219*

Cookies & Crackers ~ Brands (Cont)

Per Cookie/Cracker, Unless Indicated	C	F	Cb
Nabisco Cookies:			
Chips Ahoy!, Chocolate Chip:			
Original: 3 cookies, 1.2 oz	160	8	22
Single Serve, 1.55 oz pack	220	10	30
Mini Choc. Chips:			
Big Bag, 3 oz	420	20	57
Go Pak (14), 1 oz	150	7	20
Snak Sak, (5),1.1 oz	150	7	21
Chewy:			
Regular (2), 1.1 oz	140	6	21
Hershey's Fudge Filled (2), 1.1 oz	150	7	20
Reese's Peanut Butter (2), 1 oz	140	6	19
Soft Chunky, Original (2), 1.4 oz	180	7	28
Chunky: Original (2)	160	8	21
Choc. Chunk; Choco (2)	160	8	20
White Fudge (2), 1.2 oz	170	8	22
Golden Candy Chips, (2)	170	9	22
Reese's: Mini Pieces (2)	150	8	18
PB Cups (2)	160	9	18
Ginger Snaps, (4), 1 oz	120	3	23
Lorna Doone:			
Shorbreads: 1 oz pack	140	7	20
1.5 oz pack	210	10	29
Mallomars, Choc. Cookies (2), 1 oz	110	5	18
Newtons:			
100% Whole Grain Fig (2), 1 oz	100	2	22
Original Fig: 1 cookie, 1 oz	100	2	21
Fat-Free, 2 cookies, 1 oz	90	0	23
Strawberry, 2 cookies, 1 oz	100	2	21
Nilla Wafers: 8 Wafers, 1 oz	140	6	21
Reduced-Fat (8), 1 oz	120	2	24
Snack Pack, 1 oz	130	5	20
Vanilla (8), 1 oz	140	6	21
Nutter Butter:			
S'wich Cookies: Orig. 0.9 oz pack	120	5	17
Snack Pack, 1.9 oz	260	11	39
Bites, 1 pack, 1 oz	140	5	20
Double Nutty (2)	170	8	24
Wafers (5), 1.15 oz	160	8	18
Oreo Chocolate:			
Classics:			
Original (3), 1.2 oz	160	7	25
Double Stuf (2), 1 oz	140	7	21
Mega Stuff (2), 1.27 oz	180	9	25
Gluten Free: Regular (3), 1.2 oz	160	7	25
Double Stuf (2), 1 oz	140	7	21

Per Cookie/Cracker, Unless Indicated	C	F	Cb
Nabisco (Cont):			
Oreo Chocolate (Cont).			
Flavors: Brookie-O (2), 1.27 oz	180	9	25
Birthday Cake/Mint Flav., (2), 1 oz	140	7	21
Other Flavors, average (2), 1 oz	140	6	21
Fudge Covered: Orig. (2) 1.3 oz	190	9	25
Dark Chocolate (1), 0.85 oz	120	7	16
Thin Bites: Original, 1 oz pack	140	7	19
Mint (9), 1.2 oz	150	8	21
White Fudge Dipped (8), 1 oz	150	7	21
Thins, all flavors (4), 1 oz	140	6	21
Oreo Golden: (3), 1.2 oz	160	7	25
Double Stuf (2), 1 oz	150	7	21
Thins, all flavors (4), 1 oz	140	6	21
Teddy Grahams, all flavors, (24)	130	4	22
Crackers:			
Barnum's Animals:			
Snak-Sak (17), 1.1 oz Pack	140	4	24
Zoo Animals, 1 oz Pack	120	4	22
Good Thins (Gluten Free):			
Made w/- Cheese:			
Three Cheese (17)	130	3	23
Made with Corn: Sea Salt (38)	120	2	26
Made with Rice:			
Garden Veggie (16)	130	2	25
Simply Salt (18)	130	2	26
Made with Rice & Cheese,			
Parmesan & Garlic (17)	130	3	22
Honey Maid:			
Grahams (8) av. all varieties,	130	3	24
Low Fat, Honey (8), 1.23 oz	140	2	28
Premium: Original (5), 0.5 oz	70	2	10
Saltines (5), 0.5 oz	70	2	12
Soup & Oyster (22), 0.5 oz	60	2	11
Unsalted Tops (5)	70	2	13
Whole Grain (5), 0.5 oz	70	2	12
Triscuit, average all flavors (6), 1 oz	120	4	20
Wheat Thins:			
100% Whole Grain,1 oz	130	5	20
Original (16); Big (11), 1.1 oz	140	5	22
Reduced Fat (16), 1 oz	120	4	22
Sundried Tomato & Basil (15)	130	5	21
Other flavors, average (14)	140	5	21

Per Cookie/Cracker, Unless Indicated	C	F	Cb
Nana's: *Per Cookie*			
Gluten Free:			
Chocolate Chip (2)	130	7	18
Lemon (2)	120	5	19
Lemon Blueberry (2)	130	5	20
Snickerdoodle (2)	130	6	19
Keto: Chocolate Chip (3)	160	11	11
Lemon walnut (3)	160	12	10
Note: Carbohydrate figure contain 7 grams sugar alcohol			
Sweet Perfection:			
Chocolate Chip with Walnuts (1)	360	14	56
Double Chocolate with Walnuts (1)	360	12	60
Oatmeal Raisin (1)	360	12	58
Newman's Own Organics:			
Family Recipe: Chocolate Chip (5)	150	7	20
Double Chocolate Chip (5)	150	7	19
Fig Newmans:			
Fat Free (2)	90	0	21
Low Fat (2)	100	2	20
Plant Based (2)	100	1	21
Newman O's:			
Original (2)	130	5	19
Chocolate Creme (2)	120	5	18
Hint-O-Mint (2)	130	5	19
Peanut Butter (2)	120	5	17
Vanilla (2)	130	5	19
Nonni's:			
Biscotti:			
Original, 1 piece, 0.8 oz	90	3	14
Other varieties, 1 piece, 0.8 oz	110	4	17
Bites: Chocolate Chip (3)	100	2	17
Dark Chocolate Orange (3)	100	3	17
Limoncello (3)	120	4	20
Crackers:			
THINaddictives: *Per Pack*			
Cranberry Almond	90	3	14
Lemon Blueberry Almond	90	2	15
Mango Coconut	90	4	14
Papaya Passionfruit	90	3	14
Pistachio Almond	100	4	12
O Organics *(Albertsons)*			
Mini Chocolate Chip, 1oz Bag	140	7	19
Vanilla Animal Cookies, (8)	120	4	20
Crackers:			
Classic Rounds (8)	130	7	17
Multigrain Flatbread (3)	120	3	23
Rosemary Flatbread w/ Seasalt, 3 crackers	120	2	23
Stone Ground Wheat (5)	120	2	23

Oreo Cookies ~ *See Nabisco, Page 85*

Per Cookie/Cracker, Unless Indicated	C	F	Cb
Pepperidge Farm:			
Chunk: *Per Cookie*			
Chesapeake, Dark Chocolate Pecan	140	8	16
Lexington, Milk Chocolate, Toffee Almond	130	7	16
Montauk, Milk Chocolate	140	6	22
Nantucket, Dark Chocolate	130	7	17
Sausalito, Milk Choc. Macadamia	130	7	17
Tahoe, White Chocolate Macadamia	130	7	17
Disctinctive:			
Brussels (3)	150	7	20
Cherry Verona (3)	130	5	22
Chessmen (3)	120	5	18
Dublin Shortbread (2)	130	6	17
Gingerman (4)	130	4	22
Naples Citrus (3)	150	8	19
Milano:			
Amaretto Hot Cocoa (2)	130	7	16
Caramel Macchiato (2)	130	7	16
Coconut Flavored Chocolate	130	7	16
Dark Chocolate (2)	180	9	22
RaspberryFlavored Chocolate (2)	130	7	15
Crackers:			
Cracker Trio (3)	60	2	9
Golden Butter (4)	70	3	11
Harvest Wheat (3)	80	4	11
Goldfish Crackers (Baked):			
Original (55)	140	6	20
Cheddar Baby (89)	140	5	20
Colors (55)	140	5	20
Parmesan (60)	140	5	20
Pizza; RedHot (55)	140	5	20
Pretzel (43)	130	3	24
Flavor Blasted: Cheddar Jack'd (51)	130	5	20
Sour Cream & Onion (57)	140	5	19
Xtra Cheddar (51)	140	5	19
Xtra Cheesy Pizza (51)	140	5	21
Whole Grain: Cheddar (55)	140	5	19
Colors (55)	140	5	20
Ritz:			
Originals: Orig; Garlic Buter (5)	80	5	10
Roasted Vegetable (5)	80	4	10
Whole Wheat (5)	70	3	10
Bits: Cheese (13)	150	9	17
Peanut Butter (12)	150	8	17
Crisp & Thins, all varieties (21)	130	5	21
Fresh Stacks, Original (5)	80	5	10
Sandwich, Peanut Butter, 1.38 oz	200	11	22

Cookies & Crackers ~ Brands (Cont)

Per Cookie/Cracker, Unless Indicated

	C	F	Cb
Ritz (Cont)			
Toasted Chips: Original (13)	130	4	20
Cheddar (13)	150	6	21
Everything (13)	140	6	22
Ranch (13)	140	6	21
Sour Cream & Onion (13)	140	6	20
Shar Gluten Free ~ *See CalorieKing.com*			
Streit's:			
Flavored Wafers:			
Chocolate (3)	160	9	19
Vanilla (3)	170	11	18
Sunshine: *(Kellogg's):*			
Cheez-It Crackers:			
Original (27)	150	8	17
Reduced Fat (27)	140	6	19
Buffalo Wing (26)	150	8	19
Cheddar Jack, 1 oz pouch	150	7	18
Extra Big (14)	150	8	17
Extra Cheesy (26)	150	8	18
Extra Toasty (27)	150	8	17
Extra Toasty Cheddar Jack (26)	150	8	18
Hot & Spicy (26)	150	8	19
Italian Four Cheese (26)	150	7	19
Pepper Jack (26)	140	7	18
Duoz: Bacon & Cheese (26)	150	7	19
Jalapeno & Cheddar (26)	150	7	19
Grooves:			
Scorchin' Hot Cheddar(18)	130	6	19
Other varieties (18)	140	6	19
Puff'd, all varieties (40)	150	9	16
Snap'd: Double Cheese (20)	150	8	19
Parmesan Ranch (20)	150	8	19
Town House *(Kellogg's):*			
Crackers, Original (5)	80	5	9
Dippers, Game Day Original (4)	80	4	10
Dipping Thins:			
Black Pepper; Seasalt (7)	80	4	11
Flatbread, all varieties (8)	70	2	11
FlipSides, Original (5)	70	4	10

Per Cookie/Cracker, Unless Indicated

	C	F	Cb
Trader Joe's:			
Belgian Butter Waffle (3)	150	6	21
Crispy Crunchy Peanut Butter (6)	130	6	15
Fig (2)	150	4	28
Madeleines (2)	150	7	18
Molasses (1)	150	6	22
Raspberry Hearts (1)	130	6	17
Speculoos (4)	150	5	22
Sunflower Butter (2)	130	5	19
Vegan Cookies & Cream, Vanilla Bean Bon Bons, (1)	110	7	10
Crackers:			
Cinnamon Graham (3)	150	6	23
Everything But The Bagel (14)	140	6	20
Oganic Naan (10)	130	5	19
Rosemary Sfogliettes (12)	140	6	19
Triscuits ~ *See Page 85*			
Voortman: *Per Cookie Unless Indicated*			
Almond Crunch (2)	140	6	21
Chocolate Chip (1)	90	4	13
Coconut (1)	90	5	11
Oatmeal Raisin (2)	160	7	24
Shortbread (1)	130	5	13
Sugar Free: Almonette (1)	140	5	18
Chocolate Chip (1)	80	5	13
Note: Carb figures contain 5-6 grams Sugar Alcohol			
Wafers: Chocolate; Lemon (3)	150	7	22
Peanut Butter (3)	160	6	20
Whole Foods (365 Organic):			
Butter Shortbread (2)	150	8	17
Chocolate Chip (2)	150	8	19
Chocolate Sandwich Cremes (2)	130	5	20
Frosted Animal Cookies (5)	150	7	21
Oatmeal Raisin (2)	140	6	20

Cookie ~ Mixes

As Packaged

	C	F	Cb
Betty Crocker: *Per 3Tbsp (1 oz) Mix Unless Indicated*			
Chocolate Chip	120	3	22
Gingerbread, 1.8 oz	220	6	40
Oatmeal Chocolate Chip, 0.8 oz	90	2	18
Peanut Butter	120	4	21
Snickerdoodle, 0.8 oz	90	1	19
Sugar Cookie	110	2	23
Triple Chocolate Chunk, 1.13 oz	130	3	26
Whole Foods (365 Organic): *Per 2 Tbsp Mix*			
Chocolate Chip, 2 tbsp	110	2	23
Gluten Free, ¼ cup, 0.74 oz	80	1	13

Thaw, Bake & Serve

Per Cookie/Cracker Unless Indicated	C	F	Cb
Annie's Organic: *Per Cookie*			
Chocolate Chip, 1 oz	140	7	16
Eat Pastry Vegan *(Whole Food): Per Cookie*			
Choc. Chip Cookie Dough	50	3	6
Pillsbury Cookies:			
Eat or Bake Cookie Dough:			
Birthday Cake, 1.34 oz	160	6	23
Chocolate Chip, 1.34 oz	170	8	24
Choc. Chunk & Chip, 1.34 oz	170	7	24
Lucky Charms,1.16 oz	140	7	20
Oreo Pieces, 1.34 oz	170	8	22
Pumpkin, 1.16 oz	140	6	21
Reese's: PB, 1.34 oz	160	7	23
Pieces P'nut Butter, 1.34 oz	160	7	23
Salted Caramel Apple, 1.16 oz	140	6	21
Sugar Cookies, 1.34 oz	160	7	24
Refrigerated Sweet Buns/Rolls~ *See Page 67*			
Sweet Loren's: *Per 1 oz Raw Dough/1 Cookie*			
Pre Cut: Chocolate Chunk	120	5	18
Fudgy Brownie	110	5	17
Oatmeal Cranberry	110	4	19
Pumpkin Spice	100	4	14
Sugar	120	5	17
Less Sugar: Choc. Chunk	120	7	14
Sugar	120	6	14
Toll House *(Nestle)*:			
Edible Cookie Dough:			
Chocolate Chip, 2 T.bsp, 1.39 oz	140	5	25
Bite Size, 12 pieces, 1.05 oz	130	5	20
Funfetti, 2 Tbsp, 1.4 oz	140	4	25
Refrigerated Cookie Dough: *Per Cookie Inless Indicated*			
Chocolate Chip, 2 Tbsp, 1 oz	120	6	17
Chocolate Chip Lovers	170	8	23
Pecan Turtle Delight	170	9	21

Crispbreads

Per Crispbread Unless Indicated	C	F	Cb
Finn Crisp:			
High Fibre: Traditional	40	1	7
Round: Multigrain	50	1	8
Original	40	1	8
Snacks:			
Roasted Peppers & Chipotle, 1 oz	115	3	16
Sour Cream & Onion, 1 oz	115	3	16
Thins: Average all flavors	20	0	4
Wide Size, Original Sourdough	30	0	5
New York Flatbreads: *Per 3 Pieces*			
Everything; Sesame	140	4	22
Garlic; Poppy; Sesame	140	3	24
Poppy	140	3	22
Ryvita:			
Crispbreads: Original (3)	110	0	21
Fruit & Oats (2)	110	2	20
Sesame (4)	160	3	24
Thins:			
Caramelised Onion Flatbread (4)	120	2	21
Sweet Chilli Flatbreads (4)	110	2	21
WASA:			
Crispbread: Multigrain;	35	0	8
Sourdough (1)	30	0	7
Crisp'n light,			
7 Grains (3)	60	1	13
Gluten Free: Original (1)	45	1	10
Sesame & Sea Salt (1)	50	2	10
Thins: Rosemary & Sea Salt (2)	60	2	11
Sesame & Sea Salt (2)	60	2	10

Matzos

	C	F	Cb
Manischewitz:			
Matzos: Original (1), 1 oz	120	1	27
Egg & Onion (1), 1 oz	80	1	17
Thin: Salted(1)	120	1	26
Salted (1)	110	0	24
Crackers			
Tam Tams: Original (9), 1 oz	110	4	16
Onion (10)	140	5	20
Streit's:			
Matzos: Lightly Salted, (1)	110	1	23
Unsalted (1)	100	0	23
Moonstrips, Onion Poppy (1)	100	1	22

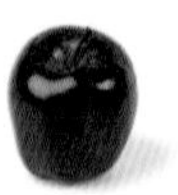
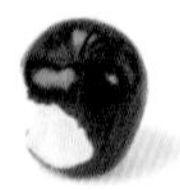
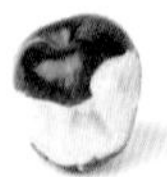
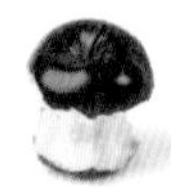
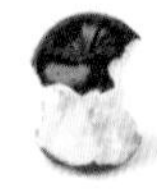
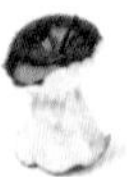
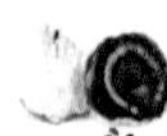

Quick Guide

	C	F	Cb
Cream			
Average All Brands			
Half & Half Cream:			
1 Tbsp, 0.5 oz	20	2	1
2 Tbsp, 1 oz	40	3	1
¼ cup, 2 oz	80	6	2
Light: Coffee/table (20% fat): 1 Tbsp	30	3	1
2 Tbsp, 1 oz	60	6	1
Sour Cream:			
Regular: 1 Tbsp, 0.5 oz	25	3	1
1 cup, 8 oz	445	45	7
Low-Fat/Light: 1 Tbsp, 0.5 oz	20	2	1
2 Tbsp, 1 oz	40	3	2
Fat-Free: Av., 2 Tbsp, 1 oz	20	0	3
Knudsen, 2 Tbsp, 1 oz	30	0	2
Kroger, 2 Tbsp, 1 oz	20	0	3
Sour Cream Substitute:			
Albertson's, 2 Tbsp, 1 oz	60	5	2
Tofutti, Sour Supreme, 2 Tbsp, 1 oz	85	5	9
Whipping Cream:			
Heavy, (37% fat):			
1 Tbsp fluid/2 Tbsp whipped	50	6	1
½ cup whipped	105	11	1
1 cup whipped	410	44	4
Light, (30% fat):			
1 Tbsp fluid/2 Tbsp whipped	45	5	1
½ cup fluid/1 cup whipped	350	37	4

Coconut Cream/Milk

	C	F	Cb
Coconut Cream, Canned:			
Plain/unsweetened: 2 Tbsp, 1 oz	75	7	3
½ cup, 4 oz	285	26	12
Sweetened:			
Coco Lopez: 1 oz	130	5	21
½ cup, 4 oz	520	20	84
Coconut Milk, Canned: *Unsweetened*			
Thai Kitchen: Lite, 2.7 fl·oz	50	5	1
Organic, 2 fl.oz	120	12	2
Regular, 2.7 l.oz	120	12	2

Whipped Toppings

	C	F	Cb
Average All Brands			
Cream (Pressurized): 2 Tbsp	20	2	1
¼ cup	40	4	2
Cream Topping, Lite, 2 Tbsp	20	1	3
Kraft: *Per 2 Tablespoons*			
Cool Whip: Original, 0.9 oz	25	2	3
Extra Creamy, 0.9 oz	25	2	2
Fat Free, 2 Tbsp, 0.9 oz	20	0	3
Dream Whip Mix, 1/16 envelope,	10	0	2

Whipped Toppings (Cont)

	C	F	Cb
Reddi-wip:			
Original, 2 Tbsp, 0.18 oz	15	1	1
Extra Creamy, 2 Tbsp, 0.18 oz	15	1	1
Fat-Free, 2 Tbsp, 0.18 oz	5	0	1
Chocolate, 2 Tbsp, 0.18oz	15	1	1
Non Dairy: Almond, 0.18 oz	10	1	2
Coconut, 0.18 oz	10	1	2

Creamers (Dairy)

	C	F	Cb
Natural Bliss: *Per Tbsp, 15 ml*			
Toasted Coconut	30	1	5
Other Flavors	35	2	5

Creamers (Non-Dairy)

	C	F	Cb
Powder:			
Coffee-Mate/Cremora/N-Rich:			
Original: 1 tsp	10	1	1
Fat Free, 1 tsp	10	0	2
Flavors: All flavors, 0.10 oz	15	1	2
Sugar Free, all flavors, 0.07 oz	15	1	1
Liquid/Refrigerated:			
Per Tablespoon			
Baileys, Coffee Creamer, all flavors, 1 Tbsp, 15ml	35	1	6
Califia Farms, all flavors, 1 Tbsp	15	0	4
Coffee-Mate: *Per Tbsp, 15 ml Unless Indicated*			
Flavors: All flavors	35	2	5
Fat-Free, all flavors	25	0	5
Sugar free, all flavors	15	1	1
Shelf Stable, all flavors	35	2	5
Unflavored: Original	20	1	2
Fat-Free	10	0	1
Natural Bliss, all flavors	30	1	5
Hood, Country Creamer, 1 Tbsp	15	1	1
International Delight: *Per Tbsp*			
Regular, all flavors	35	2	5
Fat-Free, all flavors	30	0	7
Sugar-Free, all flavors	20	2	1
Singles, all flavors, 0.4 fl.oz	30	1	5
Kroger: *Per Tbsp*			
Coffee Creamers: Original	15	1	1
Hazelnut; White Choc Mocha	30	1	5
Fat-free, French Vanilla	25	0	5
Silk:			
Almond; Oat;, all flavors	25	1	4
Soy: Original	20	2	2
Vanilla	30	2	4

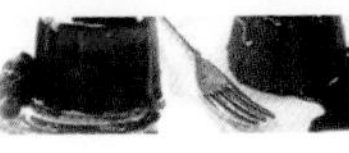

Ready-To-Serve

	C	F	Cb
Hunt's:			
Snack Pack Puddings:			
5.5 oz Container:			
Butterscotch	170	4	33
Chocolate	180	4	34
Vanilla	170	5	32
3.25 oz Container:			
Banana Cream Pie	90	3	17
Brownie Caramel Swirl	100	3	18
Butterscotch	90	3	17
Chocolate Fudge	110	2	21
Milk Chocolate	100	3	18
Tapioca	110	3	19
Vanilla	100	3	17
Sugar Free: Chocolate	70	4	14
Vanilla	60	3	11

Note: Carbohydrate figure contains 5-8 grams sugar alcohol

	C	F	Cb
Jell-O *(Kraft):*			
Cook & Serve Pudding & Pie Filling: *Dry Mix Only*			
Banana Cream, 0.77 oz	80	0	20
Butterscotch, 0.85 oz	90	0	22
Chocolate Fudge, 1 oz	100	0	25
Coconut Cream, 0.77 oz	90	3	17
White Chocolate, 0.8 oz	100	0	23
Sugar free, Fat-Free:			
Chocolate var., 0.3 oz	30	0	8
Vanilla, 0.2 oz	20	0	5
Instant: Banana Cream, ½ pkt, 0.85 oz	90	0	22
Butterscotch, 0.88 oz	90	0	22
No Bake Dessert Mix: *Dry Mix Only*			
Cheesecake: Classic, 1.83 oz	210	5	42
Strawberry, 2.43 oz	210	4	44
Oreo Dessert, 2.1 oz	260	8	47
Kozy Shack:			
Flan, Creme Caramel, 1 cup, 4 oz	150	3	27
Original Puddings: *Per ½ Cup Unless Indicated*			
Chocolate, 4.6 oz	140	3	27
Cinn. Raisin Rice, 4.6 oz	140	3	26
French Vanilla Rice, 4.6 oz	140	3	24
Original Rice, 4.6 oz	130	3	24
Tapioca, 4.6 oz	130	2	25
Simply Well Puddings,			
average all flavors, 4 oz cup	90	2	14

Ready-To-Serve (Cont)

	C	F	Cb
Kroger:			
Pudding Snacks: *Per 3.25 oz Cup*			
Chocolate	100	3	19
Vanilla	100	3	17
Swiss Miss			
Puddings: *Per 4 oz Cup*			
Butterscotch	130	4	22
Chocolate Vanilla Swirl	140	4	26
Milk Chocolate	150	4	27
Tapioca; Vanilla, aerage.	135	4	24
Triple Chocolate	150	4	2

Homemade Puddings

	C	F	Cb
Apple Tapioca, ½ cup	150	0	32
Bread Pudding, ½ cup	250	8	40
Blancmange, ½ cup	140	5	19
Chocolate, ½ cup	190	6	30
Crème Brulée, ½ cup	400	35	16
Plum Pudding, 2 oz	170	3	32
Rice, with Raisins, ½ cup	200	4	38
Sponge Pudding, 3.5 oz	340	16	45
Tapioca Cream, ½ cup	110	4	15
Trifle, ½ cup	180	7	26

Custards

	C	F	Cb
Custard Mix *(Jello/Royal Flan)*, average:			
Dry, ¼ of 2.9 oz package, 0.7 oz	80	0	19
Prepared: whole milk, ½ cup	155	4	25
2% milk, ½ cup	140	3	25
Non-Fat milk, ½ cup	125	0	25
Home Made Egg Custard:			
With Whole Milk, ½ cup	170	8	18
With 2% Milk, ½ cup	155	7	18

Gelatin • Parfait • Jell-O

	C	F	Cb
Ida Mae, Strawberry Parfait	90	2	18
Jell-O:			
Gelatin:			
Cups: All flavors, 3.4 oz	70	0	17
Sugar free, all flavors, 3.14 oz	10	0	0
Dessert Mix:			
Average all flavors, ¼ pkt	80	0	19
Sugar Free, av. all flav., 0.07 oz	10	0	0
Juicy Jels: Regular, all flavors, 3.25 oz	70	0	17
Sugar Free, all flavors, 3.14 oz cup	10	0	0
Reser's, Parfaits, Rainb.;Rasp. 3.9 oz, av.	105	2	19

Meringues

	C	F	Cb
Meringue Swirl, $^1/_2$ oz	50	0	8
Meringue Shell, 1 oz	100	0	16

Chicken Eggs

	C	F	Cb
Fresh Eggs:			
Raw:			
Small	55	4	0
Medium	65	4	0
Large	70	5	0
Extra Large	80	6	0
Jumbo	90	6	0
Egg Yolk, 1 extra large	55	5	0
Egg White, 1 extra large	17	0	0
Dried Egg Powder:			
Whole Egg: ¼ cup, 1 oz	170	12	0
1 Tbsp	30	2	0
Egg White, ¼ cup, 1 oz	105	0	0
Egg Yolk, ¼ cup, 1 oz	195	18	0

Egg Substitutes

¼ Cup (Equivalent to 1 Egg) ~ Zero Cholesterol

	C	F	Cb
All Whites *(Crystal Farms)*, 1.6 oz	25	0	0
Better 'n Eggs *(Crystal Farms):*			
Regular, 3 Tbsp	25	0	0
Egg Beaters *(ConAgra):*			
100% Egg White 3 Tbsp	25	0	0
Original, 3 Tbsp, 1.6 oz	25	0	1
Single Serve, 4 oz cup	50	0	1
Southwestern Style, 3 Tbsp, 1.6 oz	20	0	1
Egg Replacer *(Ener-g)*, 1.5 tsp	15	0	4
Naturegg *(Burnbrae Farms)*,			
Simply Egg White, ¼ cup, 2 oz	30	0	0
O-Organics *(Albertson's)*, Egg Whites	25	0	0
Vegan Egg Substitute:			
Aquafaba, ¼ cup, 2 oz	10	0	2

Liquid from cooked/canned beans or chickpeas. Replaces eggs and egg whites in recipes.
Extra Info: www.aquafaba.com

Other Eggs

	C	F	Cb
Duck, 1 large, 2.5 oz	130	10	0
Goose, 1 large, 5 oz	280	19	0
Quail, 3 eggs, 1 oz	42	3	0
Turkey, 1 large, 3 oz	135	10	0
Turtle, 1 egg, 1.75 oz	75	5	0

Omega-3 Fat Enriched

	C	F	Cb
Egg•Land's Best, 1 large	60	4	0
Horizon Organic, 1 large	70	5	0

Note: Cholesterol content is the same as regular eggs.

Cooked Eggs

	C	F	Cb
Boiled Egg: *Same as Raw Egg*			
Hard-Cooked, Small, peeled	65	4	0
Fried Egg:			
With fat: 1 large egg	105	9	1
2 small eggs	175	13	1
No fat/nonstick pan, 1 large	75	5	1
Deviled Egg, 2 halves	145	13	1
Eggs Benedict(2), on Toast or English Muffin	860	56	25
Eggs Florentine (2), on Toast or English Muffin	890	59	25
Pickled Egg, 1 large	80	6	0
Poached Egg, 1 large	65	4	0
Quiche *(Homemade):*			
Egg & Bacon, 1 slice, 5.3 oz	580	43	27
Ham & Cheese, 1 slice, 5.3 oz	475	33	29
Scotch Egg, 1 egg	300	21	16
Scrambled Eggs:			
1 large egg:			
With 1 Tbsp milk + 1 tsp fat	120	9	1
With 1 Tbsp skim milk/no fat	85	6	1
2 large eggs:			
With 2 Tbsp milk + 2 tsp fat	260	20	2
With 2 Tbsp skim milk, w/o fat	180	11	2

Omelets

	C	F	Cb
1 Egg:			
Plain (with 1 tsp fat)	125	10	1
With: ½ oz cheese	175	15	1
½ oz cheese + ½ oz ham	200	16	1
2 Eggs:			
Plain (with 2 tsp fat)	250	20	1
With: 1 oz cheese	360	29	2
1 oz cheese +1 oz ham	410	32	2
3 Eggs:			
Plain (with 1 Tbsp fat)	360	29	2
With: 2 oz cheese	580	47	3
2 oz cheese+2 oz ham	680	53	3
Extras, Tomato/Onion/Veggies, 2 oz	20	0	5
Egg Substitute *(EggBeaters):*			
2 eggs (½ cup) + 1 tsp fat	100	4	2
3 eggs (¾ cup) + 2 tsp fat	160	8	3
Extras: 1 oz Cheese	110	9	1
1 oz Ham	50	3	1

Egg Nog

	C	F	Cb
Average all Brands, ½ cup, 4 oz	170	8	18
Borden, Premium, 4 fl.oz	250	15	24
Hood, Golden, ½ cup, 4 fl.oz	180	9	22
Horizon, Low-Fat, 4 fl.oz	140	3	23

E Egg ~ Egg Dishes

Breakfast Sides

	C	F	Cb
Toast:			
Plain, 1 thick slice	85	1	13
With: 2 tsp butter/marg.	155	9	13
3 tsp/1 Tbsp fat	190	13	13
English Muffin:			
Plain, 2 oz	130	1	26
With 3 tsp fat	230	12	26
Bacon, 2 strips	70	5	0
Ham, lean, 2 oz	100	3	0
Hash Brown:			
½ cup, 3 oz	125	7	14
1 cup serving, 6 oz	250	13	28
Sausages, 2 oz link	180	16	2

Frozen Egg Breakfasts

	C	F	Cb
Jimmy Dean:			
Breakfast Sandwich: *Per Sandwich*			
Biscuit, Sausage, Egg & Cheese	410	28	27
Croissant, Sausage, Egg & Cheese	400	26	29
Muffin, Meat Lovers	480	32	30
Simple Scrambles:			
Bacon, 5.32 oz pkg	290	23	4
Meat Lovers, 5.32 oz pkg	290	22	2
MorningStar Farms,			
Breakfast Muffin Sandwich,			
Veggie Sausage, Egg & Cheese	200	8	20
Pillsbury: *Per Pastry*			
Toaster Scrambles:			
Bacon, 1.8 oz	180	10	19
Bacon & Sausage	180	10	19
Sausage	180	10	19
Red Baron:			
Biscuit Scrambles:			
Bacon (1), 5.85 oz	440	21	45
Sausage (1), 5.85 oz	410	19	46

Frozen Pancake/Waffles ~ *See Page 132*
Toaster Pastries ~ *See Page 64*

Frozen Egg Rolls

	C	F	Cb
Lotus Restaurant:			
Imperial, Chkn/Pork (1)	160	7	24
Vegetarian (1)	120	5	20
Minh:			
Mini Chicken, 3 pieces	130	5	17
Pork & Vegetables (1)	190	9	20
Pagoda Express: *Each*			
Chicken, 2.75 oz	160	4	24
Pork, 2.75 oz	180	8	20
Vegetable, 2.75 oz	130	4	21

Fast-Foods/Restaurants

	C	F	Cb
Without Any Side Options			
Arby's, Bacon, Egg & Cheese Croissant	430	26	29
Au Bon Pain, 2 Egg on Plain Bagel	390	11	51
Bob Evans:			
Omelets, Low Calorie: *Without Sides*			
Three Meat & Cheese	1130	86	22
Western	630	46	12
Bojangles: Cajun Filet Biscuit	570	27	57
Bacon, Egg & Cheese Biscuit	510	27	40
Bruegger's:			
Bagel: Egg & Cheese, 6.2 oz	430	11	60
Western, 10.5 oz	770	41	72
Burger King:			
Burrito, Breakfast Jr.	420	26	29
Croissan'wich:			
Bacon, Egg & Cheese	370	21	30
Ham, Egg & Cheese	370	19	31
Sausage, Egg & Cheese	510	34	30
Carl's Jr:			
Biscuit, Monster	830	56	47
Burrito: Bacon & Egg & Cheese	620	35	37
Big Country	620	34	49
Loaded Breakfast	650	36	50
Steak & Egg	530	26	41
Chick-fil-A, Chicken, Egg & Cheese, on Buttermilk Biscuit	550	28	48
Del Taco, Egg & Cheese B'fast Burrito	380	16	35
Denny's:			
Omelettes: Plain	340	26	2
Ultimate, with Hash Browns, & White Toast	1140	77	63
Dunkin Donuts:			
Bagel, Bacon, Egg & Cheese	520	18	67
Croissant, Sausage, Egg & Cheese	720	52	42
Eat 'N Park:			
Omelettes: Ham & Cheese	660	47	7
Meat Lovers	760	58	7
Hardee's:			
Biscuit: Loaded Omelet	630	41	46
Southwest Omelet	660	45	42
IHOP:			
Omelette: Bacon Temptation	1190	90	20
Spinach & Mushroom	950	78	20
Jack in the Box:			
Biscuit, Saussage, Egg & Cheese	530	38	27
Egg Roll	210	12	20
McDonald's:			
Biscuit, Bacon, Egg & Cheese, reg.	460	26	39
McMuffin, Egg	310	13	30
Whataburger, B'fast Bacon Platter	600	38	39

Quick Guide

	C	F	Cb
Butter			
Average All Brands			
Regular: 1 tsp, 0.2 oz	35	4	0
1 Tbsp, 0.5 oz	100	11	0
2 Tbsp, 1 oz	205	23	0
1 Stick, ½ cup, 4 oz	810	92	0
1 Pound, 2 cups, 16 oz	3255	368	0
Light: Regular, 40% Fat			
1 tsp, 0.2 oz	30	3	0
1 Tbsp, 0.5 oz	70	8	0
2 Tbsp, 1 oz	140	15	0
Whipped Butter: Regular			
1 tsp, 0.1 oz	20	3	0
1 Tbsp, 0.3 oz	65	8	0
1 Stick, 2 .7 oz	545	62	0
Whipped Light Butter *(Land O Lakes):*			
1 tsp, 0.15 oz	15	2	0
1 Tbsp, 0.4 oz	45	5	0
2 Tbsp, 0.8 oz	90	10	0
Unsalted ~ *Same as Salted*			

Flavored Butter/Spreads

	C	F	Cb
Average All Brands			
Honey Butter, (60% Fat):			
1 Tbsp, 0.5 oz	90	8	4
Downey's, 2% Fat, 1 Tbsp, 0.5 oz	60	1	11
Garlic Butter, (80% Fat):			
1 Tbsp, 0.5 oz	100	11	0
Sweet Cream Butter:			
Land O Lakes: Reguar, 1 Tbsp	100	11	0
Honey Butter Spread, 1 Tbsp	70	6	4

Butter & Butter Blends

	C	F	Cb
Per 1 Tablespoon			
Challenge: Stick, 0.5 oz	100	11	0
Tub, Whipped, 0.3 oz	70	7	0
Brummel & Brown,			
Spread Made with Yogurt, 0.5oz	45	5	1
Land O'Lakes:			
Sticks, Original, 0.5oz	100	11	0
Tubs, Butter With Olive Oil, 0.5 oz	90	10	0

Ghee (Clarified Butter)

(Example ~ Purity Farms)
Note: Ghee is 100% fat compared to regular butter (80% fat + 20% water)

	C	F	Cb
1 tsp, 0.2 oz	45	5	0
1 Tbsp, 0.5 oz	120	14	0

Light & Reduced Fat Spreads

	C	F	Cb
Per Tablespoon			
Bestlife, Buttery Spread,			
1 Tbsp, 0.5 oz	50	5	0
Benecol: Regular, 0.5 oz	70	8	0
Light, 0.5 oz	50	5	0
Blue Bonnet:			
Stick, Lactose Free, 0.5 oz	70	7	0
Tub, Orig. Soft Spread, 0.5 oz	50	6	0
Butter Buds:			
Butter Flavored: Mix, 1 tsp	5	0	2
Sprinkles, 1 tsp	10	0	2
Country Crock *(Shedd's)*: Stick, 0.5 oz	80	8	0
Tubs: Orig; Churn Spread, 0.5 oz	50	6	0
Light Spread, 0.5 oz	35	4	0
Plant Based, Almond/Avocado/Ol. Oil, 0.5 oz	100	11	0
Earth Balance, Original, 1 Tbsp	100	11	0
Fleischmann's,			
Olive Oil Spread, 0.4 oz	60	6	1
I Can't Believe It's Not Butter!:			
Tubs: Original Spread, 0.5 oz	60	6	0
Light, 0.5 oz	40	4	0
Olive Oil Spread, 1 Tbsp	60	6	0
Molly McButter, 1 tsp	5	0	1
Parkay:			
Spread: Original, 0.4 oz	60	6	0
Light, 0.5 oz	50	6	0
Stick, Original, 0.5 oz	70	8	1
Promise: Activ, Spread, 0.5 oz	45	5	0
Light Spread, 0.5 oz	45	5	0
Smart Balance:			
Tubs, Buttery Spread: Original, 0.5 oz	80	9	0
EVOO, 0.4 oz	60	7	0
Light EVOO, 0.4 oz	50	5	0
Light, with Flaxseed Oil, 0.5 oz	50	5	0
Omega 3, Light, 0.5 oz	50	5	0

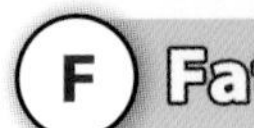

Fats ~ Spreads & Oils ◊ Mayo

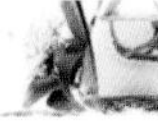

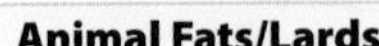

Animal Fats/Lards

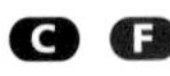

	C	F	Cb
Average All Types			
Beef Tallow/Drippings, Lard (Pork), Chicken, Duck, Goose, Turkey:			
1 Tbsp, 0.5 oz	**115**	**13**	0
2¼ Tbsp, 1 oz	**255**	**28**	0
1 cup, 7.3 oz	**1850**	**205**	0
½ pound, 8 oz	**2040**	**227**	0

Ghee/Butter/ Oil ~ *See Page 93*

Vegetable Shortening

	C	F	Cb
Average All Types			
1 Tbsp, 0.5 oz	**115**	**13**	0
2¼ Tbsp, 1 oz	**250**	**28**	0
1 cup, 7.3 oz	**1810**	**205**	0

Vegetable Oils

Includes almond, avocado, canola, corn, coconut, flaxseed, grape-seed, linseed, mustard, olive, palm, peanut, rice bran, safflower, sesame, sunflower, soybean, wheat germ. Note: Oil is 100% fat.

	C	F	Cb
1 tsp, 0.2 oz	**45**	**5**	0
1 Tbsp, 0.5 oz	**120**	**14**	0
2 Tbsp, 1 oz	**240**	**28**	0
1 cup, 7.3 oz	**1930**	**205**	0

Fish Oils

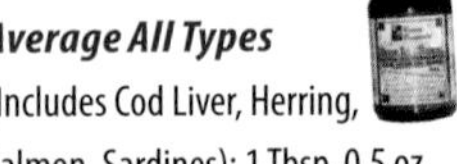

	C	F	Cb
Average All Types			
(Includes Cod Liver, Herring, Salmon, Sardines): 1 Tbsp, 0.5 oz	**125**	**14**	0

Cooking Sprays/Squeezes

Cooking Sprays: (PAM, Mazola, I Can't Believe It's Not Butter, Weight Watchers, Wesson):

	C	F	Cb
Pam: ¼ second spray	**2**	**0**	0
1-3 second spray	**6**	**1**	0
I Can't Believe It's Not Butter, Original Spray	**0**	**0**	0
Parkay, Buttery Spray	**0**	**0**	0

Olestra (Olean)

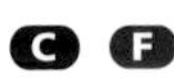

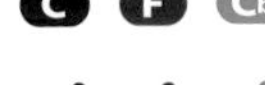

	C	F	Cb
Olestra *(Olean)*	**0**	**0**	0

Note: Olean is Proctor & Gamble's brand name for Olestra – a no-calorie cooking oil that gives snacks (like potato chips, tortilla chips and crackers) taste and texture without adding fat or calories.

Examples:

- *Frito-Lay,* Light Products *(Lays, Ruffles, Tostitos, Doritos)*
- *Pringles,* Fat-Free Potato Crisps

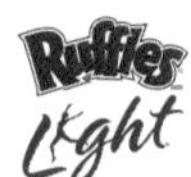

Quick Guide

Mayonnaise:	C	F	Cb
Regular: *Per 1 Tbsp, 0.5 oz Unless Indicated*			
Average All Brands	**90**	**10**	0
Best Foods; Hellman's; Kraft:			
Original/Real	**90**	**10**	0
½ cup, 4 oz	**720**	**80**	0
Hain, Safflower Mayonnaise	**100**	**11**	0
Spectrum, Canola Mayo	**100**	**11**	0
Light/Reduced Fat: *Per 1 Tbsp, 0.5 oz*			
Best Foods/Hellman's	**35**	**4**	1
Kraft, Light/Olive Oil	**35**	**3**	2
Smart Balance, Light Mayo	**50**	**5**	2
Spectrum, Light Canola Mayo, Eggless	**35**	**4**	1
Fat Free:			
Kraft: Original, 1 Tbsp	**10**	**0**	2
½ cup, 4 oz	**80**	**0**	16
Sugar Free:			
Dukes Real Mayo, 1 Tbsp	**100**	**12**	0
Vegan, Hellmann's, 1 Tbsp	**70**	**8**	0
Mayonnaise Style Dressing:			
Per 1 Tbsp, 0.5 oz			
Heinz, Original Salad Cream	**45**	**4**	3
Kraft:			
Mayo:			
Avocado Oil Mayo	**40**	**4**	1
Mayonesa	**100**	**11**	0
Mondelez:			
Miracle Whip Dressing:			
Regular	**40**	**4**	2
Light	**20**	**2**	2
Sir Kensington's, Egg/Dairy Free Classic Vegan Mayo	**90**	**10**	0

Quick Guide

Fresh Fish	C	F	Cb
Low Oil: *Less than 2.5% fat*			
White/Lightly-colored flesh. Examples: *Cod, Flounder, Haddock, Halibut, Mahi Mahi, Perch, Pike, Pollock, Snapper, Sole, Whiting.*			
Raw, without bones, 4 oz	100	1	0
Steamed, broiled, baked, 4 oz	140	2	0
Fried: Lightly floured, 4 oz	210	8	4
Breaded, 4 oz	260	12	8
In Batter, 4 oz	320	16	27
Medium Oil: *2.5-5% fat*			
Lightly-colored flesh. Examples: Bluefin Tuna, Catfish, Kingfish, Orange Roughy, Salmon (Pink), Swordfish, Rainbow Trout, Yellowtail.			
Raw, without bones, 4 oz	145	7	0
Baked/Broiled, 4 oz	195	8	0
Fried, 4 oz	230	11	8
High Oil: *Over 5% fat*			
Darker-colored flesh. Examples: Albacore Tuna, Mackerel, Salmon (Atlantic/Chinook/Sockeye), Sardines, Trout.			
Raw, without bones, 4 oz	220	14	0
Baked/Broiled, 4 oz	275	17	0
Fried, 4 oz	340	23	12

Cooking Yields (Fin Fish):

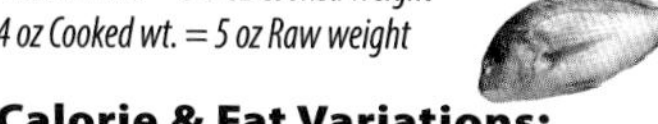

4 oz Raw wt. = 3.5 oz Cooked weight
4 oz Cooked wt. = 5 oz Raw weight

Calorie & Fat Variations:

The amount of fat/oil in fish varies with the species, season and locality. Within the same fish, fat/oil content is generally higher towards the head.

Fish & Shellfish

Edible Weights: (no bones/shell)

Item	C	F	Cb
Abalone: Raw, 3 oz	90	1	5
Fried, 3 oz	160	6	10
Ahi Tuna, grilled, 6 oz fillet (w/o fat)	235	2	0
Anchovy: Paste, 1 Tbsp, 0.5 oz	45	3	0
Canned in oil, drained, (5), 0.7 oz	40	2	0
Barracuda (Pacific), raw, 4 oz	130	3	0
Basa/Swai, raw, 4 oz fillet	70	2	0
Bass:			
Sea: Raw, 4.6 oz fillet	125	3	0
Baked, 3 oz	105	2	0
Striped: Raw, 1 fillet, 5.5 oz	150	4	0
Baked, 3 oz	105	3	0
Freshwater: Raw, 3 oz	95	3	0
Baked, 3 oz	125	4	0

Fish & Shellfish (Cont)

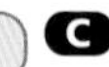

Edible Weights: (no bones/shell)

Item	C	F	Cb
Calamari/Squid:			
Raw, 4 oz	100	2	4
Baked, 1 cup	190	7	6
Fried, 3 oz	150	6	7
Catfish:			
Farmed: Raw, 1 fillet 5.6 oz	190	10	0
Baked, 1 fillet 5 oz	205	10	0
Wild: Raw, 1 fillet, 5.6 oz	150	5	0
Baked, 1 fillet, 5 oz	150	4	0
Breaded, fried, 1 fillet, 3 oz	200	12	7
Caviar, black/red, 1 Tbsp, 16g	40	3	1
Clams: Raw (4 large/9 small), 3 oz	70	1	3
Breaded, fried (20 small), 6.6 oz	380	21	20
Canned, drained, ½ cup, 2.8 oz	115	1	0
Steamed (10 small), 3.3 oz	140	2	5
Cod:			
Atlantic: Raw, 4 oz	95	1	0
Baked, 3 oz	90	1	0
Canned, solids & liquid	90	1	0
Pacific: Raw, 4 oz	80	1	0
Baked, 3 oz	70	1	0
Crab:			
Alaska King, 1 leg, cooked, 4.7 oz	130	2	0
Blue: Raw, 1 crab, 6 oz	150	1	0
Steamed, 3 oz	70	1	0
Canned, drained, 6.5 oz can	105	1	0
Dungeness: Raw, 1 crab, 5.8 oz	140	2	0
Steamed, 4.45 oz	140	2	0
Crab Cakes *(Capt. D's)*, (1), 2.8 oz	250	16	16
Crayfish:			
Farmed: Raw, 3 oz	60	1	0
Steamed, 3 oz	75	1	0
Wild: Raw 3 oz	65	1	0
Steamed, 3 oz	70	1	0
Cuttlefish, raw, 3 oz	70	1	1
Dolphinfish ~ *See Mahi-Mahi*			
Eel: Raw, 3 oz	155	10	0
Baked, 3 oz	200	13	0
Fish & Chips *(Red Lobster)*, battered, without condiments	700	33	61
Fish Sandwich *(Burger King)*, without Tartar Sauce	340	9	49
Fish Oil, 1 Tbsp, 0.5 oz	125	14	0
Flounder/Sole:			
Raw, 4 oz	80	2	0
Baked, 3 oz	75	2	0

Frozen Fish ~ *See Pages 114-122*

Fish & Shellfish (Cont)	C	F	Cb
Edible Weights: Without Bones or Shell			
Haddock: Raw, 4 oz	85	1	0
Baked, 3 oz	75	1	0
Smoked, 3 oz	100	1	0
Halibut:			
Atlantic: Raw, 4 oz	105	2	0
Baked, ½ fillet, 5.6 oz	175	3	0
Herring:			
Atlantic, raw, 4 oz	180	10	0
Canned: Plain, drained, 3 oz	130	8	0
In Tomato Sauce, 3.5 oz	140	8	2
Pickled, 2 pieces, 1 oz	75	5	3
Smoked, kippered, 4 oz	245	14	0
Jellyfish: Raw, 4 oz	30	0	0
Dried, Salted, 1 cup, 2 oz	20	1	0
Ling, raw, 4 oz	100	1	0
Lobster, Northern:			
1.5 lb Whole Lobster, edible portion:			
Raw, 6.3 oz	140	2	0
Boiled, 5 oz	140	1	0
Lobster Salads, average, ½ cup	220	13	5
Lobster Newberg, average, ¾ cup	360	20	9
Lobster Thermidor, av., 1 serving	370	22	15
Lobster Tail (Rock),			
Red Lobster, grilled/roasted	230	6	2
Lox, Regular/Nova, 2 oz	65	3	0
Mackerel, Atlantic: Raw, 4 oz	230	16	0
Baked, 3 oz fillet	225	15	0
Pacific/Jack: Raw, 4 oz	180	9	0
Baked, 3 oz	170	9	0
Spanish: Raw, 4 oz	160	7	0
Baked, 3 oz	135	6	0
Mahi-Mahi/Dolphinfish:			
Raw, 4 oz	95	1	0
Baked, 4 oz	125	1	0
Monkfish: Raw, 4 oz	85	2	0
Baked, 3 oz	80	2	0
Mullet, Striped: Raw, 4 oz	135	5	0
Baked, 3 oz	130	4	0
Mussels:			
Raw: 4 oz (edible wt)	100	3	4
1 cup, 5.3 oz (edible weight)	130	4	5
Cooked, moist heat, 3 oz	150	4	6
Ocean Perch:			
Atlantic: Raw, 4 oz	90	2	0
Baked, 3 oz	80	2	0
Octopus:			
Common: Raw, 4 oz	95	1	3
Boiled, 3 oz	140	2	4
Orange Roughy:			
Raw, 4 oz	85	1	0
Baked, 3 oz	90	1	0

Fish & Shellfish (Cont)	C	F	Cb
Edible Weights: Without Bones or Shell			
Oysters, Common, Raw, 3 oz	70	2	4
Eastern:			
Farmed: Raw, 6 medium, 3 oz	50	2	5
Cooked, dry heat, 6 med., 2 oz	45	2	5
Wild: Raw, 6 medium, 3 oz	45	2	3
Cooked, dry heat, 6 med., 2 oz	45	2	3
Breaded & Fried, 6 med., 3 oz	175	11	10
Pacific: Raw, 1 medium, 1.8 oz	40	1	3
Steamed, 1 medium, 0.8 oz	40	1	3
Perch ~ *See Ocean Perch*			
Pike: Northern: Raw, 4 oz	100	1	0
Baked, 3 oz	95	1	0
Walleye: Raw, 4 oz	105	2	0
Baked, 3 oz	100	2	0
Pollock, Atlantic: Raw, 4 oz	105	1	0
Baked, 3 oz	100	1	0
Pompano, Florida, raw, 4 oz	185	11	0
Red Snapper ~ *See Snapper*			
Roe, raw, 2 Tbsp, 1 oz	40	2	1
Sablefish: Raw, 4 oz	220	17	0
Smoked, 3 oz	220	17	0
Salmon:			
Atlantic, Farmed: Raw, 4 oz	235	15	0
Baked, 3 oz	175	10	0
Steaks: Raw, 7 oz	410	27	0
Baked, 6 oz	365	22	0
Atlantic, Wild: Raw, 4 oz	160	7	0
Baked, 3 oz	155	7	0
Steaks: Raw, 7 oz	280	13	0
Baked, 6 oz	310	14	0
Chinook: Raw, 4 oz	205	12	0
Baked, 3 oz	195	11	0
Smoked, 3 oz	100	4	0
King: Raw, 3.5 oz	185	12	0
Kippered, 3.5 oz piece	265	16	0
Smoked & canned, 3.5 oz	150	6	0
Coho:			
Farmed: Raw, 4 oz	180	9	0
Baked, 3 oz	150	7	0
Wild: Raw, 4 oz	165	7	0
Steamed, 3 oz	155	7	0
Pink/Chum: Raw, 4 oz	145	5	0
Baked, 3.5 oz	155	6	0
Canned: Drained solids, 11 oz	435	16	0
Without skin & bones, 8.5 oz	330	10	0
Sockeye: Raw, 4 oz	160	7	0
Baked, 3 oz	145	6	0
Canned, Drained solids, 3 oz	140	7	0
Smoked, 3.5 oz	205	8	0
Salmon Cake (1), 3 oz	240	15	6

Fish & Shellfish (Cont)

	C	F	Cb
Sardines: *Canned, Average all Brands*			
Drained of Oil:			
¼ cup drained, 2.2 *oz*	130	9	0
3.75 oz can, drained, 3.3 oz	190	11	0
1 large/2 medium, 3⁄5", 0.8 oz	50	3	0
in Tomato Sauce, 3.8 oz	150	8	3
Sashimi ~ *See Japanese Foods, Page 171*			
Scallops: Raw, 6 lge/15 small, 3 oz	65	1	3
Breaded, Fried (6), 5 oz	385	20	39
Steamed, 3 oz	95	1	0
Sea Bass ~ *See Bass*			
Seafood Salad, Deli Style,			
½ cup, 3.5 oz	250	21	11
Shark: Raw, 4 oz	145	5	0
Baked, 4 oz	185	7	0
Batter-dipped, fried, 4 oz	260	16	7
Shrimp:			
Raw: Small/Medium (4), 0.8 oz	15	0	0
Large (4), 1 oz	20	0	0
Breaded & Fried, 4.8 oz	395	24	27
Steamed, in shell, 3 oz	100	2	0
Canned, 1 can, 4.5 oz	130	2	0
Snapper: Raw, 4 oz	115	2	0
Baked: 3 oz	110	2	0
6 oz fillet	220	3	0
Sole: Raw, 4 oz	80	2	0
Baked, 3 oz	75	2	0
Squid ~ *see Calamari*			
Surimi, (Imitation Crab), 4 oz	110	1	17
Swai/Basa, raw, 4 oz	70	2	0
Swordfish: Raw, 4 oz	165	8	0
Medium Steak, 6 oz	250	11	0
Baked: Small Steak, 4 oz	205	7	0
Medium Steak, 6 oz	290	13	0
Tilapia: Raw, 4 oz	110	2	0
Baked: 3 oz	110	3	0
Trout, Rainbow:			
Farmed: Raw, 4 oz	160	7	0
Baked, 3 oz	145	7	0
Wild: Raw, 4 oz	135	4	0
Baked, 3 oz	130	5	0
Tuna:			
Raw: Bluefin, 4 oz	165	6	0
Skipjack, Yellowfin, av., 4 oz	120	1	0
Baked: Bluefin, 3 oz	155	6	0
Skipjack, Yellowfin, av., 3 oz	110	1	0
Canned: *in Water, drained*			
Chunk Light: 2 oz	50	1	0
3 oz can	75	2	1
5 oz can	125	3	2

Tuna (Cont): *in Water, drained (Cont)*	C	F	Cb
Solid White: 2 oz	60	1	0
5 oz can	150	2	0
7 oz can	210	2	0
in Oil, drained:			
Chunk Light: 2 oz can	80	4	0
5 oz can	200	10	0
Solid White: 2 oz can	90	4	0
6 oz can	270	12	0
Whitefish: Raw, 4 oz	150	7	0
Baked, 3 oz	145	7	1
Smoked, 3 oz	90	1	0
Whiting: Raw, 4 oz	100	2	0
Baked, 3 oz	100	2	0
Yellowtail: Raw, 4 oz	165	6	0
Grilled, 3 oz	160	6	0

Other Canned/Packaged Fish

	C	F	Cb
Bumble Bee: *Per 4 oz Drained Unless Indicated*			
Canned Salmon: *Skinless & Boneless*			
Atlantic, in Water	220	14	0
Pink, in Water	100	3	0
Canned Tuna:			
Chunk, in water	130	1	0
Prime Fillets:			
Solid White Albacore in water	140	2	0
Lemon & Pepper Yellowfin in oil	230	13	1
Pouch Tuna, Albacore, Wild Caught,			
in water, 2.5 oz	90	2	1
Chicken of the Sea: *Per 4 oz Drained*			
Canned Pink Salmon: *Skinless & Boneless*			
Pink: Wild Caught, in water	110	2	0
25% Less Sodium	110	2	0
Canned Tuna:			
Albacore: Wild Caught, in water	130	1	0
Wild Caught, in oil	170	5	0
Starkist:			
Lunch To Go Kit, Tuna Salad, 4.1 oz	260	9	25
Salmon Creations: *Per Pouch*			
Lemom Dill, 2.6 oz	70	1	1
Mango Chipotle, 2.6 oz	90	1	5
Smart Bowls: *Per Pouch*			
Tuna with Quinoa & Beans	160	4	23
Tuna w/ Pasta & Beans, Zesty Lemon	180	5	24
Tuna Creations: *Per Pouch*			
Bacon Ranch	80	1	2
Bold Thai Chili Style	90	1	7

F Flours & Grains

Flours & Grains

Food	C	F	Cb
Amaranth Flour *(Bob's Red Mill)*, ½ cup, 2.2 oz	220	4	40
Arrowroot Flour, ½ cup, 2.3 oz	230	0	56
Barley: Grain, regular, ½ cup, 2.6 oz	255	1	55
Pearled, raw, 3.5 oz	350	1	78
Buckwheat: Grain, ½ cup, 3 oz	290	3	61
Flour, whole-groat, ½ cup, 2 oz	200	2	42
Groats: Roasted, dry, ½ cup, 3 oz	285	2	62
Roasted, cooked, 3.5 oz	80	1	17
Bulgur: Dry, ½ cup, 2.5 oz	240	1	53
Cooked, ½ cup, 3.2 oz	75	1	17
Carob Flour, ½ cup, 1.8 oz	115	1	46
Coconut Flour, 2 Tbsp, 0.6 oz	60	4	10
Corn Kernels, cooked, av., ½ cup	80	1	18
Corn Bran, ½ cup, 1.3 oz	85	1	33
Corn Flour/Masa, ½ cup, 2 oz	215	3	43
Corn Grits:			
Dry, ½ cup, 2.8oz	290	1	62
Cooked, ½ cup, 4.3 oz	70	1	15
Corn Germ, toasted, ½ cup, 4 oz	100	2	22
Cornmeal, average all varieties:			
3 Tbsp, 1 oz	105	1	22
½ cup, 2.5 oz	255	1	54
Mixes, same as above	230	1	48
Cornstarch: 1 Tbsp, 0.3 oz	30	0	8
½ cup, 2.3oz	245	0	58
Couscous: Dry, 1 oz	110	0	22
Cooked, 1 cup, 5.5 oz	175	1	37
Farina: Dry, ½ cup, 3 oz	325	1	69
Cooked, ½ cup, 4 oz	55	0	12
Flaxseed: Whole, 1 T., 0.3 oz	45	4	2
Ground, 2 Tbsp, 0.3 oz	60	5	4
Garbanzo, (Chick Pea), ½ cup, 1.6 oz	180	3	27
Gluten Free Flour, 3 Tbsp	100	0	24
Hemp Flour, Wholemeal, ½ cup, 3.5 oz	300	10	5
Matzo Meal, ½ cup, 2.2 oz	230	1	48
Millet: Raw, ½ cup, 3.5 oz	380	4	73
Cooked, ½ cup, 3 oz	105	1	21
Oat Bran: Raw, ⅓ cup, 1 oz	75	2	21
Cooked, ½ cup, 3.8 oz	45	1	13
Oats, Rolled/Oatmeal:			
Dry/Groats, ½ cup, 1.5 oz	160	3	28
Cooked, ½ cup, 4.2 oz	75	1	13
Polenta ~ *See Cornmeal*			
Potato Flour, ½ cup, 2.8 oz	285	1	66
Psyllium Husks, 1 Tbsp, 0.2 oz	10	0	4
Quinoa: Dry, ½ cup, 3 oz	320	5	59
Cooked, ½ cup, 3.8 oz	130	2	24
Rice Bran, ½ cup, 2 oz	180	12	28
Rice Flour, ½ cup, 2.8 oz	290	1	63

Flours & Grains (Cont)

Food	C	F	Cb
Rice Polish, ½ cup, 3.5 oz	360	1	80
Rye Flour:			
Dark, ½ cup, 2.3 oz	210	2	44
Light, ½ cup, 1.8 oz	190	1	41
Medium, ½ cup, 1.8 oz	180	1	40
Rye Grain: ½ cup, 3 oz	280	2	59
Flakes, ¼ cup, 1 oz	100	1	21
Semolina Flour, ½ cup, 3 oz	300	1	61
Sorghum, ½ cup, 3.4 oz	325	3	72
Soy Flour:			
Defatted, 1 cup, 3.5 oz	330	1	38
Low-Fat, 1 cup, 3 oz	325	6	33
Full-Fat, 1 cup, 3 oz	365	17	29
Soy Meal, defatted, 1 cup, 4.3 oz	415	3	49
Spelt Flour, ½ cup, 2 oz	190	1	41
Tapioca Pearl:			
Dry, ½ cup, 2.7 oz	270	0	67
3 Tbsp, 1 oz	100	0	25
Teff Seed Flour, 2 oz	215	2	42
Tortilla Flour Mix, ½ cup, 2 oz	220	6	37
Triticale:			
½ cup, 3.4 oz	325	2	70
Flour, wholegrain, ½ cup, 2.3 oz	220	1	48
Wheat Bran, unprocessed, ½ cup, 1 oz	65	1	19
Wheat Flakes, ½ cup, 1.5 oz	160	1	35
Wheat Germ:			
Raw, ¼ cup, 1 oz	105	3	15
Toasted, ¼ cup, 1 oz	110	3	14
Wheat Flour:			
White, All Purpose/Self-Rising:			
1 level Tbsp, 0.3 oz	30	0	6
½ cup, 2.2 oz	230	1	48
1 cup, 4.4 oz	455	2	95
Whole Wheat, 1 cup, 4.2 oz	405	2	87

FRUIT TIME

Fruit ~ Fresh

Weights As Purchased

	C	F	Cb
Apples, all varieties, average:			
Whole, with skin:			
1 small, 4 oz	55	0	14
1 medium, 5.5 oz	75	0	19
1 large, 8 oz	110	0	28
1 extra large, 11 oz	145	0	36
Flesh only, no skin or core: 1 oz	15	0	4
Slices, 1 cup, 4 oz	55	0	14
Candy/Caramel Apple, 1 med., 6.5 oz	245	4	54
Chiquita, Apple Bites, 14 slices, 5 oz	80	0	20
Apricots: 1 small, 1.5oz	20	0	4
1 medium, 2 oz	25	0	6
1 large, 3 oz	40	0	10
1 extra large, 4 oz	50	0	12
Asian Pear, (Nashi Fruit), 1 med., 7 oz	85	0	21
Avocado:			
Fuerte (Florida) variety:			
¼ medium, 2.7 oz pulp	90	8	6
½ medium, 5.4 oz pulp	180	15	12
Mashed, 2 Tbsp, 1 oz	35	3	2
Hass variety (Californian/Mexican):			
Cubes, ½ cup, 2.5 oz	120	11	6
Mashed: 2 Tbsp, 1 oz	50	4	2
¼ cup, 2 oz	95	8	5
Pulp: ¼ medium, 1.5 oz	70	7	3
½ medium, 3 oz	140	13	7
1 medium (8.5 oz whole), 6 oz	280	26	14
Salad slices (3), 1 oz	50	4	2

Note: The fat of avocados is heart-healthy. Avocados are very low in carbs ~ most is fiber. This benefits blood sugar and cholesterol levels. Use in place of butter and other high-fat spreads.

	C	F	Cb
Banana:			
Weight with skin:			
1 baby, 3 oz	50	0	12
1 small (5″), 4 oz	65	0	16
1 medium (7″), 5 oz	80	0	20
1 large (8″), 8 oz	120	0	30
1 extra large (9″), 9 oz	135	0	34
Flesh only, weight without skin:			
Mashed, ½ cup, 4 oz	100	0	25
Slices, ½ cup, 2.5 oz	65	0	16
Green Bananas, weight with skin:			
1 medium (7″), 5 oz	75	0	18
1 large (8″), 7 oz	110	0	27
Blackberries, 1 cup, 5 oz	60	1	14
Blueberries: ¼ cup, 1 oz	15	0	4
1 cup or ½ pint ctn, 5 oz	80	0	20
1 pint container, 10 oz	160	0	40

Weights As Purchased

	C	F	Cb
Boysenberries, 1 cup, 4.5 oz	60	5	14
Breadfruit, ½ cup, 4 oz	115	0	30
Cactus Fruit:			
1 small, 2 oz	15	0	4
1 medium, 5 oz	40	0	9
1 large, 7 oz	55	0	13
Pulp, no skin, 1 cup, 5.3 oz	60	0	14
Cantaloupe: Flesh, without skin, 1 oz	10	0	2
Pieces/Balls, 1 cup, 5.5 oz	55	0	13
Slices, ½ circle, without rind:			
1 thin (buffet), ⅛″), 0.5 oz	5	0	1
1 medium (¼″), 1 oz	10	0	2
1 thick (½″), 2 oz	20	0	5
Wedges, length cut, without skin:			
1 thin, 1/16 medium, 2 oz	20	0	5
1 thick, ⅛ medium, 4 oz	40	0	9
Whole, weight with seeds and skin:			
½ small, 20 oz	195	1	46
½ medium, 28 oz	270	2	65
½ large, 2.5 lb	370	2	90
Cape Gooseberries, 1 cup, 5 oz	70	1	15
Cherimoya: Pulp, ½ cup, 3 oz	60	0	14
1 Fruit (11 oz), 8 oz edible	170	1	40
Cherries, (Red/White), sweet, raw:			
6 medium or 4 large, 2 oz	30	0	7
1 cup, 4.5 oz	75	0	18
½ lb quantity	130	0	32
Sour, red, raw, 1 cup, 4 oz	50	0	12
Clementine, 1 medium, 2.6 oz	35	0	9
Coconut, raw:			
Young, sweet,			
Pieces: 1 piece (2″ x 2″), 1.5 oz	35	2	4
½ cup, 3.5 oz	80	5	9
Mature, hard, 1 piece (2″x 2″), 1.5 oz	160	15	6
Crabapples, slices, ½ cup, 2 oz	40	0	11
Cranberries,			
fresh, ¼ cup, 1 oz	25	0	7
Custard Apple ~ *See Cherimoya*			
Dates: Medium (1), 0.3 oz	20	0	5
Large Medjool (1), 0.5 oz	40	0	10
Extra Large Medjool (1), 0.9 oz	65	0	16
Chopped, ½ cup, 3 oz	240	0	58
Dragon Fruit, (Pitahaya):			
1 medium, 4″ long, 12 oz	60	0	12
1 large, 5″long, 16 oz	80	0	18
Durian, pulp, 4 oz	165	6	31
Elderberries, ½ cup, 2.5 oz	55	1	13

Weights As Purchased	C	F	Cb
Feijoa, (Pineapple Guava), 1 medium, 2 oz	30	1	6
Figs, green/black:			
1 medium, 2 oz	40	0	10
1 large, 3 oz	60	0	15
Gooseberries, raw, 1 cup, 5 oz	65	1	15
Grapefruit, all varieties, average:			
½ fruit, 10 oz (6 oz flesh)	55	0	13
1 cup sections w/ juice, 8 oz	75	0	18
Grapes: Average, 1 cup, 5.5 oz	105	0	28
1 small bunch, 4 oz	80	0	20
1 medium bunch, 7 oz	140	0	36
1 large bunch, 16 oz	315	0	82
Granadilla, pulp, ½ cup, 4 oz	110	0	27
Guanabana, pulp, ½ cup, 4 oz	75	0	19
Guava, 1 medium, 4 oz	80	1	16
Honeydew:			
1 slice, ¾" thick, 3 oz	30	0	7
1 wedge (⅛ of 7" diameter), 12 oz (with rind)	80	0	20
Cubes/Balls, 1 cup, 6 oz	60	0	14
½ small (4½ lb whole)	180	1	42
½ medium (6 lb whole)	230	1	56
Honey Murcots, 1 only, 5 oz	45	0	11
Jaboticaba, 1 cup, 5.5 oz	55	0	14
Jackfruit, flesh, ⅛, 4 oz	105	0	27
Kiwano, ½ medium, 5 oz	35	0	8
Kiwifruit:			
1 Medium, 2.7 oz	45	0	11
1 Large, 3.2 oz	55	0	13
Langsat, Duku, 1 medium, 2 oz	25	0	5
Lemons: 1 medium, 5oz	20	0	4
1 wedge, 1 oz	5	0	1
Limes, 1 medium, 2.4 oz	20	0	7
Loganberries, frozen, ½ cup, 2.5 oz	40	0	9
Longans, 5 fruit, 0.5oz	10	0	3
Loquats, 4 fruit, 2.3 oz	30	0	8
Lychees, 4 fruit, 2.3 oz	30	0	7
Mamey Apple, cubes, 1 cup, 6 oz	85	1	20
Mandarin Orange:			
1 small, 3 oz	35	0	9
1 medium, 4 oz	45	0	11
1 large, 6 oz	50	0	13
Mango:			
Slices, ½ cup, 3 oz	55	0	14
1 small mango, 7 oz	90	1	24
1 medium: 10 oz	130	1	34
Side cheek, 4 oz	60	0	14
1 large, 17 oz	220	1	58
1 extra large, 24 oz	310	2	82
Marionberries, 1 cup, 5 oz	75	1	15

Weights As Purchased	C	F	Cb
Melons, all varieties, average, cubes/balls, 1 cup, 6 oz	60	0	14
Mulberries, 20 fruit, 1 oz	15	0	3
Nashi Fruit/Asian Pear, 1 med. 7 oz	85	0	21
Nectarines: 1 medium, 5oz	60	0	14
1 large, 7 oz	80	0	18
Oheloberries, ½ cup, 2.5 oz	20	0	5
Olives, Pickled: Green, 10 lge, 1.5 oz	60	7	2
Ripe, Greek Style, 10 medium, 1 oz	70	6	4
Ripe (Black) Californian:			
1 small/medium	5	0	0.2
1 large/extra large	6	1	1
1 jumbo	7	1	1
1 colossal	11	1	1
Oranges, all varieties, average, weights with skin:			
1 small, (2.5" diam.), 5 oz	45	0	11
1 medium (3") 7 oz	75	0	18
1 large, (3.5") 10 oz	105	0	25
1 extra large, (4"), 14 oz	130	0	30
Flesh/Pulp only, 1 cup, 6 oz	85	0	21
Peel, 1 Tbsp	0	0	0
California Navel (3"), 7 oz	70	0	17
California Valencia, 1 medium (2¾" diam.) 6 oz	60	0	14
Florida Orange, 1 med., 7 oz	70	0	17
Sunkist Navel, large, 14 oz	130	0	30
Papaya:			
1" pieces, 1 cup, 5 oz	60	0	15
1 medium, 16 oz	120	0	30
Green (unripe), ½ cup, 3.5 oz	20	0	5
Passionfruit:			
1 small, 1.5 oz	15	0	3
1 large, 2.7 oz	30	0	6
Pulp, ½ cup, 4 oz	110	0	27
Peaches: 1 baby/donut, 3 oz	30	0	7
1 small, 5 oz	50	0	12
1 medium, 6 oz	60	0	14
1 large, 7 oz	70	0	16
1 extra large, 9 oz	90	0	21
Pears, all varieties, average:			
1 mini, 2.5 oz	35	0	8
1 small, 5 oz	75	0	18
1 medium, 7 oz	100	0	25
1 large, 9 oz	130	0	33
1 extra large, 12 oz	170	0	42
Pepino, ½ medium, 4 oz	20	0	4
Persimmons: Native, 1 oz	35	0	9
Japanese (2½"d. x 2½"h), 7 oz	120	0	30
Maui, seedless, 1 medium, 5 oz	100	0	25

Weights As Purchased	C	F	Cb
Pineapple, average all varieties:			
Weights without skin:			
1 thin slice (½"), 2 oz	30	0	7
1 thick slice (¾"), 3 oz	40	0	10
1 cup, chunks, 6 oz	80	0	20
Whole fruit, wt with skin:			
Baby/Mini, 16 oz	150	0	39
Medium size, 3 lbs	450	1	118
Canned ~ *See Page 102*			
Pitanga, (Surinam-Cherry) (5), 1.2 oz	10	0	2
Plaintain:			
Fresh/Raw, weight with skin:			
1 medium, 10 oz	220	0	55
Slices, 1 cup, 5 oz	180	0	44
Cooked:			
Mashed, ½ cup, 3.5 oz	115	0	30
Slices, 1 cup, 5.5 oz	180	0	47
Fried in oil: 10 slices (¼"), 2 oz	160	6	26
1 cup, 4.2 oz	360	14	58
Plums, all varieties, average:			
1 mini/Damson, (1" diam), 0.5 oz	10	0	2
1 small (2"), 2.3oz	30	0	7
1 medium (2½"), 3.5 oz	45	0	10
1 large (3"), 5 oz	60	0	14
Plumcot, 1 medium, 6 oz	75	0	18
Pomegranate:			
1 small (3"), 5.5 oz	70	1	15
1 medium (3½"), 10 oz	125	2	27
1 large (4"), 16 oz	230	3	50
Seeds/Arils, ¼ cup, 2 oz	40	1	10
Pomelo, flesh, ½ cup, 3.5 oz	35	0	9
Prickly Pear ~ *See Cactus Fruit*			
Quince, 1 medium, 3.5 oz	55	0	14
Rambutan/Rambotang,			
Red/Yellow, 1 medium, 2 oz	15	0	4
Raspberries: ½ cup, 2 oz	30	0	7
10 raspberries, 0.8 oz	10	0	2
1 cup, 4.3 oz	65	1	15
1 pint, 11 oz	160	2	37
Sapodilla: 1 medium, 6 oz	140	2	34
Pulp, 1 cup, 8.5 oz	200	3	45
Sapote:			
Black: 1 medium, 4.5 oz	60	0	14
Pulp only, ½ cup, 4 oz	100	1	22
Mamey, piece, 1 cup, 6 oz	220	1	50
Satsuma Tangerine, 1 medium, 3 oz	45	0	11
Soursop, pulp, 1 cup, 8 oz	150	1	38
Starfruit, (Carambola):			
1 medium, (3½" long), 3 oz	30	0	6
1 large (4½"), 4.5 oz	40	0	8
Strawberries: 1 cup, 5.5 oz	50	1	12
6 medium/3 large, 2 oz	20	0	4
1 pint container, heaping, 16 oz	130	1	32
Chocolate dipped, 1 large	45	3	6

Weights As Purchased	C	F	Cb
Sugar-Apple (Sweetsop),			
pulp, ½ cup, 4 oz	120	0	28
Sugar Cane:			
Unpeeled, 1 baton (7" long), 4 oz	30	0	7
Peeled, 1 small stick (3"), 2 oz	35	0	8
Tamarillo, 1 medium, 3 oz	20	0	3
Tamarind: 1 fruit (3"x1")	5	0	2
Pulp, ½ cup, 2 oz	140	1	37
Tangelo: 1 small, 4 oz	55	0	13
1 medium, 5 oz	70	0	17
1 large, 7 oz	95	0	23
Tangerine, 1 med., (2½" diam.), 4 oz	50	0	13
Tangor, 1 medium, 4 oz	35	0	7
Tomatillos:			
3 medium, 3.5 oz	35	1	6
1lb (16 oz) quantity	160	2	27
Tomatoes:			
1 small (2¼" diameter), 3 oz	15	0	3
1 medium (2¾"), 5 oz	25	0	5
Sliced: 2 thin slices, 1 oz	5	0	1
2 thick (⅜"), 2 oz	10	0	2
Wedge, ¼, 1.3 oz	6	0	1
1 large (3½"), 8 oz	40	1	9
1 extra large (4"), 12 oz	60	1	14
Cherry: 4 medium, 2 oz	10	0	2
1 cup, 5 oz	25	0	6
Grape, 5 medium, 2 oz	10	0	2
Yellow Tear Drop, 3 medium, 1 oz	5	0	2
Canned Tomatoes/Products ~ *See Page 144*			
Tree Tomato/Tamarillo, 3 oz	20	0	5
Ugli Fruit, Tangelo type, 5 oz	40	0	8
Watermelon:			
Flesh only, weights without skin:			
1 thin slice (½"), ¼ circle, 3 oz	25	0	6
1 thick slice (1"): ¼ circle, 6 oz	50	0	12
½ circle, 12 oz	100	1	24
Buffet Slice, small, thin, 1 oz	8	0	2
Cubes or Balls, 1 cup, 5.5 oz	45	0	11
Round Seedless Melon, weight with skin:			
Medium size, 13 lb, (8" diam.):			
whole melon, 13 lb	1160	5	280
wedge, ⅛ whole, 26 oz	145	1	35
Mini size, 6 lb, (6.5" diam.):			
whole melon, 6 lb	480	3	110
wedge, ⅛ whole, 12 oz	60	0	14

Dried Fruit

	C	F	Cb
Apples, 5 rings, 1 oz	80	0	19
Apricots, 8 halves, 1 oz	65	0	16
Banana Chips, ⅓ cup, 1 oz	180	9	16
Banana Flakes, 4 Tbsp, 1 oz	80	0	20
Cranberries *(Craisins):*			
Original, ¼ cup	130	0	33
Reduced Sugar, ¼ cup	100	0	31
Chocolate Covered, ¼ cup, 2 oz	180	8	28
Dates ~ *See Dates in Fresh Fruit*			
Figs, 3 medium figs, 1 oz	90	0	23
Goji Berries, 3 Tbsp, 1 oz	100	0	21
Mango Slices, 5 pieces, 1.4 oz	25	0	6
Papaya Spears, 2 pieces, 1.4 oz	120	0	30
Peaches, 2 halves, 1 oz	60	0	15
Pears, 3 halves, 2 oz	140	1	34
Plums *(Sunsweet)*, (5), 1.4 oz	100	0	24
Prunes/Dried Plums:			
with pits, 3 medium, 1 oz	70	0	17
without pits, 4 medium, 1 oz	70	0	17
Cooked: with sugar, ½ cup, 5 oz	155	0	38
without sugar, ½ cup, 4.5 oz	135	0	33
Raisins: 2 Tbsp, 1 oz pack	85	0	22
½ cup, (unpacked), 2.5 oz	215	0	56
White Mulberries, 1 oz	90	1	22

Candied/Glazed Fruit

	C	F	Cb
Apricot, 1 medium, 1 oz	70	0	17
Cherry, Maraschino (1)	8	0	2
Citron/Fruit Peel, 1 oz	85	0	20
Ginger, 1 oz	90	0	21
Pineapple, 1 slice, 1.3 oz	120	0	29
Tamarind, dried, sweetened, 1 oz	70	0	17

Fruit Leather Rolls

	C	F	Cb
Betty Crocker: Fruit By The Foot, 1 roll, 0.8 oz	80	0	17
Fruit Gushers, 1 oz	90	1	20
Fruit Roll-Ups, 1 roll	50	1	12
Stretch Island, Leathers, 1 pouch, 0.5 oz	45	0	12

Canned/Bottled Fruit

Solids & Liquids:
Per ½ Cup, 4½ oz Unless indicated

	C	F	Cb
Apricots/Peaches/Pears:			
in juice, light	60	0	15
in heavy syrup	105	0	28
in water/diet	35	0	8
Black/Blueberries:			
in heavy syrup	120	0	30
in light syrup	110	0	26

Canned/Bottled Fruit (Cont)

	C	F	Cb
Cherries, pitted:			
in heavy syrup	105	0	27
in light syrup	85	0	22
in water	55	0	15
Maraschino, 1 oz	50	0	12
Fruit Cocktail/Salad:			
in heavy syrup	95	0	25
in juice, light	60	0	16
in water/diet	35	0	10
Gooseberries, light syrup	90	0	24
Grapefruit, in light syrup	75	0	20
Lychees, ½ cup, 4.5 oz	105	0	26
Mixed Fruit: in fruit juices/light syrup	70	0	18
in heavy syrup	90	0	24
in water/diet	40	0	10
Pineapple: in heavy syrup, 4.3 oz	110	0	26
in own juice, 4 oz	60	0	15
Prunes: with syrup, 3 oz	90	0	23
Stewed in water, ½ cup	135	0	35

Fruit Snack Cups

	C	F	Cb
Deli/Take-Out: Small, 6 oz	70	0	16
Large, 12 oz	140	0	32
Yogurt and Fruit Cup, 15 oz	380	5	75
Del Monte:			
Bubble Fruit, all flavors, 4 oz cup,	60	0	14
Fruit & Oats, average, 7 oz	185	3	36
Fruit Refreshers, average, 7 oz cup	95	0	23
Fruit Snack Cups: Average, 4 oz	70	0	17
No Sugar Added, average, 4 oz	50	0	14
Parfaits: Pineapple Coconut	180	7	31
Average other varieties, 6.25 oz	200	8	31
Dole:			
Fruit Bowls In 100% Juice:			
Diced Pears, 4 oz cup	90	0	22
Mixed Fruit, 4 oz cup	70	0	15
Fridge Packs In Juice: *Per 4.3 oz Container*			
Peach Slices	80	0	21
Pineapple Chunks	70	0	16
Other Fruits	90	0	21

Apple & Fruit Sauces

	C	F	Cb
Apple Sauce:			
Regular/sweetened, 2 Tbsp, 1 oz	20	0	6
Cranberry, Jellied, ¼ cup	110	0	25
Fruit Sauces & Purees:			
All fruit types, average: 2 Tbsp, 1 oz	25	0	6
½ cup, 4 oz	100	0	24
Mott's:			
Apple Sauce: Original, 4 oz	60	0	14
Unsweetened Mango Pineapple, 3.9 oz	50	0	13
Ocean Spray, Jellied Cranb. Sce, 2.5 oz	110	0	28

Quick Guide

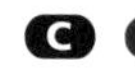 

Ice Cream

	C	F	Cb
Average all Flavors:			
Regular (10% fat):			
Examples: Dreyer's Grand, Hood, Friendly's			
½ cup, 4 fl.oz	140	7	16
1 cup, 8 fl.oz	280	14	32
1 pint, 16 fl.oz	560	28	64
Rich/Premium (16-17% fat):			
Examples: Baskin Robbins, Ben & Jerry's, Haagen-Dazs			
½ cup, 4 fl.oz	250	16	24
1 cup, 8 fl.oz	500	32	48
1 pint, 16 fl.oz	1000	64	96
Reduced-Fat/Light (5% fat):			
Examples: Breyers ½ The Fat, Friendly's Light, Hood Light			
½ cup, 4 fl.oz	140	5	21
1 cup, 8 fl.oz	280	10	42
1 pint, 16 fl.oz	560	20	84
Fat-Free:			
Example: Breyers			
½ cup, 4 fl.oz	90	0	21
1 cup, 8 fl.oz	180	0	42
1 pint, 16 fl.oz	360	0	84
Scoop Shops:			
Average all Brands			
Add extra for cone (see next column)			
Kids, 3 fl.oz	125	8	12
Regular, 6 fl.oz	250	16	24
Large, 9 fl.oz	375	24	36
Soft Serve:			
Average all Brands			
Regular: ½ cup, 4 fl.oz	255	15	25
1 cup, 8 fl.oz	510	30	50
Light: ½ cup, 4 fl.oz	145	3	25
1 cup, 8 fl.oz	290	6	50

Quick Guide

Frozen Yogurt

	C	F	Cb
Average all Brands			
Hard: Low-Fat, ½ cup	110	3	19
Non-Fat, ½ cup	110	0	24
Soft: Low-Fat, ½ cup	120	4	17
Non-Fat, ½ cup	100	0	30

Brands ~ *See Ice Cream & Novelties Section*

Quick Guide

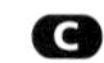  

Gelato/Ices/Frozen Custard

	C	F	Cb
Gelato: *Per ½ Cup*			
Milk base: Vanilla	160	6	25
Chocolate Hazelnut	230	15	21
Water base, ½ cup	100	0	26
Frozen Custard, Choc./Vanilla, av:			
½ cup	210	11	23
Single Scoop, 5 oz wt	300	15	38
Double Scoop, 10 oz wt	600	30	76
Fruit Ice Pops	80	0	20
Ice (Milk base): *Average all flavors*			
Hard (4% fat), ½ cup	100	3	15
Soft Serve (3% fat), ½ cup	110	2	19
Shaved Ice, average, 12 fl.oz	160	0	40
Sherbet, average, ½ cup	110	2	22
Sorbet, Fruit, fat free, ½ cup	70	0	19

Sundaes

	C	F	Cb
Dairy Queen:			
Banana split	520	14	94
Caramel Sundae, medium	430	11	72
Hot Fudge, medium	430	15	66
Strawberry	340	10	56
Toppings ~ *See Page 195*			
McDonald's:			
Sundaes:			
Hot Caramel	330	7	58
Hot Fudge	330	10	51

Ice Cream Cones & Cups

	C	F	Cb
Average all Brands			
Wafer Cone/Cup, average	20	0	4
Sugar Cone, average	50	0	14
Waffle Cone:			
Small	50	1	10
Large	90	1	19
Brands:			
Comet, Sugar Cone	50	0	11
Keebler, Sugar Cone	50	0	10
Oreo, Chocolate Cone	50	1	10

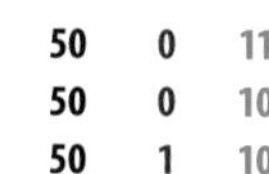

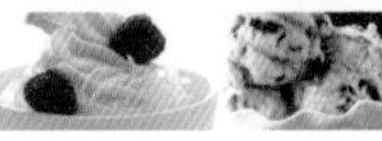

Ice Cream ~ Brands

	C	F	Cb
Baskin-Robbins ~ *See Fast-Foods Section*			
Ben & Jerry's:			
Scoop Shop Ice Cream: *Hand Scooped, 3 oz Serving*			
Americone Dream	240	13	26
Butterscotch'd	230	13	26
Cherry Garcia	200	12	22
Choc. Chip Cookie Dough	230	13	26
Chunky Monkey	240	15	25
Chocolate Fudge Brownie	210	11	26
Churray for Churros!	250	15	25
Coffee, Coffee, BuzzBuzzBuzz	220	13	23
Gimme S'more!	260	15	28
Ice Cream, 1 Pint Tubs: *Per ⅔ Cup*			
Americaone Dream	380	21	41
Cannoli	360	21	38
Caramel Chocolate Cheesecake	380	23	38
Chocolatey Love A-fair	360	21	39
Churray for Churros!	380	23	39
Half Baked	370	19	45
Ice Cream Sammie	390	22	42
Lights! Caramel! Action!	390	21	47
Milk & Cookies	380	22	39
Mousse Pie	390	24	39
Cores: Boom Chocolatta	380	23	38
Brownie Batter	350	19	41
Light Ice Cream, 1 Pint Tubs: *Per ⅔ Cup*			
Chocolate Mint	190	6	30
Chocolate Cookie EnlightenMint	190	6	30
Mocha Fudge Brownie	200	5	36
P.B. Marshmallow Swirl	230	7	34
Non Dairy: *Per ⅔ Cup*			
Change The Whirled	390	21	48
Lights! Caramel! Action!	370	18	51
Milk & Cookies	350	18	43
Mint chocolate Chance	290	14	38
Mint Chocolate Cookie	300	15	40
Topped: Bossin' Cream Pie	410	23	46
Raspberry Cheesecake	380	20	46
Fro Yo Frozen Yogurt: *Per ⅔ Cup*			
Cherry Garcia	230	4	44
Half Baked	230	4	45

Blue Bunny: *Per ⅔ Cup*	C	F	Cb
Premium Ice Cream, 1 Pint Cont:			
Bunny Tracks, 3.35 oz	250	14	29
Cherrific Cheesecake, 3.3 oz	220	10	31
Chocolate, 3.1 oz	180	9	23
Stuffed Puffs: Birthday Cake, 3.1 oz	200	7	32
Cookies 'N Creme, 3.2 oz	210	7	34
S'mores, 3.3 oz	260	12	36
Sweet Freedom:			
Double Strawberry Swirl, 3.4 oz	110	3	26
Vanilla, 3.14 oz	110	4	23
Note: Carbohydrate figures include 5-10 g sugar alcohols			
Frozen Yogurt, Vanilla Bean, 3.14 oz	140	3	25
Bars/Pops ~ *See Page 108*			
Breyers:			
Classics: *Per ⅔ Cup*			
Dble choc. Brownie Batter, 2.9 oz	180	7	29
Natural Strawb., 3.2 oz	150	7	20
Vanilla:			
Extra Creamy, 2.85 oz	140	5	24
Other Varieties, av., 3.1 oz	175	9	20
Carb Smart: Chocolate; Vanilla, 2.75 oz	110	6	17
Mint Fudge Cookie, 2.85 oz	130	7	20
Note: Carbohydrate figures include 7-8g sugar alcohol and 4g fiber			
Cookies & Candy: *Per ⅔ Cup*			
Health Toffee, 2.82 oz	190	7	28
Reeses Choc., 3.1 oz	190	9	25
Snickers, 3.3 oz	210	8	32
No Sugar Added: *Per ⅔ Cup*			
Butter Pecan, 2.7 oz	130	7	17
Vanilla, 2.6 oz	110	4	17
Vanilla Choc. Strawberry, 2.6 oz	110	4	17
Note: Carbohydrate figures include 8 sugar alcohol			
Non Dairy: *Per ⅔ cup*			
Cookies & Cream, 2.9 oz	170	7	25
Mint Choc. Chip, , 2.96 oz	190	10	24
Bruster's: *Per Small Dish*			
Ice Cream: Banana, 4.93 oz	280	14	36
Butterscotch Ripple, 4.93 oz	310	15	40
Chocolate Mudslide, 4.93 oz	340	14	49
Non Dairy:			
Banana, 2.47 oz	130	5	22
Mango, 2.47 oz	130	5	19
Peach Melba, 2.47 oz	140	4	25

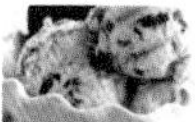
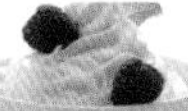

Ice Cream ~ Brands (Cont)	C	F	Cb
Carvel Ice Cream ~ *See Fast-Foods Section*			
Coldstone Creamery ~ *See Fast-Foods Section*			
Dairy Queen/Brazier ~ *See Fast-Foods Section*			
Dannon: *Per ⅔ Cup, 3.88 oz*			
Yocream:			
Premium Frozen Yogurt,			
Average all flavors	**155**	**4**	25
Low Fat Frozen Yogurt:			
Cake Batter	**140**	**2**	27
Dulce De Leche	**140**	**2**	29
Fancy French Vanilla	**130**	**1**	27
Salted Caramel corn	**140**	**2**	29
No Sugar Added Nonfat Frozen Yogurt:			
Cheesecake	**110**	**0**	24
Chocolate	**120**	**1**	26
Raspberry	**110**	**0**	23
Strawberry Banana	**110**	**0**	24
Note: Carbohydrate figure includes 5-6g sugar alcohol			
Dairy Free Sorbet:			
Choc Fudge 2.9 oz	**140**	**1**	34
Pomegranate Raspberry 2.9 oz	**130**	**0**	32
Gelato, average all flavors, 3.88 oz	**185**	**7**	26
Dippin' Dots:			
Original Dots: *Per 3 oz*			
Banana Split	**160**	**8**	20
Chocolate, 3.88 oz	**170**	**8**	22
Choc. Chip Cookie Dough, 3.5 oz	**195**	**9**	27
Cookies 'n Cream, 3.25 oz	**190**	**9**	24
Cotton Candy, 3.25 oz	**150**	**8**	18
YoDots, Strawberry Cheeesecake	**100**	**2**	20
Dreyer's/Edy's:			
Classic Ice Cream: *Per ⅔ Cup, 3 oz*			
Butter Pecan	**200**	**11**	20
Chocolate; Coffee, av.	**175**	**9**	21
Mint Choc. Chip	**200**	**11**	23
Neapolitan	**180**	**8**	20
Strawberry	**160**	**7**	20
Rocky Road Collection: *Per 3 oz*			
Chocolate Pnut Butter Park	**230**	**14**	23
Churro Caramel Crossroads	**210**	**10**	27
Cookie Cobblestone	**220**	**9**	32
Mocha Almond Avenue	**200**	**11**	23
The Original Rocky Road	**210**	**11**	24

Dreyers/Eddys (Cont):	C	F	Cb
Slow Churned Light Classics: *Per ⅔ Cup*			
Butter Pecan, 2.9 oz	**170**	**7**	24
Chocolate, 2.8 oz	**130**	**5**	22
Double Fudge Brownie, 2.8 oz	**160**	**4**	26
Slow Churned No Sugar Added: *Per ⅔ Cup*			
Fudge Tracks, 2.93 oz	**150**	**5**	23
Vanilla Bean, 2.93 oz	**130**	**4**	19
Note: Carbohydrate figure includes 5-10g sugar alcohol			
Gelati-da:			
Gelato: *Per ½ Cup, 4 oz*			
Amaretto Chocolate	**150**	**5**	23
Choc Mint Milano	**120**	**3**	22
Coffee Fudge Latte	**130**	**2**	22
Limoncello; Vanilla Marsala, average	**120**	**3**	21
Red Raspberry	**130**	**2**	25
Great Value *(Walmart): Per ⅔ Cup*			
Ice Cream: Butter Pecan, 3.1 oz	**210**	**13**	20
Chocolate, 3.1 oz	**180**	**9**	23
Choc. Chip Cookie Dough, 3.1 oz	**200**	**10**	28
Cookies & Cream, 3.14 oz	**210**	**10**	27
Mint Chip, 3.1 oz	**190**	**10**	23
Neapolitan, 3.1 oz	**170**	**8**	21
Rocky Road, 3.3 oz	**200**	**10**	27
Vanilla Bean, 3.14 oz	**180**	**9**	21
Sherbet, av. all flav., ½ cup	**110**	**0**	26
Haagen-Dazs: *Per ⅔ Cup*			
Ice Cream, 14 fl.oz Tubs:			
Bourbon Praline Pecan, 4.8 oz	**360**	**20**	40
Caramel Cone, 4.76 oz	**400**	**25**	38
Cherry Vanilla, 4.5 oz	**290**	**18**	29
Coffee Choc. Brownie, 4.8 oz	**380**	**22**	39
Creamy Mango, 4.88 oz	**330**	**17**	40
Double Belgian Choc. Chip , 4.7 oz	**420**	**27**	39
Vanilla Swiss Almond, 4.7 oz	**370**	**25**	30
White Choc. Rasp. Truffle, 4.8 oz	**360**	**20**	41
City Sweets Collection:			
Black & White Cookie, 4.88 oz	**410**	**24**	42
Coffee Chocolate, 4.8 oz	**380**	**22**	33
Summer Berry Cake Pop, 4.7 oz	**320**	**20**	31
Gluten Free: Chocolate, 4.6 oz	**330**	**21**	28
Choc. Peanut Butter, 3.3 oz	**300**	**20**	25
Coffee Chip, 4.55 oz	**340**	**22**	30
Dulce de Leche, 4.66 oz	**350**	**20**	36
Honey Salted Caramel Alm., 4.76 oz	**350**	**22**	33
Matcha Green Tea, 4.5 oz	**310**	**21**	25

Bars ~*See Page 109*

Ice Cream ~ Brands (Cont)

Hood:	C	F	Cb
Classic: *Per ⅔ Cup, 3.1 oz*			
Chocolate	190	9	24
Classic Trio	180	9	23
Coffee Cookies 'N Cream	200	10	26
Cookie Dough	210	10	28
Creamy Coffee	180	10	22
Fudge Twister	190	8	27
Golden Vanilla	190	10	22
Mint Chocolate Chip	200	11	24
Frozen Fat-Free Yogurt: *Per ⅔ Cup, 3 oz*			
Strawberry	120	0	25
Mocha Fudge	130	0	29
Vanilla Bean	120	0	26
New England Creamery ~ *www.CalorieKing.com*			
Lucerne *(Vons): Per ⅔ Cup*			
Frozen Dairy Dessert: Chocolate	130	4	22
Cookies & Cream	160	5	26
Marble Fudge	140	4	25
Neapolitan	130	4	22
Vanilla	130	4	21
Oberweis:			
Super Premium Ice Cream: *Per ⅔ Cup*			
Black Cherry, 3.8 oz	280	17	28
Brandy, 3.77 oz	280	18	24
Cookies & Cream, 3.8 oz	300	19	28
Cookie Dough P'nut Butter, 3.95 oz	370	23	37
Espresso Caramel Chip, 3.9 oz	310	18	36
Vanilla, 3.77 oz	280	19	24
Oikos ~ *see Dannon*			
Pinkberry:			
Frozen Yogurt: *Without Toppings*			
Original: Mini, 3.2 oz wt	90	0	19
Small, 4.9 oz wt	150	0	31
Medium, 8 oz wt	240	0	50
Large, 13 oz wt	390	1	81
Chocolate Hazelnut, 8 oz	360	9	59
Cookies & Cream, 8 oz	320	5	58
Passionfruit, 8 oz	240	0	50
Peanut Butter, 8 oz	390	16	49
Vanilla Latte, 8 oz	240	0	47
Dairy Free: Chocolate,8 oz	340	13	56
Coconut,8 oz	280	11	42

Red Mango (Stores):	C	F	Cb
Frozen Yogurt: *1 Cup, 8 oz, Without Toppings*			
Original	200	0	46
Banana	220	0	50
Blueberry	220	0	48
Caribbean Coconut; Vanilla Bean	260	0	58
Dark Chocolate	260	1	60
Mango	260	0	58
Milk Chocolate; Raspberry, average	260	0	61
Peanut Butter	300	10	44
Pomegranate	240	0	54
Pomegranate Dark Chocolate	240	0	54
Fro-Yo Mashups: *Per ½ Cup, 4 oz*			
Brownie Brittle; Cookie Butter, av.	140	3	24
Cake Batter; Coffee	120	1	25
NY Cheesecake; Pistachio Mustachio	130	2	27
Vanilla Latte	120	1	25
White Chocolate	140	1	29
Bars ~ *See Page 110*			
So Delicious: *Per ⅔ Cup*			
Frozen Dessert:			
Cashew Milk:			
Bananas Foster, 4 oz	240	13	29
Chocolate Cookies & Cream, 4 oz	250	13	33
Dark Chocolate Truffle, 4.1 oz	250	15	30
Salted Caramel Cluster, 4 oz	250	13	32
Snickerdoodle, 4 oz	240	11	34
Very Vanilla, 3.67 oz	190	9	26
Coconut Milk:			
Cookie dough, 4 oz	270	15	33
Mint Chip, 3.7 oz	240	15	26
Mocha Almond Fudge, 3.8 oz	250	15	28
Vanilla Bean, 3.6 oz	200	12	23
No Sugar Added:			
Mint Chip, 3.84 oz	160	11	25
Vanilla Bean, 4 oz	130	9	24
Note: Carbohydrate Figure Includes 4-5g Sugar Alcohol			
Oatmilk: Coffee Chip, 3.84 oz	230	12	29
S'mores, 3.4 oz	230	13	28
Soy Milk,			
Creamy Vanilla, 3.67 oz	160	4	31
Wondermilk: Buttery Pecan, 3.88 oz	260	16	29
Strawberry, 4 oz	220	10	29

Ice Cream ~ Brands (Cont)

Stop & Shop *(Ahold):*	C	F	Cb
Churn Style Ice Cream: *Per ⅔ Cup*			
Choc. Chip Cookie Dough	160	5	25
Cookies & Cream	160	5	27
Vanilla, Light	140	4	24
Vanilla Fudge Swirl	190	8	27
Real Ice Cream: *Per ⅔ Cup*			
Black Raspberry	180	10	22
Chocolate Chip	210	11	25
Cookies & Cream	200	10	26
Mint Chocolate Chip	200	11	24
Neapolitan	180	9	23
Strawberry	180	9	22
Vanilla	190	10	22
Vanilla Bean	190	10	22
Tasti D-Lite:			
Soft Serve: *Per 4 fl.oz*			
Vanilla: Banana	70	1	13
Birthday Cake	90	2	15
Black Cherry	70	2	14
Brownie Batter	70	2	13
Butter Pecan	70	1	12
Cappuccino	70	1	13
Chocolate Mousse	70	1	14
Cinnamon Crunch	70	1	14
Creme Brulee	70	2	14
Mango	70	1	14
Mud Pie	80	2	13
Nutella Fusion	90	3	15
Oreo Mint	80	2	15
Peanut Butter	90	4	13
Tofutti *(Milk Free):*			
Frozen Dessert Premium Pints: *Per ⅔ Cup, 3.5 oz*			
Better Pecan	250	16	24
Chocolate	200	12	21
Vanilla	260	14	32
Vanilla Almond Bark	250	15	26
Vanilla Fudge	240	14	28
Wild Berry	240	16	24

TCBY ~ *See Page 250*

Turkey Hill:	C	F	Cb
Premium Ice Cream: *Per ⅔ Cup, 3 oz*			
Black Raspberry	170	8	23
Choco Mint Chip	200	11	23
Cookies 'n Cream	190	10	25
Moose Tracks	190	8	28
Peanut Butter Ripple	170	7	23
Rocky Road	180	5	30
Vanilla Bean	170	9	21
Vanilla Chocolate Crunch	210	12	25
No Sugar Added,			
Vanilla Bean, 3.2 oz	100	0	26
Simply Natural Ice Cream: *Per ⅔ Cup*			
Belgian Style Chocolate	210	10	27
Salted Caramel	210	19	28
Strawberries & Cream	190	9	23
Vanilla Bean & Chocolate	210	11	24
Trio'politan: *Per ⅔ Cup*			
Banana Split	180	9	24
Caramel Macchiato	190	9	25
S'mores	190	10	24
Triple: Berry	130	3	24
Chocolate	160	4	28
Vanilla	160	6	24
Sherbet, Fruit Rainbow, 4 oz	160	2	36
Wawa:			
Premium Ice Cream: *Per ½ Cup*			
Butter Pecan; Mint Choc. Chip, av.	180	10	20
Chocolate; Vanilla Bean, average	160	8	20
Cookies & Cream	180	9	21
Strawberry Shortcake	160	7	22
Wegmans: *Per ⅔ Cup Unless Indicated*			
Ice Cream: Chocolate Chip	210	11	27
Chocolate Marshmallow	170	8	24
French Vanilla	200	9	26
Strawberry	180	8	25
Vanilla & Chocolate	180	9	22
Organic: Dark Chocolate	360	20	40
Vanilla & Chocolate Twist	360	22	34
Premium: Creamy Caramel	360	22	36
Dark Chocolate Flavor	340	19	39
Nutter Batter	410	26	39
Peanut Butter	470	35	32
S'mores	430	24	52
Light: *Per ⅔ Cup*			
Mint Chip	170	4	29
Pecan Praline	170	4	32
NoSugar Added: Chocolate	120	5	22
Vanilla	120	5	22

I Ice Cream Bars & Pops

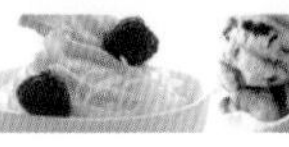

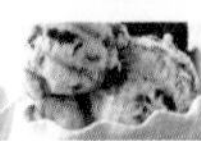

Ice Cream Bars & Pops ~ Brands

Per Bar/Serving Unless indicated	C	F	Cb
Big Bear ~ *See Klondike*			
Blue Bunny:			
Bars:			
Big Alaska Bar, (1)	250	15	27
Big Sandwich Bars:			
Bopper Sandwich	400	16	61
Vanilla Sandwich	220	6	38
Load'd: Bunny Tracks	340	19	38
Salted Caramel (1)	320	17	40
Mini Bars:			
Chocolate Cookie Crumble	140	7	19
Strawberry Shortcake	110	6	14
Vanilla Caramel Crunch	130	7	16
Single Bars:			
Chocolate Eclair	210	10	28
Cookies 'n Cream	250	12	32
Strawberry Shortcake	190	10	25
Cones:			
Caramel Lovers	310	16	38
Cookies 'n Cream	270	13	37
Big Dipper: Cookies 'n Cream	250	11	35
Vanilla	250	12	32
Twist Cones, Mint Chocolate	230	10	33
Sandwiches:			
Chips Galore	300	13	46
Chocolate Lovers	180	5	33
Neapolitan	150	4	27
Stuffed Puffs Sandwiches:			
Salted Caramel S'mores	200	5	37
S'mores	200	5	38
Breyers:			
Carb Smart, 6 Pack:			
Almond Bar, 2 oz	150	12	11
Fudge Bar, 1.7 oz	60	3	10
Vanilla Ice Cream Bar, 2 oz	140	11	11

Note: Carbohydrate figure includes 4-5g sugar alcohol

	C	F	Cb
Butterfinger Bar ~ *See Nestle Page 110*			
Diana's Bananas:			
Banana Halves:			
Milk/Dark Chocolate (1)	130	5	22
Banana Bites, Milk/Dark Chocolate, (3), 1.13 oz	80	4	11

Per Bar/Serving Unless indicated	C	F	Cb
Dove:			
Single Bars,			
Dark Chocolate, Vanilla	250	17	24
Miniatures: Variety Pack, w/ Milk/Dark Chocolate,1 piece	60	4	6
Sorbet Bars, Dark Chocolate Raspb.	150	8	19
Drumstick *(Nestlé)*:			
Classic Sundae Cones: Banana	290	15	34
Banana with Fudge	300	15	38
Original Vanilla	280	15	34
Strawberry with Fudge	300	15	38
Vanilla Caramel	300	15	39
Vanilla Fudge	300	15	38
Dipped: Choc. Cookie	280	13	38
Crushed It	270	12	38
Super Nugget: Strawberry	300	16	35
Vanilla	310	17	35
Vanilla Fudge	320	17	39
King Size: Triple Chocolate	340	14	50
Vanilla with Chocolate Swirls	350	14	52
Lil' Drums: Choc. w/ Choc. Swirls	110	5	16
Vanilla with Chocolate Swirls	110	5	16
Vanilla Fudge/Caramel	110	4	18
Simply Dipped: Mint	260	12	37
Vanilla	270	12	38
Edy's ~ *See Dreyer's*			
Eskimo Pie ~ *See Nestle*			
Fudge Bar ~ *See Nestle*			
Fat Boy:			
Cones: Chocolate Fudge Brownie	300	15	40
Cookie Dough; Caramel Praline	310	15	40
Sundae Best	310	17	34
Freeze Pops,			
Orange Cream	110	3	21
Sandwiches: Cookies 'n Cream, 3 oz	220	9	34
Mint Chocolate Chip, 3 oz	230	10	33
Old Fashioned/Premium Vanilla	210	8	32
Strawberry, 3 oz	180	7	29
Sugar Cookie	210	7	39
Sundaes: *Per 1.62 oz Bar*			
Caramel Pretzel	150	9	17
Cherry Cordial	150	10	14
Toffee Crunch	150	9	16
Vanilla Nut	150	10	14
Fudgsicle *(Breyers):*			
Fudge Bar: Original	80	3	14
Low Fat	60	2	11
No Sugar Added	80	2	18

Ice Cream Bars/Pops ~ Brands (Cont)

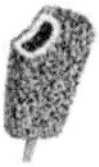

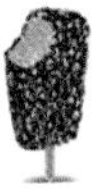

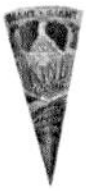

Per Bar/Serving	C	F	Cb
Good Humor:			
Dessert Bars, Singles:			
Original Vanilla, 2.8 oz	240	15	23
Chocolate Eclair, 2 oz	150	7	21
Cookies & Cream, 1.5 oz	140	7	18
Creamsicle, 2.5 oz	100	2	20
Reese's, 1.8 oz	180	11	20
Strawberry Shortcake, 2 oz	160	9	19
King Cones: *Per Cone*			
Chocolate & Vanilla, 5 oz	390	22	44
King Cone, Vanilla, 2.7 oz	230	14	25
Sandwiches:			
Single: Giant Vanilla, 3.6 oz	210	5	39
Chocolate Chip Cookie, 2.7 oz	250	10	39
Haagen-Dazs:			
Butter Cookie Cones: Coffee	280	16	29
Chocolate	300	17	33
Dark Chocolate Bar, Chocolate	270	19	22
Milk Chocolate Bars:			
Caramel Cone	260	17	24
Coffee & Almond Crunch	270	19	22
Vanilla & Almonds	270	19	20
Vanilla	250	18	20
White Chocolate Raspberry	260	16	26
Snack Size:			
Coffee & Almond Toffee runch	170	12	14
Vanilla & Almonds	180	13	13
Sorbet, Mango, 4.94 oz	200	0	50
Healthy Choice:			
Fudge Bar	100	0	22
Smoothie Bars: Mango Peach	70	1	14
Raspberry	80	1	15
Strawberry	70	1	13
Hershey's:			
Bars, Gluten Free: Banjo	120	6	15
Fudjo	110	0	25
Orange Blossom	110	3	21
Cones: Incredible	260	11	37
Moose Tracks	380	18	50
P-Nutty	200	12	25
Super cookies & Cream	190	9	26
Low fat: Cookies & Cream; Crazy, av.	140	3	25
Vanilla Chocolate Twist	140	2	23
Dessert Cups: Chocolate	230	11	29
Cotton Candy	230	11	32
Dulce de Leche	260	12	36
Midnight Caramel River	240	10	37
Ice Cups, average all flavors	120	0	30

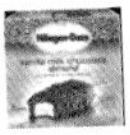

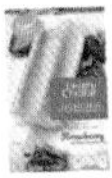

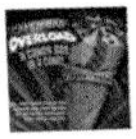

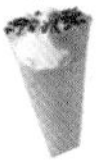

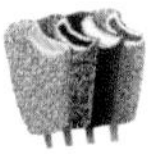

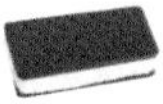

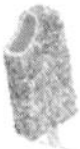

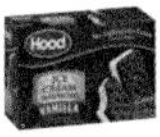

Per Bar/Serving	C	F	Cb
Hershey's (Cont):			
Sandwiches:			
Vanilla Ice Cream, 4 oz	170	6	27
Giant:			
Andes Mint	250	10	39
Vanilla	250	9	39
Mini Reduced Fat	100	2	19
Signature Bars: Banana Pudding	240	14	32
Chocolate Eclair	240	13	32
Strawberry Shortcake	240	11	32
Hood:			
Hoodsie Cups,			
Chocolate; Vanilla, 3 oz	100	5	13
Sandwich, Vanilla	170	6	27
Klondike:			
Bars:			
Single,			
Original Vanilla, 5.5 oz	290	16	33
4-Pack:			
Mint Choc. Chip, 2.8 oz	230	14	26
6 Pack: Cookies & Cream, 2.15 oz	200	10	24
Double Chocolate, 3 oz	240	14	27
Krunch, 2.65 oz	240	14	28
Mint Choc. Chip, 2.75 oz	230	14	26
Reeses, 2.71oz	250	15	26
Cones:			
Classic Chocolate	240	12	30
Cookies & Cream	230	11	32
Double Down Chocolate	230	11	30
Nuts For Vanilla	240	12	30
Unicorn Dreamin'	190	7	30
Vanilla Chillin'	220	10	31
Sandwiches:			
Cookies & Cream	190	6	33
Vanilla	180	5	31
Kroger: *Per Bar*			
Arctic Blasters:			
Orange Cream	90	1	19
Strawberry Shortcake	150	9	17
Variety Packs:			
Bar, Milk Chocolate, Vanilla	135	9	13
Cone/Sundae,			
Vanilla with P'nuts & Chocolate	240	11	33
Sandwiches, Vanilla; Snowboard	130	2	25
Luigi's: *Per 6 fl.oz cup*			
Real Italian Ice:			
Blue Raspberry Lemon Swirl	130	0	34
Cherry Lemon Swirl	110	0	29

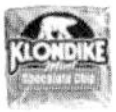

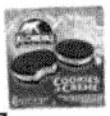

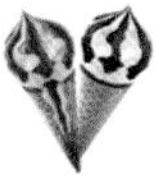

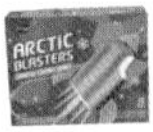

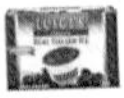

Ice Cream Bars & Pops

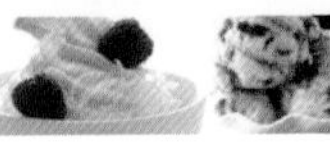

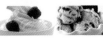

Ice Cream Bars/Pops ~ Brands (Cont)

Per Bar/Serving	C	F	Cb
M&M's:			
Cone, Single, 2.6 oz	250	12	32
Cookie Sandwiches:			
Cookies & Cream, 2.5 oz	230	9	35
Vanilla, 2.86 oz	240	10	36
Magnum:			
Bars: Caramel Duet	220	15	22
Chocolate Duet	230	15	21
Double: Caramel	270	17	29
Chocolate	260	17	27
Gold Caramel	240	14	26
Raspberry	260	16	28
Minis, Almond	150	11	13
Non Dairy: Almond	250	16	25
Hazelnut Crunch	240	15	26
Minute Maid, Juice Bars, 2.25 fl.oz	40	0	10
Nestlé:			
Bars: Butterfinger	290	17	30
Cookies N' Cream	180	11	19
Crunch	150	9	15
Crushed It: Cookies N' Cream	170	9	21
Vanilla Fudge	180	9	22
Eskimp Pie	150	5	15
Fudge Bar	110	2	20
Strawberry Shortcake	140	6	20
Dibs, Crunch, 3.3 oz container	320	21	31
Drumsticks ~ See Page 108			
Push-Up Pops, all flavors	70	1	16
Sandwiches, Vanilla	160	3	30
Popsicle:			
Fruit Pops: Strawberry	150	0	34
Average Other Fruit Flavors	165	0	40
Fruit Stacker, Banana, Orange, Strawb.	160	0	38
Fudgsicle, Low Fat	60	2	11
Scribblers, 2 Pops	60	0	14
Reeses Dessert Bar~*See Good Humor*			
Skinny Cow: *Per Item*			
Bars: Fudge; Chocolate Truffle, av.	120	3	19
Vanilla Almond Crunch	190	11	19
Cones, all flavors	170	5	28
Minis, Salted C'rmel Pretzel	90	6	9
Sandwiches, all flavors	160	4	29
Snickers:			
Bars: Milk/Dark Choc., 1.7 oz	180	11	18
2.8 oz bar	250	15	25
Cone, 2.7 oz	250	13	31
Snow Cone *(Wonder)*, av. all, 7 fl.oz	60	0	15

Per Bar/Serving	C	F	Cb
So Delicious *(Turtle Mountain):*			
Almond Based:			
Bars, Mocha Alm. Fudge	180	13	16
Sandwich, Vanilla, 1.3 oz	100	4	14
Cashewmilk:			
Dipped Bars: Dble Choc Delight, 2 oz	170	13	16
Salted Caramel Bar, 2 oz	180	13	17
Coconut Milk:			
Dipped Bar: Coconut Alm., 1.85 oz	190	14	15
Vanilla Bean, 1.8 oz	170	12	14
Fudge Bar, 2 oz	100	6	13
Sandwiches:			
Coconut, 1.3 oz	100	4	14
Vanilla Bean, 1.3 oz	100	4	14
Tampico, Freezer Pops, all var., 1.4 oz	30	0	7
Tofutti: *Per Item*			
Bars: Chocolate Fudge, 1.4 oz	30	0	6
Hooray Hooray, 1.4 oz	120	8	8
Marry Me, 1.4 oz	170	8	22
Totally Fudge Pops	95	2	19
Note: Carb figures include 0-7g sugar alcohols			
Cone, Yours Truly Sundae	170	8	22
Cuties, average all flavors	130	6	18
Toll House *(Nestle)*:			
Sandwiches:			
Chocolate Choc. Chip Cookie, 4 oz	380	16	54
Vanilla Choc. Chip Cookie, 2.1 oz	210	8	32
Mini, Vanilla	105	4	16
Turkey Hill:			
Sandwiches: Double Decker	200	8	31
Vanilla Bean	190	7	30
Reduced Fat	170	3	33
Sundae Cone, Van. Fudge	360	22	35
Twix:			
Cookies & Cream, 2.4 oz	250	14	29
Vanilla Ice Cream Bar: 3 fl.oz	250	14	28
1.6 fl.oz Bar	160	9	18
Wegmans:			
Bars: Organic Fudge	190	12	16
Chocolate Sundae Crunch	180	10	22
Strawberry Sundae Crunch	180	9	22
Sandwiches: Vanilla, 3.5 fl.oz	160	5	27
Light Vanilla, 3.5 fl.oz	160	3	29
Weight Watchers: *Per Item*			
Bars: Dark Choc. Raspberry	70	2	11
English Toffee	80	4	11
Giant Bar, Chocolate Fudge	90	1	21
Snack Bars: Cookies & Cream	90	3	15
Divine Triple Chocolate	90	3	14
Salted Caramel	90	3	14

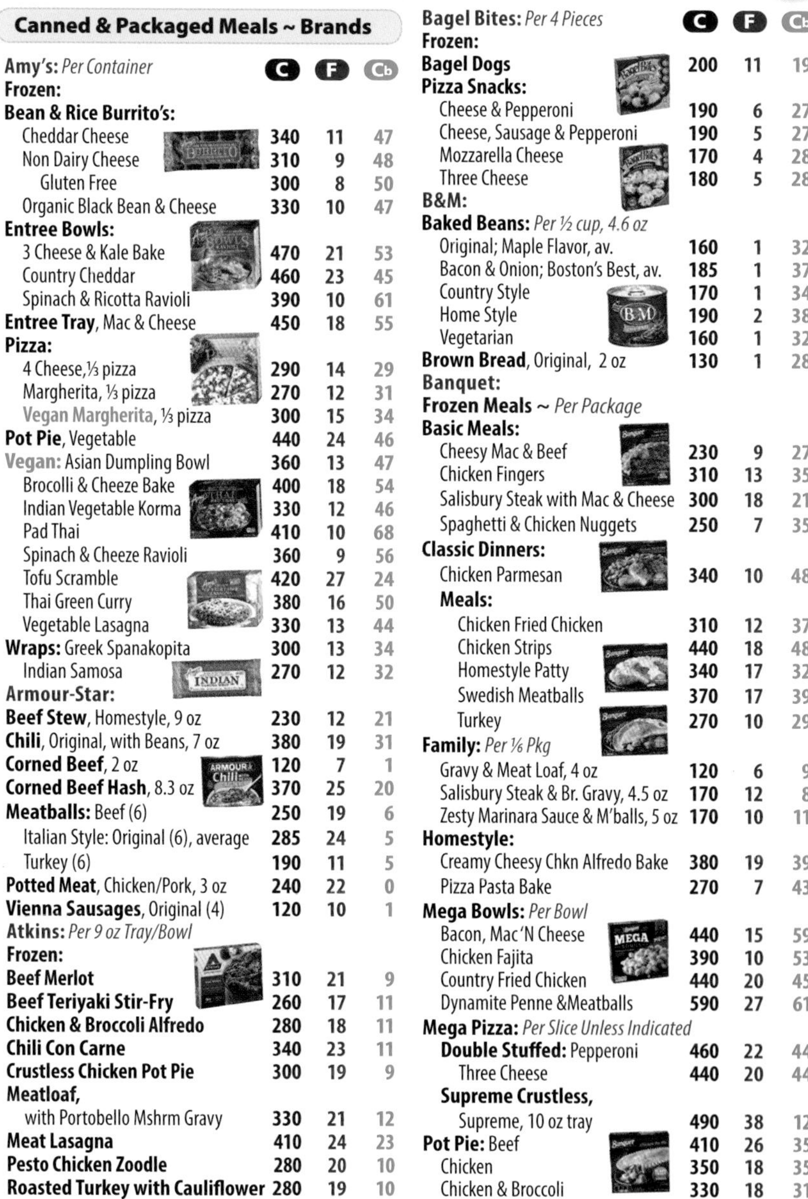

Canned & Packaged Meals ~ Brands

Amy's: *Per Container*	C	F	Cb
Frozen:			
Bean & Rice Burrito's:			
Cheddar Cheese	340	11	47
Non Dairy Cheese	310	9	48
Gluten Free	300	8	50
Organic Black Bean & Cheese	330	10	47
Entree Bowls:			
3 Cheese & Kale Bake	470	21	53
Country Cheddar	460	23	45
Spinach & Ricotta Ravioli	390	10	61
Entree Tray, Mac & Cheese	450	18	55
Pizza:			
4 Cheese, ⅓ pizza	290	14	29
Margherita, ⅓ pizza	270	12	31
Vegan Margherita, ⅓ pizza	300	15	34
Pot Pie, Vegetable	440	24	46
Vegan: Asian Dumpling Bowl	360	13	47
Brocolli & Cheeze Bake	400	18	54
Indian Vegetable Korma	330	12	46
Pad Thai	410	10	68
Spinach & Cheeze Ravioli	360	9	56
Tofu Scramble	420	27	24
Thai Green Curry	380	16	50
Vegetable Lasagna	330	13	44
Wraps: Greek Spanakopita	300	13	34
Indian Samosa	270	12	32
Armour-Star:			
Beef Stew, Homestyle, 9 oz	230	12	21
Chili, Original, with Beans, 7 oz	380	19	31
Corned Beef, 2 oz	120	7	1
Corned Beef Hash, 8.3 oz	370	25	20
Meatballs: Beef (6)	250	19	6
Italian Style: Original (6), average	285	24	5
Turkey (6)	190	11	5
Potted Meat, Chicken/Pork, 3 oz	240	22	0
Vienna Sausages, Original (4)	120	10	1
Atkins: *Per 9 oz Tray/Bowl*			
Frozen:			
Beef Merlot	310	21	9
Beef Teriyaki Stir-Fry	260	17	11
Chicken & Broccoli Alfredo	280	18	11
Chili Con Carne	340	23	11
Crustless Chicken Pot Pie	300	19	9
Meatloaf, with Portobello Mshrm Gravy	330	21	12
Meat Lasagna	410	24	23
Pesto Chicken Zoodle	280	20	10
Roasted Turkey with Cauliflower	280	19	10

Bagel Bites: *Per 4 Pieces*	C	F	Cb
Frozen:			
Bagel Dogs	200	11	19
Pizza Snacks:			
Cheese & Pepperoni	190	6	27
Cheese, Sausage & Pepperoni	190	5	27
Mozzarella Cheese	170	4	28
Three Cheese	180	5	28
B&M:			
Baked Beans: *Per ½ cup, 4.6 oz*			
Original; Maple Flavor, av.	160	1	32
Bacon & Onion; Boston's Best, av.	185	1	37
Country Style	170	1	34
Home Style	190	2	38
Vegetarian	160	1	32
Brown Bread, Original, 2 oz	130	1	28
Banquet:			
Frozen Meals ~ *Per Package*			
Basic Meals:			
Cheesy Mac & Beef	230	9	27
Chicken Fingers	310	13	35
Salisbury Steak with Mac & Cheese	300	18	21
Spaghetti & Chicken Nuggets	250	7	35
Classic Dinners:			
Chicken Parmesan	340	10	48
Meals:			
Chicken Fried Chicken	310	12	37
Chicken Strips	440	18	48
Homestyle Patty	340	17	32
Swedish Meatballs	370	17	39
Turkey	270	10	29
Family: *Per ⅙ Pkg*			
Gravy & Meat Loaf, 4 oz	120	6	9
Salisbury Steak & Br. Gravy, 4.5 oz	170	12	8
Zesty Marinara Sauce & M'balls, 5 oz	170	10	11
Homestyle:			
Creamy Cheesy Chkn Alfredo Bake	380	19	39
Pizza Pasta Bake	270	7	43
Mega Bowls: *Per Bowl*			
Bacon, Mac 'N Cheese	440	15	59
Chicken Fajita	390	10	53
Country Fried Chicken	440	20	45
Dynamite Penne &Meatballs	590	27	61
Mega Pizza: *Per Slice Unless Indicated*			
Double Stuffed: Pepperoni	460	22	44
Three Cheese	440	20	44
Supreme Crustless, Supreme, 10 oz tray	490	38	12
Pot Pie: Beef	410	26	35
Chicken	350	18	35
Chicken & Broccoli	330	18	31

Barilla:	C	F	Cb
Frozen:			
Entrees: *Per Container*			
Chicken Alfredo	310	18	22
Italian Sausage	350	7	59
Marinara/Tomato & Basil Penne, av.	310	4	59
Meat Sauce Gemelli	350	6	61
Birds Eye: *Per Frozen Weights*			
Frozen:			
Bakes: Cheddar Broccoli, 3.67 oz	100	6	7
Loaded Potato Bake, 3.74 oz	140	8	11
Cauliflower Bites:			
Loaded Bacon Cheddar Bites (4)	190	10	19
Loaded Southwest Style (4)	190	10	20
Cauliflower Wings:			
Buffalo, 4.5 oz	220	11	25
Garlic Parmesan, 4.5 oz	240	13	26
Sweet Chili, 4.5 oz	210	9	30
Sheet Pan Meals:			
Chicken:			
With Garlic Parmesan Potatoes, Cauliflower and Green Beans, 5.1 oz	150	6	14
W/- Rosemary Brown Butter Potatoes	140	5	14
Ital. Sausage with Peppers, 5.3 oz	220	14	16
Voila!:			
Alfredo Chicken, 7.6 oz	210	7	27
Beef Lo Mein, 8 oz	240	4	38
Cheesy Ranch Chicken, 6.8 oz	210	5	30
Chicken Florentine, 7.5 oz	220	6	28
Chicken Stir-Fry, 8.47 oz	250	3	41
Garlic Chicken, 6.2 oz	210	7	29
Garlic Shrimp, 6.7 oz	220	7	31
Meatless Alfredo Chick'n, 5.9 oz	170	5	20
Mongolian Style Beef, 7.73 oz	230	4	37
Sausage & Peppers, 8.2oz	280	13	29
Shrimp Scampi, 9 oz	230	4	36
Sweet & Sour Chicken, 8.15 oz	270	3	48
Teriyaki Chicken, 7.87 oz	230	3	39
Three Cheese Chicken, 6.77 oz	190	5	27
Boca:			
Frozen			
Original Veggie Crumbles, 2 oz	60	0	5
Original Chik'n Veggie Nuggets:			
4 pieces	180	8	14
Non GMO Soy, 4 pieces	180	8	13

Boca (Cont):	C	F	Cb
Frozen			
Original Veggie Patties: *Per Patty*			
All American	120	5	8
Original Chik'n	140	6	11
Spicy Chik'n	140	6	11
Vegan	80	1	7
Boston Market: *Per Package*			
Frozen:			
Bowls:			
Fr. Chicken w/- Loaded Mashed Pot.	350	14	38
Philly Cheese Steak w/ Rice & Veg.	390	17	42
Pulled Chicken with BBQ Sauce	490	21	43
Slow Cooked Beef & Red Potatoes	320	16	28
Home Style Meals:			
Boneless Pork Rib Patty	580	29	60
Chicken Bacon Ranch	540	23	51
Crustless Chicken Pot Pie	470	34	35
Hot Honey Fried Chicken	540	20	64
Meat Lovers Meatball	640	37	53
Salisbury Steak	530	32	38
Buitoni:			
Refrigerated:			
Ravioli: Impossible Beef & Chse, 9 oz	290	8	38
Impossible Italian Ssg & Chse, 9 oz	280	8	38
Tortellini: Herb Chicken, 3.9 oz	320	8	48
Mixed Cheese, 3.7 oz	310	8	45
Tortelloni, Chkn & Rstd Garlic, 9 oz	270	7	37
Dry Pasta ~ *See Page 133*			
Bush's Best: *Per ½ cup, 4.6 oz*			
Baked Beans: Original	150	1	30
Brown Sugar Hickory	160	1	33
Vegetarian	150	0	30
Black Beans	110	0	20
Chili, Pinto, mild sauce	130	1	19
Dark Red Kidney Beans	130	0	24
Garbanzo Beans (Chick Peas)	120	2	20
Grillin' Beans:			
Bourbon & Br. Sugar; Honey Chipotle, av.	170	1	35
Smokehouse; Southern Pit BBQ, av.	170	1	34
Steakhouse Recipe	190	1	39
Pinto Beans	90	0	17
Campbell's:			
Pork & Beans, 11 oz can, ½ cup, 4.6 oz serving	130	1	27
Spaghetti O's: *Per 1 Cup*			
Original, 8.9 oz	170	1	33
With Franks, 8.9 oz	220	7	29
With Meatballs, 8.9 oz	230	7	30

	C	F	Cb
Chef Boyardee:			
Canned: *Per Cup*			
Beefaroni, 8.8 oz	200	7	27
Cheesy Burger Macaroni	180	4	27
Ravioli:			
Beef in Pasta Sauce	180	5	30
Cheese, in Tomato Sauce	200	2	39
Overstuffed Italian Sausage	240	6	38
Spaghetti: With Meatballs	250	10	30
Jumbo Spag. & Meatballs	280	13	29
Microwavable Cups: *Per Cup*			
Beef Ravioli in Pasta Sauce	180	4	30
Lasagna Pasta in Meat Sauce	220	8	30
Mac & Cheese	160	4	26
Spaghetti in Tomato Sauce	130	1	26
Pizza Maker Kits: *Crust Mix & Pizza Sace Only*			
Pepperoni, ⅛ package, 4 oz	260	6	43
Traditional, ⅛ package, 4 oz	240	4	46
Pizza Sauce:			
With Cheese, ¼ cup, 2 oz	30	2	4
With Meat, ½ cup, 4.5 oz	90	4	12
Dennison's Chili: *Per Cup*			
Chili Con Carne:			
Original: With Beans	330	14	34
Without Beans	260	14	17
Chunky, with Beans	300	13	30
Hot, with Beans	330	13	34
Turkey, with Beans	220	4	32
Vegetarian, 99% fat free	170	1	31
Devour ~ *See Heinz Page 114*			
Dinty Moore *(Hormel):*			
Big Bowl (Microwave): *Approx. ½ of 15 oz Bowl*			
Beef Stew, 8.3 oz	200	10	17
Chicken & Dumplings, 8.5 oz	210	6	29
Can, Chicken & Dunplings, 8.5 oz	200	7	24
Microwave:			
Cup, Scalloped Pot, with Ham, 7.5 oz	260	16	19
Tray, Beef Stew, XL, 13 oz	330	17	29
Dr. McDougall's:			
Vegan Asian Noodle Cups:			
Pad Thai, 2 oz	200	2	43
Teriyaki, 1.87 oz	200	1	41
Spicy Kung Pao, 2 oz	200	2	38
Eden Foods (Organic): *Per Cup, 8.8 oz*			
Black Beans & Quinoa Chili	190	2	35
Great Northrn Beans Barley & Spice	190	2	38
Kidney Beans & Kamut Chil	220	2	41
Pinto Beans & Spelt Chili	200	2	40

	C	F	Cb
Farmhouse: *Per 1 Cup Prepared*			
Pasta: Fettuccine Alfredo	460	22	51
White Cheddar	380	14	51
Rice: Long Grain, Wild Herbs & Butter	250	7	43
Mexican	230	4	42
Roasted Chicken Flavor	230	4	44
French's:			
French Crispy Fried Onions:			
Original; White Cheddar:2 Tbsp	45	4	3
4 tablespoons	90	7	6
8 tablesooons	180	14	12
GardenBurger:			
Frozen			
Veggie Burger:			
Original	150	5	22
Original Steak	220	6	33
Roasted Garlic & Quinoa	230	14	22
Garden Lites: *Per Package*			
Frozen			
Cauliflower Bites: *Per Five Bites*			
Margherita	200	9	26
Mushroom & Swiss Carmelised Onion	190	8	27
Roasted Veggie & 4 Cheese	170	6	26
Cakes: Broccoli Cheddar (1)	90	6	5
Superfood Veggie (1)	80	4	8
Frittatas: *Each*			
Mushroom & 3 Cheese	80	4	6
Roasted Cauliflower	60	2	7
Spinach Egg White	70	4	5
Veggie, Bacon & Potato	80	5	6
Gorton's:			
Frozen:			
Delicious Classics:			
Clams, Crunchy Breaded, 15 pieces	230	13	21
Flounder, Crispy Batt. Fillets (2)	250	13	25
Pollock: Beer Battered Fillets (2)	230	12	23
Crispy Battered Fillets (2)	230	11	23
Crunchy Breaded Fish Sticks (4)	230	10	26
Potato Crunch Fillets (2)	230	11	24
Popcorn Shrimp, 3.5 oz	190	9	21
Everyday Gourmet:			
Cod:			
Crunchy Panko Breaded Fillets (1)	240	12	24
Crunchy Panko Fish Sticks (4)	200	10	20
Simply Bake~ Per Fillet:			
Cod, Garlic Butter	120	2	4
Haddock, Garlic Herb Butter	120	1	5
Salmon, Roasted Garlic Butter	140	5	1
Tilapia, with Seasoning	140	3	1

continued nex page...

Gorton's (Cont):	C	F	Cb
Frozen:			
Smart Solutions: *Per Fillet*			
Cod, Rstd Garlic Herb	80	2	3
Haddock, Grilled	70	1	0
Pollock, Gr. Lemon Butter	70	1	0
Tilapia: Grilled	100	4	1
Grilled Roasted Garlic Butter	100	3	1
Great Value *(Walmart)*:			
Frozen:			
Breakfast Bowls: Bacon, 7 oz	440	31	14
Sausage & Gravy, 7 oz	320	23	16
Meals: Beef Shepherd's Pie, 6.4 oz	190	10	15
Cheese Ravioli, 9.5 oz	200	6	29
Creamy Chicken & Pasta, 6.7 oz	320	17	26
Roasted Poblano Enchiladas, 9 oz	370	16	46
Spaghetti with Meat Sauce, 10 oz	360	12	48
Vegetable Lasagna, 9.5 oz	420	11	52
Healthy Choice: *Per Package*			
Frozen:			
Cafe Steamers:			
BBQ Seasoned Steak & Red Potatoes	300	4	49
Beef Teriyaki	270	4	43
Chicken Fajita	200	5	23
Crustless Chicken Pot Pie	300	6	40
Four Cheese Ravioli & Chkn Marinara	250	5	33
Grilled Chicken Marinara w/ Parm.	280	5	36
Honey Glazed Turkey & Potatoes	240	2	42
Gluten Free: Beef Merlot	180	4	24
Cajun Style Chicken & Shrimp	220	3	35
Classics: Classic Meatloaf	290	7	43
Lemon Pepper Fish	280	4	48
Power Bowls: *Per Bowl*			
Adobo Chicken	330	8	38
Chicken Feta & Farro	310	9	34
Grilled Chicken Pesto with Veggies	290	7	36
Vegan:			
Cauliflower Curry	290	4	50
Falafel & Tahini	360	13	49
Green Goddess	330	12	37
Simply Steamers: *Per Package*			
Beef & Broccoli	270	5	39
Beef Chimichurri	220	6	24
Chicken & Vegetable Stir Fry	200	5	16
Grilled Chicken & Pesto Veggies	200	5	11
Meatball Marinara	280	6	36

Heinz:	C	F	Cb
Beans, Baked in Tomato Sauce, 4.6 oz	100	0	17
Frozen:			
Devour Meals: *Per Package*			
Buffalo Chicken Mac & Cheese	670	32	68
Cajun Syle Alfredo w/ Ssg & Chkn	410	19	34
Loaded Potato with Beef & Bacon	330	14	32
Pulled Chicken Burrito Bowl	440	15	45
Smokehouse Meat & Potatoes	430	13	57
Tortellini Alfredo & Italian Sausage	560	28	55
Bowls:			
Crmy Alfredo Mac & Chse w/ Bacon	390	14	51
Sharp Cheddar Mac & Chse w/ Bacon	380	13	51
Sandwiches:			
Buffalo Chicken Grilled Cheese	500	18	59
Philly Cheesesteak Grilled Cheese	460	15	59
Hormel:			
Canned:			
Chili with Beans: *Per 8.7 oz Cup*			
Angus Beef	310	16	27
Hot	270	10	30
Turkey, 98% Fat-Free	240	7	29
Vegetarian, 99% Fat Free	200	2	35
Vegan Plant Based	180	1	28
Chili No Beans: *Per 8.3 oz Cup*			
Angus Beef	330	23	14
Chunky Beef	260	14	17
Hot	240	12	19
Turkey, 98% Fat-Free	190	3	16
100% Natural, White Chicken Chili	190	6	16
Tamales: Beef in Chile Sauce, 7.5 oz	190	9	22
Beef, Hot & Spicy in Chile Sce, 7.5 oz	180	8	22
Frozen/Refrigerated:			
Compleats: *Per 7.5 oz Package*			
Beef Pot Roast	200	6	20
Beef with Mashed Potatoes & Gravy	230	8	24
Cheese Manicotti & Meat Sauce	290	9	41
Chicken Alfredo	350	18	30
Chicken Breast & Dressing	240	5	28
Chkn Brst, Gravy & Mashed Potatoes	220	5	28
Meatloaf, Gravy & Mashed Potates	300	14	28
Roast Beef w/ Mashed Pot. & Gravy	220	7	25
Salisbury Steak	300	16	27

Hormel (Cont)...	C	F	Cb
Frozen/Refrigerated:			
Compleats (cont): *Per 7.5 oz Package*			
Chkn Brst, Gravy & Mashed Potatoes	220	5	28
Meatloaf, Gravy & Mashed Potates	300	14	28
Roast Beef w/ Mashed Pot. & Gravy	220	7	25
Salisbury Steak	300	16	27
Stroganoff	210	9	23
Swedish Meatballs	280	13	26
Turkey & Dressing	290	9	31
Side Dishes:			
Bacon Mac & Chse, 8.2 oz	340	12	42
Chipotle Chedd. Mac & Chse, 8.2 oz	340	14	41
Hot Pockets: *Per Pocket*			
Frozen:			
Big & Bold: *4 Per Pack*			
Chicken Bacon Ranch	450	17	58
Sriracha Steak	450	18	56
Crispy Buttery Crust: *5 Per Pack*			
Hickory Ham & Cheddar	270	9	39
Steak & Cheddar	320	3	39
Crispy Crust: *2 pack*			
Pepperoni Pizza	320	15	36
Croissant Crust: *2 pack*			
Hickory Ham & Cheddar	280	10	38
Garlic Buttery Crust: *12 Pack*			
Four Cheese	280	11	36
Four Meat & Four Cheese Pizza	300	13	35
Meatball & Mozzarella	290	12	38
Pepperoni Pizza	310	14	36
Seasoned Crust: *5 Pack*			
Philly Steak & Cheese	300	11	40
Breakfast: *5 Pack*			
Bacon, Egg & Cheese (1)	290	11	37
Deli Wich: *Each*			
Cheddar & Ham	240	9	29
Cheese Melt	270	12	29
Pepperoni & Mozzarella	300	14	31
Turkey & Colby	270	10	34

Hungry Jacks:	C	F	Cb
Hashbrowns,			
Original, ⅓ cup, 0.5 oz	60	0	13
Mashed Potatoes,			
Original, ⅓ cup, 0.75 oz	80	0	16
Hungry Man: *Per Package*			
Frozen:			
Dinners:			
Boneless Fried Chicken	780	39	81
Country Fried Chicken	530	27	54
Grilled Beef Patty	550	37	34
Roasted Carved White Meat Turkey	400	10	61
Salisbury Steak	590	33	52
Selects: Classic Fried Chicken	970	63	62
Mexican Style Fiesta Enchiladas	780	27	120
Smokin' Backyard Barbeque	690	24	91
Double Meat Bowls:			
Beef, Smothered Salisbury Steak	630	43	35
Chicken, Breaded Chicken Alfredo	620	27	65
José Olé:			
Burritos: *Per Burrito*			
Beef & Cheese	350	15	42
Beef & Jalapeno	320	12	40
Chimichangas: *Per Chimichanga*			
Beef & Cheese	390	20	41
Chicken & Cheese	330	13	41
Mini Tacos,			
Beef & Cheese (5)	230	11	24
Taquitos:			
Beef in Corn Tortillas (3)	240	12	26
Beef & Cheese in Flour Tortillas, (2)	260	14	26
Chicken in Corn Tortillas, (3)	200	8	26
Chicken & Chse in Flour Tortillas, (3)	220	10	26
Kid Cuisine: *Per Meal*			
All Star Chicken Breast Nuggets	450	18	56
Carnival Mini Corn Dogs	480	18	68
Level Up: Cheese Quesadillas	660	21	94
Dino Nuggets	560	24	72
Mac & Cheese Bites	540	19	81
Mini Corn Dogs	480	18	68
Popcorn Chicken	470	19	62

Kraft:	C	F	Cb
Macaroni & Cheese: *DryMix Only*			
Original (7.25 oz Box),			
2.5 oz (makes 1 cup)	250	2	49
With Added Cauliflower Pasta,			
2.5 oz (makes 1 cup)	250	2	50
Thick & Creamy (7.25 oz Box),			
2.5 oz (makes 1 cup)	260	2	50
Three Cheese (7.25 oz Box),			
⅓box (makes 1 cup)	260	2	49
White Cheddar (7.3oz Box),			
Pasta Shells, 3 oz (makes 1 cup)	320	4	59
Whole Grain (6oz Box),			
2.5 oz (makes 1 cup)	250	2	49
Microwave Cups: (4 pack)			
Orig. Cheddar, 1.9 oz	200	4	38
Triple Cheese, 2.05 oz	220	4	40
Deluxe: Original, 2.39 oz	210	8	30
White Cheddar,2.39 oz	220	8	30
Velveeta: *Per Container*			
Cheesy Potatoes, Mashed, 2 oz	180	7	24
Shells & Cheese Cups:			
Original, 2.39 oz	220	8	30
2% Milk Cheese, 2.2 oz	180	3	31
Queso Blanco, 2.39 ozz	210	7	30
Shells & Cheese Packs/Bowls/Boxes:			
Big Bowl, Bacon, 5 oz	460	18	59
Box, Broccoli, 4.5 oz	400	16	49
Kroger:			
Frozen:			
Beef Ravioli, 5 oz	280	7	44
Cheese Ravioli, 5.1 oz	280	6	43
Cheese Tortellini, 4.9 oz	270	6	46
Chicken Alfredo, 7.4 oz	270	11	28
Chinese Inspirations:			
Chicken Fried Rice, 4.23 oz	210	5	32
Vegetable Fried Rice, 1 cup, 4.23 oz	220	6	37
Flame Broiled H'style M'balls (6)	220	17	6
Italian Style Meatballs, 6 pieces	250	20	7
Meat Lasagna, Family Size, 1 cup	290	9	37
Vegetable Lasagna, 9 oz	420	24	39
Wild Mushroom Ravioli (8)	200	3	35

Kroger (Cont)	C	F	Cb
Heat & Serve:			
Chicken Fajitas, 5 oz	100	2	7
Korean Inspired Meatballs, 5 oz	430	16	58
Pulled Chicken, 4.94 oz	190	10	1
Pulled Pork, 4.94 oz	190	10	1
S'snd Pork Carnitas, 3 oz	120	6	2
Lean Cuisine:			
Frozen:			
Balance Bowls: *Per Bowl*			
Chicken Teriyaki	310	4	47
Creamy Pasta Primavera	240	4	34
Glazed Chicken	290	6	39
Lemon Garlic Shrimp Stir Fry	210	3	34
Orange Chicken	340	5	58
Roasted Eggplant with Parm & Pasta	230	5	34
Roasted Turkey & Vegetables	210	5	26
Shrimp Alfredo	300	7	40
Sticky Ginger Chicken	320	5	51
Tex Mex Rice & Black Beans	290	5	46
Cauli Bowls: *Per Bowl*			
Creamy Mac & Cheese	260	6	37
Crmy Tom. Vodka Pasta	240	7	36
Fettuccini with Meat Sauce	260	8	35
Garlic Parm Alfredo w/ Broccoli	250	9	33
Comfort Cravings: *Per Package*			
Alfredo Pasta w/ Chicken & Broccoli	280	5	39
Cheese Ravioli	250	6	39
Chicken Enchilada Suiza	300	5	54
Chicken Fried Rice	310	8	43
Fettucine Alfredo	290	5	49
French Bread Pepperoni Pizza	300	7	45
Protein Kick: *Per Package*			
Apple Cranberry Chicken	300	4	53
Baked Chicken	260	9	29
Buffalo Style Chicken	210	7	19
Butternut Squash Ravioli	300	7	49
Chicken In Sweet BBQ Sauce	240	7	29
Garlic Sesame Asian-Style Noodles with Beef	240	5	35
Grilled Chicken Caesar	270	9	27
Herb Roasted Chicken	180	5	16
Korean Style Beef & Vegetables	360	9	56
Meatloaf with Mashed Potatoes	250	7	25
Salisbury Steak with Mac. & Cheese	250	5	28
Steak Portabella	190	9	13

Pizzas ~ *See Page 137*

Lightlife (Vegan):	C	F	Cb
Smart Bacon, 2 slices	40	2	1
Smart Deli: *Per 4 slices*			
Bologna	90	3	3
Ham	90	3	3
Turkey	100	3	3
Smart Dogs: Regular, 1 link	60	2	2
Jumbo, 1 link	100	4	4
Smart Ground: *Per 1.94 oz*			
Original	70	2	4
Mexican	70	2	5
Smart Meatballs (3)	150	6	11
Smart Sausage:			
Chorizo, 1 link	130	5	5
Gimme Lean, ¼ cup, 1.87 oz	80	3	8
Italian, 1 link	130	5	7
Smart Tenders, Original Chicken (3)	150	4	11
Loma Linda (Vegan): *Per 10 oz Package*			
Bowls:			
Greek	380	10	61
Jamaican Jerk	380	10	59
Hawaiian	360	5	64
Southwest	260	2	45
Sweet Potato Harvest	480	16	70
Vegetariian Burger, 2 oz	60	1	2
Canned:			
BBQ Sauce Chik'n, 2 oz	60	1	7
Chik'n in Broth, 2 oz	40	0	4
Tuno: Lemon Pepper,5 oz	130	4	11
Spring Water, 5 oz	90	1	5
Spicy Sriracha, 2 oz	70	3	6
Thai Sweet Chili, 5 oz	150	1	22
Packaged Meals:			
Hearty Spaghetti	190	7	20
Pad Thai	260	7	36
Southwest Chunky Stew	250	5	37
Thai Green Curry	310	11	45
Thai Red Curry	240	12	22
Tikka Masala	250	6	39
Ultimate Chili, 10 oz	280	2	49
Lunchmakers (Armour):			
Cracker Crunchers w/ American Cheese:			
Chicken	200	9	21
Pepperoni	230	14	19
Turkey	210	10	22
Chips, Salsa & Cheese Nachos	210	10	28
Pepperoni Pizza	220	10	25

Marie Callender's:	C	F	Cb
Frozen:			
Bowls: *Per Bowl*			
Aged Cheddar Cheesy Chkn & Rice	380	13	46
Creamy Chicken & Dumplings	370	14	39
Four Cheese Fettuccini Alfredo	460	22	47
Garden Tomato Four Cheese Ravioli	320	13	39
Grilled Chicken Alfredo Bake	390	16	37
Grilled Chicken Pesto Cavatelli	370	9	45
New Orleans Style Chicken Alfredo	420	16	44
Red Chili Grilled Chicken Burrito	340	11	38
Shrimp Mac & Cheese	390	18	44
Slow Roasted Beef Pot Roast	220	6	26
Spicy Buffalo Style Chkn Mac & Chse	590	26	64
Traditional Lasagna with Meat Sce	430	13	51
Dinners: *Per Container*			
Beef:			
Meat Loaf & Gravy	370	15	37
Salisbury Steak	510	23	53
Steak & Roasted Potatoes	240	5	32
Chicken/Turkey:			
Country Fried Chicken & Gravy	390	17	44
Fiesta Queso Chicken	330	10	43
Roasted Turkey Breast & Stuffing	240	5	32
Sweet & Sour Chkn	550	15	88
Pasta,			
Fettuccini, Chicken & Broccoli	440	18	43
Plant Based Pot Pies: *Per Pie*			
Meatless Be'f	450	25	44
Meatless Chick'n	440	25	41
Pot Pies: *Per Pie*			
Brocc. & Cheddar Potato 10 oz	680	40	69
Chicken, 7 oz	440	26	40
Chicken w/ Cauliflower Crust, 14 oz	810	40	86
Layered:			
Beef & Bean Chili Cornbread, 11.7 oz	490	27	48
Beef Shepherd's, 11.5 oz	350	18	28
Chkn & Bacon Shepherd's, 11.7 oz	380	19	32
Kansas City BBq Sauce, Chicken & Cornbread, 11.5 oz	550	23	64
Turkey & Stuffing, 11.5 oz	260	7	33
Pub Pies: *Per Pie*			
Herb Rstd Chicken, 10 oz	760	45	69
Steak & Ale, 10 oz	790	51	62

Maruchan:	C	F	Cb
Bowls, all flavors, 3.3 oz	380	16	50
Ramen Noodle Soup, average all, 3 oz pkg	380	15	52
Instant Lunch, average, 1 container	290	11	39
Yakisoba: *Per 4 oz Pkg*			
Chicken/Teriyaki Beef Flavor, av.	500	19	69
Cheddar Cheese Flavor	540	24	68
Michael Angelo's:			
Frozen:			
Gourmeet Bowls: Chkn Cavatappi	290	7	37
Meat Lasagna Bolognese	340	14	34
Signature: Baked Ziti w/ M'balls, 11 oz	480	20	51
Chicken Parmigiana, 10 oz	430	15	49
Eggplant Parmig., 11 oz	420	26	35
Manicoti w/ Sauce, 11 oz	440	19	41
Shrimp Scampi, 10 oz	450	16	54
Three Cheese Baked Ziti, 11 oz	530	20	63
Vegetable Lasagna, 11 oz	360	11	44
Minute Rice:			
Ready To Serve: *Per 4.4 oz Container, Prepared*			
Brown Rice	210	5	39
With Quinoa	220	4	42
Chicken & Herb	230	3	44
Spanish	180	3	37
Yellow Rice	230	3	47
Morningstar Farms (Vegan/Vegetarian):			
Frozen:			
Chik'n (Vegan):			
Nuggets: BBQ (3)	200	8	20
Veggie	190	8	18
Patty, Buffalo Chicken	170	7	18
Incogmeato (Vegan):			
Chik'n Nuggets (4)	160	6	18
Chik'n Tenders (4)	230	9	20
Veggitizers (Vegan):			
Chk'n & Chse Taquito Bites (3)	200	9	21
Chorizo Nacho Bites (3)	200	9	18
Hot & Spicy Crispy Chik'n Filet (1)	200	8	17
Vegetarian Burgers: *Per Patty*			
Garden Veggie	100	3	12
Grillers: Original	130	5	8
Veggie	150	8	6
Spicy Black Bean	110	5	13
Tomato & Basil Pizza	130	7	11
Nissin:			
Chow Mein: *Per 4 oz Package*			
Chicken; Teriyaki Beef Flavors. av.	505	23	63
Shrimp Flavor	560	30	63
Cup Noodles: Curry	360	15	49
Other flavors, 1 cup	290	11	41

Nissin (Cont): *Per Pkg*	C	F	Cb
Cup Noodle Stir Fry, av. all flav.	370	13	55
Top Ramen Noodle Soup:			
Soy Sauce Flavor	380	14	53
Average otherl flavors	380	14	54
Old El Paso:			
Dinner Kits: *Incl. Shells/Tortillas, Sauce & Seasoning Mix*			
Enchilada Kit, 1 ½ Tortillas	160	4	27
Hard & Soft (2 shells)	130	5	18
Stand 'n Stuff (2 shells)	150	6	21
Refried Beans:			
Black Beans, 4.34 oz	120	2	19
Vegetarian Beans, 4.16 oz	90	1	15
Rice Mix: *Dry Mix Only*			
Cheesy Mexican Rice, 2.6 oz	270	1	59
Cilantro Lime Rice, 1.73 oz	170	1	37
Ortega:			
Canned Beans: *Per ½ cup, 4.4 oz*			
Black Beans, Original	110	0	20
Refried Beans, average	120	2	21
Meal Kits: *Incl. Shells/Burrito, Sauce & Seasoning Mix*			
Dinner Kit (2 shells)	140	6	20
Fiesta Flats (2 shells)	160	7	19
Hard & Soft Grane Kit, (2 shells)	140	6	20
Soft Taco Kit (2 tortillas)	220	3	42
Pasta Roni: *Per Cup, Prepared*			
Boxes: Angel Hair with Herbs	310	13	42
Garlic & Olive Oil Vermicelli	350	14	47
Parmesan Cheese	310	14	39
Shells & White Cheddar	290	12	39
Single Serve Cup, Chicken	190	1	41
P.F. Chang's:			
Frozen:			
Entrees: Beef with Broccoli, 9.4 oz	270	10	25
General Chang's Chicken, 10.8 oz	370	11	50
Mongolian Style Beef, 8.57 oz	230	5	31
Sesame Chicken, 10.2 oz	230	10	17
Sweet & Sour Chicken, 9.2 oz	280	6	44
Seafood: *With 2 Tbsp Sauce*			
Crispy Honey Tempura Shrimp (7)	180	5	22
Firecracker Tempura Shrimp (7)	210	12	16
Single Serve Meals: *Per Bowl*			
Chicken Pad Thai	340	6	50
Dan Dan Noodles	510	20	58

Prego:	C	F	Cb
Ready Meals: *Per Pouch*			
Creamy Three Cheese Alfedo Rotini	370	19	37
Creamy Tomato Penne	400	15	57
Marinara & Italian Sausage Rotini	350	9	55
Roasted Tomato & Vegetables Penne	300	4	55
Rice-A-Roni:			
Classic Favorites: *Per Cup, Prepared*			
Beef	310	9	51
Chicken & Broccoli	230	5	41
Chicken & Garlic	250	8	41
Mexican Style	250	7	41
Rice Pilaf	310	8	52
Single Serve Cups:			
Cheddar Broccoli	230	5	41
Chicken	190	1	41
Creamy Four Cheese	240	6	43
Rosarita:			
Black Beans, 4.5 oz	100	1	17
Pinto Beans, 4.5 oz	120	0	22
Refried Beans:			
Traditional, 4.5 oz	100	3	15
No Fat, 4.5 oz	80	0	16
Restaurant Style, 4.4 oz	90	3	13
Vegetarian, 4.5 oz	110	3	16
Safeway Select *(Albertsons):*			
Frozen:			
Signature Select:			
Chicken Teriyaki, tray	360	4	42
Chicken Tikka Masala, tray	240	5	33
Five Cheese Tortellini, 3.8 oz	240	6	37
Sweet & Sour Chicken, tray	270	5	42
S & W: *Per ½ Cup, 4.6 oz*			
Chili, average	125	1	22
Classic, average all flavors	110	0	21
Flavored Savory Side,			
Black Beans w/ jalap. & Lime,4.6 oz	130	2	22
Seapak ~ *See www.calorieking.com*			
Simply Asia: *Per Container*			
Noodles & Broth:			
Japanese:			
Ramen Noodles	200	1	42
Ramen Soy Chkn Broth	25	0	2
Udon Noodles	190	1	41
Noodle Bowls:			
Roasted Peanut	480	12	79
Sesame Teriyaki	420	4	87
Soy Ginger	440	6	86

Smart Ones *(Weight Watchers):*	C	F	Cb
Frozen:			
Smartmade: *Per Package*			
Chicken with Spinach Fettuccine	230	6	20
Grilled Sesame Beef & Broccoli	220	5	31
Mexican Style Chicken Bowl	260	5	33
Roasted Turkey & Veggies	250	3	37
Smart Ones: *Per Package*			
Angel Hair Marinara	200	2	38
Beef Pot Roast	180	4	18
Chicken Enchiladas Suiza	290	6	46
Chicken Fettuccini	300	5	44
Chicken Parmesan	280	6	35
Creamy Basil Chicken with Broccoli	170	4	15
Ham & Cheese Scramble	200	7	13
Three Cheese Ziti Marinara	300	8	43
Stagg:			
Chili with Beans: *Per Cup*			
Classic, 8.7 oz	290	13	26
Country Brand, 8.7 oz	320	17	26
Dynamite Hot, 8.7 oz	340	16	33
Laredo, 8.7 oz	300	17	23
Turkey Ranchero	260	6	32
Classic No Bean Chili, 8.32 oz	290	19	18
Vegetarian Garden 4-Bean Chili	200	2	37
Starkist:			
Chicken Creations: *Per 2.6 oz Pouch*			
Buffalo Style	90	4	3
Chicken Salad	70	2	4
Original BBQ	90	4	3
Teriyaki	80	3	3
Zesty Lemon Pepper	70	2	2
EVOO: *Per 2.6 oz Pouch*			
Wild Pink Salmon	190	15	0
Wild Yellowfin Tuna	180	12	0
Salmon Creations: *Per 2.6 oz Pouch*			
Lemon Dill	70	1	1
Mango Chipotle	90	1	5
Tuna Creations: *Per 2.6 oz Pouch Unless Indicated*			
Bacon Ranch	80	1	2
Lemon Pepper	80	1	1
Whole Grain Dijon Mustard, 3 oz	80	2	6
Tuna Smart Bowls: *Per 4.5 oz Pouch*			
Latin Citrus Quinoa & Beans	160	4	23
Spicy Pepper Rice & Beans	170	3	24
Tomato Basil Barley & Beans	160	4	21
Zesty Lemon & Pasta & Beans	180	5	24

Stouffer's:	C	F	Cb
Frozen:			
Bowl-FULLS: *For One*			
Blackened Chkn Alfredo	580	25	59
Cheesy Chicken Parm.	520	16	66
Chicken Bacon Ranch	630	25	63
Classic Pub Meatballs & Potatoes	470	20	42
Creamy Garlic Shrimp Mac & Cheese	500	18	61
Slow Roasted Steak & Potatoes	370	17	39
Lasagna: *For One*			
Cheese Lovers	350	12	43
Meat Loves	450	25	37
Veggie Lovers	400	20	41
With Meat & Sauce	360	11	42
Macaroni & Cheese: *For One*			
Macaroni & Cheese	480	21	51
Mac-FULLS: *Bowl For One*			
BBQ Pork Mac & Cheese	600	24	59
Chicken Mac & Cheese	590	22	66
Southwest Style Mac & Cheese	510	22	51
Other Entrees: *For One*			
Baked Chicken	260	11	18
Cheddar Potato Bake	510	30	44
Chicken a la King	380	13	49
Chicken Parmesan	470	19	52
Classic Meatloaf	290	12	25
Creamed Chipped Beef	340	20	19
Fish Fillet with Mac & Cheese	490	21	49
Fried Chicken	350	16	32
Rigatoni with Chicken &	410	17	40
Romano Crusted Chicken	470	19	51
Salisbury Steak	340	16	26
Spaghetti w/ Meatballs	450	13	60
Spaghetti w/ Meat Sauce	410	13	54
Swedish Meatballs	490	21	49
Tuna Noodle Casserole	390	18	38
Turkey Tetrazzini	510	27	45
White Meat Chicken Pot Pie	630	37	55
Pub Classics,			
BBQ Burger with Bacon	400	14	40

Tasty Bite (Vegetarian/Vegan):	C	F	Cb
Entrees: *Per ⅔ Cup, 4.94 oz*			
Organic Vegan:			
3 Bean Madras Lentils	140	4	19
Channa Masala	160	6	28
Chickpea Tikka Masala	170	6	22
Coconut Squash Dal	180	7	24
Indian Channa Masala	160	6	22
Jodhpur Dal	120	4	16
Vegan: Bombay Potatoes	130	5	18
Mushroom Masala	100	5	13
Punjab Eggplant	110	5	12
Spinach Dal	100	4	12
Vegetarian Entrees:			
Coconut Vegetables	130	7	13
Jaipur Vegetables	180	12	12
Kashmir Spinach	120	9	6
Mushroom Masala	100	5	13
Thai Ginger Curry	130	6	16
TGI Friday's:			
Frozen			
Angus Sliders: Classic	210	11	19
BBQ Bacon	250	14	21
Cheeseburger, with Sweet & Smokey BBQ Sce	250	13	24
Boneless Chicken Bites:			
Buffalo Style, 3 oz	160	5	18
Honey BBQ Sauce, 3 oz	150	4	18
Chicken Wings: *With Sauce*			
Buffalo Style, 3 oz	240	16	9
Honey BBQ, 3 oz	170	11	8
Restaurant Style, 3 oz	290	15	24
Mozzarella Sticks, with Marinara Sauce (3)	290	15	30
Potato Skins: Cheddar & Bacon (1)	190	10	19
Loaded	190	12	13
Spin. & Artichoke Chse Dip, 2 tbsp	30	2	2
Stuffed Jalapeno Poppers: *Per 3*			
Cheddar Flavored,	190	8	22
With Cilantro Lime Ranch Dip	220	11	25
Sweet & Smokey Meatballs (5)	320	18	23
Thai Kitchen:			
Curry & Noodle Kits (Gluten Free):			
Pad Thai	230	1	51
Rice Noodle Carts:			
Pad Thai, 9.73 oz	460	5	99
Thai Peanut, 9.77 oz	540	12	96

Trader Joe's:	C	F	Cb
Canned,			
Organic Vegetarian Chili, 8.65 oz	240	8	28
Frozen Entrees/Sides:			
Battered Fish Nuggets (4)	170	2	26
BBQ Teriyaki Chicken, 5.3 oz	240	9	11
Black Bean & Cheese Taquitos (2)	190	9	21
Breaded Shrimp, 4 oz	260	16	13
Bulgur Pilaf w/ B'nut Squash, 3.95 oz	200	10	20
Butter Chkn w/ Basmati Rice, 12.5 oz	400	13	49
Chicken Tikka Masala, 8.5 oz	360	14	39
Egg Frittata (2)	270	15	10
Hatch Chile Mac & Cheese, 6 oz	260	10	31
Jamaican Style Beef Patties (1)	440	22	45
Japchae, 6oz	190	6	34
Kalua Pork Spring Rolls (2)	290	14	33
Kung Pao Chkn with Sauce, 5.3 oz	240	10	17
Mandarin Orange Chicken, 5 oz	320	16	24
Mini Tacos: Beef (4)	270	14	23
Chicken (4)	260	13	24
Shrimp Boom Bah, 4 oz	370	30	14
S'west Style Chicken Quesadilla (1)	410	19	36
Tteok Bok Ki, 4.94 oz	280	2	61
Thai Vegetable Gyoza, 3 oz	160	5	25
Vegetable Biryani,			
with Vegetable Dumplings, 5 oz	210	6	36
Vegetable & Cheese Enchilada (2)	390	21	40
Vegan:			
Battered Fish Fillets, 3.17 oz	190	11	19
Buffalo Style Chickenless Wings (4)	270	14	21
CHICKENless Crispy Tenders (3)	170	7	14
Italian Bolognese Ravioli, 3 oz	170	6	24
Korean Beefless Bulgogi, 3.3 oz	230	11	15
Spaghetti Squash Nests			
Tyson:			
Frozen:			
Any'tizers Snacks:			
24 oz Bags Boneless Chicken Bites:			
Buffalo Style, 3 oz	190	8	18
Honey BBQ, 3 oz	190	8	18
Homestyle Chicken Fries, 3.2 oz	280	19	16
Hot Wings, Buffalo Style, 3 oz	190	13	3
Popcorn Chicken, 3 oz	170	7	14

Tyson (Cont):	C	F	Cb
Frozen:			
Breaded Chicken: *Per 3 oz Unless Indicated*			
Air Fried Breast Nuggets	160	4	15
Crispy Chicken Strips	210	10	17
Honey Battered Breast Tenders	210	13	13
Honey BBQ Chicken Strips	190	7	20
Nuggets, 3.2 oz	270	17	15
Sthrn St. Breast Tenderloins	180	9	12
Fully Cooked Steak:			
Pattie Fritters, 3.17 oz	300	21	15
Steak Fingers Shaped Patties 2.5 oz	250	18	14
Grilled Chkn Breasts: Blackened, 3 oz	110	3	1
Breast Fillets, 3.5 oz	130	5	2
Fajita Strips, 3 oz	120	4	1
Oven Roasted, Diced, 3 oz	110	3	3
Pulled	120	4	2
Refrigerated:			
Meal Kits Uncooked: *Per Kit*			
Slow Cooker:			
Beef Roast w/ Veggies	230	7	19
Pork Roast with Veggies	230	8	19
Uncle Ben's:			
Flavored Ready Rice: *Per Pouch, Unprepared*			
Butter & Garlic	220	4	42
Cheddar Broccoli	230	5	41
Cilantro Lime	240	6	41
Creamy Four Cheese,			
with Vermicelli	230	5	40
Garden Vegetable	210	3	42
Red Beans & Rice	200	3	41
Rice Pilaf	200	3	38
Roasted Chicken	210	4	41
Spanish Style	210	3	40
Van Camp's:			
Baked Beans: Orig., ½ c., 4.8 oz	150	1	30
Hickory, ½ cup, 4.8 oz	140	1	28
Beanee Weenee:			
Origina, 7.76 oz	230	6	32
Barbecue, 7.76 oz	260	6	38
Chili: No Beans, 15 oz	490	28	31
With Beans, 15 oz	490	19	55
Pork & Beans, in Tomato Sce, 4.6 oz	130	1	25

Van De Kamp's:	C	F	Cb
Frozen:			
Battered Fish: Beer Battered (2)	230	13	19
Crispy (3)	220	12	20
Crispy Haddock (2)	240	11	22
Crunchy (2)	240	11	26
Breaded Fish:			
Crunchy Sticks (6)	230	10	22
Crunchy for Sandwiches (1)	200	9	21
Whole Foods Market:			
Frozen:			
365:			
Burritos: Bean & Cheese	320	9	45
Bean & Rice, 6 oz	260	7	43
Chicken Fried Rice, 4.7 oz	160	2	28
Fish/Shrimp:			
Farmed Atlantic Salmon Fillets, 4 oz	240	15	0
Wild Caught: Gulf White Shrimp, 4 oz	100	1	0
Sockeye Salmon, 4 oz	150	5	0
Four Cheese Ravioli, 4.5 oz	280	5	42
Mac & Cheese, 7 oz	250	7	38
Organic:			
Cheese Tortellini, 4.5 oz	290	5	44
Eggplant Ravioli, 4 oz	230	5	32
Pizzas: *Per Slice*			
Cauliflower Crust, Cheese, 4 oz	220	11	16
Rising Crust: Four Cheese, 4.33 oz	300	7	42
Uncured Pepperoni, 4.44 oz	310	8	42
Thin Crust: Margherita, 5.9 oz	410	17	47
Supreme, 4.83 oz	340	15	37
Plant Based (Vegan):			
Patty (1)	80	3	7
Meatballs (6)	170	11	9
Nuggets (4)	140	6	13
Traditional Burger Patty (1)	80	3	7
Ricotta Spinach Ravioli, 4.5 oz	270	4	42
Small Bites: Mac. & Cheese (4)	210	8	27
Mozzarella Cheese Sticks (3)	320	18	24
Spanakopita (3)	190	11	16
Vegetable Egg Rolls (1)	180	6	27
Vegetable Fried Rice, 4.4 oz	140	1	29
Prepared Foods:			
Cheese Manicotti, 6.2 oz	310	9	42
Salmon Teriyaki Bowl, 14 oz	460	6	69
Spinach Minicotti, 7 oz	410	18	41
Stuffed Shells (2)	310	9	35

Yves Veggie Cuisine:	C	F	Cb
Plant Based (Vegan):			
Appetizers:			
Balls, Falafel (3)	150	7	17
Bites: Broccoli (4)	80	3	11
Kale & Quinoa (4)	90	3	13
Sweet Potato & Chickpea (4)	100	3	17
Burger Patties:			
Gluten Free Veggie (1)	110	6	5
Kale & Root Vegetables (1)	110	6	5
Deli Veggie Slices:			
Bologna (3)	60	1	2
Ham (5)	80	1	5
Pepperoni (10)	45	1	3
Salami (5)	80	1	5
Turkey (5)	80	1	4
Ground Rounds:			
Original Veggie, 1.9 oz	60	1	5
Garden Veggie Crumble, 1.9 oz	80	2	9
Veggie Dogs:			
Good Dog, 1.35 oz	45	1	2
Jumbo (1), 2.7 oz	110	2	4
The Veggie Dog (1)	50	1	2
Tofu Dog (1)	50	1	2

Other Vegan Plant Based Meals ~ See Page 124

Zatarain's:	C	F	Cb
Frozen:			
Entrees: *Per Single Serve Package Unless Indicated*			
Blackened Chicken: Alfredo	330	14	37
With Yellow Rice	510	17	70
Bourbon Chicken Pasta	460	18	52
Cajun Stule Chicken Carbonara	480	20	57
Jambalaya Flavored with Ssg	510	13	84
Sausage & Chicken Gumbo	360	14	44
Shrimp Alfredo, 1 cup, 8.64 oz	410	18	44
Rice Mixes: *Dry Mix Only*			
Black Beans & Rice, 2.32 oz	160	1	36
Black Eyed Peas & Rice, 2.32 oz	170	1	35
Bourbon Chkn Flavored Rice, 1.6 oz	160	1	36
Cajun Chicken Flavored Rice, 1.6 oz	160	1	35
Caribbean Rice Mix, 2.4 oz	250	2	53
Cilantro Lime Rice, 1.95 oz	200	1	44
Dirty Brown Rice, 1.55 oz	150	2	32
Jambalaya Rice, 1.6 oz	160	1	33
Jerk chicken, 1.6 oz	160	1	34
Spanish Rice, 1.5 oz	150	1	33
Red. Sodium: Dirty Rice, 1.34 oz	130	1	29
Jambalaya, 1.6 oz	160	1	33
Smoked Sausage: Anduille, 2 oz	170	15	1
Cajun Style, 2 oz	170	15	1

Note: Cooking reduces weight of meat by 20-45% due to water and fat losses. Average weight loss is 30%. Actual loss depends on cooking method and cooking time.

Examples:

4 oz raw weight = approx. 3 oz cooked weight

4 oz cooked weight = approx. 5½ oz raw weight

What 3 oz Cooked Meat Looks Like:

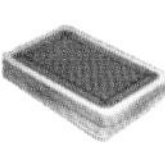

- Rectangular piece (4" x 2½" x ½" thick)
- Deck of cards (3½" x 2½" x ⅝" thick)

Quick Guide

Sirloin (Choice Grade):
External fat trimmed to ½"
Broiled, Edible Portion (no bone)

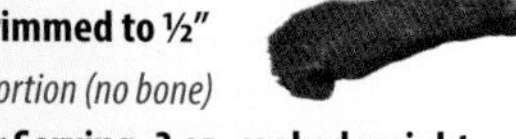

	C	F	Cb
Small/Regular Serving, 3 oz, cooked weight:			
(from 4-4½ oz raw)			
Lean + external fat (⅛"), 3 oz	**220**	**13**	**0**
Lean + marbling, 3 oz	**185**	**9**	**0**
Lean only, 3 oz	**160**	**6**	**0**
(No external fat or marbling)			
Medium Serving, 5 oz, cooked weight:			
(from approximately 7 oz raw)			
Lean + external fat (⅛"), 5 oz	**365**	**22**	**0**
Lean + marbling, 5 oz	**310**	**15**	**0**
Lean only, 5 oz	**265**	**10**	**0**
Large Serving, 8 oz, cooked weight:			
(from approximately11-12 oz raw)			
Lean + external fat (½"), 8 oz	**585**	**36**	**0**
Lean + marbling, 8 oz	**500**	**24**	**0**
Lean only, 8 oz	**425**	**15**	**0**
Extra Large Serving, 12 oz, cooked weight:			
(from approximately 16-17 oz raw)			
Lean + external fat (⅛"), 12 oz	**875**	**54**	**0**
Lean + marbling, 12 oz	**745**	**36**	**0**
Lean only, 12 oz	**640**	**22**	**0**
Pan Fried:			
Sirloin (Choice), medium serving,			
Lean + external fat (⅛"), 5 oz	**445**	**30**	**0**

Other Steaks

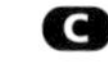  

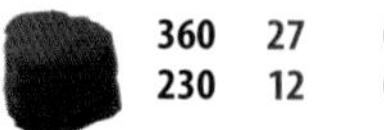

	C	F	Cb
Filet Mignon (Tenderloin):			
1 Medium steak, 6 oz raw weight:			
Broiled, with ¼" fat trim:			
Lean + fat (¼"), 4 oz	**360**	**27**	**0**
Lean only, 3.5 oz	**230**	**12**	**0**
New York/Club Steak:			
Top Loin/Short Loin:			
1 steak, regular (9.25 oz raw, ¼" fat):			
Broiled: Lean + fat (¼"), 6.3 oz	**580**	**43**	**0**
Lean + marbling, 5.5 oz	**400**	**25**	**0**
Lean only, 5.25 oz	**360**	**20**	**0**
Porterhouse Steak:			
1 Medium, 6 oz raw weight, w/out bone, broiled:			
Lean + fat (¼"), 4.3 oz	**410**	**33**	**0**
Lean only, 3.5 oz	**210**	**11**	**0**
1 Large ,12 oz raw weight, without bone, broiled:			
Lean + fat (¼") 8.5 oz cooked	**820**	**66**	**0**
Lean only, 7 oz cooked	**420**	**22**	**0**
T-Bone Steak: *Broiled or Grilled*			
Medium Size: *8 oz raw weight, without bone*			
Approximately 6 oz cooked:			
Lean + Fat (¼"), 5 oz	**400**	**28**	**0**
Lean only, 4 oz	**265**	**12**	**0**
Large Size: *12 oz raw weight*			
Approximately 9 oz cooked:			
Lean + fat (¼"), 7 oz, without bone	**560**	**39**	**0**
Lean only, 6 oz, without bone	**400**	**18**	**0**
Extra Large Size: *20 oz raw weight*			
Approximately 16 oz cooked:			
Lean + Fat (¼"), 12 oz, without bone	**960**	**66**	**0**
Lean Only, 10 oz, without bone	**660**	**30**	**0**

Also See Fast-Foods & Restaurants Section ~
Lone Star Steakhouse; Outback Steakhouse

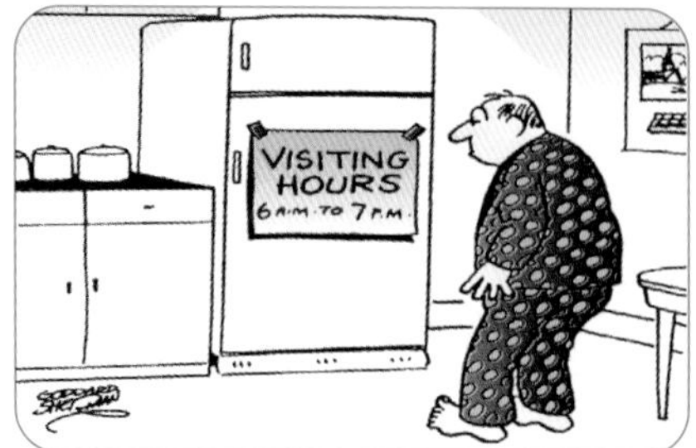

Beef – Individual Cuts

	C	F	Cb
Average All Grades			
Edible Weight, Without Bone			
Brisket, whole, braised:			
Lean + fat (¼" trim), 3 oz	**330**	**27**	0
Lean + marbling, 3 oz	**250**	**17**	0
Lean only, 3 oz	**185**	**9**	0
Chuck Blade, braised:			
Lean + fat (¼"), 3 oz	**310**	**24**	0
Lean + marbling, 3 oz	**295**	**22**	0
Lean only, 3 oz	**245**	**13**	0
Flank: Raw, 4 oz	**175**	**8**	0
Braised, 3 oz	**225**	**14**	0
Broiled, 3 oz	**155**	**6**	0
Round, bottom, braised:			
Lean + marbling, 3 oz	**190**	**8**	0
Lean only, 3 oz	**185**	**7**	0
Round, eye/tip, rstd:			
Lean + fat (¼"), 3 oz	**205**	**11**	0
Lean, w/ marbling, 3 oz	**150**	**5**	0
Round, top: *Per 3 oz, Cooked Weight*			
Braised, Lean + fat	**210**	**10**	0
Lean only	**170**	**4**	0
Broiled, Lean + fat	**180**	**8**	0
Lean only	**160**	**5**	0
Pan-fried, Lean + fat	**235**	**13**	0
Lean only	**195**	**7**	0

Beef Ribs

	C	F	Cb
Back Ribs: *7" long, visible fat trimmed to ¼"*			
10.3 oz raw w/ bone or 3.5 oz cooked, braised, w/o bone			
1 average rib	**410**	**34**	0
3 ribs	**1230**	**102**	0
Short Ribs: *2½" long, visible fat trimmed to ¼"*			
6 oz raw with bone or 2.52 oz cooked, braised, w/o bone			
1 average rib	**320**	**28**	0
3 ribs	**960**	**85**	0

Ground Beef

	C	F	Cb
Ground Beef, Raw: *Per 4 oz*			
70% lean (30% fat)	**380**	**34**	0
75% lean (25% fat)	**335**	**29**	0
80% lean (20% fat)	**290**	**23**	0
85% lean (15% fat)	**245**	**17**	0
90% lean (10% fat)	**200**	**12**	0
95% lean (5% fat)	**155**	**6**	0
Baked/Broiled: Regular (70%), 3 oz	**230**	**16**	0
Lean (80%), 3 oz	**215**	**14**	0
Extra lean (90%), 3 oz	**185**	**10**	0
Pan-Broiled:			
Regular (70%), 3 oz	**230**	**15**	0
Lean (80%), 3 oz	**210**	**14**	0
Extra lean (90%), 3 oz	**195**	**10**	0
Ground Beef Patties: *Average, 23% Fat*			
Raw, 4 oz	**330**	**25**	0
Broiled, 3 oz (from 4 oz raw)	**250**	**19**	0

Quick Guide

	C	F	Cb
Roast Beef			
Round (Eye/Tip, average): *Average All Cuts*			
Small/Regular Serving: *3 oz*			
(2 thin slices/1 thick slice)			
Lean + fat (⅛" fat trim)	**180**	**9**	0
Lean only	**145**	**4**	0
Medium Serving: *5 oz*			
(3-4 thin slices)			
Lean + fat (⅛" fat trim)	**300**	**15**	0
Lean only	**245**	**7**	0
Large Serving, 8 oz: *3 thick slices*			
Lean + fat (⅛" fat trim)	**480**	**24**	0
Lean only	**385**	**11**	0
Beef Kebab: Cooked			
Beef & Veggies, 2 oz	**160**	**10**	4
If very lean meat	**100**	**4**	4

Meat Alternatives (Vegan)

	C	F	Cb
Beyond Meat:			
Chicken Nuggets, 2.82 o	**190**	**9**	15
Crumbles: Beefy, 1.94 oz	**90**	**3**	2
Fiesty Crumbles, 1.94 oz	**90**	**3**	2
Ground Beef, 4 oz	**230**	**14**	7
Patties: Burger Patty, 4 oz	**230**	**14**	7
Steak Burger Patty,	**290**	**22**	4
Sausage, Original Brat, 2.9 oz	**180**	**11**	6
Steak, 3.1 oz	**170**	**6**	7
gardein:			
be'f: Burger, 3 oz	**130**	**5**	8
Sliders, with Bun, 2.5 oz	**130**	**3**	19
Chipotle Black Bean Slider, with Bun (1), 3 oz	**170**	**5**	26
Meatballs, (3)	**160**	**7**	9
Sliced Italian Saus'ge, 7 pieces	**110**	**6**	6
Ultimate Burgers: Black Bean (1)	**170**	**8**	15
Italian Style Chickpea (1)	**210**	**9**	21
Quorn:			
Meatless:			
ChiQin: Dippers, Original (5)	**270**	**9**	35
Pineapple Chipotle (5)	**270**	**9**	35
Diced Pieces, 3.88 oz	**120**	**3**	11
Fillets (1)	**70**	**1**	7
Tofurky:			
Burger Patty, (1), 4 oz	**250**	**16**	7
Chick'n: Barbecue, 2.65 oz	**170**	**7**	13
Lightly Seasoned, 2.65 oz	**190**	**10**	8
Roast, Ham Style w/ Ale Glaze, 3.8 oz	**220**	**7**	19

Yves Veggie Cuisine/Loma Linda ~ *See page 122*

Lamb

	C	F	Cb
Choice Grade:			
Leg (Whole), roasted:			
Lean + fat, 3 oz	220	14	0
Lean only, 3 oz	160	7	0
Leg (Sirloin Half), roasted:			
Lean + fat, 3 oz	250	18	0
Lean only, 3 oz	175	8	0
Leg (Shank Half), roasted:			
Lean + fat, 3 oz	190	11	0
Lean only, 3 oz	155	6	0
Loin Chop, broiled:			
1 chop (raw weight,4.25 oz):			
Lean + fat (2.25 oz edible)	180	12	0
Lean only (1.6 oz edible)	85	4	0
Rib Chop, broiled:			
1 chop (raw wt., 3.5 oz):			
Lean + fat (2.5 oz edible)	255	21	0
Lean only (1.75 oz edible)	105	6	0
Shoulder (Arm/Blade):			
Braised: Lean + fat, 3 oz	295	21	0
Lean only, 3 oz	240	12	0
Broiled: Lean + fat, 3 oz	240	17	0
Lean only, 3 oz	170	8	0
Roasted: Similar to Broiled			
Cubed Lamb (Leg/Shoulder):			
For stew or kebab:			
Braised, lean only, 3 oz	190	8	0
Broiled, lean only, 3 oz	160	6	0

Veal

	C	F	Cb
Edible Weights:			
Leg (Top Round):			
Braised: Lean + fat, 3 oz	180	6	0
Lean only, 3 oz	175	5	0
Pan-fried, breaded:			
Lean + fat, 3 oz	195	8	9
Lean only, 3 oz	185	6	9
Pan-fried, not breaded:			
Lean + fat, 3 oz	180	7	0
Lean only, 3 oz	155	4	0
Roasted: Lean + fat, 3 oz	135	4	0
Lean only, 3 oz	130	3	0

Veal (Cont)

	C	F	Cb
Loin Chop: *1 chop, 7 oz raw weight*			
Braised: Lean + fat, 3 oz	240	15	0
Lean only, 3 oz	190	8	0
Roasted: Lean + fat, 3 oz	185	11	0
Lean only, 3 oz	150	6	0
Rib, roasted: *Lean + fat, 3 oz*	195	12	0
Lean only, 3 oz	150	7	0
Shoulder, Arm/Blade, roasted:			
Lean + fat, 3 oz	155	7	0
Lean only, 3 oz	140	5	0
Sirloin, roasted:			
Lean + fat, 3 oz	170	9	0
Lean only, 3 oz	145	6	0
Cubed for Stew, braised:			
Leg/Shoulder, lean only, 3 oz	160	4	0
(1 lb raw yields approximately 9.25 oz cooked)			

Pork

	C	F	Cb
Fresh Pork: *Cooked Weight, without bone):* *4 oz raw weight = approx. 3 oz cooked weight*			
BBQ, Pulled:			
2 oz	90	3	10
4 oz	180	5	20
8oz	360	10	40
Blade Steak, broiled:			
Lean + fat, 3 oz	220	15	0
Lean only, 3 oz	190	11	0
Country Style Ribs, broiled/roasted:			
Lean + fat, 3 oz	280	22	0
Lean only, 3 oz	210	13	0
Spareribs, braised: *Lean & fat, 6 oz*			
(from 1 lb raw weight)	675	52	0
Leg (Ham), whole, roasted:			
Lean + fat, 3 oz	230	15	0
Lean only, 3 oz	180	8	0
Loin Chops, broiled: *Average*			
(From 1 chop: 5 oz raw weight with bone or 4 oz raw weight, without bone)			
Lean + fat, 3 oz	200	11	0
Lean only, 3 oz	165	7	0
Loin Roast, roasted:			
Lean + fat, 3 oz	210	13	0
Lean only, 3 oz	180	8	0
Rib Chops, (Boneless), broiled:			
Lean + fat, 3 oz	220	14	0
Lean only, 3 oz	185	9	0
Rib Roast:			
Lean + fat, 3 oz	215	13	0
Lean only, 3 oz	180	9	0

Pork (Cont)

	C	F	Cb
Sirloin Chop, broiled:			
Lean + fat, 3 oz	180	8	0
Lean only, 3 oz	165	6	0
Sirloin Roast, roasted:			
Lean + fat, 3 oz	175	8	0
Lean only, 3 oz	170	7	0
Tenderloin (Boneless), roasted:			
Lean + fat, 3 oz	125	4	0
Lean only, 3 oz	120	3	0
Ground Pork:			
Raw, average, 1/4 lb, 4 oz	300	24	0
Broiled, 3 oz	250	18	0
Pan-fried, drained, 3 oz	260	19	0

Bacon

	C	F	Cb
Raw: 1 med. slice, 0.75 oz	95	9	0
1 thick slice, 1.3 oz	175	17	0
(1 lb raw yields approximately 5 oz cooked)			
Broiled/Pan-Fried:			
1 medium slice, 0.3 oz	40	3	0
3 medium slices, 0.8	125	10	0
2 thin slices, 0.5 oz	75	6	0
1 thick slice, 0.9 oz	65	5	0
Canadian Bacon:			
Cooked: 1 slice, 1 oz	45	2	1
2 slices, 2 oz	90	4	1
Bacon Bits, 1 Tbsp, 0.3 oz	35	2	0
Breakfast Strips, Broiled, 1 sl., 0.4 oz	50	4	0

Ham

	C	F	Cb
Boneless Ham, cooked:			
Regular, (approximately 13% fat):			
Roasted, 3 oz	150	8	0
Extra Lean (5% fat),			
Roasted, 3 oz	125	5	0
Whole Ham, cooked:			
Lean + fat (as purchased)			
Roasted, 3 oz	210	15	0
Lean only, Roasted, 3 oz	135	5	0
Canned Ham: *Similar to boneless ham*			
Chopped, canned, 3 oz	200	16	0
Ham Patties, cooked, (1), 2.3 oz	220	20	1
Ham Steak, extra lean, 2 oz	70	2	0

Lunch Slices ~ *See Deli Meats, Page 128*

Game & Other Meats

	C	F	Cb
Bison Steak,			
lean, 6 oz (raw)	205	4	0
Boar (wild), roasted, 3 oz	140	4	0
Buffalo Steak,			
New West Foods, 4 oz	70	3	0
Caribou, roasted, 3 oz	140	4	0
Deer/Venison, roasted 3 oz	135	3	0
Goat (Capretto):			
Raw, 3 oz	95	2	0
Roasted, 3 oz	120	2	0
Ostrich:			
Blackwing Ostrich Meats:			
Sausage Patties, 4 oz	110	1	0
Strip Filet, 6 oz	160	1	0
New West Foods:			
Ground Ostrich, 4 oz	165	7	0
Ostrich Steak, 4 oz steak	130	2	0
Rabbit: Roasted, 3 oz	165	7	0
Stewed, 1 cup, diced, 5 oz	290	12	0

Variety & Organ Meats

	C	F	Cb
Brain (Lamb): Braised, 3 oz	125	9	0
Pan-fried, 3 oz	230	19	0
Chitterlings, pork, simmered, 3 oz	260	25	0
Ears, pork, simmered, 1 ear, 4 oz	185	12	0
Feet, Pork: Simmered, 3 oz	200	14	0
Cured, pickled, 3 oz	170	14	0
Hormel, 2 oz	80	6	0
Head Cheese (Pork Snouts/Ears/Vinegar/Spices)			
1 oz slice	50	4	0
Heart, Beef, braised, 3 oz	140	4	0
Jowl, pork, raw, 4 oz	750	80	0
Kidneys, braised, 3 oz	140	5	0
Liver (beef): Raw, 4 oz	150	4	4
Braised, 3 oz	140	4	3
Pan-fried, 3 oz	185	7	7
Pancreas, pork, braised, 3 oz	185	8	0
Pork Cracklins, 0.5 oz	80	6	0
Pork Hocks, 1 piece, 6 oz	340	23	0
Scrapple, pork, 2 oz	120	8	8
Spleen, pork, braised, 3 oz	130	3	0
Stomach, pork, raw, 4 oz	185	12	0
Sweetbreads:			
Beef,/Lamb, cooked, 3 oz	125	9	0
Tail, pork, simmered, 3 oz	340	31	0
Tongue: Raised Veal, 3 oz	170	9	0
Beef/Lamb/Pork, av., 3 oz	235	17	0
Tripe, beef, raw, 3 oz	85	4	0

Quick Guide

	C	F	Cb
Franks & Weiners			
Average All Brands			
Regular (Pork Mix): *Per Frank*			
Regular, 1.5 oz	140	13	1
Bun Length/Jumbo, 2 oz	185	17	2
Extra Long, 2.75 oz	255	24	2
Small/Cocktail, each	30	3	1
Beef Franks: *Per Frank*			
Regular, 1.5 oz	140	13	2
Bun Length/Jumbo, 2 oz	175	17	3
1/4 lb Dog, 4 oz	375	33	5

Franks & Weiners

	C	F	Cb
Ball Park: *Per Link*			
Angus Beef,			
Oriinal; Bun Size, 1.76 oz	160	15	2
Beef:			
Original; Bun Size, 1.87 oz	170	15	4
Grillmaster, Hearty, 2.9 oz	260	24	3
Classic: Original, Bun Size, 1.87 oz	130	11	2
Nacho Cheese, 1.87 oz	130	11	3
Prime Beef, 2.7 oz	180	20	2
Turkey, 1.76 oz	120	7	6
Foster Farms, Chicken; Turkey, 2 oz	140	12	1
Hebrew National: *Per Link*			
Beef: Regular, 1.7 oz	150	13	2
97% Fat-Free, 1.6 oz	45	1	2
All Natural, 1.73oz	140	12	2
Jumbo, 3 oz	260	23	3
Quarter Pound, ½ frank, 2 oz	170	15	2
Reduced Fat, 1.6 oz	100	8	2
Jennie-O: *PerLink*			
Turkey Franks,			
Jumbo,	120	9	2
40% Less Fat, 2 oz	120	9	2
Turkey Sausages:			
Hot Italian, 3.7 oz	150	10	0
Sweet Italian, 3.84 oz	160	10	0
Oscar Mayer: *Per Link*			
Uncured Beef Franks:			
Original, 1.48 oz	140	13	1
Jumbo; Bun Length, 1.87 oz	170	16	2
Uncured Cheese Dogs,			
Velveta, 1.6 oz	110	10	1
Shelton's: *Per Link*			
Uncured Chicken, 1.2 oz	80	7	0
Italian Turkey, 2 oz	170	15	0

Quick Guide

	C	F	Cb
Fresh Sausages			
Pork/Beef: *Average All Types*			
Small: Raw, 4" link, 1 oz	85	8	0
Broiled/Pan-fried	80	7	0
Medium: Raw, 2 oz	170	15	0
Broiled/Pan-fried	165	14	0
Large: Raw, 3 oz	255	22	0
Broiled/Pan-fried	245	21	0
Italian: Raw, 3.2 oz	315	28	1
Cooked, 2.4 oz	230	18	3
Chorizo: Beef Chorizo, 2.5 oz piece	250	23	5
Pork Chorizo, 2 oz piece	250	23	5

Note: Fat is lost in broiling/pan frying. Cooked weight = approx. 60-70% raw weight

Smoked Sausages

	C	F	Cb
Per 2 oz Link:			
Butterball, Turkey	90	6	5
Eckrich:			
Original, Natural Casing	200	17	4
Skinless: Beef Rop	190	15	5
Cheddar	190	16	5
Jalapeno & Cheddar	190	15	5
Hillshire Farm:			
Basil Pesto Chicken	110	7	3
Beef	170	14	3
Cheddarwurst	180	16	2
Chicken	100	7	3
Hot Smoked	180	16	3
Johnsonville ~ *See CalorieKing.Com*			

Breakfast Sausages/Patties

	C	F	Cb
Butterball: *Fully Cooked*			
Turkey, Sausage Links (3), 2 oz	110	7	0
Jimmy Dean: *Fully Cooked*			
Heat 'N Serve Sausage Links:			
Original (3), 2 oz	220	19	2
Pork (3), 2.4 oz	270	26	1
Turkey (3), 2 oz	130	8	2
Heat 'N Serve Sausage Patties:			
Pork, Original (2), 1.8 oz	210	20	1
Turkey (2), 1.8 oz	120	8	1
Maple Pork, 2 oz	215	19	2
Sage Pork, 2 oz	210	19	2
Breakfast Sandwiches ~ *See Page 92*			
Jones Dairy Farm:			
Golden Brown Sausages: *Fully Cooked*			
Mild/Maple Pork (3), average, 2 oz	250	24	2

Vegetarian Patties:

Boca ~ *See Page 112*
GardenBurer ~ *See Page 113*

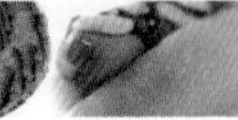

Bagel, Corn & Hot Dogs

	C	F	Cb
Hot Dogs, Ready-To-Go:			
Includes Ketchup/Relish			
Regular, 1.5 oz frank, 1.5 oz bun	260	15	22
Bun Length, 2 oz frank, 1.5 oz bun	290	18	21
Jumbo Dog, 2 oz frank, 2 oz bun	360	20	36
¼ lb Beef Dog, 2 oz bun	480	15	36
Mile Long Dog, 2.6 oz dog, 1.5 oz bun	360	24	23
Corn Dogs:			
Beef/Pork Frank, average, 2.6 oz	170	10	16
Foster Farms:			
Corn Dogs:			
Honey Crunchy:			
Regular (1), 2.7 oz	190	9	18
Mini (4), 2.7 oz	220	13	19
Gluten Free, 2.7 oz	180	9	20
Jumbo, 4 oz	280	14	27
Schwanns,			
Yelloh!, Mini Corn Dog, (4), 2.7 oz	200	10	23
State Fair: *Per Dog*			
Beef Corn Dog, 2.7 oz	240	13	26
Classic Corn Dog: Regular, 3.3 oz	220	11	23
Mini (5), 3.3 oz	230	14	18
Bagel Dogs:			
Hebrew National,			
Beef Bagel Dogs, 4 pieces, 2.75 oz	240	13	22
Schwanns,			
Yelloh!, Bagel Dogs w/ Cheese (1)	360	15	38
Vienna Beef,			
Mini Bagel Dogs (5), 4.6 oz	310	18	31
Hot Dog Toppings/Extras:			
American Cheese, 1 slice, 1 oz	110	9	1
Chili Con Carne, ¼ cup	50	2	6
Ketchup, 1 Tbsp	15	0	4
Mustard, 1 Tbsp	20	0	1
Onions, chopped, 1 Tbsp	5	0	1
Pickle Relish, 1 Tbsp	20	0	5
Sauerkraut, ½ cup	20	0	5

Deli/Lunch Meats & Sausage

	C	F	Cb
Beef Jerky/Meat Snacks,			
Berliner (pork/beef), 1 oz	65	5	1
Beerwurst (Beef):			
Small (2¾"diam), 1/16" slice	20	2	0
Large (4" diam), ⅛" slice	75	7	1
Beerwurst (Pork):			
Small (2.75"diameter), 1/16" slice	15	1	0
Large (4"diameter), ⅛" Slice	55	4	1
Blood Sausage, 1 oz	100	9	1

Deli/Lunch Meats & Sausages (Cont)

	C	F	Cb
Bologna:			
Beef Bologna: 1 slice, 1 oz	90	8	0
Light, 1 slice, 1 oz	60	4	2
Oscar Mayer, Regular, 1 oz	90	8	1
Chicken & Pork Bologna,			
Oscar Mayer, with added Beef, 1 oz	80	7	0
Pork Bologna: 1 Slice, 1 oz	65	6	1
Fat-Free, 1 slice, 1 oz	20	0	2
Pork & Beef,			
Boar's Head, 2 oz	150	13	1
Turkey Bologna, av., 1 oz	60	5	1
Oscar Mayer, 1 oz	50	4	1
Bratwurst, average, 1 oz	80	7	1
Braunschweiger, (Pork/Liver/Sausage),			
Oscar Mayer, Liver, 2 oz	190	14	1
Chicken, average:			
1 thick or 2 thin slices, 1 oz	30	1	1
2 oz slice	60	2	2
Hillshire Farm,			
Rotisserie S'snd Chicken Breast, 2 oz	60	1	1
Corned Beef, average, full fat, 1 oz	60	5	1
Ham, Sliced: *Per 1 oz Slice*			
Baked/Broiled	35	1	1
Honey/Brown Sugar, average	35	1	1
Oscar Mayer,			
Honey Ham, 2.26 oz	70	2	3
Prosciutto, average	70	5	0
Ham & Cheese Loaf, average, 1 oz	70	5	1
Oscar Mayer, 1 oz	70	6	3
Italian Sausage, 2.6 oz	250	20	3
Kielbasa: Polish Sausage, 2 oz	65	5	1
Beef, 2 oz link	190	17	1
Knockwurst, av., 1 oz	90	8	1
Linguica *(Gaspar's),* Mild, 2 oz	130	9	1
Liverwurst, 1 oz	65	5	2
Liver Pate, fresh, average, 1 oz	90	8	1
Mortadella: 1 oz	105	9	0
Boar's Head, 6 slices	160	14	0
Olive Loaf: Average, 1 oz	70	5	3
Oscar Mayer, 1 oz	80	6	3
Pancetta, *Boars Head, 0. 5 oz slice*	50	5	0

Deli/Lunch Meats & Sausages (Cont)

	C	F	Cb
Pastrami (Beef):			
Boar's Head:			
1st cut Pastrami Brisket, 2 oz	90	4	2
Top Round Pastrami, 2 oz	80	3	1
Hillshire, Deli Select, Ultra Thin. 2 oz	60	2	1
Peppered Beef, 1 oz slice	40	2	1
Pepperoni, 5 slices, 1 oz	140	13	0
Pickle Loaf, average, 1 oz	70	5	5
Pickle & Pepper Loaf, *Boars Head,* 2 oz	150	13	2
Proscuitto/Proscuitti, av., 1 oz	70	5	1
Roast Beef, Lean, 1 oz	40	2	0
Salami:			
Beef, average, 1 oz	80	7	1
Beef Chicken Pork,			
Oscar Mayer: Cotto, 1 slice, 1 oz	50	4	0
Beer Salami, average, 1 oz	50	4	1
Pork: Genoa, sliced, average, 1 oz	100	8	1
Boarshead, 2 oz	190	15	1
Fortuna's Stick, 1 oz	110	8	1
Pork & Beef:			
Dry, Hard, av., 1 oz	100	8	1
Boar's Head, 1 oz	110	9	1
Oscar Mayer, Hard, 1 slice, 0.95 oz	100	8	1
SPAM (Hormel): *Per 2 oz*			
Classic: 2 oz serving	180	16	1
7 oz can	630	56	4
12 oz can	1080	96	6
Spam Lite: 2 oz	110	8	1
12 oz can	660	48	6
Other Varieties: *Per 2 oz Unless Indicated*			
Hickory Smoke Flavor	180	16	1
Hot & Spicy	160	14	1
Maple Flavored	180	16	3
Oven Roasted Turkey	80	5	1
Spam Spread	160	12	5
Spam with Bacon	180	16	1
25% Less Sodium	180	16	1
Spam Singles: *Per 3 oz*			
Classic, 2.5 oz package	210	18	2
Lite, 2.5 oz package	130	9	2

Deli/Lunch Meats & Sausages (Cont)

	C	F	Cb
Summer Sausage:			
Beef:			
Armour, 2 oz	190	17	2
Hillshire Farm, 2 oz	190	16	1
Old Wisconsin, 2 oz	180	14	2
Treet *(Armour),* Luncheon Loaf, Original, 2 oz	140	11	4
Turkey, average: 1 oz slice	30	1	1
0.8 oz slice	22	1	1
Turkey Breast:			
Butterball, Roasted: 1 slice 1 oz	50	1	1
Hillshire, Oven Roasted, Thin Sliced, 2 oz	50	1	2
Turkey Ham, 1 slice, 1 oz	35	2	1
Turkey Loaf, 1 oz	30	1	1
Turkey Pastrami, 1 oz	35	2	1
Turkey Roll, 1 oz	40	2	1

Vegetarian Deli ~ *See Page 118*

Meat Spread

	C	F	Cb
Average All Brands:			
Chicken, white meat, 2oz	140	11	2
Corned Beef, 2 oz	140	11	1
Ham, Deviled, 2 oz	180	15	1
Liverwurst, 2 oz	160	13	4
Roast Beef, 2 oz	130	10	2
Turkey, 2 oz	110	7	2
Underwood: *Per 2.1 oz*			
Deviled Ham	180	15	1
Liverwurst	160	13	4
Roast Beef	140	10	2
White Meat Chicken	130	8	3

Paté

	C	F	Cb
Les Trois Petit Cochons: *Per 2 oz*			
Pate: au Poivre Noir	210	19	2
de Campagne	250	24	0
Mousse: de Foie De Canard Au Porto	170	15	3
Du Perigord	160	14	3
Truffle	170	14	2
Vegan, Garden Vegetable Terrine	50	3	4
Old Wisconsin Pate, Braunschweiger, 2 oz	210	18	3

Nuts

Per 1 oz Unless Indicated	C	F	Cb
Acorns, raw 1 oz	110	7	12
Almonds: Dried/Dry Roasted:			
Whole: 12 medium size, 0.5 oz	85	8	3
23-25 medium size, 1 oz	170	15	6
½ cup, 2.5 oz	420	37	13
Ground, 1 cup, 3.4 oz	545	47	20
Sliced, ½ cup, 1.6 oz	260	22	10
Slivered, ½ cup, 2 oz	310	27	12
Chocolate Coated (5-6), 1 oz	150	10	15
Honey Roasted, 1 oz	170	14	8
Oil Roasted (*Blue Diamond*), 1 oz	170	16	5
Brazil Nuts, 8 medium, 1 oz	185	19	3
Cashews, dry or oil roasted:			
14 large/18 med./26 small: 1 oz	165	14	9
½ cup, 2.4 oz	375	31	20
Honey Roasted, 1 oz	165	13	10
Chestnuts:			
Average, dried, 1 oz	105	1	22
Raw/Fresh, 5-6 nuts, 1 oz	60	0	13
Canned, water chestnuts, sliced/whole/drained, 1 oz	30	0	7
Coconut, Fresh:			
1 piece, 2"x2"x ½ ", 1 oz	185	18	7
Shredded, fresh, ½ cup, 1.4 oz	140	13	6
Dried (Desiccated):			
Sweetened: Shredded, 1 oz	145	10	14
Grated, ½ cup, 1.3 oz	185	13	18
Unsweetened, 1 oz	185	18	7
Cream (canned), ½ cup, 5.2 oz	285	26	12
Milk (canned), unsweetened, ¼ cup, 2 fl.oz	100	10	3
Water (center liquid), ½ cup, 4.3 oz	25	0	5
Filberts or Hazelnuts:			
Shelled, 18-20 nuts	180	17	5
Chopped, ¼ cup, 1 oz	180	18	5
Ground, ¼ cup, 0.6 oz	120	12	3
Ginkgo Nuts, canned, 14 med., 1 oz	32	1	7
Hickory, 30 small nuts, 1 oz	200	18	5
Macadamia Nuts, Shelled:			
Raw or Dry Roasted, avg:			
12 small or 8 med., 1 oz	200	21	4
6-7 large, 1 oz	200	21	4
½ cup, 2.3 oz	480	51	10
Mixed Nuts: Raw, 18-22 nuts, 1 oz	170	15	7
Oil Roasted, all types	170	16	6
Sweet Roasts, 26 pieces, 1 oz	160	12	10
Planters, Dry Roasted/Honey, 1 oz	150	11	11
Nut Toppings, chopped, 1 Tbsp, 0.3 oz	40	4	2

Per 1 oz Unless Indicated	C	F	Cb
Peanuts:			
Dry or oil roasted, average:			
Small handful, ¾ oz	125	10	4
⅕ cup, 1 oz	165	14	6
½ cup, 2.5 oz	415	35	15
3 oz bag	500	42	18
7 oz bag	1160	98	42
Raw: Shelled, 1 oz	160	14	5
In shell, 1 oz	115	110	3
Planters:			
Cocktail, all varieties	170	14	5
Honey Roasted	160	13	7
Spanish Redskins	170	15	4
Sweet N' Crunchy	140	8	15
Japanese Style Peanuts, Coated in Crunchy Shell	150	8	13
Pecans, roasted:			
10 halves, 0.5 oz	95	10	2
20 Halves, 1 oz	195	20	4
1 cup, halves, 3.5 oz	680	71	14
Pilinuts, dried, 1 oz	215	24	1
Pine Nuts, dried, 1 Tbsp, 0.3 oz	70	7	2
Pistachios, raw:			
Shelled, 45 nuts, 1 oz	160	13	8
Unshelled, 2 oz	165	14	7
Lance, Roasted, 1.5 oz	120	9	6
Sesame Nut Mix, 1 oz	160	13	9
Soy Nuts: Dry Roasted	130	6	9
½ cup, 3 oz	390	18	28
Revival, Chocolate Covered, 2 oz	200	12	20
Trail Mix *(Planters):*			
Dessert Mixes: Banana Sundae, 1 oz	150	10	13
Oatmeal Raisin Cookie, 1 oz	140	7	17
Turtle Sundae, 1 oz	160	11	13
Energy Mix, 1.4 oz	240	19	14
Peanut Butter Chocolate, 1.15 oz	180	12	13
Spicy Nuts & Cajun Sticks, 1 oz	150	11	11
Sweet & Salty, 1.1 oz	150	9	15
Tropical Fruit, 1.1 oz	150	9	15
Walnuts, average all types:			
7-10 halves, 0.5 oz	90	9	2
15-20 halves, 1 oz	175	17	3
Chopped, ½ cup, 2.2 oz	380	36	6
Ground, ¼ cup, 0.7 oz	130	13	3

Quick Guide

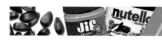

	C	F	Cb
Peanut Butter: *Average All Brands*			
1 level tsp, 0.2 oz	35	3	1
1 level Tbsp, 0.6 oz	100	9	4
1 oz Quantity	165	14	6
½ cup, 5 oz	835	72	29

Peanut Butter ~ Brands

	C	F	Cb
Jif: *Per 2 Tbsp*			
Creamy, 1.2 oz	190	16	8
Regular: With Honey, 1.2oz	190	15	10
No Added Sugar, 1.16oz	200	17	7
Reduced Fat, all varieties, 1.27 oz	190	12	15
Laura Scudder's: *Per 2 Tbsp*			
Natural: Smooth; Nutty, 1.13 oz	190	16	7
Smooth, Unsalted, 1.13 oz	190	16	7
Organic, Nutty, 1.13 oz	180	16	5
Peter Pan: *Per 2 Tbsp*			
Creamy/Crunchy, 1.13 oz	200	16	7
Honey Roast Creamy, 1.2oz	200	14	
Natural, Creamy, 1.16 oz	210	17	6
Planters, Creamy/Crunchy, 2 Tbsp	180	15	8
Smucker's, Goober, Grape/Srawberry, av., 3 Tbsp. 2 oz	220	11	30
Skippy: *Per 2 Tbsp*			
Blended w/ Plant Protein, 1.16 oz	210	16	6
Creamy, 1.16 oz	190	16	6
No Sugar AddedVarieties, 1.16 oz	210	18	4

Peanut Butter & Jelly Sandwich

	C	F	Cb
1 sandwich: *With 2 oz Bread*			
Thin Spread, 1 Tbsp Peanut Butter + 1 Tbsp Jelly	310	10	48
Thick Spread, 2 Tbsp Peanut Butter + 2 Tbsp Jelly	480	19	67

Nut & Chocolate Spread

	C	F	Cb
Nutella:			
1 Tbsp, 0.7 oz	110	6	11
2 Tbsp, 1.3 oz	200	11	22

Note: Nutella contains approx. 50% sugar & 13% hazelnuts

Other Nut & Seed Butters

Per 1 Tbsp, 0.5 oz	C	F	Cb
Almond Butter	100	10	4
Cashew Butter	95	8	5
Hazelnut Butter; Pecan Butter	110	10	2
Pistachio Butter	90	7	5
Sesame Butter (Tahini)	90	8	3
Soy Nut Butter	75	5	4

Seeds

	C	F	Cb
Alfalfa Seeds, sprouted, ½ cup, 0.5 oz	5	0	1
Caraway/Fennel, 1 tsp	7	1	1
Chia Seeds: 1 Tbsp, 0.4 oz	45	3	4
3 Tbsp, 1 oz	140	9	12
Cottonseed Kernels, roasted, 1 Tbsp	50	4	2
Flaxseeds, 3 Tbsp, 1 oz	140	9	9
Hemp Seeds, 3 Tbsp, 1 oz	160	14	3
Lotus Seeds, dried, ½ cup, 0.5 oz	55	1	10
Poppy Seeds, 1 tsp	15	1	1
Pumpkin/Pepita Seeds, whole:			
Roasted/Tamari: 1 oz	150	12	4
½ cup, 4 oz	590	48	15
Dried (hulled), ¼ cup, 1 oz	155	13	5
Safflower Kernels, dried, 1 oz	150	11	10
Sesame Seeds:			
Dried, 1 Tbsp, 0.3 oz	50	5	2
Roasted/Toasted, 1 oz	160	14	8
Sunflower Kernels/Seeds:			
Dried, ¼ cup w/out hulls, 0.3 oz	200	18	7
Dry Roasted: 1 Tbsp, 0.3 oz	45	4	2
¼ cup, 1 oz	165	14	7
Oil Roasted, ⅕ cup, 1 oz	170	14	7
Watermelon Seeds, dried, ¼ cup, 1 oz	150	13	4

Nut eaters are healthier and live longer, say scientists.

Nuts are a nutritious source of protein, vitamins, minerals, fiber, healthy fats, and antioxidants.

The fat and fiber of nuts can help reduce blood cholesterol. Their protein and fiber also promotes meal satiety (fullness) and reduces hunger levels – of benefit in weight control.

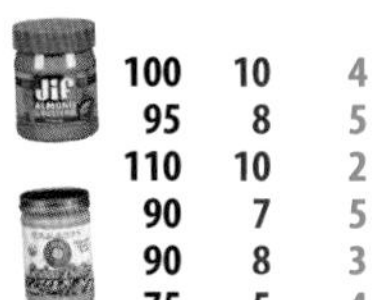

Eat nuts instead of high-sugar snacks, candy and soft drinks. Add chopped nuts to breakfast cereals.

Quick Guide

	C	F	Cb
Pancakes:			
Plain: *Average All Types*			
Small (3" diameter), 0.8 oz	50	2	6
Medium (4" diameter), 1.3 oz	85	4	11
Large (6" diameter), 2.5 oz	175	8	22
Add Extra for Syrups/Butter			
Pancake Syrup: Regular, 1 Tbsp	50	0	12
¼ cup, 4 Tbsp	185	0	49
Lite, 1 Tbsp	25	0	7
¼ cup, 4 Tbsp	100	0	27
Butter/Margarine:			
Regular, 1 Tbsp	100	11	0
Whipped, 1 Tbsp	65	8	0
Waffles:			
Homemade, 7" waffle, 2.5 oz	220	11	25
Frozen + Toasted, (4" diam.), 1 oz	105	3	16

Pancake Brands

	C	F	Cb
Prepared as Directed			
Bisquick: *Prepared with Water*			
Pancake/Waffle Mix: *Per 1.4 oz*			
Original Pancake & Baking Mix	140	2	30
Hungry Jack: *Just Add Water*			
Complete Pancake Mix: *Makes 3 x 4" Pancakes*			
Buttermilk, 1.34 oz	130	1	28
Chocolate Chip, 1.34 oz	130	2	27
Extra Light & Fluffy, 1.34 oz	130	1	28
Kodiak: *Just Add Water*			
Power Cakes Flapjack & Waffle Mix:			
Original, 1.87 oz	180	4	29
Carb Consious, Buttermilk, 1.87 oz	220	11	21
Northern Pines, Just Add Water,			
Premium Mix (3), prepared	200	4	38
Pearl Mining: *Prepared*			
Mixes: *Makes 4" Pancakes*			
Original (2)	190	6	28
Buttermilk (2)	180	6	26
Complete, Apple Cinnamon	160	2	33
On The Go, average, 2 oz mix	225	5	42

Frozen Breakfasts

	C	F	Cb
Eggo *(Kellogg's):*			
French Toaster Sticks:			
Original (2)	210	6	37
Cinnamon (2)	220	5	40
Mini Toast:			
Berry Blast, 3.25 oz	260	8	43
Cinnamon, 3.25 oz	290	10	47
Pancakes:			
Blueberry (3)	250	7	44
Buttermilk (3)	250	8	40
Chocolatey Chip (3)	260	8	44
Minis, Buttermilk Pancakes, (11)	270	8	44
Pillsbury:			
Pancakes:			
Homestlye, (3)	240	4	45
Mini, Funfetti Buttermilk(11)	250	5	45

Frozen Waffles

	C	F	Cb
Eggo *(Kellogg's):*			
Blueberry; Strawberry (2)	180	6	29
Buttermilk (2)	180	6	28
Chocolatey Chip (2)	200	7	32
Homestystyle (2)	180	5	30
Grab & Go Liege Style:			
Buttery Maple Flavored (1)	230	10	30
Strawberry (1)	230	10	30
Vanilla Bean (1)	230	10	29
Thick & Fluffy:			
Original (1)	160	7	23
Cinnamon Brown Sugar (1)	170	6	25
Double Chocolately (1)	170	6	27
Nature's Path:			
Buckwheat Wildberry (2)	190	6	33
Chia Plus (2)	190	7	31
Dark Chocolate Chip (2)	180	6	33
Flax Plus (2)	200	8	30
Homestyle (2)	200	7	33
Pumpkin Spice (2)	180	6	31
Van's:			
Gluten Free: Original (2)	180	7	28
Apple Cinnamon (2)	220	7	33
Blueberry (2)	220	8	35
Multigrain (2)	140	5	20
Protein: Original (2)	200	7	26
Blueberry (2)	210	7	27
Chocolate Chip (2)	250	9	30

Spaghetti/Pasta

- Pasta includes all shapes and sizes; (e.g. spaghetti, fettuccini, elbows, shells, twists, sheets, cannelloni, linguini, tubes, ziti).
- All regular pasta products have the same cals/fat/carbs on a weight basis.
- 1 oz Dry = approximately 2.5 -3 oz cooked.

Dry Spaghetti/Pasta

	C	F	Cb
1 oz quantity	105	1	21
1lb box/pkg, 16 oz	1685	7	339
Elbows, 1 cup, 4 oz	380	2	80
Shells, small, 1 cup, 3.3 oz	330	2	69
Spirals, 1 cup, 3 oz	305	2	64
Barilla:			
Blue Box: Angel Hair, 2 oz	200	1	42
Fettuccini, 2 oz	200	1	42
Other varieties, 2 oz	200	1	42
Great Value:			
Angel Hair, 2 oz	200	1	41
Penne Rigate, 2 oz	200	1	42
Rigatoni, 2 oz	200	1	41

Cooked Spaghetti/Pasta

	C	F	Cb
Plain, All Types (no added fat):			
Firm/Al Dente (8-10 minutes), 1 oz	42	1	8.5
Medium (11-13 minutes), 1 oz	37	1	7.5
Tender (14-20 minutes), 1 oz	32	1	7
Longer cooking increases water absorbed			
Spaghetti: ½ cup, 2.5 oz	90	1	18
Medium serving, 1 cup, 5 oz	225	2	44
Large serving, 2 cups, 10 oz	450	3	88
Extra large, 3 cups, 15 oz	675	5	132
Elbows/Spirals, 1 cup, 5 oz	220	2	43
Small Shells, 1 cup, 4 oz	180	1	36
Protein-fortified:			
Dry, 1 c., 3.4 oz	350	2	63
Cooked, 1 cup, 5 oz	230	1	45
Spinach/Vegetable:			
Dry, 1 cup, 3 oz	310	1	61
Cooked, 1 cup, 5 oz	180	1	38
Whole-wheat:			
Dry, 1 cup, 3.8 oz	365	2	79
Cooked, 1 cup, 5 oz	175	1	37

Fresh Pasta (Refrigerated)

	C	F	Cb
Average All Brands:			
Plain/Spinach/Tomato:			
As purchased, 4.5 oz	370	3	70
Cooked, 1 cup, 5 oz	185	2	35
Home-made, w/o egg, cooked, 1 c. 5 oz	175	1	35
Buitoni:			
Cut Pasta:			
Angel Hair, 2.8 oz	220	2	45
Fettuccine/Linguine, av., 3 oz	235	2	46
House Foods:			
Tofu Shirataki Noodles:			
Angel Hair/Fettuccini, Macaroni/Spaghetti, 4 oz	20	1	6
Nasoya,			
Shirataki Spaghetti, Pasta Zero, ⅔ cup, 4 oz	15	0	4

Macaroni & Cheese

	C	F	Cb
Packaged (Kraft) ~ *See Page 116*			
Restaurant: *Average*			
Side Serve, 6 oz	265	13	26
Medium serve, 1 cup, 9 oz	350	17	34
Large serve, 2 cups, 18 oz	700	34	68

Noodles

	C	F	Cb
Plain/Egg: Dry, 1 oz	110	2	20
1 cup, 1.4 oz	145	2	27
Cooked: ½ cup, 2.8 oz	110	2	20
1 cup, 5.5 oz	220	4	40
Stir-Fried: 1 cup, 5.5 oz	270	9	40
2 cup serving, 11 oz	540	18	80
Low Carb Noodles, (Konjac/Shiritaki), 4 oz	5	0	2
Note: Carbs are from glucomannan fiber			
Yolk Free (Cooked):			
Manischewitz, Yolk Free, 2 oz	200	1	41
Chinese: Cellophane/Rice, dry, 1 oz	100	0	25
Chow Mein/hard, dry, 1 oz	150	9	16
Japanese: Soba: Dry, 1 oz	95	1	21
Cooked, 1 cup, 4 oz	115	1	24
Somen: Dry, 1 oz	100	1	21
Cooked, 1 cup, 6 oz	230	1	49
Japanese Style Pan Fried, Yaki-Soba (*Maruchan's*), av., 5.6 oz	260	3	50
Ramen Noodles ~ *See Page 118*			
Rice Noodles: Dry, 3.5 oz	365	1	83
Cooked, 1 cup, 6.2 oz	190	1	44
Annie Chun's, 2 oz	190	0	43
Simply Asia/Thai Kitchen ~ *See Pages 119 & 121*			

Egg Roll/Won Ton Wrappers

	C	F	Cb
Egg/Spring Roll (1), 0.8 oz	65	0	15
Won Ton Wrapper (1), 0.3 oz	20	0	4

Quick Guide

	C	F	Cb
Fruit Pies: *Average All Brands, 9" Pie*			
Apple; Blueberry; Cherry:			
Small Serving, ⅛ pie, 4.8 oz	350	16	49
Medium Serving, ⅙ pie, 6.5 oz	465	22	65
Large Serving ¼ pie, 9.5 oz	700	33	98
Whole Pie (9"), 38 oz	2800	131	392
Other Pies: *Per Serving, ⅙ of 9" Pie*			
Chocolate Cream Pie	345	22	38
Custard: Egg Pie	220	12	22
Coconut Pie	330	18	35
Lemon Meringue Pie	305	10	53
Peach Pie	260	12	39
Pecan Pie	440	23	57
Pumpkin Pie	315	14	41
Shoo-Fly Pie	400	13	70

Dessert/Fruit Pies ~ Brands

	C	F	Cb
Hostess:			
Apple, 4.5 oz	450	19	65
Cherry Pie, 4.5 oz	480	20	69
Marie Callender's:			
Key Lime Pie, 4.5 oz	490	19	72
Lattice Cherry Pie, 4.5 oz	380	16	56
Peach Cobbler Pie, 4 oz	330	16	43
Peanut Butter Pie, 4.7 oz	620	46	43
Southern Pecan Pie, 4 oz	530	30	60
Turtle, 4.7 oz	560	36	55
Mrs Smith's:			
Cobblers: Blackberry, 4 oz	240	8	38
Peach, 4 oz	240	8	39
Flaky Crust: *Per ⅛ Pie*			
Apple, 4.6 oz	330	18	41
Cherry, 4.4 oz	340	17	43
Peach, 4.6 oz	330	18	41
Sara Lee: *Per Slice*			
Creme Pies:			
Chocolate, ⅕ pie, 3.9 oz	440	27	46
Coconut, ⅙ pie, 4.5 oz	370	20	44
Key Lime, ⅕ pie, 4.8 oz	410	17	59
Fruit Pies: Apple, 4.27 oz	320	13	44
Cherry, 4.27 oz	310	14	44
Peach, 4.27 oz	300	13	42
Raspberry, 4.27 oz	320	13	48
Seasonal Pies: Pumpkin, 4.27 oz	260	11	38
Sweet Potato, 4.27 oz	260	9	43
Tastykake: Baked Apple Pie (1)	300	12	45
Orange Kream-Cicle Pie (1)	320	15	42

Croissants

	C	F	Cb
Average all Brands			
Plain/Butter/Cheese: Mini, 1 oz	115	6	13
Small, 1.5 oz	170	9	19
Medium, 2 oz	230	12	26
Large, 2.5 oz	290	15	32
Sweet Croissants:			
Almond Filled, 3 oz	330	18	39
Chocolate Filled, 3 oz	360	19	43
Dunkin' Donuts, Plain Croissant	340	19	37

Croissant Sandwiches ~ *See Page 165*

Pastry & Pie Crust

	C	F	Cb
Pie Crust, Baked, 9" diameter shell:			
1 Pie Shell, 6.5 oz	970	64	87
2-crust Pie, 9", 11.3 oz	1660	109	150
Filo Pastry: 4 sheets, 2.5 oz	210	3	40
Athens, Phyllo Dough, 5 sheets, 2 oz	180	1	36
Puff:			
Pepperidge Farms: Sheets, 1.5 oz	160	10	16
Bake & Fill Shells, 1.7 oz	180	11	18
Arrowhead Mills,			
Graham Cracker Pie Crust, ⅛ of 9"	110	5	15
Keebler:			
Ready Crust: *Per ⅛ of 9" Crust*			
Chocolate	100	5	14
Graham	100	5	13
Low Fat	100	4	15
Shortbread Crust	100	5	14
Marie Callenders,			
Pastry Pie Shell, ⅛, 1 oz	130	8	13
Mrs Smith's,			
Deep Dish Pie Crust, ⅛ pie, 1 oz	130	8	14
Nabisco:			
Honey Maid,			
Graham Cracker Crust, ⅛ pie, ¾ oz	110	5	14
Nilla, Pie Crust, ⅛ of Pie, 0.75	100	3	16
Pillsbury, Pie Crusts, Refrigerated, ⅛ pie, 0.9 oz	100	6	12
Trader Joe's, Pie Crust, ⅛ pie, 1.37oz	190	13	17

Pie Fillings ~ Canned

	C	F	Cb
Apple/Blueb./Cherry/Strawb., average:			
Sweetened: ⅓ cup, 3.2oz	90	0	22
1 cup, 9.5 oz	270	0	66
1 can, 21 oz	600	0	150
Light/Lite, ⅓ cup, 3.2 oz	60	0	15
Unsweetened, ⅓ cup, 3.2 oz	35	0	8
Lemon Crm/Creme, ⅓ cup, 3.2 oz	130	2	28

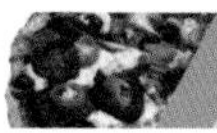

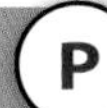

Pizzas ~ Ready to Eat

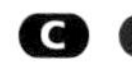 

Figures Based On Pizza Hut

Cheese

Medium Size (12"):	C	F	Cb
Hand Tossed Crust:			
⅛ Pizza (1 slice)	210	7	26
½ Pizza (4 slices)	840	28	104
Whole Pizza (8 slices)	1680	56	208
Original Pan: ⅛ Pizza (1 slice)	240	10	28
½ Pizza (4 slices)	960	40	112
Whole Pizza (8 slices)	1920	80	224
Thin 'N Crispy Crust:			
⅛ Pizza (1 slice)	180	7	22
½ Pizza (4 slices)	720	28	88
Whole Pizza (8 slices)	1440	56	176

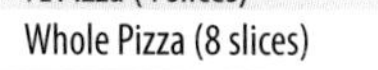

Meat Lover's

Figures Based On Pizza Hut

Medium Size (12"):	C	F	Cb
Hand Tossed Crust:			
⅛ Pizza (1 slice)	280	15	26
½ Pizza (4 slices)	1120	60	104
Whole Pizza (8 slices)	2240	120	208
Original Pan: ⅛ Pizza (1 slice)	310	17	28
½ Pizza (4 slices)	1240	68	112
Whole Pizza (8 slices)	2480	136	224
Thin 'N Crispy Crust:			
⅛ Pizza (1 slice)	280	16	22
½ Pizza (4 slices)	1120	64	88
Whole Pizza (8 slices)	2240	128	176

Pepperoni

Figures Based On Pizza Hut

Medium Size (12"):	C	F	Cb
Hand Tossed Crust:			
⅛ Pizza (1 slice)	220	9	25
½ Pizza (4 slices)	880	36	100
Whole Pizza (8 slices)	1760	72	200
Original Pan: ⅛ Pizza (1 slice)	250	11	28
½ Pizza (4 slices)	1000	44	112
Whole Pizza (8 slices)	2000	88	224
Thin 'N Crispy: ⅛ Pizza (1 slice)	200	9	22
½ Pizza (4 slices)	800	36	88
Whole Pizza (8 slices)	1600	72	176

Veggie Lover's

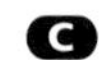  

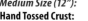

Figures Based On Pizza Hut

Medium Size (12"): *With Marinara Sauce*	C	F	Cb
Hand Tossed Crust:			
⅛ Pizza (1 slice)	190	6	27
½ Pizza (4 slices)	760	24	108
Whole Pizza (5 slices)	1520	48	216
Original Pan: ⅛ Pizza (1 slice)	230	9	29
½ Pizza (4 slices)	920	36	116
Whole Pizza (8 slices)	1840	72	232
Thin 'N Crispy Crust:			
⅛ Pizza (1 slice)	170	5	24
½ Pizza (4 slices)	680	20	96
Whole Pizza (8 slices)	1320	40	192

Large Pizzas

Figures Based On Domino's

Large (14")	C	F	Cb
Hand Tossed Crust:			
ExtravaganZZa: ⅛ Pizza (1 slice)	410	20	39
½ Pizza (4 slices)	1640	80	156
MeatZZA: ⅛ Pizza (1 slice)	400	19	38
½ Pizza (4 slices)	1600	76	152
Pacific Veggie: ⅛ Pizza (1 slice)	330	13	38
½ Pizza (4 slices)	1320	52	152

Extra Large NY, Single Slice

Figures Based On Sbarro: ⅙ 17" Pizza	C	F	Cb
Cheese	460	16	57
Classic Hawaiian	480	15	62
Sausage	590	27	59
Spinach & Tomato	475	18	59

Individual Personal Pan Pizzas

Pan (6"): Figures Based On Pizza Hut	C	F	Cb
Backyard BBQ Chicken	720	24	100
Cheese	600	24	68
Pepperoni	600	28	68
Supreme	640	28	72
Veggie Lovers	560	20	72
Chicago-Style Deep Dish: *Per Individual, 6 slices*			
Figures Based On Uno Pizzeria			
Cheese & Tomato	1680	78	108
Chicago Classic	2160	156	114
Prima Pepperoni	1680	190	108

Frozen Pizzas

	C	F	Cb
Amy's: *Per ⅓ Pizza Unless Indicated*			
Cheese	290	12	33
Margherita	270	12	31
Mushroom & Olive	260	11	31
Spinach	300	12	36
Vegan: Margherita	300	15	34
Meatless Pepperoni, gluten free	320	15	40
Supreme	290	12	37
Veggie Crust, Spinach	250	10	32
California Pizza Kitchen: *Per ⅓ Pizza*			
Cauliflower~Gluten Free:			
Artisanal Style Cheese	280	12	29
Pepperoni, Mushroom & Sausage	300	15	29
Crispy Thin Crust: BBQ Recipe Chkn	290	11	33
Four Cheese; Margherita, average	310	16	29
Sicilian Recipe	350	17	31
Signature Pepperoni	330	17	29
White Recipe	280	11	31
Gluten-Free:			
BBQ Recipe Chicken, ½ pizza	290	9	37
Margherita, ⅓ pizza	190	8	21
Celeste: *Per Pizza*			
Pizza For One: Original 4 Cheese	380	17	48
Deluxe	370	16	47
Pepperoni	370	17	46
Sausage	370	17	47
Daiya *(Vegan):*			
Gluten Free Thin Crust: *Per ⅓ Pizza Unless Indicated*			
Cheeze Lovers, 5,22 oz	400	15	60
Fire Roasted Veggie, ¼ pizza, 4.34 oz	300	11	46
Meatless:			
Meat Lovers, ¼ pizza, 5.53 oz	340	14	48
Pepperoni, 5.53 oz	410	17	61
M'shrm & Rstd Garlic, ¼ pizza, 4.23 oz	290	11	45
Supreme, ¼ pizza, 4.87 oz	310	11	45
DiGiorno:			
Bacon & Cheese Stuffed Crust: *Per ¼ Pizza*			
Bacon Me Crazy, 5.4 oz	410	21	34
Chicken Baon Ranch, 5.47 oz	380	17	37
Cheese Stuffed Crust: *Per ⅕ Pizza*			
Five Cheese, 4.44 oz	310	15	28
Pepperoni, 4.44 oz	320	16	28
Supreme, 5.3 oz	360	19	30

DiGiorno (Cont):	C	F	Cb
Crispy Pan: *Per ⅕ Pizza*			
Four Cheese, 5.33 oz	430	22	40
Pepperoni, 5.2 oz	430	22	39
Three Meat, 4.73 oz	390	21	33
Croissant Crust: *Per ⅕ Pizza*			
Four Cheese, 5.1 oz	370	18	36
Pepperoni, 5 oz	380	20	35
Three Meat, 5.1 oz	410	22	36
Hand Tossed Crust: *Per ¼ Pizza*			
Four Cheese	300	10	39
Pepperoni	320	12	39
Supreme	340	14	39
White Pizza	270	7	40
Hand Tossed Traditional Crust:			
Personal: Chicken	640	22	86
Chicken Alfredo	640	23	83
Rising Crust: *Per ⅙ Pizza*			
Four Cheese, 4.7 oz	300	10	37
Hawaiian, 4.76 oz	280	8	39
Italian Sausage, 5 oz	340	14	38
Freschetta: *Per Slice*			
Brick Oven:			
5 Cheese, 5.2 oz	370	17	39
Pepperoni, 4.55 oz	330	17	32
Spinach & Roasted M'shrms, 4.5 oz	270	10	34
Three Meat, 4.6 oz	340	18	32
Naturally Rising:			
4 Cheese, 5 oz	370	14	48
Canadadian Style,			
Bacon Pineapple, 4.5 oz	290	9	41
Pepperoni, 4.55 oz	330	13	40
Supreme, 5.2 oz	350	15	41
Great Value *(Walmart):*			
Cauliflower Crust: Margherita, 5.9 oz	370	18	38
Pepperoni, 4 oz	280	15	26
Rising Crust:			
Cheese, 4.6 oz	300	10	41
Pepperoni, 5.3 oz	350	11	49
Supreme, 5.1 oz	330	12	42
Three Meat, 4.6 oz	320	12	42
Thin Crust, Pepperoni, 5.43 oz	410	22	35

Frozen Pizzas (Cont)

	C	F	Cb
Kroger:			
3 Minute Microwave: *Per 7.2 oz Pizza*			
Cheese	480	18	62
Pepperoni	540	25	63
Self Rising Crust: *Per 1/6 pizza*			
Double Bacon	310	10	41
Four Cheese	300	9	42
Supreme	340	13	43
Three Meat	330	12	42
White Chicken	310	11	41
Lean Cuisine:			
Favorites: *Per Package*			
French Bread Pepperoni	310	7	46
Features: *Per Package*			
Four Cheese	370	8	54
Pepperoni	390	10	53
Spinach & Mushroom	360	9	51
Supreme	350	8	52
Red Baron:			
Brick Oven: *Per 1/4 Pizza*			
Cheese Trio, 4.4 oz	320	14	34
Meat-Trio, 4.6 oz	320	15	34
Pepperoni, 4.5 oz	330	17	33
Supreme, 4.66 oz	300	14	34
Classic Crust: *Per 1/4 Pizza*			
Four Cheese, 5.25 oz	380	17	40
Four Meat, 4.37 oz	300	14	32
Pepperoni, 5.15 oz	380	17	40
Sausage & Pepp.,4.4 oz	320	15	32
Deep Dish Singles: *Per Pizza*			
Cheese, 5.6 oz	410	16	51
Meat-Trio, 5.6 oz	400	18	47
Supreme, 5.75 oz	420	19	47
French Bread Singles,			
Pepperoni (1)	380	15	46
Fully Loaded: *Per 1/6 Pizza*			
Five Cheese	350	16	38
Pepperoni	380	19	37
Stuffed Crust: *Per 1/4 Puzza*			
Four Cheese, 5.2 oz	380	17	39
Meat-Trio, 5.47 oz	400	19	39
Pepperoni, 5.2 oz	390	18	39
Thin & Crispy Crust: *Per 1/3 Pizza*			
Bacon Lovers, 5.11 oz	380	18	38
Five Cheese, 5 oz	350	16	38
Pepperoni, 5.3 oz	400	20	38
Supreme, 4.4 oz	300	15	29

Signature Select *(Albertsons):*	C	F	Cb
Rising Crust: *Per 1/6 Pizza*			
Five Cheese	330	12	41
Pepperoni	380	17	41
Supreme	360	15	41
Ultra Thin Crust: *Per 1/3 Pizza*			
Five Cheese	340	18	27
Margherita	300	18	23
Supreme	340	19	27
Three Meat Sicilian	320	17	26
Smart Ones *(Weight Watchers):*			
Thin Crust: Cheese, 4.37 oz	270	7	36
Pepperoni Pizza, 4.37 oz	280	9	36
Stouffer's:			
French Bread Pizzas: *Two Per Boz*			
Cheese (1)	360	16	40
Deluxe (1)	410	21	42
Extra Cheese (1)	410	18	43
Pepperoni (1)	400	20	41
Three Meat (1)	460	25	40
Tombstone:			
Original: *Per 1/4 Pizza*			
Canadian Bacon, 4.9 oz	300	12	33
Deluxe, 5.4 oz	350	16	35
Five Cheese, 4.83 oz	370	18	33
Hamburger, 5.1 oz	340	15	34
Pepperoni, 4.83 oz	360	18	34
Pepperoni & Sausage, 4.87 oz	340	16	34
Sausage; Sausage & Mushroom	350	16	35
Supreme, 5.12 oz	340	16	35
Tony's: *Per 1/4 Pizza*			
Cheese, 4.73 oz	330	13	39
Meat Trio, 5 oz	350	16	39
Pepperoni, 4.7 oz	330	14	38
Supreme, 5.1 oz	350	15	39
Totino's:			
Crisp Crust Party Pizza: *Per 1/2 Pizza*			
Combination, 5.36 oz	350	18	37
Supreme, 5.47 oz	340	17	37
Triple Cheese, 4.9 oz	320	16	37
Triple Meat, 5.3 oz	340	17	37
Trader Joe's:			
Cauliflower Crust Cheese, 1/3 pizza	250	12	24

Quick Guide

	C	F	Cb
Chicken			
From 3lb ready-to-cook chicken			
Breast/Wing Quarter:			
Roasted: with skin	300	15	0
without skin	185	5	0
Fried, batter dipped	530	30	17
Leg Quarter:			
Thigh & Drumstick:			
Roasted: with skin	270	16	0
without skin	185	8	0
Fried, batter dipped	435	25	15
KFC ~ *See Fast-Foods Section*			

Per 4 oz Edible Portion

	C	F	Cb
Average of Light Meat: *Per 4 oz without Bone*			
Roasted: with skin	250	12	0
without skin	175	5	0
Stewed: with skin	230	12	0
without skin	180	5	0
Fried: Batter-dipped, with skin, 4 oz	315	17	11
Flour-coated, with skin, 4 oz	280	14	2
Average of Dark Meat: *Per 4 oz without Bone*			
Roasted: with skin	290	18	0
without skin	235	11	0
Stewed: with skin	265	17	0
without skin	220	10	0
Fried: Batter-dipped, with skin, 4 oz	340	21	11
Flour-coated, with skin, 4 oz	325	19	5

Chicken Parts

	C	F	Cb
Broilers or Fryers: *Edible Weights (no bone)*			
Breast: *Per ½ Breast*			
Raw: with skin, 5 oz	250	14	0
without skin, 4.25 oz	140	3	0
Roasted: with skin, 4 oz	195	8	0
without skin, 3 oz	140	3	0
Stewed: with skin, 4 oz	200	8	0
without skin, 3.3 oz	145	3	0
Fried: Batter-dipped, w/ skin, 5 oz	365	19	13
Flour-coated, with skin, 4 oz	220	9	2
Drumstick: *Per Drumstick*			
Roasted: with skin, 2 oz	115	6	0
without skin, 2 oz	75	3	0
Stewed: with skin, 2 oz	115	6	0
without skin, 2 oz	80	3	0
Fried: Batter-dipped, w/ skin, 3 oz	195	11	6
Flour-coated, with skin, 1.8 oz	120	7	1

Chicken Parts (Cont)

	C	F	Cb
Broilers or Fryers (Cont): *Edible Weights (no bone)*			
Thigh Portion:			
Raw: with skin, 3.3 oz (4¼ oz with bone)	200	14	0
without skin, 2.4 oz	80	3	0
Roasted: with skin, 2.3 oz	155	10	0
without skin, 2 oz	110	6	0
Stewed: with skin, 3 oz	160	10	0
without skin, 2 oz	105	5	0
Fried: Batter-dipped, with skin 3 oz	240	14	8
Flour-coated, with skin, 2.3 oz	165	9	2
Wing: *Per Wing, Bone In*			
Raw Weight, 3.2 oz			
Raw: with skin	110	8	0
without skin	35	1	0
Roasted: with skin	100	7	0
without skin	45	2	0
Fried: Batter-dipped, with skin	160	11	5
Flour-coated, with skin	105	7	1
Stewed, with skin, 4 oz	100	7	0
Buffalo Wings ~ *See Fast-Foods Section*			
Neck: Simmered, with skin	95	7	0
without skin	30	2	0
Skin Only: *Skin from ½ Chicken*			
Raw skin, 3 oz	275	26	0
Roasted skin, 2 oz	255	23	0
Stewed skin, 3 oz	260	24	0
Fried, flour-coated, 2 oz	280	24	5
Fried, batter-dipped, 6.8 oz	750	55	44
Roasters: *Average of Light & Dark Meat*			
Roasted: with skin, 4 oz	250	15	0
without skin, 4 oz	190	8	0
Dark Meat, without skin	200	10	0
Light Meat, without skin	175	5	0
Stewing Chicken: *Per 4 oz, average of Light & Dark Meat*			
Stewed: with skin	325	22	0
without skin	270	14	0
Dark Meat, without skin	290	17	0
Light Meat, without skin	240	9	0
Capon Chicken:			
Roasted: with skin, 4 oz	260	13	0
½ Chicken, with skin, 23 oz	1460	74	0
Chicken Offal & Stuffing:			
Giblets: Simmered, 1 cup	230	7	1
Fried, flour-coated, 1 cup	400	20	6
Gizzard, simmered, 1 cup	210	4	0
Heart, simmered, 1 cup	270	12	0.2
Liver: Raw, 4 oz	130	6	0
Simmered, 1 cup	215	9	1
Liver Pate, fresh, 1 Tbsp, 1 oz	30	2	1
Stuffing, average, ½ cup	180	9	22

Chicken Products

	C	F	Cb
Bumble Bee:			
Chicken In Water: *Per 2 oz Drained*			
Premium White, Chunk	70	2	1
Premium Breast	70	1	1
Foster Farms:			
Chicken Breast Strips, grilled, 3 oz	100	2	1
Wings, Bone In:			
Honey BBQ Glazed, 3 wings, 3 oz	170	11	6
Hot 'n' Spicy, 3 wings, 3 oz	170	12	3
Tyson:			
Anytizers, Frozen:			
Bites: Buffalo Style, 3 oz	190	8	18
Honey BBQ, 3 oz	190	8	18
Wings:			
Hot Wings, Buffalo Style (3)	190	13	3
Honey BBQ Seasoned (3)	190	12	8

Duck, Goose, Quail

	C	F	Cb
Duck, Roasted:			
with skin, 3 oz	290	24	0
without skin, 3 oz	170	10	0
½ duck, with skin, 14 oz	1290	108	0
Goose: Roasted with skin, 3 oz	260	19	0
without skin, 3 oz	200	11	0
Pheasant, cooked, 3 oz	210	10	0
Quail, cooked, 1 whole, 6 oz	385	24	0

Turkey

	C	F	Cb
Fryer-Roasters: *Per 3 oz Serving*			
Roasted:			
Light Meat: with skin	140	4	0
without skin	120	1	0
Dark Meat: with skin	155	6	0
without skin	140	4	0
½ of Whole Turkey: (Approx. 3.3 lbs raw weight without neck and giblets; 1.8 lbs cooked weight)			
Roasted: with skin	1650	74	0
without skin	1125	31	0
Ground Turkey, raw: (4 oz raw wt. = 3 oz cooked wt.)			
85% lean, regular, 4 oz	170	10	0
93% lean: Average, 4 oz	160	8	0
Jennie-O, 4 oz	170	8	0
Trader Joe's, 4 oz	150	8	0
94% lean, *Foster Farms*, 4 oz	150	7	0
Breast, no skin, 4 oz	115	1	0
Patties: Small, 3 oz	130	7	0
Medium, 4 oz	170	10	0

Turkey Parts

	C	F	Cb
Roasted, Edible Weights, without bone:			
Breast, (½), (from 17.3 oz raw weight with bone):			
with skin, 12 oz (no bone)	525	11	0
without skin, 10.8 oz	415	2	0
Back (½): with skin, 5 oz	265	13	0
without skin, 4 oz	165	6	0
Leg (Thigh & Drumstick): (from 1 lb raw weight with bone)			
with skin, 9 oz (without bone)	410	13	0
without skin, 7.8 oz (w/out bone)	355	9	0
Wing: (From 7.3 oz raw weight)			
with skin, 3 oz (without bone)	185	9	0
without skin, 2 oz (w/out bone)	100	2	0
Neck: Simmered, 1 neck, 9 oz (with bone)	275	11	0
Giblets, simmered, 1 cup, 5 oz	240	7	3

Young Hens (Roasted)

	C	F	Cb
Light Meat:			
with skin, 3 oz	175	8	0
without skin, 3 oz	135	3	0
Dark Meat: with skin, 3 oz	200	11	0
without skin, 3 oz	165	7	0

Young Toms ~ *Similar to Young Hens*

Turkey Products

	C	F	Cb
Foster Farms:			
Raw & Skinless: Breast Tenders, 4 oz	100	1	0
Ground Turkey, 85% lean, 4 oz	230	17	0
Tenderloins, 99% fat free	130	2	0
Hormel, Canned Turkey Breast, 97% Fat Free, in water, 3 oz	70	2	0
Jennie-O:			
Cooked, Slow Rstd Dark Turkey, 3 oz	140	9	2
Raw: Bacon, raw, 1 slice, 1 oz	30	3	0
Burgers: 93% Fat Free, 4 oz	160	8	0
All White, 8.8 oz	250	15	0
Seasoned, 4 oz	160	8	0
Spam, Oven Roasted Turkey, 2 oz	80	5	1
Valley Fresh, 100% Natural, Canned White Turkey Breast, in water, 2 oz	50	1	0

R Rice & Rice Dishes

White Rice

	C	F	Cb
Raw:			
Glutinous, 1 cup, 7 oz	685	1	151
Long Grain, 1 cup, 7 oz	675	1	148
Short Grain, 1 cup, 7 oz	715	1	158
Wild Rice, 1 cup, 6 oz	570	2	120
Cooked Rice: *Boiled/Steamed*			
Short/Medium Grain:			
½ cup, 3.3 oz	140	0	30
1 cup (½ Pint), 7.2 oz	265	1	59
2 cups (1 Pint), 13 oz	480	1	106
Long Grain: ½ cup, 2.8 oz	100	0	22
1 cup, 6 oz	205	1	44
Glutinous/Sticky, 1 cup, 6 oz	170	1	37
Parboiled, ½ cup, 3 oz	105	1	22
Precooked/Instant:			
Dry, ½ cup, 4 oz	380	1	82
Cooked, ½ cup, 3 oz	95	1	21
Wild Rice,			
Cooked, 1 cup, 5.8 oz	165	1	35

Brown Rice

Average of Short or Long Grain

	C	F	Cb
Raw/Dry: ½ cup, 3.3 oz	340	3	71
1 cup, 7 oz	685	6	143
Cooked: ½ cup, 4 oz	110	1	22
1 cup, 7 oz	220	2	46

Rice Dishes

	C	F	Cb
Chinese Fried Rice:			
½ cup, 3 oz	140	5	21
1 cup, (½ Pint), 5 oz	280	9	42
2 cups, (1 Pint), 10 oz	565	18	84
Mexican Style Rice:			
Taco Time, Seasoned, 4.6 oz	200	3	40
Rice-A-Roni ~ *See Page 119*			
Rice with Raisins/Pinenuts, 1 cup	400	11	60
Rice Pilaf: Restaurant, 1 cup	275	8	46
O'Charley's, side dish, 1 portion	160	4	27
Rice Pudding,			
Kozy Shack, Original, 1 pudding cup	130	3	24
Risotto, 1 cup	420	12	70
Saffron Rice, 4 oz	175	7	25
Spanish Rice: 1 cup, 5 oz	390	9	72
El Pollo Loco, Small, 5 oz	160	2	32
Sticky Rice, 1 cup, 5 oz	155	1	34
Sushi Rice: 1 Tbsp	25	0	5
1 cup, 5.2 oz	390	0	77
Other Packaged Rice Products:			
Uncle Ben's / Zatarain's ~ *See Page 121*			

Deli Salads

Average All Outlets	C	F	Cb
Antipasto Salad, ½ cup	135	8	13
3-Bean Salad, ½ cup	90	5	12
Bulgur Salad, ½ cup	70	2	12
Caesar Salad, Classic, 1 cup	200	14	15
Side Salad, without Dressing	25	0	6
Carrot Raisin: with Dressing, ½ cup	135	12	6
without Dressing, ½ cup	20	0	5
Chef's Salad: Regular, w/o Dressing	620	37	8
with 2 oz Thousand Island Drssng	860	61	8
Chicken Salad, ½ cup/scoop, 4 oz	280	21	2
Coleslaw: Traditional, ½ cup	150	8	18
w/ Low Cal Dressing, ½ c.	50	2	8
Corn, Mexican, ½ cup	240	12	33
Cucumber: Non-Oil Dressing, ½ cup	60	0	14
with Oil Dressing, ½ cup	140	12	8
Eggplant Salad, ½ cup	75	5	7
Fettucini, with veges, ½ cup	135	6	16
Garden Salad, without Dressing, 1 cup	10	0	2
Greek Salad, 1 cup	105	8	7
Greek Vegetables, 1 cup	110	8	6
Lobster Salad, ½ cup, 4 oz	250	21	11
Macaroni Salad, ½ cup, 5 oz	360	26	26
Nicoise, 1 cup	450	32	18
Pasta Salad, ½ cup	200	11	19
Potato Salad: Dijon, 3 oz	120	7	13
with Mayonnaise, ½ cup, 4 oz	215	15	17
Lowfat, ½ cup	110	2	21
Rice Salad, ½ cup	150	10	13
Saffron Rice, 4 oz	175	7	25
Spinach Salad, 1 cup	180	13	13
Tabouli, ½ cup	125	7	13
Three Bean Salad, ½ cup	90	5	12
Tomato & Mozzarella, ½ cup	180	14	10
Tortellini, with Basil Pesto, ½ cup	150	9	15
Waldorf, with Mayo, ½ cup	110	7	12
Signature Salads: *Per 6 oz Serving* (Supplied to Deli's and Institutions)			
Antipasto Salad	510	50	4
Artichoke Salad, marinated	400	41	8
California Medley	120	7	15
Cheese Agnolotti	250	8	23
Chicken Salad	420	33	11
Crabmeat Flavored	450	38	20
Egg Salad	300	23	14
Fresh Button Mushroom	190	16	6

Signature Salads (Cont): *Per 6 oz*	C	F	Cb
Fresh Button Mushroom	190	16	6
Ham Salad	400	32	14
Prima Pasta Salad	360	30	18
Seafood Pasta Del Mar	170	10	21
Seafood, Crab & Shrimp	420	34	20
Shrimp Salad	360	32	8
Tuna Salad	450	36	14

~ *Also See Fast-Foods & Restaurants Section*

Fresh Salad Packs

Pre-Packaged (Supermarkets):	C	F	Cb
Dole:			
Kits: *Per 3.5 oz, with Dressing*			
Caesar: Classic	140	12	8
Light	90	6	8
Chopped Kits:			
Applewood Bacon	120	7	11
Buffalo Ranch	140	11	8
Sesame Asian	130	9	12
Salad Blends: *Per 3 oz, Without Dressing*			
American	15	0	3
Arugula; Baby Spinach	20	0	3
Field Greens; Very Veggie	20	0	4
Fresh Express:			
Chopped Salad Kits: *Per3.5 oz*			
Pomegranate	150	9	17
Poppyseed	140	7	18
Twisted Asian Caesar	190	14	13
Twisted Lemon Caesar	170	15	5
Salad Greens: *Per 5 oz Package*			
Butter Supreme	25	0	4
Spinach & Arugua	35	1	5
Ready Pac:			
Bistro Bowls: *Per Container with Dressing*			
Chicken BLT	260	22	6
Cranberry Walnut	200	9	24
Salad Kits: *Per 3.5 oz with Dressing*			
Bacon Caesar	160	14	5
Kale Cranb. Pecan Crunch	200	14	17
Mediterranean Crisp	140	10	11

Salad Toppings

	C	F	Cb
Bac'n Pieces, *McCormick,* 1Tbsp, 0.3 oz	30	1	2
Bacon Bits *(Hormel)*, 1Tbsp	25	2	0
Bac-Os, Bits *(Betty Crocker)*, 1 Tbsp	30	1	2
Chow Mein Noodles, dry, ½ cup	120	7	13
Croutons, 2 Tbsp, 0.3 oz	40	1	7
Salad Toppins, *McCormick*, 4 tsp	35	2	3
Sunflower Seeds, 1 Tbsp, 0.3 oz	45	4	2
Toasted Sliced Almonds, 2 T., 1 oz	85	7	3

S Salad Dressings

Quick Guide

Salad Dressings

Average All Brands: *Per 2 Tbsp, Approx 1 fl.oz*	C	F	Cb
Balsamic Vinaigrette:			
Regular	90	9	3
Light, 2 Tbsp	45	4	2
Fat Free, 2 Tbsp	25	0	6
Blue Cheese: Regular, 2 Tbsp	145	15	2
Regular, 1/4 cup, 2 oz	280	30	3
Light, 2 Tbsp	30	1	4
Caesar: Regular, 2 Tbsp	165	17	1
Regular, 1/4 cup, 2 oz	310	34	2
Light, 2 Tbsp	35	2	6
Coleslaw: Regular, 2 Tbsp	125	11	8
Regular, 1/4 cup, 2 oz	245	21	15
Light, 2 Tbsp	110	7	14
French: Regular	145	14	5
Regular, 1/4 cup, 2 oz	260	25	9
Light, 2 Tbsp	65	4	9
Fat/Oil-Free, 2 Tbsp	40	0	10
Italian: Regular, 2 Tbsp	85	9	3
Regular, 1/4 cup, 2 oz	165	16	6
Light, 2 Tbsp	55	6	2
Fat/Oil-Free, 2 Tbas	15	0	3
Ranch: Regular, 2 Tbsp	145	16	2
Regular, 1/4 cup, 2 oz	290	30	4
Light, 2 Tbsp	60	4	7
Fat-Free, 2 Tbsp	35	1	8
Thousand Island: Reg., 2 T.	115	11	5
Regular, 1/4 cup, 2 oz	210	20	9
Light, 2 Tbsp	60	4	7
Fat-Free, 2 Tbsp	40	1	10

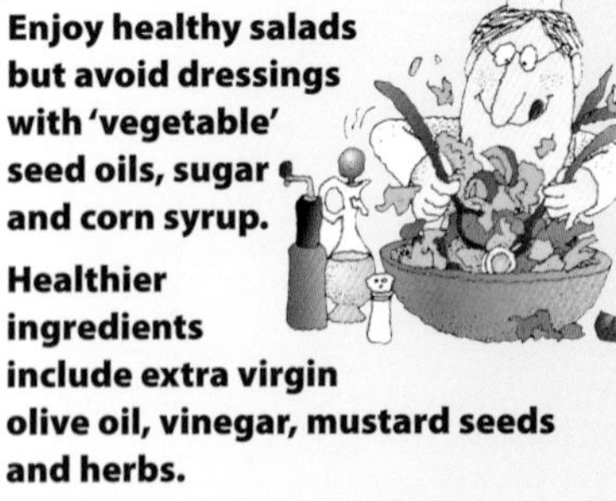

Enjoy healthy salads but avoid dressings with 'vegetable' seed oils, sugar and corn syrup.

Healthier ingredients include extra virgin olive oil, vinegar, mustard seeds and herbs.

Home-made is the best choice.

Annie's Naturals: *Per 2 Tbsp*	C	F	Cb
Organic: Caesar	100	11	2
French	110	10	3
Goddess	120	12	2
Green Goddess	100	11	1
Lite, Goddess	60	6	1
Vinaigrettes:			
Organic Balsamic	100	10	2
Sesame Ginger	90	8	4
Shiitake & Sesame	130	13	2
Bernstein's: *Per 2 Tbsp*			
Cheese & Garlic Italian	80	8	2
Cheese Fantastico	90	9	1
Italian Dressing & Marinade	90	9	2
Restaurant Recipe Italian	100	11	1
Light Fantastic, Cheese Fantastico	25	2	3
Best Foods: *Per 1 Tbsp Unless Indicated*			
Avocado Oil Mayo	60	7	1
Real Mayonnaise: Orig.	90	10	0
Extra Creamy	100	11	0
Light	35	4	1
Spicy Chipotle	100	11	0
Vegan Dressing & Spread	70	8	1
Cardini's: *Per 2 Tbsp*			
Caesar:			
Original	140	15	1
Light	80	8	1
Garlic Lemon	150	16	1
Three Cheese	140	15	1
Balsamic Vinaigrette:			
Regular	100	8	5
Lite Greek	50	5	2
Great Value *(Walmart): Per 2 Tbsp Unless Indicated*			
Blue Cheese	120	13	1
Buttermilk Ranch	110	11	2
French Style	90	6	9
Traditional Italian	80	7	5
Mayo: Whole, 1 Tbsp	90	10	0
Light	35	4	1
Hidden Valley: *Per 2 Tbsp*			
Coleslaw	150	15	4
Ranch: Original	130	13	1
Light	60	5	4
Plant Based	110	12	1
Other Flavors: Avocado	90	9	2
Buttermilk	130	13	2
Greek Yogurt	60	5	3

Brands ~ Salad Dressings (Cont)

	C	F	Cb
Kraft: *Per 2 Tbsp*			
Aged Balsamic Vinaigrette	80	7	4
Regular Dressings:			
Asian Toasted Sesame	80	6	7
Buttermilk Ranch	110	12	2
Classic: Catalina	70	6	4
Caesar	120	12	2
Creamy Italian	80	8	2
Honey Mustard	80	5	8
Peppercorn Ranch	110	11	2
Ranch with Bacon	120	12	2
Roka Blue Cheese	120	12	1
Thousand Island	130	12	4
Tuscan House	60	5	3
Zesty Italian	60	5	3
Fat Free:			
Classic Ranch	50	0	11
Zesty Italian	10	0	1
Lite: Catalina	60	1	11
Raspberry Vinaigrette	30	1	5
Zesty Italian	25	1	3
Marie's: *Per 2 Tbsp*			
Classics:			
Chunky Blue Cheese	160	18	1
Creamy: Caesar	120	13	1
Italian Garlic	180	19	1
Ranch	180	19	1
Original Coleslaw	150	13	7
Thousand Island	160	16	4
Plant Based: Creamy Dill Ranch	45	4	1
Meyer Lemon Basil	50	4	4
Sesame Ginger Vinaigrette	50	4	4
Smoked Black Pepper Caesar	45	5	1
Specialty: Avocado Poblano	80	8	1
Honey Mustard	140	13	6
Poppy Seed	150	13	8
Vinaigrette: Blue Cheese	120	11	4
Garlic Parmesan Italian	110	11	2
Italian	80	8	3
Raspberry	50	3	6
White Balsamic Shallot	110	11	3

	C	F	Cb
Marzetti's: *Per 2 Tbsp*			
Classic Refrierated:			
Honey French	140	10	11
Ranch	140	15	1
Signature Blue Cheese	130	14	1
Supreme Caesar	130	13	1
Slaw: Regular	150	14	6
Light Original	90	6	
Country French	160	14	7
Italian	90	8	4
Poppyseed	170	14	11
Simply:			
Balsamic Vinaigrette	50	5	3
Blue Cheese	50	4	2
Creamy Caesar	50	4	2
Ranch	50	4	3
Vinaigrette: Balsamic	50	3	5
Olive Oil & Vinegar	100	10	1
Roasted Garlic Italian	90	8	2
Newman's Own: *Per 2 Tbsp*			
Balsamic Vinaigrette	110	11	2
Creamy Caesar	160	18	1
Family Recipe Italian	120	13	1
Honey Mustard	90	7	7
Parmesan & Roasted Garlic	110	11	2
Poppy Seed	140	13	5
Raspberry Walnut	70	5	7
Light: Balsamic Vinaigrette	45	4	2
Caesar	70	6	2
Italian	60	6	0
Wish-Bone: *Per 2 Tbsp*			
Creamy: Buffalo Ranch	130	13	2
Caesar	110	11	2
Cheddar Bacon Ranch	130	13	2
Chunky Blue Cheese	110	11	2
Fat Free	30	0	7
French	120	11	5
Ranch	130	13	1
Thousand Island	110	11	4
Light: Chunky Blue Cheese	60	6	2
Italian	80	7	5
Parmesan Peppercorn Ranch	60	5	2
Vinaigrettes:			
Balsamic	60	5	4
Champagne	130	14	1
Garden Herb	40	4	2
Jalapeno Lime	80	8	3
Red Wine	60	5	5

Gravy

	C	F	Cb
Homemade Gravy, average:			
Thin, little fat, 2 Tbsp, 1 oz	20	1	3
Thick: 2 Tbsp, 1.3 oz	50	2	9
¼ cup, 3 oz	100	4	18
McCormick:			
Brown, 1 Tbsp	20	1	4
Turkey, 1 Tbsp	20	1	4

Gravy-In-Jars

	C	F	Cb
Boston Market,			
Classic Beef, ¼ cup, 2 fl.oz	30	1	4
Campbell's,			
Beef/Chicken/Turkey, ¼ cup, 2 fl.oz	30	1	4
Heinz: *Per ¼ cup, 2 fl.oz*			
Homestyle: Bistro Au Jus	15	0	2
Classic Chicken	30	2	3
Mushroom; Pork	20	1	3
Roasted Turkey	25	2	3
Savory Beef	25	1	3
Safeway, Chicken, ¼ cup, 2 fl.oz	40	3	3

Tomato Products

	C	F	Cb
Whole/Chopped/Crushed/Diced:			
Regular: 1 cup, 9 oz	50	0	10
In Aspic, ½ cup	50	0	12
with Green Chili, 1 cup, 9 oz	60	0	16
Stewed, ½ cup, 1.7 oz	40	2	7
Wedges in Tomato Juice, 1 cup	70	1	18
Salsa, average, 2 Tbsp, 1 oz	25	0	6
Tomato Ketchup:			
Regular: 1 Tbsp, 1 oz	15	0	4
Single Serve, 1 packet	10	0	3
Heinz, Simply Heinz 1 Tbsp, 1 oz	15	0	4
Tomato Paste:			
Regular: 2 Tbsp, 1 oz	25	0	6
¾ cup, 6 oz	140	1	32
Tomato Puree, ½ cup, 5 oz	50	0	10
Tomato Sauce:			
Regular, ½ cup, 4.4 oz	50	0	11
Spanish Style, ½ cup, 4.3 oz	40	0	9
with Mushr., ½ cup, 4.3 oz	45	0	10
with Onions, ½ cup, 4.3 oz	50	0	12
Tomato Seasoning, 3 tsp	20	0	4
Sundried Tomatoes:			
Natural, 5-6 pieces, 0.4 oz	20	0	5
In Oil, drained, 6 pieces, 1 oz	40	3	4

Sauces ~ Brands

	C	F	Cb
A-1 *(Kraft):*			
Marinade:: *Per Tbsp, ½ oz*			
Chicago Steakhouse	20	1	3
Classic	15	0	4
New Orleans Cajun	20	0	5
Texas Mesquite Marinade	15	0	4
Sauce: Original	15	0	3
Bold & Spicy	20	0	5
Smoky Black Pepper	30	0	7
Spicy Chipotle	30	0	7
Sweet Chili Garlic	25	0	6
Sweet Hickory	25	0	5
Barilla:			
Pesto: Creamy Genovese, ¼ cup	300	26	12
Rustic Basil	200	19	5
Roasted Garlic	50	1	12
Tomato & Basil	50	1	10
Traditional	50	1	10
Bertolli:			
Alfredo Sauce: *Per ¼ Cup*			
Alfredo with Parm. Chse	110	11	2
Creamy Basil w/ Parmesan	100	10	2
Garlic with Parmesan	100	10	2
D'Italia: Alfredo with White Wine	100	10	2
Cacio e Pepe Alfredo	60	5	2
Four Cheese	110	10	2
Rustic Cut Marinara, with Traditonal Vegetables	70	4	9
Traditional: *Per ½ Cup*			
Five Cheese w/ Ricotta, Romano & Parmesan	90	3	12
Portobello Mushroom	70	3	9
Vodka	140	10	10
Buitoni: *Per ¼ Cup Unless Indicated*			
Pasta Sauce:			
Alfredo	140	13	3
Marinara, ½ cup	70	4	9
Meat, ½ cup	125	8	7
Pesto: Basil	300	28	5
Reduced Fat	220	18	8
Bull's-Eye: *Per 2 Tbsp*			
BBQ Sauce: Original	60	0	14
Hickory Brown Sugar	70	0	16
Hickory Smoke	60	0	14
Smoky Mesquite	45	0	10
Catelli: *Per ½ Cup*			
Garden Select Pasta Sauce:			
Country Mushroom	45	1	9
Garlic & Onion	45	1	9
Parmesan Romano	60	2	9
Meat Sauce	50	2	8

Sauces ~ Brands (Cont)

	C	F	Cb
Cento:			
Arrabbiata, ½ cup	60	4	6
Italiano, ¼ cup	25	0	6
Marinara, ½ cup	70	4	6
Porcini, ½ cup	70	4	7
Rustica Passata, ¼ up	35	1	5
Vodka, ½ cup	110	9	6
Classico:			
Alfredo: *Per ¼ Cup*			
Creamy, 2 oz	50	4	3
Roasted Garlic, 2 oz	45	4	3
Family Favorites: *Per ½ Cup*			
Meat, 4.4 oz	60	1	10
Parm. & Romano, 4.4 oz	70	2	10
Traditional, 4.4 oz	80	3	13
Contadina: *Per ¼ Cup*			
Pizza Sauce: Sweet Tomato Basil	35	0	8
with Pepperoni, canned	40	1	7
Tomato Sauce, canned	20	0	4
Crosse & Blackwell:			
Meat: Ham Glaze, 1 Tbsp	25	0	6
Mint Sauce, 1 tsp	5	0	2
Mincemeat: *Per ¼ Cup*			
Regular	140	0	35
Rum & Brandy	140	0	36
Seafood: *Per ¼ Cup*			
Cocktail Sauce, 3 oz	90	0	21
Shrimp Sauce, 3 oz	90	0	21
Dave's Gourmet:			
Pasta Sauce: *Per ½ Cup*			
Butternut Squash	100	4	16
Creamy Parmesan Romano	120	8	9
Organic: Hearty Marinara	70	4	8
Organic Red Heirloom	70	3	9
Roasted Garlic & Sweet Basil	50	2	8
Spicy Heirloom Marinara	70	3	9
Vegan Bolognese	80	4	8
Del Monte:			
Pasta Sauces: *Per ½ Cup*			
Four Cheese; Traditional, av.	60	1	12
Mushroom	60	1	11
Average other varieties	60	1	13
Sloppy Joe Sauce: *Per ¼ Cup*			
Original	60	0	13
Emeril's:			
Alfredo, Four Cheese Sauce, ¼ cup	60	5	4
Pasta Sauces: *Per ½ Cup*			
Homestyle Marinara	90	3	14
Kicked Up Tomato	80	4	11
Marinara	90	3	14
Roasted Gaaahlic	80	4	12
Roasted Red Pepper	70	4	9
Vodka Sauce	110	7	12
Francesco Rinaldi:			
Alfredo, all flavors, ¼ cup	60	5	3
Cheese,			
Three Cheese, ½ cup	60	1	13
Garden, average., ½ cup	50	1	11
Meat Flavored, ½ cup	60	2	11
Pizza, ¼ cup	20	0	4
Traditional, ½ cup	60	1	11
French's,			
Worcestershire Sauce, 1 tsp	0	0	0
Heinz: *Per 1 Tbsp*			
57 Steak Sauce	20	0	4
Chili Sauce	20	0	4
Cocktail Sauce, Original, ¼ cup, 2.2 oz	80	0	17
Dill Relish	0	0	0
Texas Bold & Spicy BBQ	45	0	10
Tomato Ketchup: Regular	20	0	5
Sweet Ketchili	60	0	15
Worcestershire Sce, tsp	0	0	0
House of Tsang:			
Bangkok Peanut, 1.16 oz	80	5	8
Classic Stir Fry, 0.6 oz	25	1	5
Ginger Sriracha, 1.23 oz	20	0	5
General Tso, 0.67 oz	45	1	10
Green Thai Curry, 1.1 oz	60	4	6
Korean BBQ, 0.67 oz	25	0	6
Oyster Flavored, 0.63 oz	30	0	7
Saigon Sizzle, 0.63 oz	40	1	7
Sweet & Sour, 0.63 oz	30	0	7
Hunt's:			
Ketchup, all varieties, 1 tbsp	20	0	5
Pasta Sauce: *Per ½ Cup*			
Four Cheese	50	0	10
Garlic & Herb	35	0	7
Mushroom	40	0	8
Zesty & Spicy	40	1	8

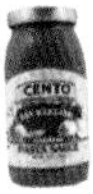

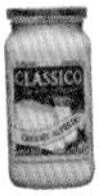

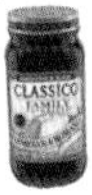

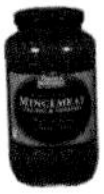

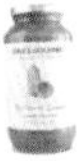

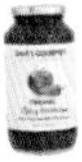

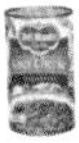

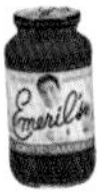

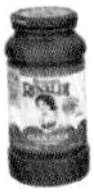

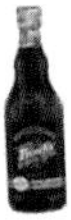

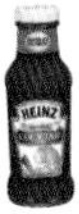

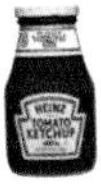

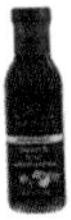

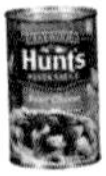

Brands (Cont)

	C	F	Cb
Kikkoman: *Per Tablespoon*			
Cooking Sauces: Hoisin,	90	0	21
Oyster Flavored, Gluten Free	25	0	6
Soy Sauces: Double Fermented Shoyu	15	0	1
Gluten Free Soy	10	0	1
Organic Soy	10	0	1
Smooth Aromatic Shoyu	10	0	1
Teriyaki Sauces: Original	15	0	2
Gluten Free	20	0	4
Roasted Garlic	20	0	3
Takumi: Original	30	0	6
Garlic & Green Onion	35	1	6
Gochujang Spicy Miso	45	1	9
Knorr:			
Classic Sauce Mix: Alfredo, 1 tbsp	25	1	4
Bearnaise, 1 tsp	10	0	2
Creamy Pesto, 1 tbsp	25	0	5
Garlic & Herb, 1 tbsp	50	1	9
Hollandaise, 1 tsp	10	0	2
Pesto, 1 tbsp	15	0	3
Kraft: *Per 2 Tablespoons*			
Horseradish	100	9	4
Original Barbecue	60	0	14
Sweet Honey Barbecue	60	0	14
Las Palmas: *Per ¼ Cup*			
Green Enchilada Sauce, all varieties, 2 oz	25	2	3
Red Chili Sauce	15	1	3
La Victoria,			
Red/Green Enchilada Sauce, av., 2 oz	25	2	3
Lawry's:			
30 Minute Marinade: *Per Tbsp*			
Baja Chipotle	10	0	2
Caribbean Jerk with Papaya	15	0	4
Chipotle Molasses	30	0	7
Hawaiian w/ Tropical Fruit Jce	20	0	4
Herb & Garlic; Lemon Pepper	10	0	2
Honey Bourbon	25	0	5
Hickory Brown Sugar	25	0	6
LemonPepper with Lemon	10	0	2
Mediterranean Herb & White Wine	10	0	2
Mesquite, w/ Lime Juice	10	0	2
Sesame & Ginger	25	0	5
Steakhouse	10	0	2
Teriyaki with Pineapple Juice	15	0	3
Steak & Chop	5	0	1

	C	F	Cb
Lea & Perrins:			
Marinade, Cracked Peppercorn, 1 Tbsp.	15	0	4
Tradtn'l Steak Sauce, 1 Tbsp	20	0	5
Worcestershire Sauce:			
Original,1 tsp, 5 ml	5	0	1
Reduced Sodium, 1 tsp, 5 ml	5	0	1
Mrs. Dash:			
Marinades: *Per 1 Tbsp*			
Garlic Herb	15	0	3
Lime Garlic	15	0	3
Sweet Teriyaki	35	0	9
Newman's Own: *Per ½ Cup Inless Indicated*			
Pasta Sauce:			
Marinara	80	2	12
Organic: Marinara	90	4	11
Olive Oil, Basil & Garlic	90	4	11
Roasted Garlic	70	3	11
Sockarooni	70	2	12
Tomato & Basil	70	2	11
O Organics *(Von's): Per ½ Cup Unless Indicated*			
Enchilada, Red/Green, ¼ cup	20	0	4
Pasta: Alfredo, ¼ cup	70	7	3
Arrabiata	60	2	10
Marinara	60	2	11
Portobello Mushroom	45	2	7
Roasted Garlic Alfredo	70	7	3
Old El Paso:			
Creamy: Queso, 1 Tbsp	20	2	2
Salsa Verde, 1 Tbsp	40	4	1
Enchilada Sauce:			
Green Chile, 2.15 oz	25	2	3
Red, all, 2.1 oz	20	0	4
Taco Sauce, all,1 Tbsp	5	0	1
Zesty Ranch, 1 tablespoon	20	2	2
Pace: *Per 2 Tbsp*			
Nacho Cheese Sauces, ¼ cup	50	3	5
Picante Sauce, all varieties	10	0	2
Prego: *Per ½ Cup, Unless Indicated*			
Alfredo, Four Cheese, ¼ cup	50	4	3
Basil Pesto Italian, ¼ cup	200	19	4
Classic Italian: Creamy Vodka	120	6	13
Cremini Pomodoro & Roasted Garlic	70	2	12
Fire Roasted Tomato	70	2	11
Fresh Mushroom, Italian			
Hidden super Veggies Traditional	70	2	12
Italian: Fresh Mushroom	60	1	12
Tomato Flavored with Meat	70	2	12
Marinara	60	2	10
Premier Japan, Hoisin;Teriyaki, 1 T.	15	0	3

Brands (Cont)

	C	F	Cb
Ragu:			
Cheese Sauces: *Per ¼ Cup*			
Classic Alfredo	90	9	2
Creamy Basil Alfredo	90	8	3
Double Cheddar	100	9	3
Roasted Garlic Parmesan	90	8	3
Chunky Sauces: *Per ½ Cup*			
Garden Combination	90	3	14
Mama's Special Garden	90	3	15
M'shrm & Green Peppers	80	2	13
Parmesan & Romano	80	3	13
Six Cheese	90	3	14
Super Chunky Mushroom	80	2	14
Old World Style: *Per ½ Cup*			
Flavored with Meat	90	4	12
Marinara; Mushroom, av.	75	3	11
Traditional	60	1	11
Pizza, Homemade Style, ¼ cup	30	1	5
Simply Sauces: *Per ½ Cup*			
Roasted Garlic	60	2	10
Traditional	70	1	12
Signature Select *(Safeway): Per ½ Cup Unless Indicated*			
Cocktail Sauce, ¼ cup	70	0	17
Enchilada Sauce, medium, ¼ cup	25	2	4
Kung Pao, 2 tablespoons	50	1	10
Pasta Sauce: Arrabbiata	130	8	13
Four Cheese	80	4	12
Marinara	70	2	11
Tomato Basil	80	3	12
Traditional with Meat	70	2	11
Steak Sauce, tablespoon	10	0	2
Taco Bell, Creamy Jalapeno Sauce, 1 Tablespoon, 1 oz	70	7	1
Tony Roma's:			
Original, 2 Tbsp	50	0	12
Carolina Honey BBQ Sce, 2 Tbsp	70	0	18
Trader Joe's,			
Organic Kansas City Style BBQ Sauce, 2 Tbsp	45	0	11
Walnut Acres,			
Organic Pasta Sauces, average all var., ½ cup, 5 oz	50	1	10

Seasonings & Flavorings

	C	F	Cb
Auromatic Bitters *(Angostua)*, 1 tsp	15	0	4
Bacon Bits, average, 1 Tbsp	35	2	2
Bacon Chips *(Durkee)*, 1 Tbsp	30	1	2
Bac-Os *(Betty Crocker)*, 1Tbsp	30	2	2
Blends *(Mrs Dash)*, 1 tsp	0	0	0
Butter Buds, 1 tsp	5	0	2
Flavor Enhancer *(Accent)*, 1 tsp	0	0	0
Flavor Sprinkles *(Molly McButter)*, Natural/Cheese, 1 tsp	5	0	1
Garlic Bread Sprinkle, 1 tsp	8	1	1
Garlic Salt, 1 tsp	2	0	0
Italian Seasoning, 1 tsp	4	0	1
Lemon Pepper Seasoning, 1 tsp	7	0	1
Meat Tenderizer, av., 1 tsp	7	0	1
Salad Crunchies *(McCormick)*, 1 tsp	10	1	2
Salt, Reg., Sea Salt, Lite Salt	0	0	0
Seasoning *(Old Bay)*, ¼ tsp	0	0	0
Seasoning Mix *(Vegit)*, ¼ tsp	0	0	0
Seasoning Mixes, av., ¼ pkg	70	1	9
Taco Seasoning, av., ¼ pkg	30	1	4
Bragg's, Liquid Aminos	0	0	0
Old El Paso: Chili Season. Mix, 1 Tbsp	8	1	2
Cheesy Taco Seasoning Mix, 1 Tbsp	10	1	2
Taco/Burrito Seasoning Mix, 2 tsp	15	0	4
Fajita Seasoning Mix, 1 tsp	5	0	2

Spices & Herbs

	C	F	Cb
Average all types, 1 tsp	5	0	1
All Purpose, 1 tsp	0	0	0
Allspice, ground	5	0	1
Chili Powder	8	0	1
Cinnamon, ground	6	0	2
Curry Powder	6	0	1
Garlic Powder	9	0	2
Nutmeg, ground	12	0	1
Onion Powder	7	0	2
Parsley, dried	4	0	1
Pepper, average	6	0	1
Saffron	2	0	0
Salt-Free Blends, 1 tsp	0	0	0
Tumeric, ground	8	0	1
Seeds: Fenugreek	12	1	2
Mustard, Poppyseed	15	1	1
Other varieties, average	7	0	1

Home-Popped Popcorn

	C	F	Cb
Popping Corn Kernels,			
2 Tbsp, 1 oz	110	1	26
(makes approximately 5 cups)			
Air-popped, without oil: Plain, 1 oz	110	1	22
1 cup, 0.2 oz	20	0	5
Oil-popped: Plain, 1 oz	145	8	16
1 cup, 0.4 oz	55	3	6
Popcorn Oil, 1 Tbsp	120	14	0

Microwave Popping Corn

	C	F	Cb
Act II Popcorn: *Unpopped*			
Butter: 2 tablespoons, 1.2oz	130	6	19
2.75 oz bag	315	15	46
Butter Lovers, 2 Tbsp, 1.2 oz	140	7	20
Movie Theatre Butter/ Buttery Kettle Corn:			
2 Tablespoons, 1.2 oz	150	8	19
Bag, 2.75oz	410	22	52
Xreme Butter,			
2 tablespoons, 1.27oz	160	9	20
BodyKey *(Amway)*, Slim Popcorn,			
Sea Salt, 1 bag, 0.7 oz	110	7	10
Jolly Time: *Popped*			
Blast O Butter, 1 cup	45	3	4
Crispy 'n White Light, 1 cup	25	1	4
Xtra Butter: 1 cup	40	3	4
4 cups	160	10	16
Newman's Own: *Unpopped*			
Microwave:			
Butter Flavor, 1.05 oz	150	8	16
Sea Salt, 1.05 oz	150	9	16
Organic Butter, 1.16 oz	150	5	23
Orville Redenbacher's: *Unpopped*			
Butter:			
2 Tablespoons, 1.23 oz	170	12	17
Light, 3 Tbsp, 1.48 oz	160	6	27
Movie Theater,			
2 Tablespoons, 1.2 oz	170	12	16
Ultimate Butter, 2 Tbsp, 1.23 oz	170	11	17
Naturals, 2 Tablespoons 1.23 oz	170	11	18
Smartpop!, Butter, 3 Tbsp, 1.3 oz	120	2	26
Pop Secret: *Popped*			
Double Butter, 1 cup	30	2	3
Extra Butter,1 cup	30	2	3
Skinnygirl *(Orville Redenbacker's)*,			
Butter/ Lime & Sea Salt,			
unpopped, 1.5 oz	160	6	28

Bagged Popcorn

	C	F	Cb
Average All Brands (Ready-to-Eat)			
Regular/Plain: ½ oz package	80	5	8
1 oz package	160	10	16
4 oz package	640	40	64
2 oz Box (store/airport)	320	16	32
3 oz Bag (9" high x 5" wide)	480	24	48
Caramel Popcorn,			
with nuts, 1 cup, 2 oz	230	12	39

Bagged Popcorn ~ Brands

	C	F	Cb
Boston's, Lite, 3½ cups, 1 oz	140	5	20
Cracker Jack: Original, 1 cup, 2 oz	240	4	46
Chocolate & Caramel, 1 cup, 2 oz	220	1	50
Crunch 'N Munch:			
Buttery Toffee: ⅔ cup, 1.1 oz	150	5	24
1 cup, 1.65 oz	225	8	36
Caramel: ⅔ cup, 1.1 oz	160	7	22
1 cup, 1.65 oz	240	10	33
fiddle faddle:			
Butter: ⅔ cup	130	2	26
1 cup	195	3	39
Caramel: ⅔ cup	120	2	24
1 cup, 2 oz	180	3	36
Popcorn Indiana:			
Kettlecorn,			
Sweet & Salty, 1 oz	130	7	16
Popcorn:			
Classic White Cheddar, 1 oz	150	9	15
Himalayan Pink Salt	150	9	15
Movie Theater, 1 oz	140	11	11
Sea Salt, 1 oz	150	9	15
Poppycock:			
Bags: Cashew Lovers, ½ cup, 1 oz	150	6	21
Pecan Delight, ½ cup, 1 oz	150	6	22
Cannisters, Orig./Pecan Delight, av:			
½ cup, 1.1 oz	155	7	21
1 cup, 2.2 oz	310	14	42
Skinny Pop,			
Aged White Cheddar, 3 cups	140	8	14

Movie Theater Popcorn

	C	F	Cb
Small, (7 cups): Plain	385	21	44
with Butter (3 pumps, 0.8 oz)	570	42	44
Medium, (15 cups): Plain	825	45	94
with Butter (4 pumps, 1 oz)	1075	73	94
Large, (20 cups): Plain	1100	60	124
with Butter (6 pumps, 2 oz)	1485	102	124
Butter: 1 Pump, 0.3 oz	65	7	0
4 Pumps (2 Tbsp), 1 oz	250	28	0

Corn & Tortilla Chips

	C	F	Cb
Average All Brands			
Corn Chips:			
Average all types: 1 oz	150	8	18
8 oz bag	1200	64	144
Fritos, Original, 32 chips, 1 oz	160	10	16
Tortilla Chips: Average, 1 oz	140	7	18
(1 oz = approx. 12 chips or 13 strips)			
Doritos: Original, 1 oz	140	7	18
Nacho Chse; Salsa Verde, av., 1 oz	145	8	18
Popchips: Barbecue, 1 oz	130	5	20
Buffalo Ranch, 1 oz	120	4	20
Snyder's:			
El Restaurante, all flavors, 1 oz	150	8	17
Yellow Corn/White, av., 1 oz	135	5	21
Tostitos:			
Average all flav., 1 oz	145	7	19
Baked! Scoops, 1 oz	120	3	22
Utz, Bar-B-Q Flavor Corn Chips	150	9	16

Potato Chips/Crisps

	C	F	Cb
Average All Brands			
Regular:			
Plain or flavored, (4 chips)	30	2	3
1 oz package (20 chips)	150	10	15
4 oz quantity	600	40	60
14 oz package	2100	140	210

Chips/Crisps ~ Brands

	C	F	Cb
Hippeas, Chick Pea Puffs, average all flavors, 0.78 oz	100	4	15
Lay's *(Fritolay):*			
Classics, Wavy Original, 1 oz	160	10	15
Kettle Cooked, Original, 1 oz	150	9	17
Pringles:			
All Flavors: 1 oz	150	9	16
Large can, 6 oz	900	54	96
Reduced Fat, Original, 1 oz	140	7	18
Ruffles: Original, 1 oz	160	10	15
Ridge Twists, all flavors1 oz	140	8	18
Simply7: Lentil Chips, all flavors	140	7	17
Quinoa, average all flavors, 1 oz	140	7	19
Sun Chips: Original, 16 crisps, 1 oz	140	6	19
Whole Grain, Harvest Cheddar, 1 oz	140	6	19

Pretzels

	C	F	Cb
Average All Brands			
Hard-Baked Pretzels: *Each*			
1 oz quantity	110	1	23
Sticks, thin, 2¼" (9/oz)	12	0	3
Twists, thin, ¼" thick, (5/oz)	25	0	5
Dutch (2¾"x 2⅝"), 1 oz	55	1	11
Snyders, Sourdough, 1 oz	110	0	23
Soft Pretzel Twists, average: *Each*			
Plain: Small, 2 oz	210	2	43
Medium, 4 oz	390	4	80
Large, 5 oz	485	5	100
Big Cheese, 1.8 oz	130	3	22
New York Street Vendors, 7 oz	660	6	135
Trader Joe's, Peanut Butter filled, 1 oz	140	8	14
Snyder's: Milk Chocolate Dips, 1 oz	150	7	20
White Creme Dips, 1 oz	140	6	21

Pretzels ~ Brands

	C	F	Cb
Flipz: Milk Choc, 8 pieces, 1 oz	140	5	21
White Fudge, 7 pcs, 1 oz	140	5	21
Rold Gold *(Frito-Lay):*			
Braided Twists,			
Honey Wheat (8), 1 oz	110	1	23
Heartzels, Orig., 0.7 oz pkt	80	1	16
Rods, Original (3), 1 oz	110	1	22
Thins, Original (9), 1 oz	110	1	23
Tiny Twists, Cheddar, (20), 1 oz	110	2	22
Snyder's of Hanover: *Per 1 oz*			
Braided Twists, Sea Salt	110	2	21
Butter Snaps, 1 oz	120	1	25
Chocolate Covered, Jalapeno Ranch	130	5	18
Gluten Free, Sticks	120	3	24
Rounds, Butter	110	2	21
Sourdough Nibblers	120	0	25
Sticks	110	1	23
SuperPretzel:			
6 Count Soft, Original (1), 2.3 oz	160	0	34
Bites (3), 2 oz	160	5	21
Softstix (2), 1.76 oz	130	3	20
Utz:			
Nuggets, 1 oz	100	0	22
Sourdough Pretzels, Extra Dark, 1 oz	110	2	21

Snacks

Note: Actual weight of packaged snacks is usually 5-10% more than label Net Wt. For accuracy, weigh snack and allow extra calories, fat and carbs for any extra weight.

Snacks	C	F	Cb
Apple Chips *(Seneca)*, av., 1 oz	140	7	20
Bagel Crisps *(N.Y. Style)*, 6 crisps, 1 oz	130	6	17
Baguette Chips, 1 oz	130	5	19
Banana Chips *(T.Joe's)*, ¼ cup, 1 oz	160	9	19
Beef Jerky *(Jack Link's)*, av., 1 oz	80	1	6
Beef Sticks:			
Slim Jim, Monster, Original, 1.94 oz	260	19	10
Jack Link's, Original (1), 1.84 oz	240	18	12
Beet Chips *(Rhythm)*, Sea Salt, 1.4oz	160	3	29
Trader Joes, 3 Seed Crackers(17)	150	8	18
BodyKey *(Amway)*:			
Zesty Protein Snack, 1 oz	120	4	15
Bugles, Orig.; Nacho Cheese, 1 oz	150	7	18
Cheese Balls *(Utz)*, 1 oz serving	150	9	14
Cheese Bites *(Trader Joes)*, 1 oz	160	12	1
Cheese Nips *(Nabisco)*, (29), 1 oz	150	6	19
Cheese Puffs, average, 1 oz	160	10	15
Cheetos:			
Crunchy: Av. all flavors, 1 oz	165	10	15
4 oz package	640	40	60
Baked!;, average, 1 oz	135	5	20
Fantastix!, average, 1 oz	130	5	20
Simply Puffs, Wh. Cheddar, 1 oz	160	9	16
Cheez-It *(Sunshine)*:			
Snack Mix: Classic, ½ cup, 1 oz	130	5	20
Double Cheese, ½ cup, 0.9 ozz	130	6	18
Chester's: Fries, Flamin' Hot, 1 oz	150	8	18
Puffcorn, Cheese, 1 oz	160	11	13
Chex Mix *(General Mills)*:			
Cheddar, 1/2 cup, 1.06 oz	130	4	22
Traditional, 1.06 oz	120	4	22
Chicharrones ~ *See Pork Skins*			
Crackers *(Tr. Joes)*, Mini Edamame (28)	120	2	21
Churro Trail Mix *(Great Value)*, 1.06 oz	170	11	14
Combos, Crackers, av., ⅓ cup, 1 oz	140	6	18
Cool Cuts, Carrot & Ranch, 2.3 oz	60	5	6
Corn Chips ~ *See Page 149*			
Corn Nuts: Av all flav., 1 oz	130	5	20
1.7 oz bag	210	8	34
Edamame,			
Seapoint Farms, Dry Roasted, 1 oz	130	5	9
Fritos,			
Corn Chips, Orig.; Flamin' Hot, 1 oz	160	10	16

Snacks (Cont)

Snacks (Cont)	C	F	Cb
Fruit Snacks ~ *See Page 102 & 151*			
Funyuns, Onion Flavored, 1 oz	140	6	19
Goldfish, Crackers, av., 1 oz	140	5	20
Gold-n-Chees *(Lance)*:			
Snack Crackers, 1 oz	140	6	18
Gripz *(Sunshine)*, Mighty Tiny (1)	120	6	15
Flamin Hot Peanuts *(Munchies)*, 1 oz	170	15	5
Kale Chips *(Rhythm)*:			
Kool Ranch, 1 oz	160	12	8
Zesty Nacho, 1 oz	160	12	8
Lance ~ *See Sandwich Crackers Page 151*			
Munchies *(Frito-Lay)*,			
Snack Mix, all flavors, 1 oz	140	7	18
Munchos *(Fritolay)*, all flavors, 1 oz	160	10	16
Nutella, w/ Breadsticks/Pretzels, av.	265	13	35
Nutter Butter, Sandwich Cookies:			
2 Cookies	130	5	20
Bites, 1 pack	130	5	20
Wafers (5), 1.2 oz	160	8	18
Oreo Cookies, all Creme Fillings:			
Double Stuf (2), 1 oz	140	7	21
Mini: 1 Pack, 1 oz	140	5	21
Snak-Sak (9), 1 oz	140	6	21
Oriental Mix Rice Snacks, 1 oz	125	4	21
Peanut Butter Nuggets, (10), 1 oz	140	6	15
Pepitas, dried or roasted, ¼ cup, 1 oz	155	14	3
Pirate's Booty,			
Aged White Cheddar, 1 oz	140	6	18
Pita Chips *(Stacy's)*, (10), 1 oz	130	5	19
Plaintain Chips *(Goya)*, 1 oz	150	8	19
PopChips Ridges, av., 1 oz	130	5	19
PopCorners, Kettle, 1 oz	125	4	20
Popcorn ~ *See Page 148*			
Pork Cracklins, 1 oz	160	12	0
Pork Skins/Rinds: 1 oz	160	10	0
Baken-ets, Traditional, 1 oz	80	5	0
Mission, Chiccarones, 4 oz package	640	45	0
Potato Chips ~ *See Page 149*			
Potato Skins Chips *(TGI Friday)*,			
all flavors, 16 chips, 1 oz	140	8	16
Puffed Wheat,			
Sabritones, Chili & Lime, 1 oz	140	8	16
Pretzels ~ *See Page 149*			

Snacks (Cont)

	C	F	Cb
Rice Cakes:			
Lundberg: Honey Nut (1)	80	1	19
Thin Stackers, Brown Rice (4), 1 oz	110	1	24
Quaker:			
100% Whole Grain, lightly salted (1)	35	0	7
Chocolate (1)	60	1	12
Rice Chips,			
Lundberg, average, 1 oz	135	6	18
Sandwich Crackers:			
Austin, Cheese Sandwich Crackers:			
w/ Cheddar, 0.9 oz	130	6	16
w/ Peanut Butter, 1.37 oz	190	9	24
Cheese Crackers, with PB, 0.9 oz	130	6	15
Lance: Nekot Lemon Creme, 1pkg	240	11	35
Toasty, PB, 1 pkg	180	9	21
Toast Chee, PB, 2 oz	220	10	25
Ritz Bits: Cheese (13), 1 oz Pkg	160	9	18
Peanut Butter, 1 oz	150	8	17
Sesame Sticks, Salted,			
SunRidge Farm, 1 oz	170	12	14
Smart Puffs,			
Pirates Booty, 1 oz	140	7	17
Soybeans in Pods,			
AFC, ½ cup, 3.2 oz	90	5	3
Soy Crisps, average, 1 oz	120	3	17
Soy Nuts: Dry Roasted, 1/4 cup, 1 oz	130	6	9
Choc-Coated, 1 oz	140	7	13
Sun Chips,			
Fritolay, average, 1 oz	140	6	19
Takis, Crunchy Fajitas, 1 oz	150	8	17
Tings *(Robert's)*, 2 oz bag	300	16	36
Toasted Chips (*Ritz*), av. all, 1 oz	130	5	21
Tortilla Chips, White,			
Garden of Eatin, Touch of Lime, 1 oz	130	7	17
Trail Mix (Nuts/Seeds/Dried Fruit):			
Regular, 3 Tbsp, 1 oz	140	9	13
Tropical, 3 Tbsp, 1 oz	130	7	16
Turkey Jerky: Teriyaki, 1 oz	80	1	8
Trader Joe's, Original, 1 oz	60	0	6
Veggie Braided Twists,			
Snyder's, 1 oz	110	2	21
Wheat Thins *(Nabisco)*, av. all, 1 oz	135	5	21
Woats, Oatsnack, av., 1/4 cup, 1 oz	120	5	17
Yogurt Pretzels *(Larissa Veronica)*,			
5 pieces, 1 oz	150	8	20
Yogurt Raisins, Vanilla,			
Sun-Maid, 1 oz	120	5	20

Fruit Snacks

	C	F	Cb
Betty Crocker:			
Fruit Gushers, Strawb. Splash, 0.9 oz	90	2	20
Fruit by the Foot, 1 roll, 0.8 oz	80	1	17
Fruit Roll Ups, 1 roll, 1 oz	50	1	12
Sunkist:			
Fruit Lover's Trail Mix:			
Pineapple Coconut Blend, 1 oz	120	5	18
Straweberry Banana, 1 oz	110	4	19

Fruit Snack cups ~ See Page 102

Vending Machines

	C	F	Cb
Bugles, Nacho Cheese, 1 oz	150	9	18
Cheese Balls *(Utz)*, 1 oz	150	9	16
Cheetos, Crunchy, av., 1 oz	165	10	15
Cheeze-It, Classic Snack Mix, 1 oz	140	5	20
Chester's, Flamin' Hot Fries, 1 oz	150	8	17
Choc Chip Cookies:			
Chips Ahoy, 2 oz pkg	280	14	38
Famous Amos, 1.2 oz pouch	170	8	23
Grandma's, (1), 1.4 oz	200	10	25
Chocolate Bars:			
Hershey's, Milk Choc.,2 oz	220	13	26
Kit Kat, 1.5 oz	210	11	28
Snickers, 1.86 oz bar	250	12	32
Donut, plain cake, 1.4 oz	160	9	18
Doritos, av. all flavors, 1 oz	145	8	18
Fritos, Corn Chips, Orig., 2.75 oz	440	28	44
Fruit Pie,			
Hostess, Apple, 5 oz	430	17	67
Granola/Cereal Bars, av., 1 oz	140	3	26
M & M's:			
Milk Chocolate, 2 oz	280	10	40
Peanuts, 2 oz	280	14	34
Oreo Cookies, (3), 1.2 oz	160	7	25
Peanut Butter cups,			
Reese's, 2 oz	210	12	24
Popcorn, plain, 1 oz	160	10	16
PopChips Ridges, 1 oz	130	5	19
Pork Skins, 2 oz	240	15	0
Potato Chips: 1 oz	150	10	15
Baked! (*Ruffles*), Orig.,1 oz	120	3	22
Potato Skins Chips *(TGI Friday's)*,			
all flavors, 1 oz	140	8	16
Pretzels *(Snyder's)*, Olde Tyme, 1 oz	120	1	24
Raisins, 1 oz package	45	0	11
Rice Krispies Treat, Original, 0.78 oz	90	2	17
Skittles, Original,1 oz	110	1	26
Starburst, Fruit Chews, Orig., 1 oz	120	3	24
Tortilla Chips, 1 oz	140	7	18

S Soups

Homemade & Restaurant

Restaurant & Take-Out:	C	F	Cb
Average All Recipes: ***Per 1 Cup, 8 fl oz***			
For 12 fl.oz Serving: Add 50% of figures			
For 16 fl oz Serving: Double the figures			
Bean Medley	200	3	34
Beef Consomme	30	0	2
Borscht, w/ Sour Cream	130	8	14
Bouillabaisse	400	15	10
Chicken & Corn	290	14	20
Chicken & Wild Rice	80	4	9
Chicken Consomme	50	0	2
Chicken Curry	180	8	18
Chicken Jambalaya	160	7	8
Chicken Noodle	80	2	12
With Chicken	160	4	12
Chicken Soup	80	2	6
Chili with Beans	250	12	25
Clam Chowder	240	15	17
Corn & Crab	120	3	18
Corn Chowder	150	8	16
Cream of Broccoli	200	12	20
Cream of Potato	150	7	17
Cream of Mushroom	200	13	15
Fish Chowder	220	15	6
French Onion	420	15	25
Gazpacho	50	0	5
Lentil Soup	250	9	28
Lobster Bisque	320	15	10
Matzo Ball Soup	180	7	24
Minestrone	125	3	20
Mulligatawny	300	15	8
Pea & Ham	240	10	25
Potato & Bacon	170	7	19
Pumpkin, Creamy	210	10	26
Shark Fin Soup	100	4	8
Spicy Shrimp Soup, 1 bowl	160	7	10
Split Pea Soup	180	3	30
Vegetable (Fat Free)	75	0	18
Vegetable Beef	80	2	10
Vichyssoise	200	9	15
Watercress	90	4	13

Other Soups ~ *See International & Fast-Foods Sections (Arby's, Au Bon Pain, Boston Market, Dunkin' Donuts, Denny's, Schlotzsky's, Sizzler, Souplantation, Sweet Tomatoes, Zoup!)*

Homemade Soups: *Calculate calories, fat and carbohydrates from recipe ingredients.*

Bouillon Cubes & Powders

Bouillon Cubes: *Average all types*	C	F	Cb
Regular, 1 cube	5	0	1
Extra Large, 1 cube	20	1	1
Powders, average, 1 tsp	10	0	1
Herb-Ox:			
Instant Broth & Seasoning,			
Beef, 1 envelope, 0.14 oz	5	0	1
Chicken, 1 envelope, 0.14 oz	5	0	1

Soup ~ Brands

	C	F	Cb
Amy's:			
Heat & Serve (Organic): *Per 1 Cup,*			
Alphabet	110	2	21
Black Bean Vegetable	210	4	35
Chunky Vegetable	80	2	5
Carrot Ginger	200	13	18
Cream of Mushshroom, ¾ cup	150	11	11
Lentil Vegetable	160	4	24
Rustic Italian Vegetable	190	8	24
Southwestern Vegetable	130	5	18
Split Pea	120	1	20
Thai Coconut	210	14	15
Thai Curry Sweet Pot. Lentil	280	20	20
Tortilla with Rstd Sweet Pot.	130	5	18
Campbell's:			
Chunky: *Per Cup, Unless Indicated*			
Baked Potato w/ Ched. & Bacon Bits	190	9	22
Baked Potato with Steak & Cheese	200	10	21
Beef with Country Vegetables	110	2	16
Chicken & Sausage Gumbo	140	4	21
Chicken Corn Chowder	140	3	22
Chipotle Chkn & Corn Chowd.	180	8	20
Classic Chicken Noodle	120	3	14
Creamy Chkn & Dumplings	170	9	14
Hearty Bean & Ham, Smoked	150	2	27
Jambalaya Chkn, Ssg & Ham	140	4	20
Sirloin Steak & Hearty Vegetables	120	3	18
Manhattan Clam Chowder	110	3	15
Old Fashioned Potato Ham Chowder	180	9	17

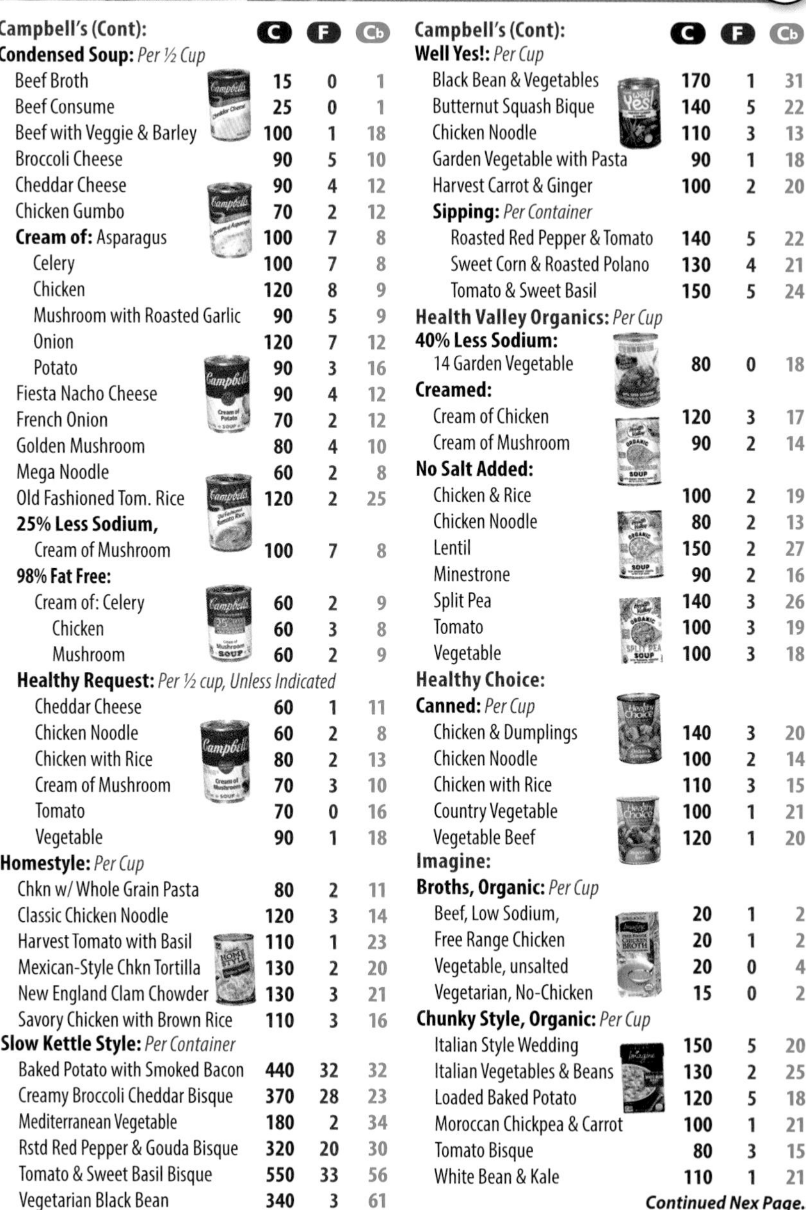

Campbell's (Cont):

Condensed Soup: *Per ½ Cup*	C	F	Cb
Beef Broth	15	0	1
Beef Consume	25	0	1
Beef with Veggie & Barley	100	1	18
Broccoli Cheese	90	5	10
Cheddar Cheese	90	4	12
Chicken Gumbo	70	2	12
Cream of: Asparagus	100	7	8
Celery	100	7	8
Chicken	120	8	9
Mushroom with Roasted Garlic	90	5	9
Onion	120	7	12
Potato	90	3	16
Fiesta Nacho Cheese	90	4	12
French Onion	70	2	12
Golden Mushroom	80	4	10
Mega Noodle	60	2	8
Old Fashioned Tom. Rice	120	2	25
25% Less Sodium,			
Cream of Mushroom	100	7	8
98% Fat Free:			
Cream of: Celery	60	2	9
Chicken	60	3	8
Mushroom	60	2	9
Healthy Request: *Per ½ cup, Unless Indicated*			
Cheddar Cheese	60	1	11
Chicken Noodle	60	2	8
Chicken with Rice	80	2	13
Cream of Mushroom	70	3	10
Tomato	70	0	16
Vegetable	90	1	18
Homestyle: *Per Cup*			
Chkn w/ Whole Grain Pasta	80	2	11
Classic Chicken Noodle	120	3	14
Harvest Tomato with Basil	110	1	23
Mexican-Style Chkn Tortilla	130	2	20
New England Clam Chowder	130	3	21
Savory Chicken with Brown Rice	110	3	16
Slow Kettle Style: *Per Container*			
Baked Potato with Smoked Bacon	440	32	32
Creamy Broccoli Cheddar Bisque	370	28	23
Mediterranean Vegetable	180	2	34
Rstd Red Pepper & Gouda Bisque	320	20	30
Tomato & Sweet Basil Bisque	550	33	56
Vegetarian Black Bean	340	3	61

Campbell's (Cont):

Well Yes!: *Per Cup*	C	F	Cb
Black Bean & Vegetables	170	1	31
Butternut Squash Bique	140	5	22
Chicken Noodle	110	3	13
Garden Vegetable with Pasta	90	1	18
Harvest Carrot & Ginger	100	2	20
Sipping: *Per Container*			
Roasted Red Pepper & Tomato	140	5	22
Sweet Corn & Roasted Polano	130	4	21
Tomato & Sweet Basil	150	5	24
Health Valley Organics: *Per Cup*			
40% Less Sodium:			
14 Garden Vegetable	80	0	18
Creamed:			
Cream of Chicken	120	3	17
Cream of Mushroom	90	2	14
No Salt Added:			
Chicken & Rice	100	2	19
Chicken Noodle	80	2	13
Lentil	150	2	27
Minestrone	90	2	16
Split Pea	140	3	26
Tomato	100	3	19
Vegetable	100	3	18
Healthy Choice:			
Canned: *Per Cup*			
Chicken & Dumplings	140	3	20
Chicken Noodle	100	2	14
Chicken with Rice	110	3	15
Country Vegetable	100	1	21
Vegetable Beef	120	1	20
Imagine:			
Broths, Organic: *Per Cup*			
Beef, Low Sodium,	20	1	2
Free Range Chicken	20	1	2
Vegetable, unsalted	20	0	4
Vegetarian, No-Chicken	15	0	2
Chunky Style, Organic: *Per Cup*			
Italian Style Wedding	150	5	20
Italian Vegetables & Beans	130	2	25
Loaded Baked Potato	120	5	18
Moroccan Chickpea & Carrot	100	1	21
Tomato Bisque	80	3	15
White Bean & Kale	110	1	21

Continued Nex Page...

Imagine (Cont):	C	F	Cb
Creamy: *Per 8 fl.oz Cup*			
Butternut Squash	100	2	20
Broccoli	70	1	14
Garden Tomato, Light Sodium	80	1	16
Potato Leek	90	3	14
Portobello Mushroom	80	3	12
Tomato; Tomato Basil, av.	85	1	16
Kettle Cuisine: *Per 8 fl.oz Cup*			
Albondigas Meatball Soup	150	7	17
Beef, Barley & Vegetable	110	3	13
Broccoli Cheddar	310	25	13
Buffalo Chicken	240	15	14
Carrot Ginger	110	4	18
Chicken Tortilla	110	4	14
Chipotle Sweet Potato	150	6	24
Classic Gazpacho	50	2	8
Coconut Curry Chicken	190	8	20
Cream of Crab	290	23	15
Hungarian Mushroom	230	16	18
Lobster Bisque	260	18	18
Maryland VegetableCrab	90	2	15
Minestrone	80	2	14
North Atlantic Haddock Chowder	250	17	13
Organic Split Pea & Kale	80	2	13
Portuguese Kale with Linguica	160	7	21
Knorr:			
Cubes: *Per ½ Cube, 1 Cup, Prepared*			
Beef; Chicken, average, 0 .2 oz	17	1	1
Homestyle Stock: *Per 1 Tsp*			
Beef	10	1	1
Chicken	10	1	1
Lipton:			
Cup-a-Soup: *Per Cup*			
Chicken varieties, average	70	2	14
Spring Vegetable	50	1	9
Recipe Secrets: *Dry Mix*			
Golden Onion, 1 ⅔ Tbsp	50	1	10
Onion Mushroom, 1⅔ Tbsp	30	0	7
Average other flavors, 1 Tbsp	25	0	6
Soup Secrets, Dry Mix, av. all flav., 2 T.	65	1	11
Manischewitz:			
Dry Soup Mix:			
Matzo Ball, 1 oz	45	0	8
Canned: *Per 1 cup*			
Condensed Chicken Broth, 4.3 oz	15	0	2
Maruchan:			
Instant Lunch, average all flavors, 1 pkg	290	12	38
Ramen, all flavors, 1 pkg, 3 oz	380	14	52

Nissin:	C	F	Cb
Soup'd Up Cup Noodles: *Per Package*			
Roasted Chicken Flavor, 37 oz	330	12	46
Savory Shrimp Flavor, 37 oz	330	13	45
Souper Meal, Beef, 1.45 oz pkg	550	22	77
Pacific Foods:			
Condensed: *Per Container*			
Cream of Chicken	190	6	23
Cream of Mushroom	190	8	27
Creamy: *Per 1 Cup*			
Cumin Carrot Oat Milk	100	3	14
Moroccan Sweet Potato	130	5	19
Tomato Basil	90	2	13
Hearty Organic: *Per 1 Cup*			
Cashew Carrot Ginger Bisque	140	5	22
Chicken Noodle	80	1	12
Thai Sweet Potato	160	7	22
Other Soup Varities ~ See CalorieKing.com			
Progresso: *Per Cup*			
Broths: Beef	15	0	1
Classic Chicken	5	0	0
Vegetable	5	0	1
Light: *Per 1 cup*			
Beef Pot Roast	70	1	9
Broccoli Cheese	120	6	11
Chicken Noodle	60	1	9
New Eng. Clam Chowder	100	3	16
Rich & Hearty:			
Beef Pot Roast w/ Country Vegetables	110	2	16
Broccoli Cheese with Bacon	180	13	10
Chicken & Homestyle Noodles	110	3	14
Chkn Pot Pie w/ Dumplings	130	4	17
Lasagna Style w/ Ital Ssg	170	7	20
New Eng. Clam Chowder	170	7	23
Steak & Vegetables	100	2	16
Rhree Cheese Tortellini	110	10	16
Traditional: *Per 1 Cup*			
Cheese Tortellini Garden Vegetable	100	1	20
Chickarina	110	4	12
Chicken & Rotini	90	2	13
Italian-Style Wedding	120	4	15
Manhattan Clam Chowder	100	2	17
Potato, Broccoli & Cheese	210	13	19
Vegetable Classic: *Per 1 Cup*			
Creamy Mushroom	130	9	12
Green Split Pea w/ Bacon	150	2	29
Minestrone	110	2	20
Tuscan-Style White Bean	130	2	23
Other Soup Varities ~ See CalorieKing.com			

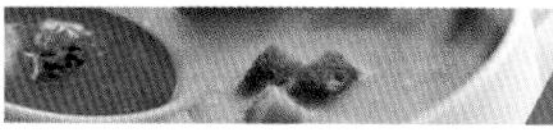

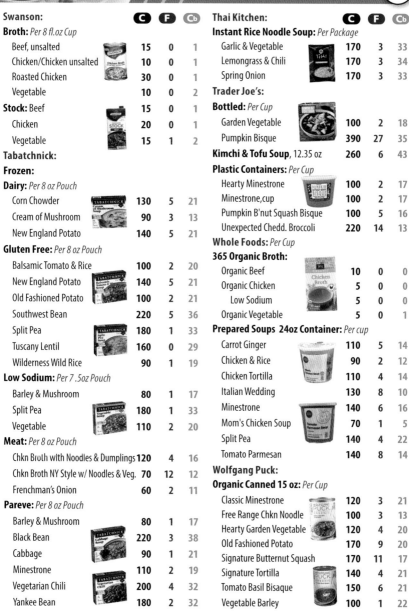

Swanson:	C	F	Cb
Broth: *Per 8 fl.oz Cup*			
Beef, unsalted	15	0	1
Chicken/Chicken unsalted	10	0	1
Roasted Chicken	30	0	1
Vegetable	10	0	2
Stock: Beef	15	0	1
Chicken	20	0	1
Vegetable	15	1	2
Tabatchnick:			
Frozen:			
Dairy: *Per 8 oz Pouch*			
Corn Chowder	130	5	21
Cream of Mushroom	90	3	13
New England Potato	140	5	21
Gluten Free: *Per 8 oz Pouch*			
Balsamic Tomato & Rice	100	2	20
New England Potato	140	5	21
Old Fashioned Potato	100	2	21
Southwest Bean	220	5	36
Split Pea	180	1	33
Tuscany Lentil	160	0	29
Wilderness Wild Rice	90	1	19
Low Sodium: *Per 7 .5oz Pouch*			
Barley & Mushroom	80	1	17
Split Pea	180	1	33
Vegetable	110	2	20
Meat: *Per 8 oz Pouch*			
Chkn Broth with Noodles & Dumplings	120	4	16
Chkn Broth NY Style w/ Noodles & Veg.	70	12	12
Frenchman's Onion	60	2	11
Pareve: *Per 8 oz Pouch*			
Barley & Mushroom	80	1	17
Black Bean	220	3	38
Cabbage	90	1	21
Minestrone	110	2	19
Vegetarian Chili	200	4	32
Yankee Bean	180	2	32

Thai Kitchen:	C	F	Cb
Instant Rice Noodle Soup: *Per Package*			
Garlic & Vegetable	170	3	33
Lemongrass & Chili	170	3	34
Spring Onion	170	3	33
Trader Joe's:			
Bottled: *Per Cup*			
Garden Vegetable	100	2	18
Pumpkin Bisque	390	27	35
Kimchi & Tofu Soup, 12.35 oz	260	6	43
Plastic Containers: *Per Cup*			
Hearty Minestrone	100	2	17
Minestrone,cup	100	2	17
Pumpkin B'nut Squash Bisque	100	5	16
Unexpected Chedd. Broccoli	220	14	13
Whole Foods: *Per Cup*			
365 Organic Broth:			
Organic Beef	10	0	0
Organic Chicken	5	0	0
Low Sodium	5	0	0
Organic Vegetable	5	0	1
Prepared Soups 24oz Container: *Per cup*			
Carrot Ginger	110	5	14
Chicken & Rice	90	2	12
Chicken Tortilla	110	4	14
Italian Wedding	130	8	10
Minestrone	140	6	16
Mom's Chicken Soup	70	1	5
Split Pea	140	4	22
Tomato Parmesan	140	8	14
Wolfgang Puck:			
Organic Canned 15 oz: *Per Cup*			
Classic Minestrone	120	3	21
Free Range Chkn Noodle	100	3	13
Hearty Garden Vegetable	120	4	20
Old Fashioned Potato	170	9	20
Signature Butternut Squash	170	11	17
Signature Tortilla	140	4	21
Tomato Basil Bisaque	150	6	21
Vegetable Barley	100	1	22

S Soy Products & Tofu

Soybean Products

Soybean Products	C	F	Cb
Cheeses (Soy) ~ *See Page 78*			
Miso Soy Bean Paste:			
Cold Mountain: Light Yellow, 1 tsp	10	0	1
Mellow Red, 1 tsp	15	0	3
Red, 1 tsp	10	0	1
Miso Soup (dry mix):			
1 Tbsp., dry mix	35	1	5
1 cup, prepared	35	1	5
Natto, ½ cup, 3 oz	160	7	14
Okara (Tofu fiber residue), ½ c., 2 oz	47	1	8
Tempeh: 1 piece, 3 oz	180	8	12
Fried, 3 oz	250	14	14
Seitan *(Westsoy)*, Strips, 3 oz	120	2	4
Soybean Protein *(TVP)*, 1 oz	95	0	8
Soy Bean Paste, 1 tsp	10	0	2
Soy Beans ~ *See Page 160*			
Soy Drinks ~ *See Page 49*			

Tofu ~ Brands

Tofu ~ Brands	C	F	Cb
Azumaya Tofu:			
Extra Firm; Firm, av., 3 oz	75	4	2
Firm (Silken), 3 oz	45	2	1
House Foods: *Per 3 oz*			
Organic: Grilled, Super Firm	70	4	3
Medium Firm	50	3	2
Soft	50	3	2
Super Firm, cubed	70	4	3
Premium: Firm	70	4	2
Extra Firm	80	5	2
Soft	60	3	2
Mori-Nu Tofu: *Per 3 oz*			
Extra Firm	45	2	1
Firm Silken	50	2	1
Lite Silken	30	1	0
Organic Silken	45	2	1
Plus, Fortified Extra Silken	80	6	4
Soft	45	2	1
Nasoya: *Per 3 oz*			
Organic: Extra Firm	90	5	3
Firm	80	4	2
Silken	40	2	1
Organic Tofubaked: *Per 4 oz*			
Sesame Ginger	150	8	5
Teriyaki	140	7	6
Organic Toss'ables,			
Garlic & Herb, 3 oz	150	8	5

Supplements

Supplements	C	F	Cb
Aloe Vera Juice, undiluted, 2 fl.oz	5	0	1
Flakes, 1 heaping Tbsp, 0.3 oz	30	1	4
Powder, 1 heaping Tbsp, 1 oz	50	1	6
Tablets, 2 tabs	4	0	`
Calcium Chews: *CVS*, 1 chew	20	0	3
Trader Joe's, Chocolate,1 chew	20	1	3
Cod Liver Oil, 1 Tbsp	125	13	0
Fiber Choice, 2 tabs	15	0	4
Fiber,			
Fibersure, 1 heaping tsp	25	0	6
Fish Oil Capsules, (1), av.	10	1	0
Flax Oil:			
Capsules (2)	10	1	0
Barlean's, softgels (3)	110	11	0
Garlic Tablets/Capsules, each	3	0	0
Glowelle:			
Beauty Drink, 8 fl.oz	100	0	24
Powder Stick (1)	50	0	12
Lecithin Granules, 1 Tbsp	55	4	1
Metamucil, Powder:			
Orange (Smooth Texture), 1 rounded Tbsp	45	0	12
Sugar-Free, 1 rounded tsp	20	0	5
Pink Lemonade, Sugar-Free, 1 rounded tsp	20	0	5
Capsules: Heart & Digestive (6)	10	0	3
Strong Bones (5)	10	0	3
Meta, Fiber Wafers (2)	100	5	16
Protein, Powders, av., 1 oz	100	1	0
Seaweed: Dried, 1 oz	85	1	22
Soaked, drained, 1 oz	15	1	3
Spirulina, 1 tablet	2	0	1
Vitamins/Minerals: Tabs/Caps (1)	2	0	0
Vitamin E Capsules, each	5	1	0
Viactiv Chews, Choc. (1)	20	1	4

Cough & Pharmaceutical

Cough & Pharmaceutical	C	F	Cb
Antacids: Av., 1 tablet	4	0	1
Liquid, 1 Tbsp	6	0	1
Antacid Sodium Counts ~ *See Page 280*			
Cough/Cold Syrups:			
Regular: With sugar, 1 Tbsp	35	0	9
With alcohol, 1 Tbsp	46	0	9
Diabetic Tussin, Sugar Free, 1 T.	0	0	0
Cough Drops/Lozenges ~ *See Page 75*			
Sudafed, Syrup 1 tsp	14	0	3
Tylenol, Liquid: Child, 1 tsp	17	0	4
Extra Strength, 1 tsp	11	0	3

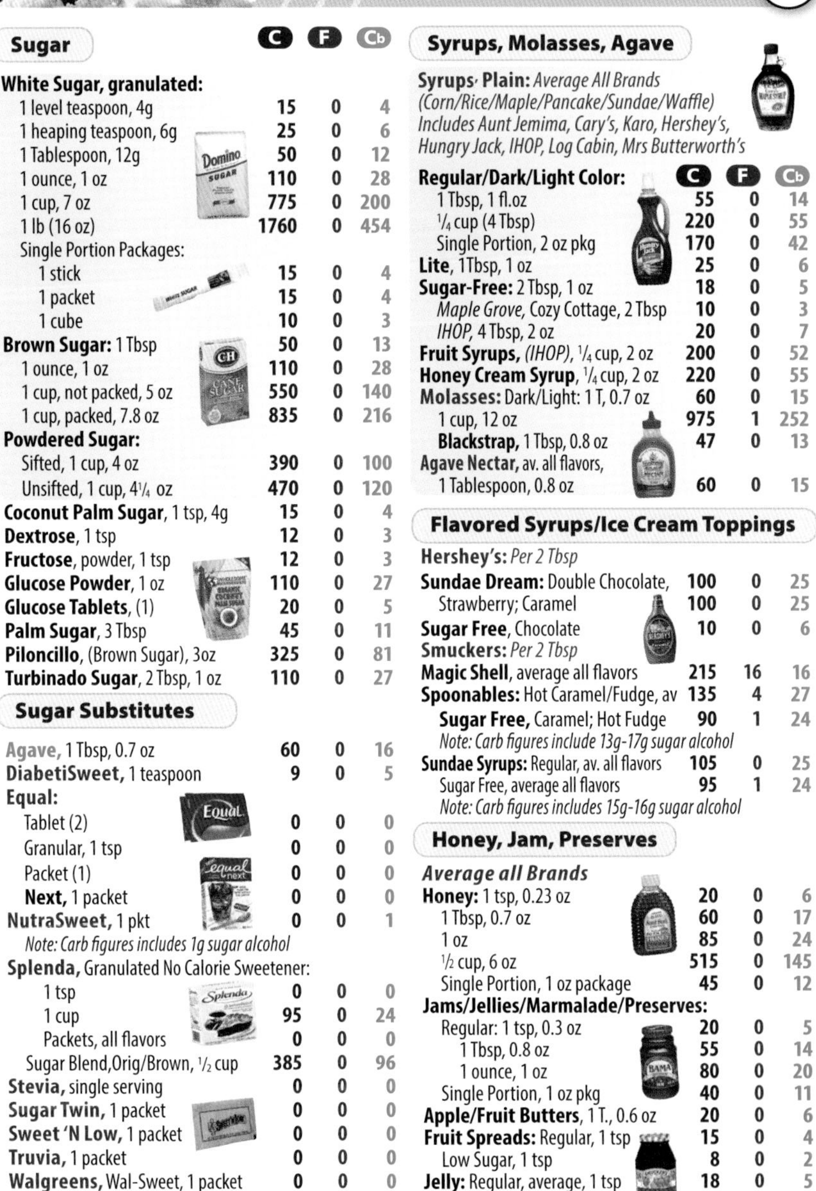

Sugar

	C	F	Cb
White Sugar, granulated:			
1 level teaspoon, 4g	15	0	4
1 heaping teaspoon, 6g	25	0	6
1 Tablespoon, 12g	50	0	12
1 ounce, 1 oz	110	0	28
1 cup, 7 oz	775	0	200
1 lb (16 oz)	1760	0	454
Single Portion Packages:			
1 stick	15	0	4
1 packet	15	0	4
1 cube	10	0	3
Brown Sugar: 1 Tbsp	50	0	13
1 ounce, 1 oz	110	0	28
1 cup, not packed, 5 oz	550	0	140
1 cup, packed, 7.8 oz	835	0	216
Powdered Sugar:			
Sifted, 1 cup, 4 oz	390	0	100
Unsifted, 1 cup, 4 1/4 oz	470	0	120
Coconut Palm Sugar, 1 tsp, 4g	15	0	4
Dextrose, 1 tsp	12	0	3
Fructose, powder, 1 tsp	12	0	3
Glucose Powder, 1 oz	110	0	27
Glucose Tablets, (1)	20	0	5
Palm Sugar, 3 Tbsp	45	0	11
Piloncillo, (Brown Sugar), 3oz	325	0	81
Turbinado Sugar, 2 Tbsp, 1 oz	110	0	27

Sugar Substitutes

	C	F	Cb
Agave, 1 Tbsp, 0.7 oz	60	0	16
DiabetiSweet, 1 teaspoon	9	0	5
Equal:			
Tablet (2)	0	0	0
Granular, 1 tsp	0	0	0
Packet (1)	0	0	0
Next, 1 packet	0	0	0
NutraSweet, 1 pkt	0	0	1
Note: Carb figures includes 1g sugar alcohol			
Splenda, Granulated No Calorie Sweetener:			
1 tsp	0	0	0
1 cup	95	0	24
Packets, all flavors	0	0	0
Sugar Blend, Orig/Brown, 1/2 cup	385	0	96
Stevia, single serving	0	0	0
Sugar Twin, 1 packet	0	0	0
Sweet 'N Low, 1 packet	0	0	0
Truvia, 1 packet	0	0	0
Walgreens, Wal-Sweet, 1 packet	0	0	0
Whey Low, 1 tsp	4	0	1

Syrups, Molasses, Agave

Syrups, Plain: *Average All Brands (Corn/Rice/Maple/Pancake/Sundae/Waffle) Includes Aunt Jemima, Cary's, Karo, Hershey's, Hungry Jack, IHOP, Log Cabin, Mrs Butterworth's*

	C	F	Cb
Regular/Dark/Light Color:			
1 Tbsp, 1 fl.oz	55	0	14
1/4 cup (4 Tbsp)	220	0	55
Single Portion, 2 oz pkg	170	0	42
Lite, 1Tbsp, 1 oz	25	0	6
Sugar-Free: 2 Tbsp, 1 oz	18	0	5
Maple Grove, Cozy Cottage, 2 Tbsp	10	0	3
IHOP, 4 Tbsp, 2 oz	20	0	7
Fruit Syrups, *(IHOP)*, 1/4 cup, 2 oz	200	0	52
Honey Cream Syrup, 1/4 cup, 2 oz	220	0	55
Molasses: Dark/Light: 1 T, 0.7 oz	60	0	15
1 cup, 12 oz	975	1	252
Blackstrap, 1 Tbsp, 0.8 oz	47	0	13
Agave Nectar, av. all flavors, 1 Tablespoon, 0.8 oz	60	0	15

Flavored Syrups/Ice Cream Toppings

	C	F	Cb
Hershey's: *Per 2 Tbsp*			
Sundae Dream: Double Chocolate,	100	0	25
Strawberry; Caramel	100	0	25
Sugar Free, Chocolate	10	0	6
Smuckers: *Per 2 Tbsp*			
Magic Shell, average all flavors	215	16	16
Spoonables: Hot Caramel/Fudge, av	135	4	27
Sugar Free, Caramel; Hot Fudge	90	1	24
Note: Carb figures include 13g-17g sugar alcohol			
Sundae Syrups: Regular, av. all flavors	105	0	25
Sugar Free, average all flavors	95	1	24
Note: Carb figures includes 15g-16g sugar alcohol			

Honey, Jam, Preserves

Average all Brands

	C	F	Cb
Honey: 1 tsp, 0.23 oz	20	0	6
1 Tbsp, 0.7 oz	60	0	17
1 oz	85	0	24
1/2 cup, 6 oz	515	0	145
Single Portion, 1 oz package	45	0	12
Jams/Jellies/Marmalade/Preserves:			
Regular: 1 tsp, 0.3 oz	20	0	5
1 Tbsp, 0.8 oz	55	0	14
1 ounce, 1 oz	80	0	20
Single Portion, 1 oz pkg	40	0	11
Apple/Fruit Butters, 1 T., 0.6 oz	20	0	6
Fruit Spreads: Regular, 1 tsp	15	0	4
Low Sugar, 1 tsp	8	0	2
Jelly: Regular, average, 1 tsp	18	0	5
Imitation, Low Calorie, 1 tsp	4	0	1

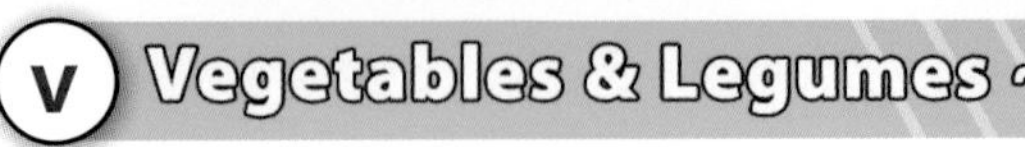

V Vegetables & Legumes ~ Fresh

Vegetables	C	F	Cb
Alfalfa Sprouts, ½ cup, 1 oz	5	0	1
Anaheim Pepper, raw, 3 oz	20	0	4
Artichokes, Globe/French:			
1 medium, 5 oz	60	0	13
1 large, 5.7 oz	75	0	17
Artichoke Heart, plain, 2 pieces	15	0	3
Asparagus, raw/frozen:			
Cuts & Tips, ½ cup, 4.3 oz	20	0	3
Spears, 3 medium	10	0	2
Bamboo Shoots, cooked, ½ cup, 2 oz	7	0	1
Beans, Green/Snap/String:			
10 beans (4" long), 2 oz	20	0	4
Pieces, ½ cup, 3 oz	30	0	7
Dried Beans (Kidney, Brown, Lima, Navy, Pinto, White):			
Raw: 2 Tbsp, 1 oz	95	1	18
1 cup, 7 oz	665	3	126
Cooked: 1 oz	35	0	7
½ cup, 3 oz	105	0	21
Bean Sprouts, average, ½ cup, 2 oz	15	0	4
Beets (Beetroot):			
Raw, 1 beet (2" diam.), 4 oz	35	0	8
Cooked, 1 cup, slices, 3 oz	35	0	8
Canned ~ *See Page 161*			
Beet Greens, cooked, ½ cup, 3 oz	20	0	4
Bell Pepper ~ *See Peppers*			
Bitter Melon/Gourd, 1 cup, 2 oz	15	0	2
Blackeye Peas, cooked, ½ cup, 3 oz	100	1	18
Bok Choy (Chinese Chard), cooked, 3 oz	10	0	2
Breadfruit, ¼ small fruit, 3 oz	100	0	26
Broadbeans (Fava Beans):			
Green, raw, (in pod): 4 pods (4 oz with shells, 1.2 oz beans)	30	0	6
1 cup beans, without shell, 5 oz	110	1	22
Mature Seeds: Raw, 1 cup, 5.3 oz	510	3	87
Cooked, ½ cup, 3 oz	95	0	17
Broccoflower, ⅕ head, 4 oz	35	0	7
Broccoli: Raw, chopped,1 cup, 3 oz	30	0	6
3 Florets, 3 oz	25	0	5
1 Spear (5" long), 1.oz	10	0	2
1 Whole, Medium, 14 oz	135	2	26
1 Head (no stalk), 11 oz	105	1	21
1 Stalk, small (5" long), 5.3 oz	50	1	10
Brocco Sprouts, ½ cup, 1 oz	15	0	2
Brussels Sprouts:			
Cooked, ½ cup, 2.8 oz	30	1	6
2 Sprouts, 2 oz	15	0	3
Butterbeans, cooked, ½ cup, 3 oz	90	0	16
Cabbage, average other flavors:			
Raw: 1 leaf, large, 1 oz	5	0	2
Shredded, 1 cup, 3 oz	15	0	4
½ large head (7" diam), 22 oz	150	1	35
Cooked, shredded, ½ cup, 3 oz	15	1	4

Vegetables (Cont)	C	F	Cb
Cactus Leaf (Nopales):			
1 leaf, 5 oz	20	0	4
1 cup (slices), 3 oz	15	0	3
Carrots, regular thick variety:			
1 small, 4 oz	45	0	11
1 medium, 6 oz	70	0	16
1 large, 8 oz	95	0	22
Chopped, 1 cup, 5 oz	50	0	12
Grated, 1 cup, 4 oz	45	0	11
Slices, 1 cup, 5 oz	50	0	12
Sticks (4"), 4-5, 2 oz	20	0	4
Long thin variety, 1 medium, 2.2 oz	25	0	6
Baby: Snack size, 3 medium, 1 oz	10	0	3
Snack Pack, 3 oz	30	0	7
Cassava, raw, 1 cup, 3 oz	330	1	78
Cauliflower, raw:			
Pieces, 1 cup, 4 oz	25	0	5
½ medium head, 10 oz	70	0	15
Cooked, 3 florets, 2 oz	10	0	2
Celeriac, ½ cup, raw, 2.8 oz	35	0	7
Celery: 1 large stalk, 11", 2.2 oz	10	0	2
4 Strips, thin sticks, 1 oz	5	0	1
Chopped, 1 cup, 4 oz	15	0	3
Chard (Swiss), ½ cup, cooked, 3 oz	20	0	4
Chayote Squash:			
1 medium, 7 oz	40	0	9
Pieces, 1 cup, 5 oz	25	0	6
Chickpeas, (Garbanzo Beans):			
Dry, 1 cup, 7 oz	730	12	121
Cooked, 1 cup, 5.8 oz	270	4	45
Chicory Greens, 1 cup, 1 oz	7	0	2
Chili Peppers ~ *See Peppers*			
Chinese Long Bean, slices, 1 cup, 3.2 oz	45	0	8
Chives, chopped, 1 Tbsp	1	0	0
Choy Sum, 3 oz	15	0	3
Cilantro, (Coriander), 1 cup	5	0	1
Collards, cooked, ½ cup, 3 oz	25	0	5
Corn, Yellow/White:			
Raw: Kernels, ½ cup, 3 oz	80	1	19
Ear (5"x 1¾"), 6 oz	155	1	37
Cooked: Kernels, ½ cup, 3 oz	77	1	18
Cob, small, 2.3 oz	60	1	14
Ear, large, 6 oz	120	1	28
Cress, garden, raw, 1 cup, 1.8 oz	15	0	3
Cucumber, average other flavors:			
Slices, ½ cup, 2 oz	10	0	2
Green, 1 medium (9"), 11 oz	45	0	11
Persian, 1 medium (8"), 6 oz	25	0	5
Daikon Radish, ½ cup, slices, 2 oz	9	0	2
Dandelion Greens, raw, ½ cup, 1 oz	10	0	3
Edamame, (Immature green soybeans):			
Shelled, ½ cup, 2.6 oz	110	5	8
With shells, 10 pods, 1.3 oz	30	1	3

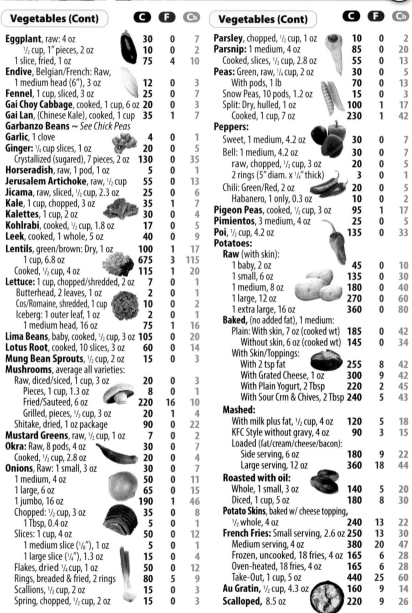

Vegetables (Cont)	C	F	Cb
Eggplant, raw: 4 oz	30	0	7
½ cup, 1" pieces, 2 oz	10	0	2
1 slice, fried, 1 oz	75	4	10
Endive, Belgian/French: Raw,			
1 medium head (6"), 3 oz	12	0	3
Fennel, 1 cup, sliced, 3 oz	25	0	7
Gai Choy Cabbage, cooked, 1 cup, 6 oz	20	0	3
Gai Lan, (Chinese Kale), cooked, 1 cup	35	1	7
Garbanzo Beans ~ *See Chick Peas*			
Garlic, 1 clove	4	0	1
Ginger: ¼ cup slices, 1 oz	20	0	5
Crystallized (sugared), 7 pieces, 2 oz	130	0	35
Horseradish, raw, 1 pod, 1 oz	5	0	1
Jerusalem Artichoke, raw, ½ cup	55	0	13
Jicama, raw, sliced, ½ cup, 2.3 oz	25	0	6
Kale, 1 cup, chopped, 3 oz	35	1	7
Kalettes, 1 cup, 2 oz	30	0	4
Kohlrabi, cooked, ½ cup, 1.8 oz	17	0	5
Leek, cooked, 1 whole, 5 oz	40	0	9
Lentils, green/brown: Dry, 1 oz	100	1	17
1 cup, 6.8 oz	675	3	115
Cooked, ½ cup, 4 oz	115	1	20
Lettuce: 1 cup, chopped/shredded, 2 oz	7	0	1
Butterhead, 2 leaves, 1 oz	2	0	1
Cos/Romaine, shredded, 1 cup	10	0	2
Iceberg: 1 outer leaf, 1 oz	2	0	1
1 medium head, 16 oz	75	1	16
Lima Beans, baby, cooked, ½ cup, 3 oz	105	0	20
Lotus Root, cooked, 10 slices, 3 oz	60	0	14
Mung Bean Sprouts, ½ cup, 2 oz	15	0	3
Mushrooms, average all varieties:			
Raw, diced/siced, 1 cup, 3 oz	20	0	3
Pieces, 1 cup, 1.3 oz	8	0	1
Fried/Sauteed, 6 oz	220	16	10
Grilled, pieces, ½ cup, 3 oz	20	1	4
Shitake, dried, 1 oz package	90	0	22
Mustard Greens, raw, ½ cup, 1 oz	7	0	2
Okra: Raw, 8 pods, 4 oz	30	0	7
Cooked, ½ cup, 2.8 oz	20	0	4
Onions, Raw: 1 small, 3 oz	30	0	7
1 medium, 4 oz	50	0	11
1 large, 6 oz	65	0	15
1 jumbo, 16 oz	190	1	46
Chopped: ½ cup, 3 oz	35	0	8
1 Tbsp, 0.4 oz	5	0	1
Slices: 1 cup, 4 oz	50	0	12
1 medium slice (⅛"), 1 oz	5	0	1
1 large slice (¼"), 1.3 oz	15	0	4
Flakes, dried ¼ cup, 1 oz	50	0	12
Rings, breaded & fried, 2 rings	80	5	9
Scallions, ½ cup, 2 oz	15	0	3
Spring, chopped, ½ cup, 2 oz	15	0	3

Vegetables (Cont)	C	F	Cb
Parsley, chopped, ½ cup, 1 oz	10	0	2
Parsnip: 1 medium, 4 oz	85	0	20
Cooked, slices, ½ cup, 2.8 oz	55	0	13
Peas: Green, raw, ¼ cup, 2 oz	30	0	5
With pods, 1 lb	70	0	13
Snow Peas, 10 pods, 1.2 oz	15	0	3
Split: Dry, hulled, 1 oz	100	1	17
Cooked, 1 cup, 7 oz	230	1	42
Peppers:			
Sweet, 1 medium, 4.2 oz	30	0	7
Bell: 1 medium, 4.2 oz	30	0	7
raw, chopped, ½ cup, 3 oz	20	0	5
2 rings (5" diam. x ¼" thick)	3	0	1
Chili: Green/Red, 2 oz	20	0	5
Habanero, 1 only, 0.3 oz	10	0	2
Pigeon Peas, cooked, ½ cup, 3 oz	95	1	17
Pimientos, 3 medium, 4 oz	25	0	5
Poi, ½ cup, 4.2 oz	135	0	33
Potatoes:			
Raw (with skin):			
1 baby, 2 oz	45	0	10
1 small, 6 oz	135	0	30
1 medium, 8 oz	180	0	40
1 large, 12 oz	270	0	60
1 extra large, 16 oz	360	0	80
Baked, (no added fat), 1 medium:			
Plain: With skin, 7 oz (cooked wt)	185	0	42
Without skin, 6 oz (cooked wt)	145	0	34
With Skin/Toppings:			
With 2 tsp fat	255	8	42
With Grated Cheese, 1 oz	300	9	42
With Plain Yogurt, 2 Tbsp	220	2	45
With Sour Crm & Chives, 2 Tbsp	240	5	43
Mashed:			
With milk plus fat, ½ cup, 4 oz	120	5	18
KFC Style without gravy, 4 oz	90	3	15
Loaded (fat/cream/cheese/bacon):			
Side serving, 6 oz	180	9	22
Large serving, 12 oz	360	18	44
Roasted with oil:			
Whole, 1 small, 3 oz	140	5	20
Diced, 1 cup, 5 oz	180	8	30
Potato Skins, baked w/ cheese topping,			
½ whole, 4 oz	240	13	22
French Fries: Small serving, 2.6 oz	250	13	30
Medium serving, 4 oz	380	20	47
Frozen, uncooked, 18 fries, 4 oz	165	6	28
Oven-heated, 18 fries, 4 oz	165	6	28
Take-Out, 1 cup, 5 oz	440	25	60
Au Gratin, ½ cup, 4.3 oz	160	9	14
Scalloped, 8.5 oz	220	9	26

Vegetables (Cont)

Item	C	F	Cb
Pumpkin:			
Raw, 1" cubes, 1 cup, 4 oz	30	0	7
Cooked:			
Baked, without fat, 4 oz	90	7	9
Mashed: 1 scoop, 2 oz	10	0	2
½ cup, 4.3 oz	25	0	6
Pumpkin Flowers, 1 cup, 1.2 oz	5	0	1
Purslane: Cooked, ½ cup, 2 oz	10	0	2
Raw, 1" cubes, 1 cup, 2 oz	5	0	2
Radicchio: 2 leaves, 1 oz	5	0	1
Shredded, 1 cup, 2 oz	20	0	4
Radishes: 1 small	0	0	0
10 medium/5 large, 1.6 oz	5	0	1
Slices, ½ cup, 2 oz	10	0	2
Rhubarb, raw, ½ cup, 2 oz	15	0	3
Rutabaga, cubes, cooked, ½ cup, 3 oz	30	0	7
Salsify, cooked, slices, ½ cup, 3 oz	50	0	11
Sauerkraut, ½ cup, 3 oz	15	0	3
Seaweed: Dried, 1 oz	5	0	2
Soaked, drained, 1 oz	15	0	4
Nori/Laver, dried, 6 sheets, 1 oz	35	0	5
Shallots, chopped, 1 Tbsp, 1 oz	5	0	1
Sorrel, raw, ½ cup, 4 oz	20	0	4
Soybeans: Dry, ½ cup, 3.3 oz	390	18	28
Mature, dry, 1 oz	120	6	9
Cooked, ½ cup, 3 oz	150	8	8
Soy Products/Tofu/Tempeh ~ *See Page 156*			
Spinach: Cooked, ½ cup, 3 oz	20	0	4
Creamed, av., ½ cup, 5 oz	190	15	8
Raw: 3 leaves,1 cup, 1 oz	7	0	1
1 Bunch, 12 oz	80	2	12
Baby Spinach, 1 cup, 1 oz	5	0	1
Squash:			
Summer: Raw, ½ cup, 3 oz	10	0	2
Cooked, slices, ½ cup, 3 oz	15	0	3
Winter, cooked:			
Acorn: Cubes, ½ cup, 4 oz	35	0	9
½ medium (10 oz raw weight)	115	0	30
Butternut: Cubes, ½ cup, 4 oz	40	0	10
¼ medium (9 oz raw weight)	115	0	30
Spaghetti, ½ cup, 1.8 oz	15	0	3
Succotash, cooked, ½ cup, 3.3 oz	110	1	23
Sweetcorn ~ *See Corn*			
Sweet Potatoes:			
Cooked with skin (w/o fat), 1 medium, 4 oz	105	0	24
Without skin, mashed, ½ cup, 6 oz	125	0	29
Fries (Alexia, Julienne syle), approximately 12 pieces, 3 oz	140	5	24

Vegetables (Cont)

Item	C	F	Cb
Swiss Chard, cooked, chopped,1 c., 6 oz	35	0	7
Taro, cooked, ½ cup, 2.3 oz	95	0	23
Tomatoes: 1 small (2¼" diam.), 3 oz	15	0	3
1 medium (2¾" diameter), 5 oz	25	0	5
1 large (3½" diameter), 8 oz	40	1	9
1 extra lge (4" diam.), 12 oz	60	1	14
Chopped, 1 cup, 7 oz	35	1	7
Tomatillo: 1 medium, 1.2 oz	10	0	2
1lb quantity for recipe	135	5	27
Turnip: Cooked, ½ cup, 2.8 oz	15	0	4
Greens, cooked, ½ cup, 3 oz	15	0	3
Water Chestnuts: 5-6 nuts, 1 oz	56	1	13
Raw, slices, ½ cup, 2.3 oz	60	0	15
Canned, 1 oz	15	0	3
Watercress, 10 sprigs, 1 oz	3	0	1
Yams: Cooked, steamed, ½ cup, 3 oz	80	0	19
Baked:			
1 medium (6") 8 oz	265	1	63
1 large (9") 12 oz	400	1	94
Yardlong Bean, 1 pod, 1 oz	5	0	1
Yucca Root, raw, ½ cup, 4 oz	165	0	39
Zucchini: Raw, 1 medium, 7 oz	30	1	7
1 large, 12 oz	60	1	12
Cooked, slices, ½ cup, 3 oz	15	0	4

Frozen Vegetables

Item	C	F	Cb
Birds Eye:			
Seasoned:			
Asian Medley, 2.71 oz	50	2	8
Brown Sugar Sweet Potatoes, 9 oz	320	8	58
Garlic Baby Peas & Mushrooms, 3 oz	70	2	11
Garlic Cauliflower, 3.1 oz	40	2	5
Ranch Broccoli Florets, 2.9 oz	50	2	6
Steakhouse Green Beans, 2.93 oz	60	3	7
Steamfresh:			
Asparagus Spears (6)	20	0	3
Brussels Sprouts, 2.7 oz	40	0	6
Cut Green Beans, 3 oz	30	0	5
Mixtures: Brocc. Cauliflower, 3 oz	25	0	4
Brocc., Cauliflower, Carrots, 2.75 oz	30	0	5
Brocc. , Carrots, Sugar Snap Peas, & Water Chestnuts, 3.1 oz	35	0	7
Roasted Red Potato Blend, 2.65 oz	50	0	11
Power Blends:			
California Style, 10.8 oz bag	350	6	61
Italian Style, 11.5 oz	350	6	56
Quinoa & Spinach, 10 oz	310	7	52
Southwest Style, 12.07 oz	380	3	69

Frozen Vegetables (Cont)

	C	F	Cb
Green Giant: *Per Frozen Weight*			
Mashed Cauliflower: Original, 4.2 oz	80	5	7
Cheddar & Bacon, 4.4 oz	90	6	6
Riced Veggies:			
Creamy Alfredo Cauliflower, 1 cup	50	3	5
Rainbow Cauliflower, ¾ cup	20	0	4
Sauced/Lightly Sauced:			
Cheesy Riced Cauliflower, 1 cup	40	2	5
Cheesy Riced Cauli. & Broccoli, 1 cup	40	2	5
Creamed Spinach, ⅔ cup	80	3	11
Garden Vegetable Medley, 1¼ cups	80	1	17
Riced Cauliflower w/ Green Beans, Fried Onions & Mshroom Sce, 1 cup	110	7	10
Simply Steam:			
Backyard Grilled Potatoes, 1 cup	120	3	20
Cut Green Beans, 3 oz	30	0	6
Honey Roasted Sweet Corn, 3 oz	80	2	14
Restaurant Style,			
Garlic Parmesan green Beans, 3 oz	60	2	8
Veggie Tots: Brocc. & Cheese, 2.7 oz	170	8	20
Cauliflower, 2.7 oz	150	7	20
Sweet Potato & Cauliflower, 2.7 oz	170	7	24
Ore-Ida: *Per 3 oz Unless Indicated*			
Extra Crispy Fries:			
Fast Food Fries	130	7	17
Crinkles	140	7	17
Seasoned Crinkles	140	8	17
Golden Fries: Crinkles	100	5	14
Crispers	200	14	15
Fries	90	4	14
Steak Fries	90	3	14
Twirls	110	6	15
Hash Browns:			
Golden Patties (1)	100	7	10
Shredded Hash Brown Potatoes	60	0	15
Mashed Potatoes,			
Homestyle Steam 'n' Mash, 3.35 oz	70	0	17
Tater Tots: Golden, 8 pieces	130	8	14
Mini Tater Tots, 19 pieces	150	9	14

Canned/Bottled

	C	F	Cb
Solids & Liquid			
Artichoke Hearts:			
Fancifoods: Plain, 1 oz (1)	8	0	1
Marinated, ¼ bottle, 1 oz	25	2	2
Asparagus: Drained, 3 spears	10	0	2
Pieces, ½ cup, 4.3 oz	25	1	3
Bamboo Shoots, 1 cup, 5 oz	25	0	4
Bean Salad, ½ cup, 4.4 oz	90	0	20
Beans: Baked, ½ cup, 5 oz	120	1	27
Butter, ½ cup, 5 oz	90	0	16
Green, ½ cup, 3 oz	15	0	3
Italian, ½ cup, 5 oz	30	0	6
Kidney, ½ cup 4 oz	105	1	19
Lima, ½ cup, 5 oz	80	0	15
Pinto, ½ cup, 5 oz	105	1	18
Beets: Sliced, ½ cup, 3 oz	25	0	6
Crinkle/Pickled, ½ cup	80	0	20
Carrots: Sliced, ½ cup, 3 oz	20	0	4
Del Monte, Honey Glazed, ½ cup	75	0	18
Corn: Kernels, ½ cup, 5 oz	80	1	18
Creamed style, ½ cup, 5 oz	90	1	23
Garbanzo/Chick Peas, ½ c, 4.2 oz	145	2	27
Hearts of Palm, (1), 1.2 oz	7	0	1
Mushrooms: ½ cup, 3 oz	20	0	4
In Butter Sauce, 2 oz	20	1	2
Onions: Cocktail (1)	0	0	0
Pickled, 1 medium, 1 oz	10	0	2
Peas, ½ cup, 3 oz	60	1	10
Peppers: Hot Chili, Jalapeno (1), 1 oz	5	0	1
Red/Green, 1 oz	5	0	1
Sweet, undrained, 3 oz	13	0	3
Jalapeno, with liquid, ½ cup chopped	20	1	3
Fried, drained, 2 Tbsp, 1 oz	60	5	3
Salsa, average all varieties, 2 Tbsp	10	0	2
Sauerkraut, drained, 1 cup, 5 oz	25	0	6
Spinach, ½ cup, 4 oz	25	1	4
Succotash: Cream Style, ½ cup	100	1	23
w/ whole kernels, undrained, ½ cup	80	1	18
Sweetcorn ~ *See Corn*			
Sweet Potato, ½ cup, 4 oz	90	0	24
Tomatoes, Sundried: Nat., 5-6 pieces	20	0	5
In Oil, drained, 6 pieces, 1 oz	40	3	4
Tomato Products ~ *See Page 144*			
Vegetables, mixed, ½ cup, 4 oz	45	0	8
Yams: In Light Syrup, ½ cup, 4 oz	105	0	25
Candied, ½ cup, 5 oz	170	0	46
Zucchini, in Tomato Sauce, ½ cup, 4 oz	30	0	8

Quick Guide

	C	F	Cb
Yogurt: *Average All Brands: Per 8 oz Container*			
Plain Yogurt: Whole	140	8	10
Low-Fat	145	4	16
Fat-Free	125	1	17
Fruit Flavored: Whole	225	8	32
Low-Fat	230	3	43
Fat-Free, regular	215	1	43
Fat-Free, no sugar added	80	0	15
Yogurt Parfait/Deli Cups:			
With Fruit Pieces: (2/3 Yogurt + 1/3 Fruit)			
Small, 8 oz cup	140	3	20
Large, 12 oz cup	210	5	30
With Fruit + Granola:			
Small, 8 oz cup (+ 0. 75 oz Granola)	235	7	30
Large, 12 oz cup (+ 1.3 oz Granola)	400	13	58

Yogurt ~ Brands

	C	F	Cb
Activia:			
Probiotic Yogurts:			
60 Calorie, all flavors, 4 oz	60	0	10
Dairy Free, all flav., 5.3 oz	120	4	18
With Fiber, Strawberry & Pinepaple, 4 oz	90	2	18
Axelrod:			
32 oz Ctn: Regular Plain, 8 oz	160	8	15
Lowfat Plain, 6 oz	100	3	11
Fat Free, Plain, 6 oz	80	0	11
6 oz Containers:			
Low Fat, Fruit flavors, av.	180	2	36
NonFat Vanilla	90	0	17
Brown Cow:			
Cream Top: *Per 5.3 oz Cup*			
Whole Milk: Plain	130	7	11
Apricot Mango	150	5	23
Blueberry	160	5	26
Cherry Vanilla	160	5	26
Chocolate	180	6	28
Coffee; Vanilla	150	6	19
Maple	150	6	20
Peach; Raspberry; Strawberry	160	5	25
32oz Containers:			
Plain, 6 oz	140	8	12
Maple, 6 oz	180	7	23
Vanlla, 6 oz	170	7	21
Cabot:			
Greek Style: *Per 6 oz Serving*			
Whole Milk, Plain	230	16	9
Lowfat (2%): Plain	130	4	8
Strawberry; Vanilla Bean	180	3	26
Triple Cream, Vanilla Bean	260	13	26
Nonfat, Plain, 8 oz	80	0	13
Chobani: *Per 5.3 oz Unless Indicated*			
Greek Yogurt:			
Blended: Coffee Cream	160	5	19
Mixed Berry	140	3	17
Flip: Per 5 oz			
Almond Coco Loco, 5 oz	190	8	24
Coffee Brownie Bliss	160	4	23
Cookies & Cream	160	4	22
Key Lime Crumble	170	5	22
Peanut Butter Dream	180	6	20
Salted Caramel Crunch	160	4	23
S'mores S'mores	160	4	22
Less Sugar, 5.3 oz, av.	120	3	10
Nonfat, Plain	80	0	6
On The Bottom:			
Mango	130	2	15
Strawberry Banana	130	3	16
Non Fat, all flavors	110	0	15
Plain, 32 oz Ctn:			
Lowfat, 6 oz	120	3	7
Nonfat, 6 oz	90	0	6
Whole Milk, 6 oz	170	9	7
Zero Sugar, all flavors, 5.3 oz	60	0	5
Dannon:			
Activia ~ *See Activia*			
Creamy, Strawberry, 4 oz	70	0	14
Creamy Classic, Fruit Flavors, 4 oz	100	2	17
Fruit On The Bottom, all flavors, 5.3 oz	130	2	25
Lowfat: Plain, 5.3 oz	100	3	12
Coffee; Vanilla, 5.3 oz	140	2	24
Plain, 32 oz Ctn:			
Lowat, 6 oz	110	3	12
Nonfat, 6 oz	80	0	13
Whole Milk, 6 oz	110	6	7
Fage Greek Yogurt:			
Best Self, Plain, 5.3 oz	110	3	5
Total: *Per 6 oz Serving*			
Plain, 5% Milk Fat	140	8	5
Plain, 2% Milk Fat	100	3	5
Plain, 0% Milk Fat, 6oz	80	0	5
Total Blended, Fruit Flav., av., 5.3 oz	100	0	13
Total Split Cups, 2% Milkfat, Average Fruit Flavor, 5.3 oz	120	3	13
Forager ~ Organic *(Dairy Free)*: *Per 5.3 oz*			
Cashewmilk: Strawberry	160	6	20
Unsweetened Plain	130	9	9

Yogurt Brands (Cont)

	C	F	Cb
Great Value *(Walmart):*			
Greek, Nonfat: *Per 6 oz*			
32 oz Ctn: Plain	90	0	7
Vanilla	140	0	21
Greek Light: Fruit flavors, 5.3 oz	80	0	7
Vanilla, 6 oz	100	0	9
Greek Whole Milk, Honey Van., 6 oz	200	8	25
Lowfat Tubes, all flavors, 2 oz	50	1	10
Original Lowfat,av. fruit flavors, 6 oz	135	2	26
Kemps: *Per 6 oz*			
5 lb Containers:			
Lowfat, Plain, Sweeetened	120	2	13
Nonfat: Fruit Flavors, av.	125	0	26
Vanilla	130	0	28
kite hill (Dairy Free): *Per 5.3 oz Cup*			
Almondmilk: Plain	140	9	12
Unsweetened	140	10	9
Other Flavors, average	150	8	19
Kroger:			
Light Nonfat, Strawberry, 5.3 oz	90	0	8
Lowfat: CarbMaster, Fruit Flav., 6 oz	70	2	5
Fruit On Bottom, average, 6 oz	150	2	27
Whole Milk, Blended Vanilla, 6 oz	180	5	26
La Yogurt: *Per 6 oz Container*			
Probiotic Low Fat:			
Original; Fruit Flavors, av.	155	2	30
Rich & Creamy, Fruit Flav., av.	180	2	33
Probiotic Nonfat, Fruit Flav., av.	90	0	16
LaLa:			
Blended Low Fat: Fruit Flavors, 6 oz	150	1	28
Pina colada	150	2	29
Lavva (Dairy Free): *Per 5.3 oz*			
Pili Nut Yogurt: Original	185	14	11
Average other flavors	150	11	11
Lucerne *(Safeway):*			
Greek Nonfat, Plain, 6 oz	100	0	10
Low-Fat, Blueberry Flav., 6 oz	170	2	34
Light Nonfat, Fruit Flav., 6 oz	100	0	18
Whole Milk, Vanilla, 6 oz	180	5	28
Mountain High: *Per 8 oz*			
32 oz Containers:			
Whole Milk Original: Plain	170	7	15
Strawberry; Vanilla, av.	200	7	27
Lowfat: Plain	130	3	16
Vanilla	170	3	28
Fat Free: Plain	110	0	16
Vanilla	160	0	28
Nancy's:			
Greek Probiotic: Nonfat, Plain, 6 oz	120	0	8
Wholemilk, Plain, 6 oz	160	6	7
Oatmilk: Plain, 6 oz	120	6	11
Fruit Flavors, 5.3 oz	140	5	19
Vanilla, 5.3 oz	130	5	17

	C	F	Cb
Oikos *(Dannon):*			
Blended Greek Nonfat: *5.3 oz Cups:*			
Plain	90	0	6
Fruit Flavors	100	0	13
32 oz Tubs: Plain, 6 oz			
Vanilla Bean, 6 oz	120	0	14
Pro, all flavors, 5.3 oz cup	140	3	8
Triple Zero, fruit l flavors, 5.3 oz cup	90	0	7
O Organics *(Safeway):*			
Greek, Nonfat Strained, Plain, 6 oz	100	0	6
Open Nature:			
Coconut, Plain, 6 oz	120	9	9
Greek Strained Nonfat:			
Fruit On Bottom, average, 5.3 oz	120	0	18
Oui (Dairy Free ~ *Yoplait)***:** *Per 4.97 oz Jar*			
Coconut Milk: Plain; Vanilla	150	8	19
Fruit Flavors, average	145	7	19
Whole Milk: Creamy Rasp. & Choc.	210	12	23
Fruit Flavors; Honey; Maple, av.	170	8	22
Siggi's:			
Coconut Milk: Fruit Flavors, average	175	10	11
Toasted Coconut	190	11	12
Skyr: *Per 5.3 oz Unless Indicated*			
0%: Plain	90	0	6
Other Flavors	110	0	13
2%: Coconut	160	5	14
Other Flavors	140	3	14
4%, all flavors, 4.4 oz	130	5	11
Rich & Creamy, av., 4 oz	140	6	12
Silk (Dairy Free): *Per 5.3 oz Cups Inless Indicated*			
Almondmilk: Dark Choc. Coconut	190	11	20
Strawberry	180	11	18
Vanilla	180	15	10
Greek Style Coconut,			
all flavors	190	11	13
Soy Yogurt: Fruit flavors, average	125	4	18
Vanilla	140	4	21
32 oz Tubs: Plain, 6 oz	110	4	10
Vanilla, 6 oz	150	4	23
So Delicious (Dairy Free):			
Coconut Milk: *Per 5.3 oz*			
Plain: Regular	110	5	17
Unsweetened	80	5	8
Blueberry; Chocolate, av.	140	4	24
Vanilla	130	4	22
Average other fruit flavors	135	4	24
Stonyfield Organic:			
0% Fat: Plain, 5.3 oz	70	0	11
Vanilla, 5.3 oz	110	0	20
Greek:			
Whole Milk: Plain, 6 oz	150	6	7
Vanilla Bean, 6 oz	170	5	18
Nonfat: Plain, 6 oz	90	0	7
Vanilla Bean, 6 oz	130	0	18

...continued next page

Yogurt Brands (Cont)

	C	F	Cb
Stonyfield Organic (Cont): *Per 6 oz Unless Indicated*			
Greek (cont):			
Grass Fed, Whole Milk, Plain, 6 oz	150	6	7
High Protein Parfaits, av., 7 oz	260	8	30
Low Fat, Fruit flavors, av., 4 oz	70	1	12
Trader Joe's: *Per 6 oz Unless Indicated*			
Cultured Organic Cashew,			
Plain, Unsweetened	140	9	11
Fruit Flavored Whole Milk,			
Rasp/Strawb. & Cream, 4 oz	140	6	18
Greek, with Honey	230	15	20
Voskos:			
Greek:			
Nonfat: Plain, 8 oz	140	0	9
Exotic Fig, 5.3 oz cup	160	0	28
Vanilla Bean, 5.3 oz cup	130	0	21
Nonfat Fruit On Bottom			
Apricot Mango, 5.3 oz	110	0	15
Wild Strawberry, 5.3 oz	120	0	18
Nonfat Real Fruit: Blueb., 6 oz	140	0	19
Pineapple, 6 oz	150	0	21
Whole Mik: Original Plain, 8 oz	280	20	15
Original Honey, 8 oz	290	14	32
Wallaby Organic: *Per 6 oz Unless Indicated*			
Greek:			
Lowfat, Plain	120	3	8
Nonfat, Plain	100	0	8
Whole Milk: Plain	160	8	8
Strawberry	190	6	22
Vanilla Bean	190	6	23
No Sugar Added, Strawb., 5.3 oz	120	5	9
Whole Milk: Plain	130	6	10
Vanilla	160	5	23
Wegmans: *Per 6 oz Uness Indicated*			
Coconutmilk: Plain	200	14	14
Vanilla	230	12	29
Greek Nonfat: Plain, 5.3 oz	80	0	5
Fruit flavors, av., 5.3 oz	125	0	18
Vanilla, 5.3 oz	110	0	13
Organic Lowfat, Vanilla, 6 oz	140	3	23
Whole Foods (365 Organic):			
Greek:			
Nonfat, Plain, 6 oz	100	0	7
Whole Milk, Plain, 6 oz	150	6	7
Lowfat, Vanilla, 6 oz	110	2	19
Whole Milk: Plain, 6 oz	120	6	9
Vanilla, 6oz	150	5	20
YoCrunch:			
4 oz Lowfat Vanilla:			
M&M's Peanut	140	4	21
Average Other Flavors	130	3	21
6 oz Lowfat Vanilla,			
Kellogg's Granola, 6 oz	180	2	35

Yogurt Brands (Cont)

	C	F	Cb
Yooga (Dairy Free): *Per 4.4 oz Cup*			
Coconut Milk: Sea Salt Chocolate	150	11	10
Other Flavors, average	140	11	10
Yoplait:			
Single Serve Cups: *Per 6 oz*			
Original: Chery w/ Chocolate	170	3	31
Real Fruit, average	140	2	28
Strawberry Smoothie	150	1	30
Lactose Free, all flavors av., 6 oz	140	2	26
Light, all flavors, 6 oz	80	0	15
Whips!: *Per 4 oz*			
Coconut Crème; Choc., average	160	4	25
Average other flavors	140	3	25
Greek 100 Protein, av. all flav., 5.3 oz	100	0	10
Go-Gurt Dunkaroos,			
Strawb.; Vanilla B'Day Cake, 2.2 oz	130	3	22
Kid Cup: Original, all flavors, 4 oz	100	1	21
Cinn. Toast Crunch, Vanilla, 4.27 oz	130	2	26
Cocoa Puffs, Vanilla, 4.27 oz	130	1	27
Trix, Strawberry, 4.27 oz	130	1	27

Yogurt Drinks & Probiotics

	C	F	Cb
Activia *(Dannon):*			
Probiotics:			
Dailies, all flavors, 3.1 fl.oz	70	2	11
Drinks, av. all flavors, 7 fl oz	160	4	25
Immune System, av. all flav., 7 fl.oz	65	2	10
Dannon:			
DanActive Dailies, all flav., 3.1 fl.oz	75	1	13
Danone:			
Danimals Smoothies: All flavors, 3.1 fl.oz	50	0	11
Pouches, all flavors, 4 fl.oz	80	1	13
Glen Oaks, Probiotics, all flav., 6 fl.oz	150	3	27
Lifeway: *Per 8 fl.oz Unless Indicated*			
Kefir:			
Functional Shots: All flavors, 4 fl.oz	60	1	9
Probiotics, all flavors, 4 fl.oz	140	2	18
Nonfat, Plain, unsweetend	90	0	9
Traditional, Original	150	8	12
Mushroom Oat, all flavors, 4 fl.oz	60	1	10
Organic Whole Milk Kefir:			
Plain	150	8	9
Average Other Flavors	190	8	18
Organic Lowfat Kefir: Plain	110	2	12
Other flavors	140	2	20
Organic Oat, all flavors, 4 fl.oz	140	2	25
Probugs, Strawnana; 4 fl.oz	80	3	8
Stonyfield:			
Probiotic Low Fat Smoothies:			
6 fl.oz Bottle, average	110	2	17
10 fl.oz bottle, average	180	3	29
Yakult: Regular, 2.7 fl.oz bottle	50	0	12
Light, Nonfat, 2.7 fl.oz	25	0	6

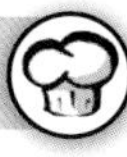

Cafeteria-Style Foods

Average All Preparations:	C	F	Cb
Beef Stroganoff, 5 oz	195	13	7
Beef Stroganoff, with 4 oz noodles	350	14	36
Chicken Lasagna, 1 piece	300	11	32
Chicken Chop Suey, with 4 oz rice	245	4	37
Deep Dish Burrito, 7 oz	265	13	20
Ground Beef Casserole, 2 scps, 6 oz	245	13	17
Italian Meat Sce, for Spaghetti, 5 oz	150	9	9
with 5 oz Spaghetti	350	10	49
Lasagna, 1 piece	275	11	25
Meatloaf, 3 oz	205	13	4
Ranch Beans, 2 scoops, 6 oz	350	11	45
Red Beans & Rice, 7 oz	280	9	37
Scalloped Potato/Ham, 2 scoops, 6 oz	160	6	20
Stuffed Shells in Sauce, (1)	105	3	17
Swedish Meatballs, (3)	205	12	9
Sweet & Sour Pork/Rice, 9 oz	240	3	40
Swiss Steak, w/ Mushroom Gravy, 6 oz	280	11	4
Tator Tot Casserole, 2 scoops, 6 oz	260	15	20
Tenderloin Tips/Mshrm Gravy: 5 oz	210	13	3
With 5 oz noodles	395	15	38
Tuna Noodle Casserole, 2 scoops, 6 oz	180	6	17
Turkey Tetrazzini, 2 scoops, 6 oz	195	7	17
Vegetable Lasagna, 1 piece	250	13	21

Croissants

	C	F	Cb
Unfilled, medium 1.5 oz	180	10	21
Filled: With Ham (2 oz), garnish	280	14	24
With Ham (2 oz), Cheese (2 oz)	470	30	20
With Chick (2 oz) Cheese (2 oz)	470	30	20
With Turkey/Ham/Cheese (2 oz ea.)	580	36	20
Au Bon Pain: Ham & Cheese	390	21	35
Spinach & Cheese	290	17	28

7-Eleven ~ *See Page 236*

Bagels

	C	F	Cb
Plain: Large, 4 oz (without filling)	320	2	65
With 2 oz Cream Cheese	500	27	54
With 2 oz Lox (Smoked Salmon)	400	4	65

Also see Bagels Section ~ *Page 56*
Fast-Foods Restaurants ~ *Page 175*
Au Bon Pain ~ *Page 178*
Bruegger's ~ *Page 185*
Einstein Bros Bagels ~ *Page 199*

Sandwiches

No Spreads Unless Indicated: Includes 2 Slices Bread ~ 3 oz	C	F	Cb
BLT, (5 strips Bacon, 2 Tbsp Mayo)	600	40	46
Breaded Chicken & Garnish	540	28	46
Chicken Salad, with Mayo., 5 oz	580	30	49
Chopped Liver, Egg Mayonnaise	630	25	44
Corned Beef with Mustard, 5 oz	560	28	44
Egg Salad, with Mayonnaise	570	29	49
Egg Salad Club, with Bacon & Mayo,	780	53	49
Grilled Cheese, (3 oz)	540	30	44
Ham, (4 oz), Cheese (4 oz), & Mayo.	910	56	44
Lobster Salad, (4 oz), w/ Mayo.	530	25	45
Overstuffed Tuna Salad, (7 oz)	870	39	75
Philly Cheese Steak Sandwich	550	23	42
Reuben, (6 oz Beef/Pastrami, 2 oz Cheese, 2 Tbsp Dressing)	920	60	28
Roast Beef, (4 oz), with Mustard	460	12	45
Roast Pork, (4 oz), with Apple Sauce	500	16	55
Shrimp Salad Club, w/ Bacon & Mayo	800	57	48
Sloppy Joe with Sauce, (7 oz)	600	30	45
Steak Sandwich, (5 oz cooked)	680	32	41
Triple Cheese Melt, (4 oz)	720	45	46
Tuna Salad, (5 oz), with Mayonnaise	610	30	49
Turkey Breast, (5 oz), w/ Mayo.	460	18	44
Turkey Breast, (5 oz,) with Mustard	360	7	44
Turkey Club, with Bacon & Mayo.	830	38	31
Vegetarian, with Avocado & Cheese	820	49	72

7-Eleven ~ *Page 236*
Schlotzsky's ~ *Page 237*
Subway ~ *Page 245*

Wraps & Roll-Ups

Average All Types **Meat/Chicken/Fish/Veggie:**	C	F	Cb
Small, approximately 9 oz	500	25	48
Regular, approximately 15 oz	830	40	80
Large, approximately 22 oz	1400	70	134

Fast-Foods Restaurants ~ *Page 175*
Au Bon Pain ~ *Page 178*
Sonic Drive-In ~ *Page 241*
Subway ~ *Page 245*
WAWA ~ *Page 254*

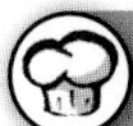

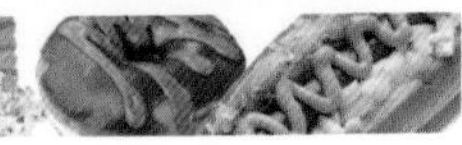

Fair & Carnival Foods

Food	C	F	Cb
Barbeque Chicken/Meats:			
Chicken, ½ chicken, 15 oz	740	24	34
Grilled Chicken Pita, with dressing	680	19	82
Teriyaki Chicken, on stick, w/ dress.	250	6	4
Pork Ribs, 18 oz	1360	68	21
Turkey Leg: Regular, 19 oz	1135	54	0
Caveman (2lb Turkey Leg, with 1lb Bacon)	2360	177	3
Bacon: Fried, on-a-stick, with syrup	230	16	5
Choc-covered Bacon, 4.5 oz dish	640	43	30
Beef Stew over Rice, 2 cups	440	14	61
Butter Balls, deep fried, 4 Balls	460	38	24
Cheese Curds, Breaded & fried, *Culver's*, 6.7 oz	670	38	54
Corn Dogs: Regular, 4 oz	250	14	23
Jumbo, 6 oz	375	21	36
Pretzel-Wrapped Dog	300	16	30
Papa Pup, on-a-stick	400	24	32
Pronto Pup, on-a-stick	170	9	16
Corn On The Cob, 8" (1), 16 oz	200	1	42
Finger Foods:			
Artichoke, fried, 9 pieces	250	14	24
Chicken Nuggets, (6)	340	17	26
Chicken Strips, (4), 4.5 oz	445	21	33
Onion Rings, 3 rings	310	13	40
Onion Flower	1320	72	140
Shrimp, Fried, 10-12 pieces, 5 oz	555	30	36
Spam, deep-fried in batter, 2 pieces	330	24	18
Gator:			
Big Gator, Nuggets/Hushpuppies	550	31	54
Stick Gator, 1 sausage	250	20	4
Greek:			
Baklava, 2" square	245	13	32
Falafel, 11.6 oz	660	27	85
Greek Salad, 14 oz	520	48	17
Gyro, 7.5", 12 oz	680	40	55
Spanakopita, 8 oz	200	8	23
Hamburgers:			
⅓ Pound Burger, 7.5 oz	670	41	26
Cheeseburger, 6 oz	550	36	25
Hot Dogs: *With Bun*			
Regular: No extras	215	14	28
With Chili, 6 oz	450	32	32
With Chili & Cheese, 7.3 oz	500	36	31
⅓ Pound Hot Dog	550	41	31
Foot Long Hot Dog	470	26	41
Jumbo, Bratwurst/Kielbasa, average	800	60	28

Fair & Carnival Foods (Cont)

Food	C	F	Cb
Mexican:			
Burrito, with Bean/Beef, 17 oz	1100	41	104
Carne Asada, 14.5 oz	820	44	58
Cheese Quesadilla, 1.8 oz	480	27	40
Chicken Taco, 3.3 oz	210	12	16
Fish Taco, 5 oz	270	13	31
Jalapeno Pepper, choc-covered (3)	270	15	31
Nachos with Cheese, 9" plate	860	59	70
Tamale, 3.5 oz	180	8	21
Taquito, 5 oz	370	17	43
Pizza:			
Pizza Bread, Pepperoni, ½ loaf, 12 oz	1115	32	151
Pizza on-a-stick, 1 piece	535	28	55
Personal Pizza: *Per 7"*			
Cheese	670	24	80
Pepperoni	795	35	80
Ham & Pineapple	800	31	87
Potatoes & Fries:			
Australian Battered Potatoes	1290	66	155
Baked Potato, 14 oz	435	1	100
Fries: French, 7 oz	560	24	79
Cheese Fries, 10 oz	645	38	62
Chili Fries, 10 oz	700	36	83
Curly Fries, 7 oz	620	30	78
Jamaican Jerk Fries, 7 oz	640	34	77
Sweet Potato, baked, 14 oz	405	1	97
Tornado, on-a-stick	210	15	18
Salads/Sides:			
Chili, 1 cup	280	11	24
Cole Slaw, 5 oz	350	21	37
Pickle, whole (6")	30	0	8
Potato Salad, 5 oz	290	15	35
Sandwiches: *7½" Roll*			
Ham, 11 oz	645	39	47
Hot Pastrami, 9 oz	760	17	62
Roast Beef, 11 oz	620	36	46
Philadelphia Cheese Steak, 13 oz	680	36	49
Turkey, 11 oz	665	24	65
Drinks:			
Icee, 16 fl.oz	235	0	59
Shakes, average, 16 fl.oz	690	33	85
Slushies: Horchata, 16 fl.oz	280	8	50
Lemonade, 18 fl.oz	210	0	52
Orange Julius, 20 fl.oz	490	10	96
Strawberry Julius, 20 fl.oz	430	0	98
Soft Frozen Lemonade, 12 fl.oz	300	0	78
Smoothies, Berry Flavors, 16 fl.oz	350	1	80

Fair & Carnival Foods (Cont)

	C	F	Cb
Cakes Pastries:			
Funnel Cake, Plain (1)	760	44	80
Toppings:			
Apple Cinnamon, 2 oz	85	3	16
Cinnamon & Sugar, 2 tsp	40	0	10
Strawberry & Cream, 2 oz	70	0	16
Cheesecake on-a-stick, 6 oz	655	47	56
Churro, (1), 9", 1.6 oz	170	8	22
Cream Puff, 4.3 oz	500	43	22
Fried Twinkie, (1)	420	34	45
Puff-on-a-Stick, (4), 8.6 oz	995	86	44
Strawberry Crepe, 4.3 oz	280	14	36
Twinkie Dog, (Sundae)	500	14	89
Candied Apple, 7 oz	330	0	80
Cookies:			
Sweet Martha, (1), 0.8 oz	90	4	14
Deep Fried: Oreos, tray (5)	890	48	108
Cookie Dough on stick, 3 pieces	670	32	89
Cotton Candy:			
Small, 1 oz	110	0	27
Large, 2.3 oz	250	0	62
Family Size, 5.5 oz	610	0	151
Dirt Dessert, 1 cup, 9.3 oz	405	12	69
Donuts, Jumbo Twist, (1), 7.5 oz	905	49	109
Fried Dough/FryBread:			
Plain: 7", 3.7 oz	390	19	47
9", 4¾ oz	510	25	61
Toppings: Cinnamon Sugar, 2 tsp	40	0	10
Butterscotch; Caramel, 2 Tbsp	115	0	29
Hot Fudge, average, 2 Tbsp	110	4	22
Cheese Powder, 2 tsp	70	3	2
Honey, 1 Tbsp, 0.8 oz	65	0	17
Fudge, 1.5 oz	200	11	25
Ice Cream & Frozen Treats:			
Deep-fried Klondike Bar, w/ syrup	430	16	18
Dippin' Dots Ice Cream, 6 oz cup	380	20	46
Frozen Banana, choc. coated, 5 oz	240	4	53
Frozen Yogurt, in sugar cone, 14 oz	475	2	94
Ice Cream: Small, sugar cone, 10 oz	775	42	83
Large, sugar cone, 14 oz	935	54	96
Sherbet, 8 oz	270	4	59
Snow Cone, with 3 oz syrup	270	0	68
Strawberry, Choc. Dipped, 1 piece	125	7	15
Popcorn:			
Plain: Small, 3 oz	450	24	48
Large, 6 oz	900	48	96
Kettle Corn: Small, 5 oz	600	15	110
Large, 10 oz	1200	30	220
Pretzels, Soft, 4.5 oz	340	2	70
S'more, on stick	275	16	27

Stadium Foods

	C	F	Cb
Burgers:			
Bacon Burger, 8.3 oz	470	25	34
Cheeseburger, 8.3 oz	450	23	33
Hamburger, 7.8 oz	400	19	33
French Fries, 6.4 oz	470	34	39
Fruit Cup, 6 oz	80	0	20
Hot Dogs:			
Chili Dog, 7.7 oz	520	29	45
Hot Dog, 6.4 oz	465	21	50
Jumbo Dog, 6 oz	440	25	38
Kraut Dog with Sauerkraut, 7.8 oz	490	27	41
Individual Pan Pizza (6"): *Per Pizza*			
BBQ Chicken	630	24	71
Cheese	630	27	71
Pepperoni	660	30	70
Nachos, 40 chips, with 4 oz cheese	1100	59	132
Sandwiches:			
Chicken: With Bacon, 8.3 oz	530	31	41
With Cheese, 8.3 oz	510	29	40
Without Cheese, 7.7 oz	460	25	40
Polish Sausage Sandwich, 7 oz	565	33	46
Snacks:			
Brownie, 2.5" x 4.5"	360	18	44
Cheese Sauce, 1.3 oz	100	8	4
Cheetos, 2.8 oz package	440	28	42
Chocolate Chip Cookie, 2.3 oz	280	12	40
Churro, (1), 10", 2 oz	210	10	26
Doritos, Nacho, 2.8 oz package	390	20	48
King Size Candy:			
Butterfinger, 3.8 oz	480	18	75
Nestle Crunch, 2.8 oz	390	21	85
Lay's, Chips, 2.8 oz package	440	28	42
Peanuts, in shell, 8 oz	930	80	24
Popcorn: Small (9 cup size)	575	35	56
Large (15 cup size)	950	58	93
Pretzel, Soft, Reg., 5.5 oz	490	4	101
Red Vines, 5 oz box	500	0	117
Snow Cone: With 3 oz syrup	270	0	68
With 6 oz syrup	540	0	136
Beverages:			
Orange Juice, 12 fl.oz	180	0	2
Beer:			
Heineken, 16 fl.oz	200	0	16
Miller: Draft, 16 fl.oz	195	0	17
Lite, 16 fl.oz	125	16	4
Jack Daniels, Punch, 12 fl.oz	235	0	34
Wine, White, 9 fl.oz	190	0	6
Soda, (with ½ ice), average:			
20 fl.oz	160	0	40
32 fl.oz	260	0	65
Starbuck's, Coffee, Frappuccino, 9.5 fl.oz	200	3	37

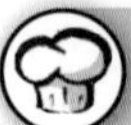

Restaurant & International Foods

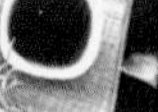

Asian & Chinese Dishes

	C	F	Cb
Appetizers:			
Crab Cake, 2.3 oz	125	10	1
Dumplings: *Per Dumpling*			
Pork: Steamed	80	5	5
Fried	90	6	5
Vegetable, steamed	35	1	5
Egg Rolls, Mini, 3 rolls	100	3	11
Spring Roll:			
Small, 1.5 oz	85	4	9
Medium, 3 oz	170	8	17
Large, 5 oz	290	15	29
Wonton, 1 only	75	4	5
Soup: Egg Flower, bowl 12 oz	90	2	16
Hot & Sour Soup, bowl 12 oz	110	4	14
Rice: Plain,1 cup, 6.5 oz	320	2	66
2 Cups, 13 oz	640	4	132
Fried: 1 cup, 5 oz	365	11	55
Large dish, 16 oz	950	28	67
Noodles, Chinese Egg, cooked, 1 cup	200	4	37
Entrees & Mains: *Per Serving*			
Almond Chicken, 6 oz	270	10	21
BBQ Pork, 5.5oz	440	23	15
Beef in Black Bean Sauce, 8.5 oz	390	17	17
Broccoli Beef, 6 oz	370	21	13
Chicken & Broccoli, 5.5 oz	160	8	10
Chicken Skewers, 3 oz	210	9	18
Chop Suey:			
Chicken, 5 oz	140	9	2
Pork, 5 oz	170	12	3
Chow Mein, Beef/Chicken, 8 oz	390	12	59
Crab Puff/Rangoon, 1 dumpling	190	11	13
Crispy Fried Chicken, 8 oz	485	33	12
Egg Drop Soup: With Noodles, 1 cup	110	3	16
Without Noodles, 1 cup	60	3	4
Egg Foo Yung with Sauce, 1 cup	270	15	16
Kung Pao Chicken, 5.5 oz	240	15	12
Lemon Chicken, 5 oz	525	21	57
Lo Mein, stir-fried, 8 oz	705	42	49
Omelet, Chicken/Shrimp, 16 oz	990	82	10
Orange Chicken, 5.5 oz	500	27	42
Steamed Whole Fish,			
½ Sockeye Salmon	646	36	23
Sweet & Sour:			
Fish, 20 oz	1160	58	106
Pork, 5.5 oz	400	23	35
Vegetable Combo, with oil, 6 oz	367	5	66
Vegetables, Steamed, without oil, 6 oz	135	1	29
Sauces: Mandarin Sauce 1.5 oz	70	0	17
Potsticker Sauce, 1.5 oz	35	0	8
Bubble Tea, average, 12 fl oz	280	1	68
Fortune Cookie, each	32	1	7

Cajun & Creole

	C	F	Cb
Alligator, cooked, 4 oz	160	2	0
Baked Herb Chicken, 1 serving	850	53	2
Bouillabaisse	400	15	10
Cajun Fried Turkey, 1 serving	630	25	0
Cocktail Sauce, 2 Tbsp	30	0	6
Couche-Couche, ½ cup	80	0	17
Crawfish Bisque, 1 serving	500	10	10
Crawfish, cooked, 2 oz	45	1	0
Creole Jambalaya, 1 serving	550	30	15
Frog Legs, steamed (2)	45	0	0
Guinea Fowl, flesh, 4 oz, cooked	160	4	0
Hogshead Cheese, ¼ cup	80	6	0
Jambalaya, Shrimp & Crabmeat	520	14	12
Red Beans & Rice, 1 serving	400	17	52
Roasted Quail, with Bacon, on Toast	550	25	15
Remoulade Sauce, 2 Tbsp, 1 oz	110	11	2
Shrimp Creole, 1 serving	450	20	10
Stuffed Smothered Steak, with 1 cup Rice	890	50	50
Turtle, cooked, 3 oz	120	3	0

Canadian Foods

	C	F	Cb
Bagels, Montreal-Style:			
Plain, 100g/3.5 oz	300	2	60
Poppyseed, 100g/3.5 oz	310	4	58
Sesame, 100g/3.5 oz	320	6	56
Bannock: Plain 33g/1.2 oz	120	3	20
With currants/raisins, 85g/3 oz	215	9	32
Meals:			
Baked Beans in Maple Syrup, 1 cup, 250g/8.8 oz	320	1	62
Donnairs (*Pizza Delight*):			
Famous, regular, 250g/8.8 oz	510	21	60
Super, regular, 310g/11 oz	685	34	62
Poutine:			
Boston Pizza Ca, Classic, 400g/14 oz	590	28	68
Harvey's Ca, Classic, 308/10.86 oz	700	36	73
McDonald's Ca, 1 serving	870	37	113
Swiss Chalet, Chalet -Style, 381g/13.44 oz	820	48	78
Shish Taouk:			
Chicken: 1 skewer, 200g/7 oz	270	25	9
Wrap, 455g/16 oz	1150	12	195
Tassot:			
Beef, 283g/10 oz	430	28	12
Goat, 100g/3.5 oz	360	36	9
Toutiere, 170g/6oz	600	42	35

Canadian (Cont)

	C	F	Cb
Pastries:			
Beaver Tails:			
Cheese & Garlic, 80g/2.8 oz	390	30	28
Cinnamon & Sugar, 80g/2.8 oz	315	13	30
Butter Tart, mini, 1 tart	120	3	16
May West,			
Original, 54g/1.9 oz	240	11	34
Nanaimo Bar, 56g/2 oz	270	16	30
Snacks: Maple Syrup Taffy, 40g/1.4 oz	130	0	33
Potato Chips: Dill Pickle Flav., 40g	160	10	15
Ketchup Flavor, 50g/1.8 oz	260	16	26

French Foods

	C	F	Cb
Blanquette d' Agneau, (Lamb Stew)	800	30	17
Brioche, 1 cake	280	14	34
Bouillabaisse	400	15	10
Coq au Vin, leg/thigh	700	28	31
Coquilles St. Jacques	320	13	36
Crème Brulée, 1 serving	460	40	21
Baguette, 3 slices, 2.2 oz	150	1	35
Creme Caramel, (Caramel Custard)	260	10	38
Crepe Suzette, 1x6" crepe with sauce	220	10	13
Duck a l'Orange, ¼ duck, 22 oz	970	44	19
Escargot, (Snails), in garlic butter (6)	200	10	4
Frog Legs, fried, 4 medium pairs	400	20	10
Lamb Noisettes, fried, 2 chops	500	40	1
Potage Creme Crecy, (Carrot Soup)	360	18	14
Salade Nicoise, (Tuna/Olives/Vegs)	450	13	14
Veal Cordon Bleu, (Veal/Ham)	650	25	18
Vichyssoise, (Potato /Leek Soup), 1 c.	200	9	15

Baguette & French Stick ~ *Page 54*

German Foods

	C	F	Cb
Beef: Goulash with Veggies	520	20	46
Weiner Schnitzel, 1 medium	750	35	38
Chicken: Fried, Viennese-style	530	20	28
Livers with Apple/Onion, 6 oz	460	28	10
Herring, pickled: Rollmops, 4 oz	260	16	3
With Sour Cream, 4 oz	310	20	3
Pork, Sauerbraten (Pot Roast)	650	35	15
Sausage: Bratwurst, grilled, 6 oz	450	37	2
Hot Sausage Curry	300	7	6
Cakes:			
Black Forest, 1 slice	380	16	30
Bavarian Bread Dumpling, 3 small	330	10	28
Kugelhupf Cake, 1 large slice, 4 oz	400	23	40
Torte: Linzer (Almond/Raspb. Jam)	430	18	58
Sacher (Chocolate/Apricot Jam)	260	12	23

Greek Foods

	C	F	Cb
Baklava Pastry: Small	240	13	32
Large, 3.8 oz	400	21	45
Calamari, deep fried, 1 cup	300	13	17
Chicken Kebob Plate	345	13	8
Dolmades, 2 rolls, 6 oz	200	5	13
Galactobureko, 1 only			
(Filo, Custard, Pastry in Syrup)	360	15	48
Greek Chicken Salad	400	18	9
Gyros: 6" Pita, 8 oz	475	32	35
7½" Pita, 12 oz	680	40	55
Hummus & Pita, 4 oz	260	12	30
Kataifi, (Filo, Nut, Pastry in Syrup)	350	11	56
Moussaka: Small serving, 8 oz	350	22	22
Large serving, 16 oz	700	44	44
Soup, Avgolemono (Egg & Lemon			
with Chicken & Rice), 1 cup	85	6	5
Souvlaki, (Lamb), each, 2 oz	120	6	1
Stuffed Tomatoes, (2)	250	12	17
Taramosalata, 1 T., 0.5 oz	40	3	2
Tyropita, (Filo/Egg/Cheese Pastry)	350	26	31

Hawaiian

	C	F	Cb
Ahi Tuna, grilled w/o fat, 6 oz fillet	220	2	0
Chicken Long Rice, 1 cup, 7 oz	240	14	12
Gyoza, 1 only	55	2	6
Haupia, (Coconut Pudd.), 1 pce, (4"x 2½")	120	6	17
Hawaiian Sweet Bread, ½" slice, 2 oz	180	4.5	29
Kalua: Chicken, 4 oz	280	16	0
Pork, 4 oz	350	24	0
Kim Chee, (pickled cabbage), ½ cup, 4 oz	20	0	5
Kulolo, (Taro Pudding), 1 slice	125	5	19
Lau Lau:			
Chicken (1), 7 oz	280	21	3
Pork (1), 7 oz	320	26	5
Loco Moco, (rice/burger/egg/gravy)	650	27	63
Lomi Salmon, ¼ cup, 4 oz	20	1	2
Malasadas, (Donut), 2 oz	240	13	26
Manapua, (Char Siu Pork Bun), 2.3 oz	180	8	25
Poi ,(mashed cooked taro), 1 cup., 8.5 oz	270	1	65
Poke, average all types, 3 oz	90	1	0
Portuguese Sausage, 2 oz	180	15	2
Potato Salad, ½ cup, 5 oz	170	10	17
Shave Ice, *(Matsumoto)*, all flavors:			
With Ice Cream, 1 large	300	4	64
With Beans, 1 large	290	0	72
Spam Musubi:			
With Regular Spam	265	11	34
(4 oz rice+1.3 oz Spam/7-Eleven Hawaii)			
Homemade, w/ Lite Spam (50% less fat)	220	5	34
Taro Pancake Mix, ⅓ cup (makes 2)	140	2	26

Hawaiian (Cont)

	C	F	Cb
Plate Lunches:			
Chicken Katsu, (9 oz:) With Rice	1110	48	108
+ Macaroni Salad, ¾ cup	1360	68	123
or Tossed Salad + 2 T. French Dress.	1240	61	111
Hamburger, (5 oz): With Rice	710	24	81
Gravy + Macaroni Salad	1135	49	112
Mahi Mahi, (7 oz): With Rice	650	12	90
+ Macaroni Salad + Tartar Sce	1150	58	109
or Macaroni Salad, w/o Tartar ce	935	34	108
or Tossed Salad + 3 Tbsp Fr. Dress.	815	27	96
or Tossed Salad, without dressing	670	12	93
Teri Beef, (5 oz): With 2 scoops Rice	790	23	94
+ Macaroni Salad, ¾ cup	1095	47	113
or Tossed Salad, without dressing	800	23	95

Indian & Pakistani

Per Serving, Meat dishes allow 4 oz meat/serving

	C	F	Cb
Aloo Samosa, each	155	12	12
Alu Gosht Kari, (Meat/Potato Curry)	600	40	23
Chicken Korma	500	35	6
Chicken Pilaf	700	53	50
Chicken Tikka	260	16	2
Chicken Vindaloo	400	20	8
Chapati/Roti, 7″ diameter, 1 piece	60	1	11
Dahl, (Lentil Puree):			
1 cup, without oil	230	1	37
1 Tbsp Tadka (oil topping)	120	13	0
Dhakla, (Lentil Dish), 1″ square, 1 oz	105	5	13
Dhansak, ½ cup	105	4	11
Gosht Kari	460	25	17
Lamb Pilaf	520	35	40
Lassi, (Sweet or Mango), 1 cup, 8 oz	160	4	24
Masala Gosht, (Beef/Tomato/Gravy)	400	25	18
Mulligatawney Soup	300	15	8
Murgh Tikka, 1 cup	300	4	7
Naan Flatbread, 2 oz	160	4	29
Pappadum, 1 large/2 small	50	3	5
Pesrattu, (Lentil Crepe), 9″, 2.6 oz	130	5	15
Pork Vindaloo Curry, without Rice	620	47	3
Rajmah, 1 cup	225	5	35
Rogan Josh,			
without Rice/Potatoes	500	30	3
Shahi Korma, (Braised Lamb)	430	28	3
Tandoori Chicken:			
Breast	260	13	5
Leg/Thigh portion	300	17	6

Italian Dishes

	C	F	Cb
Entrees:			
Baked Ziti: Small	370	27	32
Regular	575	42	49
Breadstick , 2 oz piece	120	3	25
Broccoli Fettucine Alfredo, regular	815	23	125
Bruschetta, 2 slices	380	17	53
Calzones, av. all varieties	840	34	101
Cannelloni, 1 tube, 6 oz	280	15	18
Cheese Breadstick, 2.4 oz piece	180	8	20
Cheese Ravioli, with sauce	495	17	65
Chicken Alfredo	775	29	82
Chicken Parmigiana, 11 oz	520	22	16
Chicken Scallopine, dinner	1110	71	68
Eggplant Parmigiana	900	39	78
Fettucine Alfredo: Lunch, 9 oz	885	65	63
Dinner, 15 oz	1475	108	104
Linquine & Seafood, dinner	1130	71	79
Manicotti Formaggio	800	38	57
Meat Lasagne:			
Small, 10 oz	440	23	39
Large, 16 oz	700	36	60
Meat Ravioli	725	22	102
Minestrone Soup, 1 bowl	110	2	18
Penne Rustica: Lunch	1300	71	76
Dinner	1540	80	101
Ravioli, over-stuffed, average	990	67	57
Panini Sandwich:			
Chicken, 16 oz	900	38	81
Meats, average, 18 oz	940	39	81
Vegetarian, 15 oz	750	31	83
Pizza, Ready-To-Eat ~ *See Page 135*			
Spaghetti & Meatballs:			
With Tomato Sauce: Kids	500	20	58
Medium/Lunch	1080	63	89
Large/Dinner	1430	81	119
With Meat Sauce: Kids	550	25	56
Medium/Lunch	1300	79	84
Large/Dinner	1700	103	110
Veal Marsala, dinner	1320	66	132
Veal Parmigiana, dinner	1270	65	116
Vegetable Primavera	610	8	116
Salad,			
Caprese , 11 oz	445	34	10
Desserts:			
Gelato: Vanilla (Milk Base), ½ cup	200	15	18
Choc. Hazelnut (Milk), ½ cup	370	29	26
Water Base, ½ cup	100	0	25
Lemon Ice,	180	0	45
Tiramisu, 1 piece, 5 oz	400	29	30

Further listings ~ *See Fast-Foods Section*

Japanese

	C	F	Cb
Sashimi: (Sliced Raw Seafood/Beef)			
Ika (Squid), 4 oz	**105**	2	0
Hamachi (Yellowtail), 4 oz	**165**	6	0
Maguro (Yellowfin Tuna), 4 oz	**120**	1	0
Niku (Beef), 5 oz	**200**	10	0
Saba (Mackerel), 4 oz	**160**	7	0
Suzuki (Sea Bass), 4 oz	**110**	1	0
Tako (Octopus), 4 oz	**95**	1	0
Sushi Rice: Cooked, 1 Tbsp	**25**	0	5
1 cup, 5.3 oz	**380**	3	82
Sushi (Maki) Rolls: *Per Piece*			
Average all types (California Rolls; Cream Cheese with Crab; Eel; Salmon; Shrimp; Tuna; Yellowtail; Vegetable)			
Small (1.2" diam. x 1.2" high), 0.8 oz	**25**	1	3.5
Medium (1¾" diam. x 1¾" high), 1.6 oz	**50**	1	7
Large (2¼" diam. x ⅞" high), 2 oz	**60**	2	9
Sushi Packs: *Per Pack*			
Average all types: 6 large pieces	**370**	5	55
9 medium pieces	**360**	6	60
12 small pieces	**265**	3	45
Futomaki (thick roll), 6 pieces	**380**	5	72
Hand Roll (Cone), 4 oz	**120**	2	18
Inari (rice filled soybean pocket), 4 pces	**420**	9	73
Sushi-Nigiri, (fish on rice), average all varieties, 1 piece	**70**	1	12
Sushi Plate, Assorted: 6 pieces	**420**	3	36
Combination (Sushi & Sushi Rolls) 2 Sushi + 6 small & 3 medium rolls	**400**	7	72
Dipping Sauces: Average, 2 Tbsp	**30**	0	7
Ginger Vinegar Dressing, 2 Tbsp	**20**	0	5
Edamame: (young green soybeans):			
Boiled beans (no pods), 4 oz	**160**	7	12
Steamed (in pods), 4 oz	**60**	3	5
Katsu-don, Pork with Rice	**1100**	39	141
Miso Soup, with Tofu pieces, 1 cup	**85**	3	11
Sake Wine, (16% alcohol), 3 fl.oz	**115**	0	7
Seaweed Salad, 1.5 oz	**20**	2	0
Sukiyaki, (Beef/Tofu/Veggies), 8 oz	**400**	24	32
Tempura:			
3 large shrimp & veggies	**320**	18	25
1 shrimp only	**60**	4	3
Teppan Yaki, (Steak, Seafood & Veggies), 10 oz serving	**470**	30	15
Teriyaki: Beef, 4 oz	**350**	25	4
Chicken, 4 oz	**260**	9	7
Salmon, medium, 6 oz	**270**	8	3
Yakatori, 1 skewer, 2.5 oz	**140**	5	1

Kosher/Deli Foods

	C	F	Cb
Bagel/Bialy, 1 small, 2 oz	**160**	2	32
Beiglach, (Cheese Knish)	**350**	17	35
Blintzes: Average, 1 only	**120**	1	25
With Sour Cream & Preserves	**370**	10	30
Borscht, (Without Sour Cream): 1 cup	**85**	3	14
Diet/Reduced Calorie, 1 cup	**30**	1	7
Cabbage Rolls, (meat/rice), 5 oz	**170**	6	21
Chicken Broth: 1 cup	**80**	8	0
With vegetables	**100**	8	5
With noodles	**150**	9	16
Lowfat, plain, 1 cup	**25**	1	0
Cholent, 1 medium serving, 1 cup	**350**	16	48
Chopped Liver: 1 serving, 3 oz	**110**	6	5
With Egg Salad, ¼ cup	**100**	7	3
Farfel, dry, ½ cup	**90**	1	21
Gefilte Fish Balls:			
Regular, 2 oz	**55**	2	4
With Jelled Broth	**80**	2	6
Cocktail size, 1 oz	**30**	1	2
Sweet: Medium, 2 oz	**65**	2	4
With Jelled Broth	**95**	2	9
Hallah, (Yeast Bread), 1 slice, 1 oz	**85**	2	14
Herring: Smoked, 2 oz	**120**	8	0
In Sour Cream, 2 oz	**150**	10	0
Kasha, cooked, ½ cup	**100**	1	20
Kipfel, (Vanilla/Almdond Cookie), 1 pce	**60**	2	7
Knaidlach ~ *See Matzo Balls*			
Knish: Kasha/Potato, 1 only	**130**	4	22
Cheese, 1 only	**350**	17	35
Kreplach, beef, 1 piece	**40**	1	6
Kugel, potato/noodle, 1 serving	**300**	20	25
Latkes, (Potato Pancake): 2 oz	**200**	11	22
3 Latkes w/ Sour Cran Apple Sauce	**750**	25	95
Lochshen: Plain, 1 cup	**130**	2	26
Pudding, 1 cup	**380**	13	48
Lox, (Smoked Salmon), 2 oz	**65**	2	0
Mandelbrot, (Almond Bread), 1 slice, ¼" thick	**45**	2	5
Matzo, 1 oz board	**110**	1	21
Matzo Balls: 2 small, or 1 large, 2"	**90**	3	12
Extra large ball, 3"	**180**	6	24
Matzo Ball Soup:			
Cup w/ 2 small or 1 large ball	**150**	5	27
Bowl w/ Chkn & Noodles	**325**	13	34
Jerry's Deli, large bowl	**560**	17	56
NY Cheesecake, 4 oz	**350**	24	26
Pierogi, potato/cheese, 1 piece	**90**	4	11
Reuben S'wich, w/ ½ lb Corned Beef	**920**	60	28
Schmaltz, (Rend'd Chicken Fat), 1 T.	**90**	10	0

Korean Food

Korean Food	C	F	Cb
Bibimbab, (Veg. & Beef on Rice), 1 cup	565	15	89
Bulgogi, (Barbeque Beef), 3.5 oz	325	12	15
Galbi (Short Ribs), 16 oz	975	61	16
Gujeolpan, (Pancake with Meat & Vegetables), 1 cup with 1 pancake	340	11	39
Japchae, (Noodle w/ Veggies & Meat), 1¼ cups	365	19	34
Sides:			
Kimchee, (Cabbage Relish), ½ cup	30	0	6
Namool, (Assorted Vegetables), 1 cup	125	6.5	9
Soups: *Per Serving*			
Muguk, (Radish & Chive Soup), 6 oz	105	7	6
Samgyetang, (Ginseng Chkn Soup):			
Without Chicken Skin, 1 cup	520	11	60
With Chicken Skin, 1 cup	725	35	60
Yuk Gae Jang, (Spicy Beef Soup), 1¼ cups	180	13	5

Lebanese/Middle East

Lebanese/Middle East	C	F	Cb
Baba Ghannouj, 2 Tbsp, 1 oz	70	6	2
Baklava, (Pastry, Nuts, Syrup), 1 pastry, 1¾ oz	245	18	18
Cabbage Rolls, (Cabb. Leaf, Meat, Rice), 1 roll, 3 oz,	100	3	12
Cous Cous, (Semolina, Milk, Fruit, Nuts), 1 cup	400	21	43
Falafel, (Chick Pea Fritter), Fried, 1 medium, 1 oz	60	4	4
Hummus, ¼ cup, 2.2 oz	105	3	5
Fried Kibbi, (Wheat, Meat Pinenuts), 1 piece, 3 oz	180	8	15
Kafta, (Ground Lamb, Ssge on Skewer), 1 skewer, 1.5 ozoz	85	5	2
Kibbeh Naye, (raw Lamb, Bulgur & Spice) 1 cup, 9 oz	450	18	28
Lebanese Omelet, 1 serving, 4 oz (Egg, Spinach, Pinenuts, Onion)	200	12	13
Pilaf, (Rice, Onion, Raisins, Apr., Spice) 1 cup	400	11	60
Shawourma, (Spit-Roast Beef), 4 oz serving	280	15	2
Shish Kabob, 1 stick, 2.5 oz	130	7	2
Spinach Pie, 1 piece, 3.5 oz	290	21	20
Sweet Almond Sanbusak, (Pastry, Almonds, Spices), 1 piece	200	15	11
Tabouli, 1 serving, 4 oz	125	7	13
Tahini Sauce, average, 1 Tbsp	90	8	2

Mexican Food

Mexican Food	C	F	Cb
Burritos *(Taco Bell):* Bean	370	10	56
Supreme Beef	420	16	53
Chili, plain, ¼ cup	90	6	8
Chili con Carne: With Beans, 1 cup	310	17	15
Without Beans, 1 cup	370	28	10
Chimichangas, Beef, 5 oz	400	19	43
Chorizo Sausage, 2 oz	265	23	0
Churro, (1), 1.5 oz	150	8	18
Corn Chips, ½ cup, 1 oz	160	10	17
Enchilada, average	330	10	49
Fajitas, Chicken	200	7	20
Guacamole, average, 2 Tbsp, 1 oz	45	4	2
Horchata: *(Don Jose)*, 1 cup, 8 fl.oz	140	4	25
Cacique, 1 pint bottle, 16 fl.oz	320	7	62
Margarita, with 1.5 oz Tequila	160	0	6
Masa, (Pre-mixed for Tamales), 1 oz	80	5	9
Menudo:			
With Hominy, 1 cup	240	9	19
Without Hominy, 1 cup	170	9	2
Nachos: With cheese, peppers, 1 portion, 6-8 nachos, 7 oz	600	33	60
With cheese, beans, beef, peppers, 1 portion, 6-8 nachos, 9 oz	570	31	56
Del Taco: Regular, 4 oz	300	19	30
Macho Nachos, 17 oz	1000	56	94
Taco Bell, BellGrande®, 10.8 oz	780	40	84
Nopal Cactus Salad, 1 cup	130	9	11
Papas Fritas, (1), 6 oz	325	18	40
Piloncillo, (Brown Sugar):			
1 Tbsp, 0.5 oz	50	0	13
Cone, small, 3", 3 oz	325	0	81
Quesadilla, Cheese	490	28	39
Queso Fresco, ¼ cup	80	5	8
Refried Beans, ¾ cup, 6 oz	160	3	26
Rice Pudding, (Arroz Con Leche), 4 oz	140	3	24
Soup, Black Bean, 1 bowl	200	3	34
Tacos *(Taco Bell):*			
Crunchy: Regular	170	10	12
Supreme	200	12	15
Soft: Crispy Potato	270	13	31
Grilled Steak	250	14	19
Taco Salad with Salsa	840	52	85
Taco Sauce, average, ¼ cup	15	0	3
Taco Shell, regular	50	2	8
Tamales, Beef/Chicken, av. 4.5 oz	250	11	27
Taquitos, Beef & Cheese, 4.5 oz	330	15	36
Tostada (*Taco Bell*)	250	10	29
Tortilla, Corn, 6" diameter	70	1	14
Tortilla Chips, 1 oz	150	8	18
Soup, Black Bean, 1 bowl	200	3	34

Extra Food Listings ~ See Fast Food Section (Examples: Del Taco, Taco Bell, Taco Cabana, Taco Time)

Mexican (Cont)

	C	F	Cb
Breads:			
Bolillos, 1 roll, 3.5 oz	240	4	42
Mexican Cornbread, 4″ square	210	11	19
Pan de Leche, 1 roll, 1.3 oz	110	3	20
Telera, 2 oz	150	2	19
Cakes, Cookies, Pastries Pan Dulce:			
Banderilla, 1 piece	140	10	8
Bigotes, 7″	570	22	44
Capirotada, (Bread Pudding), 10 oz	810	38	107
Cinnamon Cookies, 2	125	8	13
Concha, av. all varieties:			
Small (3″ diameter), 2.5 oz	250	8	38
Medium (4″ diameter), 3.5 oz	350	11	53
Large (5″ diameter), 5.5 oz	550	18	84
Cream Puff, with Custard, 4.3 oz	255	14	25
Cuernos, (Horns), 3 oz	340	17	41
Donut, large, 4″, 3.5 oz	440	21	58
Elotes, 3.5 oz	450	24	51
Empanadas, average all varieties:			
Medium, 3 oz	300	14	42
Large, 4 oz	400	19	56
Fiesta Cookie, (1), 2.3 oz	280	8	47
Galletas Mixtas:			
Small, 1 oz	100	3	16
Medium, 2 oz	200	5	32
Large, 3 oz	300	8	48
Guayaba, 3.3 oz	360	14	53
Jelly Roll, (1), 3.3 oz	240	4	46
Mantecadites, 4.5 oz	670	42	64
Mini Cupcake, (1),1.8 oz	180	8	25
Muffins/Nino Enbuelto, large, 6 oz	465	11	48
Nuez, 3.3 oz	380	17	52
Ojo de Buey, 4 oz	360	15	55
Orejas, 1 medium, 3 oz	310	15	38
Pan Dulce, 1 bun	330	10	45
Panquecitos, 2.5 oz	260	11	36
Piedras, 4 oz	470	15	76
Polvorones: Small, 1.5 oz	180	9	24
1 large, 3 oz	370	18	48
Pound Cakes, mini, 3.5 oz	380	16	52
Puerquitos, 3.5 oz	350	12	55
Rebanadas, 3.5 oz	390	18	51
Roles De Canela, (Cinn. Roll), 4.5 oz	490	15	81
Roscas, 1 piece, 2.8 oz	360	18	44
Semitas *(Bimbo)*, 1 piece, 2.2 oz	210	6	33
Sopapillas, (flaky pastry puffs): 1 piece	100	7	10
With Honey & Cream	200	14	18
Strawberry Crema Roll, 2.5 oz slice	240	5	45

Extra Food Listings ~ *See CalorieKing.com*

Polish

	C	F	Cb
Cabbage Rolls, w/ Sour Cream, 2 small	220	10	30
Chicken Casserole, w/ Mshrms, 1 cup	520	27	5
Kielbasa, (Sausages, Onions, fried), 2 large	350	28	2
Meatballs, in sour cream, 3 x 1½″ balls	300	16	11
Pierogi, Fruit/Vegetables, 3″ ball	80	2	15
Pork Goulash, (Pork/Vegetable Stew)	550	21	38
Pot Roast, with Vegetables	630	21	28

Soul Foods

	C	F	Cb
Breakfast Sausage, fried, 2 patties	250	17	0
Brunswick Stew, 1 cup, 8.5 oz	320	14	19
Cornbread, homemade, 3 oz	200	7.5	28
Fatback, 0.5 oz	110	11	0
Ham Hock, pickled, 3 oz	200	12	0
Hog Maw, 1 oz	70	5	0
Hominy, cooked, ¾ cup	110	1	25
Hush Puppies, 5 pieces	260	12	35
Kale, cooked, ½ cup	20	0.5	4
Opossum, roasted, without bone, 3 oz	190	9	0
Oxtail, cooked, without bone, 2 oz	85	5	0
Pig's Ear, ¼ ear	50	3	0
Pig's Foot, ½ foot	70	5	0
Pig's Tail, ⅓ tail	115	10	0
Poke Salad, cooked, ½ cup	16	1	3
Pork Brains, braised, 3 oz	115	8	0
Pork Chitterlings, simmered, 3 oz	260	25	0
Pork Cracklings, 0.5 oz	80	6	0
Pork Neck Bones, cooked, no bone, 2 oz	100	5	0
Pork Skin, 1 cup	70	5	0
Pork Tongue, ⅓ tongue	75	6	0
Sousemeat, 1 oz	60	5	0
Succotash, ½ cup	80	1	17
Sweet Potato Pie, ⅛ of 9″ pie	250	12	34
Tripe, 2 oz	55	2	0
Vienna Sausage:			
2 small, 1 oz	90	8	1
1 small, 0.5 oz	45	4	1

OLD McDONALDS FARM
128 FOR PEOPLE WHO WANT BETTER
Brooklyn

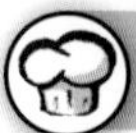

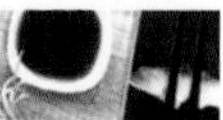

Spanish

Food	C	F	Cb
Arroz Abanda, (Fish with Rice)	340	8	31
Arroz Con Pollo, (Rice/Chkn Salad)	500	23	50
Clams Marinara, 8 clams	330	16	22
Cochifrito, (Lamb with Lemon/Garlic)	650	25	5
Cochinillo Asado, (Rst Suckling Pig), 2 slices	300	15	3
Cocido Madrileno, (Madrid-Style Boiled Dinner)	450	27	18
Flan de Leche, (Caramel Custard)	325	9	52
Fritadera de Ternera, (Sauteed Veal)	450	27	2
Gazpacho, 1 bowl	60	0	15
Mole Poblano, ½ cup	205	14	16
Paella a la Valenciana, (Chicken & Shellfish Rice)	900	42	70
Pollo a la Espanola, (Chicken)	475	30	4
Ternera al Jerez, (Veal with Sherry)	660	29	6
Zarzuela, (Fish & Shellfish Medley)	530	27	40

Thai Foods

Food	C	F	Cb
Appetizers: Satay Pork, 1 oz	100	4	2
Spring Roll, 1.3 oz	110	6	13
Soups, Tom Yam (Hot & Sour):			
Spicy Shrimp/Seafood:			
1 cup	100	4	6
1 bowl	160	7	10
Vegetarian, 1 cup	50	0	11
Curries: Chicken with Ginger, 1 cup	390	34	4
Thick Red Curry with Beef, 1 cup	600	50	7
Thai Chicken Curry, 1 cup	340	23	4
Massaman Curry, 1 cup	680	57	8
Green Curry with Pork, 1 cup	480	44	5
Pad Thai, large serving, 18 oz	990	38	125
Fish: Steamed with Spicy Thai Sce	450	8	46
Crispy Fried, 5 oz	290	15	9
Spicy Chicken, stir-fry	450	22	14
Spicy Garlic Tofu, stir-fry	340	18	18
Sticky Thai Rice: Plain 1 cup, 6 oz	170	1	36
With Coconut & Sesame Seeds, 1 cup	880	28	120
Stir-fried Rice Noodles, 1 cup 5.5 oz	270	9	40
Stir-fried Vegetables, 1 cup	100	3	18
Salads: Green Papaya Salad	160	0	40
Spicy Prawn, 9 shrimp	170	3	15
Thai Beef Salad, 1 serving	260	9	15
Thai Chicken, 1 serving	330	9	17
Thai Noodle, 1 serving	410	13	45
Satay Chicken & Peanut Sauce, 1 satay stick	390	24	20
Sauce, Peanut Satay, ½ cup, 4 oz	160	10	13

Vietnamese

Food	C	F	Cb
Banh Cuon, (Steam Rice w/ Pork), 1 roll	105	7	8
Bo Nuong, (Beef Satay), 2 sticks	265	9	4
Bo Xao Dau Phong, (Ginger Beef with Onion, Fish Sce)	750	30	10
Ca Chien Gung, (Whole Snapper/Ginger)	600	16	6
Canh Chay, (Vegetable/Tofu Soup)	80	3	13
Cari Chicken, 1 cup	475	29	16
Cari Chicken, with Rice Noodle, 1 cup curry & 1 cup noodles	660	29	60
Cari Chicken, with Steamed Rice, 1 cup curry & 1 cup rice	650	29	55
Cuu Xao Lan, (Curried Lamb and Veggies in Coconut)	900	40	80
Ga Chien, (Crisp Chick + Plum Sauce)	900	40	105
Ga Nuong, (Chicken Satay + Sauce)	240	10	4
Ga Xao Rau, (Marinated Chicken Braised with Vegetables)	800	26	100
Gio Lua, (Lean Pork Pie), ⅙ of pie	245	12	0
Goi Cuon, (Cold Spring Rolls), 1 roll	60	1	7
Rau Cai Xao Chay, (Stir Fried Veggies)	400	15	65
Thit Bo Vien, (Beef Balls), 6 balls	225	14	2
Thit Heo Goi Baup Cai, (Spicy Cabb. Rolls with Pork), 1 roll	200	7	11
Soup: *Per Bowl, ½ Cup*			
Bun Bo Hue, (Hot & Spicy Soup):			
Without Pork Feet	340	9	35
With Pork Feet	830	45	35
Chicken & Rice Noodle Soup	400	3	55
Pho Bo, (Beef Noodle Soup)	410	7	59
Pho Ga, (Chicken Noodle Soup)	460	6	58
Pho Tai, (Rare Beef & Noodle Soup)	440	7	73
Salad, Goi Du Du, (Green Papaya), ½ cup	155	3	29
Sauce, Nuoc Cham (Hot Sauce)	5	0	1

Gourmet & Miscellaneous

Food	C	F	Cb
Ants Eggs/Larvae, 1 Tbsp	20	0	0
Ants, chocolate coated, 3 Tbsp	140	7	2
Bee Maggots, canned, 3 Tbsp	65	2	0
Caviar, black/red, 1 Tbsp	40	3	0
Caterpillars, canned, 2 oz	60	2	0
Frog Legs, fried, 1 pair (large)	125	7	0
Haggis, boiled, 4 oz	350	24	22
Locusts, roasted, 1 oz	35	1	0
Silkworms, raw, 1 oz	60	2	0
Snails in garlic butter, 6 large	200	10	4
Snake, roasted, 4 oz	160	6	0

Nutritional data is based on U.S. outlets

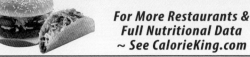

For More Restaurants & Full Nutritional Data ~ See CalorieKing.com

A&W® (Oct '23)

Burgers:	C	F	Cb
Original Bacon Cheeseburger:			
Single	460	23	40
Double	650	36	41
Cheeseburger	400	16	42
Double Cheeseburger	590	29	42
Hamburger	350	11	41
Mushroom & Onion Melt: Single	400	17	38
Double	580	29	39
Papa Burger: Single	450	22	42
Double	640	35	42
Sandwiches: Crispy Chicken	480	20	51
Club	540	25	52
Grilled: Chicken	410	12	38
Chicken Club	470	17	39
Chicken Tenders,			
breaded, 3 pcs	260	9	5
Corn Dog Nuggets, 10 pieces	540	26	40
Hot Dogs: Plain	310	18	28
Coney	320	19	26
Coney Cheese Dog	360	22	29
Footlong Hotdog	610	34	52
Fries: Chili Cheese Fries, 7 oz	410	18	51
French Fries:			
Small/Kids, 2.5 oz	210	8	29
Regular, 4 oz	310	13	45
Large, 5.5 oz	430	17	61
Onion Rings, 5.1 oz	280	4	53
Dipping Sauces: *Per 1 oz Cup*			
BBQ	40	0	10
Buttermilk Ranch	130	14	1
Honey Mustard	45	0	10
Spicy Papas	130	12	6
A&W Root Beer Float:			
Regular: 16 oz Cup	310	5	61
20 oz Cup	340	5	68
32 oz Cup	610	11	119
Diet Root Beer, 16 oz	160	5	24
Cones: Chocolate, regular, 5.5 oz	290	7	51
Root Beer, regular, 5.5 oz	260	8	41
Freeze:			
Root Beer: 16 oz	380	9	68
20 oz	520	12	92
Diet Root Beer, 16 oz	270	9	41
Polar Swirls: M&M, 12 oz	810	29	123
Oreo, 12 oz	660	17	100
Reese's Peanut Butter Cup, 12 oz	690	29	95
Shakes: Chocolate/Vanilla, av., 16 oz	540	17	87
Strawberry, 16 oz	520	17	81
Sundaes: Chocolate, regular	360	11	61
Hot Fudge/Hot Caramel, reg., av.	385	13	63

Applebees® (Oct '23)

Appetizers: *As Served*	C	F	Cb
Brew Pub Pretzels & Beer Chse Dip	1160	49	146
Chipotle Lime Chicken Quesadillas	1120	69	78
Chicken Wonton Tacos	600	26	58
Crunchy Onion Rings	1320	60	180
Mozzarella Sticks	860	43	77
Neighborhood Nachos, Chicken	1830	117	118
Spinach & Artichoke Dip	980	61	89
White Queso Dip & Chips	920	53	83
Wings: Boneless Wings, plain	630	31	50
Dressings: Bleu Cheese	200	22	1
Ranch	160	16	2
Garlic Parmesan	390	41	5
Honey BBQ Wings	190	0	48
Honey Pepper	230	0	59
Sweet Asian Chile	260	3	56
Bowls:			
Southwest Chicken	820	29	90
Tex-Mex Shrimp	710	27	91
Burgers: *With Classic Fries*			
Classic	1120	66	90
Classic Bacon Chseburger	1330	83	92
Classic Cheeseburger	1220	74	91
Quesadilla	1590	105	94
Whisky Bacon	1630	102	117
Chicken: *With Menu Set Sides*			
Bourbon Street Chicken & Shrimp	790	43	47
Chicken Tenders Plate	1080	62	95
Chicken Tenders Platter	1410	80	123
Fiesta Lime Chicken	1170	60	98
Pasta: *As Served, with Breadstick*			
Broccoli Blackened Shrimp Alfredo	1290	75	103
Classic Broccoli Chicken Alfredo	1390	76	102
Four Cheese Mac & Cheese,			
w/ Honey Pepper Chicken Tenders	1350	54	160
Three Cheese Chicken Penne	1320	69	99
Sandwiches & More: *With Fries, without Customizing or Dressing*			
Bacon Ranch Gr. Chicken S'wch	1120	58	91
Bacon Ranch Crispy Chicken S'wich	1260	72	110
Chicken Fajita Rollup	1390	75	116
Clubhouse Grille	1450	80	128
Sweet & Spicy Crispy Chkn S'wich	1350	62	159
The Prime Rib Dipper	1380	72	123

Applebees® cont... (Oct '23)

Seafood: With Fixed Sides	C	F	Cb
Blackened Cajun Grilled Salmon	600	28	47
Double Crunch Shrimp	1150	50	143
Hand Battered Fish & Chips, with Tartar Sauce	1470	95	115
***Steaks & Ribs:** With Fixed Sides*			
Steak: 6 oz Top Sirloin	550	23	43
8 oz USDA Sirloin	620	26	45
12 oz USDA Ribeye	850	45	44
Bourbon Street Steak	820	47	48
Double Glazed Baby Back Ribs:			
Full Rack	1440	91	68
Half Rack	850	51	53
Riblets:			
Plate, without sauce	910	52	55
Platter, without sauce	1350	80	71
Shrimp & Parmesan Sirloin	900	51	49
***Salads:** Includes Fixed Salad Dressing*			
Caesar: with Blackened Shrimp	680	51	31
with Grilled Chicken	790	53	29
Crispy Chicken Tender	1020	72	57
Oriental Grilled Chkn	1250	82	79
Strawberry Balsamic Chicken	670	42	31
Soup: Chicken Tortilla	280	15	25
French Onion	370	22	26
Tomato Basil	210	12	22
Fries & Sides:			
Baked Potato:			
With Sour Cream & Whipped Butter	530	31	59
Loaded	590	35	59
Breadstick	180	7	25
Classic Fries	400	18	53
Crunchy Onion Rings	560	30	66
Four-Cheese Mac & Cheese w/ Bacon	390	18	38
Garlic Mashed Potatoes	260	11	37
Garlic Mashed Potatoes, loaded	430	26	40
Garlicky Green Beans	150	12	8
Steamed Broccoli	100	8	5
Waffle Fries	480	24	58
***Desserts:** As Served*			
Brownie Bite	330	15	48
Sizzlin' Butter Pecan Blondie	1040	59	116
Sugar Dusted Donut Dippers	1520	54	247
Triple Chocolate Meltdown	850	37	125

Arby's® (Oct '23)

Sandwiches:	C	F	Cb
Beef 'n Cheddar: Classic	450	20	45
Double	630	32	48
½ Pound	740	39	48
Chicken: Buffalo Crispy Chicken	500	23	48
Chicken Bacon Swiss	610	30	51
Classic Crispy Chicken	510	25	48
Roast Beef: Classic	360	14	37
Double	510	24	38
½ Pound	610	30	38
Smokehouse Brisket	560	29	42
Chicken Nuggets:			
4 pieces	210	10	12
6 pieces	310	15	18
9 pieces	470	23	28
Chicken Tenders:			
3 pieces	370	18	28
5 pieces	610	30	47
Dipping Sauces: Buffalo, 1 oz	10	1	2
Honey Mustard, 1 oz	130	13	5
Ranch, 1 oz	100	10	1
Tangy BBQ , 1 oz	45	0	10
Market Fresh: Greek Gyro	700	44	55
Corned Beef Reuben	680	31	62
Roast Beef Gyro	540	29	48
Turkey, Ranch & Bacon Sandwich	810	35	79
Wraps: Buffalo Chicken	790	45	61
Crispy Chicken Club	880	49	64
Sliders: Buffalo Chicken	260	12	26
Chicken	230	9	25
Jalapeno Roast Beef	180	7	16
Roast Beef	170	7	16
Crinkle Cut Fries: Small	250	12	32
Medium	390	19	49
Large	530	26	68
Curly Fries: Small	250	13	29
Medium	410	22	49
Large	550	29	65
***Sides:** Without Sauce*			
Jalapeno Bites: 5 pieces	290	17	31
8 pieces	470	27	50
Mozzarella Sticks: 4 pieces	440	23	37
6 pieces	650	35	56

continued next page...

Arby's® cont... (Oct '23)

Kids Menu:	C	F	Cb
Fries: Crinkle cut, small	250	12	32
Curly, small	250	13	29
Nuggets: 4 pieces	210	10	12
6 pieces	310	15	18
Sliders: Buffalo Chicken Slider	260	12	26
Chicken Slider	230	9	25
Jalapeno Roast Beef Slider	180	7	16
Roast Beef Slider	170	7	16
Beverages: Lowfat White Milk	90	2	10
Lowfat Chocolate Milk	150	3	26
Breakfast: *Per Serving*			
Biscuits: Bacon	340	17	36
Bacon, Egg & Cheese	470	28	37
Chicken	390	18	44
Ham	340	16	37
Ham, Egg & Cheese	460	24	38
Sausage	500	33	36
Sausage, Egg & Cheese	630	44	39
Croissants: Bacon, Egg & Cheese	430	26	29
Ham, Egg & Cheese	410	23	30
Ssge, Egg & Cheese	580	43	30
Potato Cakes: 2 Cakes	250	14	23
3 Cakes	370	21	35
4 Cakes	490	28	46
Sourdough Sandwiches:			
Bacon, Egg & Cheese	470	22	46
Ham, Egg & Cheese	460	18	47
Sausage, Egg & Cheese	630	38	47
Wraps: Bacon, Egg & Cheese	490	26	41
Ham, Egg & Cheese	470	23	43
Sausage, Egg & Chse	620	40	42
Sauces: Arby's, 0.5 oz	15	0	3
Bronco Berry, 1 oz	60	0	15
Cheddar Cheese, 1.5 oz	50	4	4
Horsey, 0.5 oz	60	5	3
Ketchup, 0.3 oz	10	0	3
Marinara, 1 oz	20	0	4
Spicy Three Pepper, 0.5 oz	25	1	3
Tangy BBQ, 1 oz	45	0	10
Desserts:			
Apple Turnover	430	18	65
Cherry Turnover	390	13	65
Salted Caramel & Chocolate Cookie	430	18	63
Shakes: *Per Regular*			
Chocolate; Jamocha, average	540	17	87
Vanilla	480	17	70
Blueberry Lemonade, regular	160	0	41

Atlanta Bread Co® (Oct '23)

Breakfast Bagel Sandwiches:	C	F	Cb
Egg & Cheese	525	17	69
Egg, Cheese & Bacon	455	11	69
Egg, Cheese & Ham	505	13	69
Side, Breakfast Potatoes	170	9	20
Paninis: Chicken Pesto	735	30	76
Cuban	845	41	75
Steakhouse	725	33	68
Sandwiches: Chicken Salad	745	42	57
Grilled Caprese	700	36	64
Roast Beef	475	16	52
Roasted Turkey	510	16	58
Tuna Salad	720	38	60
Salads: *Per Full Size, with Dressing, without Bread*			
Balsamic Blue	605	44	40
Caesar	790	55	60
Chopstix Chicken	855	46	80
Cobb	355	17	32
Greek	700	51	40
Sides, Black Beans & Corn	190	9	24

Au Bon Pain® (Oct '23)

Bagels: *Per Bagel*	C	F	Cb
Asiago Cheese, 4 oz	310	5	54
Cinnamon Raisin, 3.7 oz	270	1	57
Everything, 3.6 oz	270	2	54
Plain, 3.5 oz	260	1	53
Sesame Seed, 3.6 oz	280	2	54
Whole Wheat Skinny , 1.6 oz	90	1	21
Breakfast Sandwiches:			
2 Eggs on a Bagel	400	11	54
with Bacon	480	17	55
with Bacon & Cheese	530	22	55
Egg Whites On Skinny Wheat Bagel:			
Cheddar	210	7	22
Cheddar & Avocado	360	23	25
Smoked Salmon & Avocado	470	16	62
Classic Oatmeal, 12 oz	260	5	47
Fruit Cup, large, 12 oz	140	1	36
Yogurt Parfait:			
Blueb. Yog. & Wild Blueberry, 10.2 oz	370	9	65
Greek Van. Yog. & Wild Blueb., 10.2 oz	320	8	44
Sandwiches: *Per Whole Sandwich*			
Cafe: Extra Bacon BLT	600	31	58
Tuna Salad on Croissant	480	23	34
Turkey Club	590	27	48
Signature: Chipotle Turkey & Avoc.	770	43	59
Caprese	620	31	56

Au Bon Pain® cont... (Oct '23)

Harvest Hot Bowls:	C	F	Cb
Mayan Chicken	560	11	85
Mediterranean Chicken	670	26	76
Roasted Vegetarian	640	32	75
Soups: *Per 12 fl.oz*			
Baked Stuffed Potato	390	24	34
Broccoli Cheddar	340	24	20
Chicken Noodle	120	3	15
Clam Chowder	350	20	32
Italian Wedding	160	7	15
Lemon Orzo Chicken	230	12	20
Lobster & Corn Bisque	280	16	25
Vegetarian Minestrone	120	1	22
Specialty: Macaroni & Cheese	880	43	92
Turkey Chili	330	9	44
Salads: *Without Dressing*			
Chicken Caesar Asiago	260	8	21
Chicken Cobb with Avocado	430	24	16
Chef	280	13	10
Mediterranean	350	24	24
Southwest Chicken	310	9	31
Dressings: *Per 1.5 fl.oz*			
Balsamic Vinaigrette	100	9	5
Caesar	220	24	1
Chili Lime Vinaigrette	120	10	8
Green Goddess	210	22	3
Ranch	200	20	4
Cake, Cookies, Croissants, Danish:			
Cake, Iced Lemon Pound, 4.5 oz	470	21	66
Cinnamon Swirl Roll, 5.2 oz	490	19	73
Cookies:			
Chocolate Chip, 2.8 oz	370	18	54
Oatmeal Raisin, 2.2 oz	290	11	46
Croissants: Almond, 4 oz	490	25	59
Apple, 3.3 oz	280	14	34
Chocolate, 3.9oz	470	25	55
Maple Pecan, 3.45 oz	410	27	37
Plain, 2.4 oz	280	16	28
Danish, Sweet Cheese, 4.9 oz	500	23	63
Muffins: Blueberry, 4.3 oz	420	21	53
Chocolate Chip, 4.2 oz	490	25	61
Triple Berry, 4.2 oz	420	21	53
Scone, Cinnamon Chip, 3.7 oz	460	25	50
Beverages: *Per 16 fl.oz*			
Hot: Caffe Latte	140	7	12
Caramel Macchiato	270	8	41
Chocolate	350	12	51
Iced: Mocha Latte	300	9	49
Vanilla Latte	230	7	35
Strawberry Banana Smoothie	290	0	68

For Complete Items ~ See CalorieKing.com

Auntie Anne's® (Oct '23)

Pretzels: *With Butter*	C	F	Cb
Cinnamon Sugar	470	12	84
Jalapeno	330	5	63
Original	340	5	65
Pepperoni	480	16	65
Roasted Garlic & Parm.	380	8	68
Sour Cream & Onion	380	8	68
Sweet Almond	390	6	74
Dips:			
Caramel, 1.7 oz	170	2	37
Cheese, 1.4 oz	90	8	2
Hot Salsa Cheese, 1.4 oz	90	8	2
Light Cream Cheese, 1.25 oz	80	6	1
Marinara, 2 oz	45	1	7
Melted Cheese, 2 oz	150	12	6
Sweet Glaze, 1.7 oz	150	0	39
Sweet Mustard, 1.5 oz	90	3	14
Pretzel Dogs: *With Butter*			
Original	360	20	33
Cheese	370	20	33
Jalapeno Cheese	370	20	34
Mini Pretzel Dogs (10)	630	35	56
Pretzel Nuggets, Orig., w/ Butter, 16 oz	390	5	75
Smoothies: Mango, 16 fl.oz	230	0	20
Strawberry; Strawb. Banana, 16 fl.oz	220	0	54

Back Yard Burgers® (Oct '23)

Black Angus Burgers: *On Brioche Bun*	C	F	Cb
Back Yard Burgers: *Without Cheese Unless Indicated*			
Classic	760	47	49
Double Classic	1210	84	49
Black Jack w/ Pepper Jack Cheese	920	63	46
Black & Bleu w/ Blue Cheese Crumbles	940	65	46
Chipotle w/ Beef, Bacon & Cheddar	1000	67	56
Mushroom Swiss with Swiss Cheese	850	56	44
Chicken Sandwiches: *On Brioche Bun*			
Blackened Chicken w/out cheese	620	27	51
Black Jack Club with Bacon, Chicken & Pepperjack Cheese	710	37	47
Grilled Chicken without cheese	460	11	46
Hawaiian Chicken without cheese	530	11	64
Specialties: *Without Cheese*			
Breaded Chicken Tender Basket, w/o Toppings, Sauce or Bread	540	36	27
Veggie Burger, Brioche Bun	430	10	68
Turkey Burgers: *On Brioche Bun*			
Classic without cheese	540	28	42
Club with Swiss Cheese	660	38	43
Wild with Pepper Jack Cheese	610	33	44

continued next page ...

Back Yard Burgers® cont... (Oct '23)

Fries:	C	F	Cb
Chili Cheese Fries, seasoned, reg.	790	59	52
Seasoned Fries: Regular, 4.5 oz	480	36	38
Large, 6 oz	640	47	50
Sweet Potato Fries, regular, 6 oz	450	29	40
Waffle Fries: Reg., 6 oz	820	56	66
Large, 8 oz	1100	75	88
Sides: Back Yard Chili	310	18	15
Creamy Cole Slaw	200	16	15
Loaded Baked Potato	420	21	45
Panko Onion Rings, regular, 4 oz	340	13	47
Salads: *With Set Ingredients, without Dressing*			
Back Yard:			
Blackened Chicken without Cheese	450	21	22
Grilled Chicken without Cheese	350	10	21
Cranberry Pecan w/ Blackend Chkn	770	41	52
Side Salad w/o Meat, with Ched. Chse	140	6	14
Dressings:			
Bleu Cheese	220	24	1
Caesar	260	26	4
Gorgonzola Vinaigrette	170	15	6
Honey Mustard	200	20	7
Ranch, Homestyle	150	16	1
Dessert/Cobblers: Apple or Cherry	390	16	58
Apple or Cherry Cobbler A La Mode	540	24	78
Peach	350	12	57
Ice Cream, A La Carte	150	8	20
Milk Shakes: *With Whole Milk & Whipped Topping*			
Chocolate: Vanilla, av.	745	35	98
Chocolate Oreo	850	40	115
Peanut Butter	830	51	79

Baja Fresh® (Oct '23)

Burritos: *Base Ingredients Only*	C	F	Cb
Baja	650	37	58
Diablo	830	49	74
Fajita	820	44	82
Impossible	640	26	84
Mexicano	490	19	71
Nacho	860	46	84
Ultimo	810	42	82
Nachos: Base Ingredients Only	1430	87	113
Nachos Queso	1120	61	115
Tacos: *With Standard Toppings*			
Americano Taco: Carnitas	290	13	25
Chicken	250	13	21

Baja Fresh® cont... (Oct '23)

Salads: *Without Dressing*	C	F	Cb
Baja:			
BBQ Chicken (includes chicken)	360	15	37
Ensalada Base Only	110	4	17
Tostada Base Only	670	40	62
Tacos: *Base Ingredients Only*			
Americano	180	8	21
Baja	100	3	17
Grilled:			
Shrimp with Corn Tortilla	180	7	21
Wahoo with Corn Tortilla	230	9	27
Impossible	300	13	39
Wahoo Crispy	290	18	24
Add Protein: Carnitas	180	5	11
Chicken	150	7	1
Shrimp	170	8	2
Steak	190	9	1
Veggies	50	2	9
Wahoo: Crispy	360	21	18
Grilled	220	14	1
Add Rice & Beans: Black Beans	150	1	26
Pinto Beans	160	1	29
Rice	130	5	19
Sides: Guacamole, 8 oz	3190	34	24
Queso, 8 oz	4580	46	16
Rice & Black Beans, 17.4 oz	580	13	91
Rice & Pinto Beans, 17.4 oz	600	13	96
Tortilla Chips, 5 oz	710	28	99

For Complete Nutritional Data ~ see CalorieKing.com

Baskin Robbins® (Oct '23)

Cones:	C	F	Cb
Cake	25	0	5
Fancy Waffle Cone, with Sprinkles	310	13	46
Fresh-Baked Waffle	150	4	29
Sugar	50	1	10
Ice Creams: *Per 2.5 oz Scoop*			
Classic Flavors: Baseball Nut	170	9	21
Cherries Jubilee	150	7	20
Chocolate	170	9	20
Chocolate Chip	150	10	15
Chocolate Fudge	150	9	17
Coffee Shop Cold Brew	170	8	20
Cotton Candy	150	7	18
Gold Medal Ribbon	150	8	18
Icing On The Cake	200	11	18
Jamocha Almond Fudge	160	9	17
Made with Snickers	180	9	23

Baskin Robbins® cont... (Oct '23)

Ice Creams (Cont): Per 2.5 oz Scoop	C	F	Cb
Classic Flavors Cont:			
Mint Chocolate Chip	105	10	14
Nutty Coconut	190	12	18
Old Fashioned Butter Pecan	180	11	16
Oreo Cookies 'n Cream	170	9	20
Oreo 'n Cold Brew	200	11	22
Peanut Butter 'n Choc.	200	13	19
Pistachio Almond	170	12	13
Pralines 'n Cream	170	9	20
Reese's Peanut Butter Cup	190	11	20
Rocky Road	180	9	22
Strawberry Cheesecake	160	8	18
Triple Mango	130	5	22
Vanilla	150	10	13
World Class Chocolate	180	10	20
No Sugar Added:			
Caramel Turtle Truffle	120	5	24
Pineapple Coconut	100	4	18
Note: Carbohydrate figures include 9-16 grams sugar alcohol			
Non Dairy: Daiquiri Ice	90	0	22
Lemon Sorbet	80	0	21
Mint Chocolate Chunk	170	9	24
Ice Cream Quarts: *Per ⅔ Cup, 3.46 oz*			
Chocolate/ Mint Chocolate Chip, av.	230	14	24
Chocolate Chip Cookie Dough	250	13	31
Gold Medal Ribbon	230	11	29
Jamocha Almond Fudge	250	13	28
Oreo Cookies 'n Cream	240	13	28
Peanut Butter 'n Choc.	280	18	27
Vanilla	230	14	23
Very Berry Strawberry	190	9	24
Novelty, Mango Chamay Bar	90	0	23
Sundaes:			
Premium Layered:			
Choc. Chip Cookie Dough	1130	48	164
Oreo	920	44	122
Reese's P'nut Butter Cup	1250	85	106
Bakery, Brownie, 2.2 oz	240	9	36
Beverages: *Per 16 fl.oz*			
Milkshakes:			
Chocolate Chip Cookie Dough	760	36	95
Mint Chocolate Chip	690	36	78
Peanut Butter 'n Chocolate	790	46	82
Vanilla	680	37	74
Very Berry Strawberry	610	26	80

Big Apple Bagels® (Oct '23)

Bagels:	C	F	Cb
Asiago Melt; Swiss Melt, av.	370	6	65
Cinnamon Sugar	370	2	78
Everything	340	3	66
Plain or Salt	320	2	64
Cream Cheese: *Per 1.5 oz*			
Cheddar & Bacon	140	13	2
Plain/Salsa/Scallion, average	135	12	2
Plain, Lite	100	9	2
Strawberry	130	11	5
Tomato-Basil/Lox/Dill Garlic, av.	140	13	3
Muffins: *With Whole Egg*			
Mini: Blueberry; Lemon Poppyseed	90	5	12
Cinnamon Swirl Cheesecake	90	5	9
Large:			
Blueberry	590	28	78
Choc. Cheesecake, 6 oz	650	38	70
Breakfast Sandwiches:			
French Toast with Egg:			
on BAB Bagel	1020	55	107
On MFM Bagel	1060	55	117
Salads:			
Caesar, with Caesar Dressing	450	34	19
Chicken Club, with Ranch Dressing	760	59	18
Mediterranean Bread Salad, with Balsamic Vinaigrette	740	41	63
Beverages: *Per Medium, 16 fl.oz*			
Hot Chocolate	440	12	71
Mocha; White Chocolate Latte, av.	380	8	66
Vanilla Creme Latte	310	7	50

Biggby Coffee® (Oct '23)

Hot Drinks: *Per Tall, 16 fl.oz, without Whipped Cream*	C	F	Cb
Cafe au Lait: with 2% Milk	100	4	9
with Nonfat Milk	65	0	9
with Soy	90	3	11
Caffe Latte: with 2% Milk	160	5	19
with Nonfat Milk	115	0	16
with Soy	160	5	19
Cappuccino: with 2% Milk	105	4	10
with Nonfat Milk	70	0	10
with Soy	95	3	11
Chai Latte: with 2% Milk	315	8	51
with Nonfat Milk	255	0	51
Dark Hot Chocolate: w/ 2% Milk	320	9	50
with Non-Fat Milk	260	2	50
Creme Freeze Smoothies: *Per 16fl.oz w/out Wh. Crm*			
Banana Berry	405	6	89
Mango	540	5	118
Nutty Mocha Caramel, 2% Milk	560	18	94
Raspberry Zinger	385	5	85

BJ's Restaurant® (Oct '23)

Shareable Appetizers: Full Order	C	F	Cb
Ahi Poke	500	20	44
Chicken Pot Stickers	400	11	59
Crispy Calamari	670	26	62
Mozzarella Sticks	810	39	76
Root Beer Glazed Ribs	560	17	83
Sliders	840	30	81
Spinach & Artichoke Dip	1050	54	111
***Loaded Burgers:** With French Fries*			
Bacon Cheeseburger	1350	80	98
Bacon-Guacamole Deluxe	1420	85	102
Bistro	1350	76	105
Classic	1180	66	97
Crispy Jalapeno	1430	87	105
Hickory Brisket & Bacon	1620	90	124
Mushroom Swiss	1600	105	102
***Specialty Entrees:** Includes Menu Set Sides*			
Cauliflower & Quinoa Power Bowl	530	23	66
with Chicken	770	28	71
Cherry Chipotle Glazed Salmon	580	26	40
Lemon Thyme Chicken	630	19	52
Mediterranean Chicken Pita Tacos with Bistro Grains	690	22	81
New Orleans Jambalaya	1330	76	70
Spicy P'nut Chkn w/- Sobda Noodles	940	52	74
***Pasta:** Includes Garlic Knot*			
Deep Dish Ziti	1400	91	99
Grilled Chicken Alfredo	1610	85	133
Italiano Veggie Penne	780	34	94
Jumbo Spaghetti & Meatballs	1590	82	161
Shrimp Scampi	1650	99	130
***Deep Dish Pizza:** Per Large Slice*			
BBQ Chicken	340	10	42
Classic Combo; Pepp. Extreme, av.	375	18	38
Gourmet Five Meat	400	20	39
Sweet Pig; Vegetarian, average	295	10	40
***Tavern Crust Pizza:** Per Slice (1/12 Pizza)*			
Brewhouse; Italian Market, average	115	6	9
Garlic Chicken Pesto	100	5	9
Spicy Pig	90	4	9
***Sandwiches:** With French Fries*			
Brewhouse Philly	1460	86	110
California Chicken Club	1310	69	91
Classic Prime Rib Dip	1590	119	105
***Steaks & Slow Roasted Favorites:** Without Sides*			
Baby Back Pork Ribs, half rack, with Peppered BBQ Sce	710	34	74
Classic Rib-Eye	1080	67	5
Dble Bone In Pork Chop	610	38	13
Prime Rib Dinner	1290	103	6
Soups: Chicken Tortilla, Bowl	280	12	30
Clam Chowder: Bowl w/ Crackers	510	31	37
Sourdough Loaf with Crackers	1470	42	219

BJ's Restaurant® cont...(Oct '23)

Salads: With Dressing & Toppings	C	F	Cb
BBQ Chicken Chopped Salad	930	47	64
Caesar Salad	810	64	44
Honey-Crisp Chicken Salad	1360	103	75
Santa Fe	1040	61	58
Tri-Tip Wedge Salad	1300	91	68
Sides: Broccoli	40	0	6
Classic Baked Potato	590	28	70
French Fries	350	19	40
Honey Sriracha Brussels Sprouts	160	4	23
Rice Pilaf	230	6	39
Sweet Potato Fries	330	12	52
White Cheddar Mashed Potatoes	330	18	33
Desserts: Monkey Bread Pizookie	1380	67	182
Salted Caramel Pizookie	1380	56	204
Soda Floats, Black Cherry/Or. Crm	535	19	83

Blimpie® (Oct '23)

Subs:

Per Regular, 6" White Sub, with Standard Menu Board Toppings Unless Indicated

	C	F	Cb
Blimpie Best	455	15	53
BLTA	580	32	51
Club	430	14	54
Ham & Swiss	420	13	53
Italian Beef	540	21	49
Meatball Parmigiana	730	36	58
Philly Cheesesteak	560	24	50
Roast Beef & Provolone	440	13	53
Sicilian with Ciabatta	520	20	58
Spicy Italian	460	19	53
The Blimp	810	48	63
Tuna	470	21	48
Turkey Reuben with Ciabatta	520	21	58
Ulltimate Club with Ciabatta	570	27	58
Spicy Hawaiian Pizza Sub	520	18	55
Soup: Chicken Noodle	160	4	22
Cream of Broccoli with Cheese	210	14	12
Crm of Potato w/ Bacon	220	11	23
Tomato Basil	180	12	18
Vegetable Beef with Barley	200	7	30
Breakfast:			
Biscuits: Bacon, Egg & Cheese	420	22	37
Sausage, Egg & Cheese	560	36	37
Bluffin, Egg & Cheese	240	8	29
Burritos: Ham, Egg & Cheese	570	27	51
Sausage, Egg & Cheese	710	43	50
Croissant, Bacon, Egg & Cheese	380	21	30

Bob Evans® (Oct '23)

Burgers:	C	F	Cb
Big Farm Burgers:			
Bacon Cheeseburger	720	44	40
Cheeseburger	590	29	52
Rise & Shine	1200	70	98
Steakhouse	870	57	47
Sandwiches:			
All American BLT	680	35	64
Double Cheese Pot Roast Dip	1090	68	56
Farmhouse: Grilled Chicken	670	34	42
Homestyle Chicken	820	44	51
Dinners: *With Menu Set Side Dishes & Gravy/Sauce Unless Indicated*			
Comfort Food Classics:			
Chicken-N-Noodle Deep Dish	570	22	55
Fork-Tender Pot Roast	950	62	62
Slow Roasted Turkey & Dressing	820	45	84
Dinner Bell Plates:			
Down-Home Country Fried Steak	800	47	68
Grilled Chicken Breast	460	26	25
Hand Breaded Chicken Breast	670	35	49
Hickory Smoked Ham Steak	440	24	39
Farmhouse Kitchen Chicken: *Without Sides*			
Grilled to Perfection Chicken Breasts (2)	270	4	2
Hand Breaded Fried Chkn Breasts (2)	580	27	19
Homestyle Fried Chicken Strips (3)	640	36	46
Honey Butter Chkn, Biscuit & Butter	940	48	58
Sizzling Steak & Seafood: *Without Sides*			
Fried Shrimp & Cocktail Sauce	350	3	65
Great Alaskan Cod with Tartar Sauce	640	39	39
Lemon Pepper Sole Fillets (2)	380	18	25
Sirloin Steak w/ Gr. Onions & Mshrms	660	45	10
Sirloin Steak & Shrimp with C'tail Sce	710	36	39
Salads: *With Menu Set Dressing Unless Indicated*			
Cranberry Pecan Chicken	920	59	55
Farmhouse Garden Side Salad, without dressing	110	5	13
Grilled Chicken Cobb without Avocado	790	57	18
Wildfire: Grilled Chicken	670	30	62
Fried Chicken Tenders (2)	970	52	92

Bob Evans® cont... (Oct '23)

Lunch/Dinner Sides:	C	F	Cb
Bread & Celery Dressing	340	15	42
Broccoli, with Butter	110	10	5
Carrots	90	5	13
Dinner Rolls	380	17	50
French Fries	330	14	47
Fesh Cut Fruit	90	0	22
Green Beans with Ham	30	2	4
Hashbrowns	220	12	28
Homefries	250	17	24
Mac & Cheese	250	12	25
Mashed Potatoes w/ Chicken Gravy	210	14	19
Soups: *Per Bowl, w/ 4 Saltine Crackers*			
Cheddar Baked Potato	390	21	32
Chicken N Noodles	290	15	26
Hearty Beef Vegetable	230	5	36
Breakfast:			
Bowls & Skillets:			
Double Meat Protein Bowl	1020	78	36
Sunshine Skillet w/o Bread or Biscuit	660	17	107
Country Biscuit, w/o eggs or sides	520	36	29
Everything, with Hash Browns	1130	73	63
Sausage Gravy & Biscuits (2)	660	38	67
Western Omelet	650	50	11
Griddle & More: *With Set Toppings & Syrups*			
Brioche French Toast (2)	810	20	142
Hotcakes: Buttermilk (4)	1150	28	209
Double Blueberry (4)	1090	23	203
Double Chocolate (4)	1120	27	199
Breakfast Sides:			
Banana Nut Bread	260	8	30
Biscuits with Margarine (2)	520	31	53
Eggs: Egg White	60	0	1
Freshly Cracked	200	16	1
Scrambled	160	11	1
Homefries	250	17	24
Grits with butter, bowl	390	32	25
Hardwood Smoked Bacon (3)	190	14	1
Hashbrowns	200	12	28
Hickory-Smoked Ham	100	3	2
Sausage Links (3)	320	29	1
Sausage Patties (2)	320	26	2
Turkey Sausage Links (2)	140	7	2
Dessert: Choc. Peanut Butter Pie, 1 sl.	640	42	69
Double-Crust Apple Pie, 1 slice	600	28	82
Holy Ciow Chocolae Cake	610	29	86

Bojangles® (Oct '23)

Biscuit:	C	F	Cb
Bacon, Egg & Cheese	510	27	40
Cajun Filet	570	27	57
Country Ham & Egg	460	25	38
Gravy Biscuit	430	21	49
Sausage	470	28	38
Sausage & Egg	550	34	38
Southern Filet	550	27	54
Steak	620	40	48
Biscuit Add Ons: American Cheese	40	4	1
Egg	80	6	0
Chicken: Breast (1)	540	29	24
Leg (1)	190	13	8
Thigh (1)	240	10	14
Wing (1)	150	8	8
Homestyle Tenders, 4 pieces	490	24	39
Roasted Chicken Bites, 6.7 oz	350	14	9
Supremes, 4 pieces	500	25	33
Sandwiches: Bo's Chicken	670	36	95
Grilled Chicken	570	33	36
Grilled Chicken Club	690	39	39
Fixins': *Per Individual Size, Unless Indicated*			
Bo-Tato Rounds, medium	390	24	40
Cole Slaw	170	11	20
Green Beans	20	0	5
Macaroni & Cheese	280	18	21
Mashed Potatoes 'N Gravy	120	3	18
Seasoned Fries: Small	360	21	39
Medium	450	26	49
Picnic	670	38	73
Salads: *Without Dressing or Croutons*			
Chicken Supreme	490	28	28
Garden	120	9	3
Grilled Chicken	270	14	4
Dressings: Blue Cheese, 1.5 fl.oz	230	24	2
Buttermilk Ranch, 1.5 fl. oz	200	20	2
Honey Dijon, 1.5 fl.oz	120	7	14
Sweets: Bo-Berry Biscuit (1)	370	17	49
Cinnamon Twist (1)	380	24	38
Sweet Potato Pie	350	20	41

Boston Market® (Oct '23)

Sandwiches: *Per Whole Sandwich, with Standard Ingredients*	C	F	Cb
Chkn Avocado Club on Ciabatta Roll	1110	66	75
Chkn Salad Carver on Multigr. Roll	870	51	63
Rotiss. Chicken Carver on Ciab. Roll	980	53	73
Sthwest Chkn Carver on Ciabatta Roll	1110	65	76
Individual Meals: *Without Sides or Corn Bread*			
Meatloaf, regular	470	33	17
Parmesan Rotisserie Half Chicken	590	28	12
Roasted Garlic & Herb Half Chkn	650	35	13
Rotisserie Prime Rib, 8 oz	630	47	0
Sesame Half Chicken	630	30	18
Turkey Pot Pie	710	38	64

Boston Market® cont...(Oct '23)

Salad Bowls: *With Dressing*	C	F	Cb
Chicken Caesar	770	51	33
Southwest Cobb	760	53	30
Sides: Cornbread	160	3	31
Creamed Spinach	240	17	12
Fresh Steamed Veggies	60	4	7
Fresh Vegetable Stuffing	220	10	28
Garlic Dill New Potatoes	100	2	20
Macaroni & Cheese	310	10	41
Mashed Potatoes	270	11	37
Steamed Brocoli	35	0	6
Sweet Corn	160	7	20
Sweet Potato Casserole	460	12	87
Soup, Chicken Noodle	240	9	20
Kid's: *Without Sides or Corn Bread*			
Chicken: Dark, 1 thigh, 1 drumstick	230	13	1
White, 1 breast, 1 wing	270	11	0
Meatloaf	240	16	9
Turkey	80	3	0
Sauce: Cranberry Walnut Relish	140	2	31
Gravy, Beef/Au Jus/Chicken	10	0	2
Horseradish	60	3	6
Zesty BBQ	40	0	10
Desserts:			
Apple Pie, 1 slice	560	32	66
Chocolate Brownie (1)	340	14	53
Chocolate Cake, 1 slice	570	33	66
Chocolate Chunk Cookie (1)	370	18	53

For Complete Nutritional Data ~ see CalorieKing.com

Boston Pizza® (Oct '23)

Starters: *Without Sauce*	C	F	Cb
Classic Nachos, half size	1050	59	81
Classic Poutine	590	28	68
Garlic Fingers	800	30	112
Spinach & Artichoke Dip	1260	58	137
Burgers: *Without Sides*			
Boston Brute	800	24	108
Boston-Sized	1040	77	49
Plant Based, Vegan	710	44	59
Gourmet Pasta: *Per Full Order*			
Creamy Mushroom & Spinach Bake	1410	75	145
Jambalaya Fettuccini	1370	61	144
Parmesan Shrimp Alfredo	1180	45	146
The Hungry Carnivore	1450	79	126
Mains: *As Served, Without Extra Side Choice*			
Chicken Parmesan	980	31	128
NY Strip Loin Steak	1040	67	76
Slow Roasted Pork Back Ribs, half	670	44	36

Boston Pizza® (Oct '23)

Pizzas: Per Medium Slice	C	F	Cb
Boston Royal	220	8	26
Bourbon BBQ Chicken	260	11	27
Deluxe	200	6	25
Vegetarian	170	5	26
Sandwiches: *Without Sides*			
Grilled Chicken Clubhouse	1040	44	98
Honey Dill Fried Chicken	760	37	74
Kick'n Memphis Chicken	1210	75	86
Montreal Smoked Meat	910	59	40
N Y Steak	560	38	35
Salads: *Entree Size with Dressing*			
Chicken Caesar	680	49	13
Crispy Chicken Pecan	950	72	50
Desssert:			
Chocolate Brownie Addiction	1000	47	133
NY Cheesecake	580	37	54

Braum's® ~ *see CalorieKing.com*

Bruegger's® (Oct '23)

Bagels:	C	F	Cb
Blueberry, 4.1 oz	310	1	65
Cinnamon Sugar, 4.9 oz	380	2	83
Everything, 4.4 oz	330	3	64
Five Cheese, 4.4 oz	360	10	51
Onion, 4.2 oz	310	1	63
Plain, 4.1 oz	290	1	59
Rosemary Olive Oil, 4.1 oz	340	5	63
Sesame, 4.5 oz	380	9	61
Cream Cheese: *Per 1.5 oz*			
Bacon Scallion; Jalapeno, av.	140	12	5
Light Herb Garlic/Plain	100	6	4
Plain; Jalapeno, av.	135	12	5
Smoked Salmon; Strawberry	135	12	4
Breakfast Bagel S'wiches: *With Standard Toppings*			
Egg, Cheese & Bacon	530	19	62
Egg, Cheese & Ham	470	13	62
Egg, Cheese & Turkey Sausage	510	17	61
Egg, Cheese & Pork Sausage	610	28	60
Deli Sandwiches: *Plain Bagel With Standard Toppings*			
BLT	540	23	64
Garden Veggie	360	2	72
Ham	400	7	65
Turkey	440	7	67
Signature & Bagel Sandwiches: *W/ Standard Toppings*			
Herby Turkey on Sesame Bagel	570	15	75
Hot Pastrami on Everything Bagel	580	18	65
Leon. da Veggie on Asiago Parm. Bagel	520	16	67
Turkey Chipotle Club on Evrythng Bagel	710	32	74
Western Brisket on Five Cheese	840	52	57

Bruegger's® cont... (Oct '23)

Salads: Without Dressing	C	F	Cb
Blue Apple	360	18	30
Chicken Caesar	200	8	14
Dressings: Balsamic Vinaigrette, 1 oz	60	6	3
Caesar, 1 oz	80	7	2
Champagne Vinaigrette, 1 oz	130	14	1
Ranch, 1 oz	90	10	1
Sides, Twice Baked Hashbrowns	170	11	11
Soup, Chicken & Wild Rice, 8 oz	270	20	11
Dessert, Blueberry Muffin, Main St.	490	28	54

For Complete Menu & Data ~ see CalorieKing.com

Burgerville® (Oct '23)

Burgers: With Standard Ingredients	C	F	Cb
Bacon Chseburger on Non Seeded Bun	640	38	37
Colossal on Non Seeded Bun	540	28	40
½ lb Colossal On Non Seeded Bun	790	46	40
Double Cheeseburger on Plain Bun	520	29	32
Original: Cheeseburger on Plain Bun	400	21	32
Hamburger on Plain Bun	350	17	32
Northwest Cheeseburger on Non Seeded Bun	590	33	38
Number 6 ½lb Burger on Brioche Bun	770	46	30
Chicken & Chips, without sauce	780	43	78
Halibut Fish & Chips, w/out sauce	700	33	80
Sandwiches: *On Brioche Bun, Without Cheese*			
Best Coast: Crispy Chicken	580	33	54
Grilled Chicken	410	17	29
Blazin' Hot Pepper: Crispy Chicken	620	35	55
Grilled Chicken	440	19	31
Sides: *Without Sauce*			
Classic Fries: Small, 2.8 oz	260	12	35
Regular, 5 oz	410	19	57
Large, 6.5 oz	510	24	70
Fried Asparagus	270	15	32
Fried Pickle Chips	480	32	43
Farm Salad: *Without Dressing*			
with Blue Cheese Crumblies	120	8	3
with Grilled Chicken Breast	100	2	4
with Smoked Salmon	90	3	3
Dressing, Ranch	190	20	2
Bliss Shakes (Non Dairy): *Per 16 oz w/out Wh. Cream*			
Chocolate	840	31	143
Chocolate Hazelnut	1040	57	130
Fresh Strawberry	880	38	132
Vanilla	970	37	156
Add Coconut Whipped Cream	90	4	12
Ice Cream Milkshakes: *Per 16 oz with Whipped Cream*			
Chocolate Hazelnut	1080	72	98
Portland Cold Brew	910	55	89
Vanilla	770	42	90

Burger King® (Oct '23)

Flame Grilled Burgers:	C	F	Cb
Bacon Cheeseburger	340	16	31
Double	440	24	32
Bacon King	1200	81	58
Big King	490	30	34
Cheeseburger	290	13	31
Double	400	21	32
Hamburger	250	10	29
Impossible King	550	22	57
Rodeo	340	13	41
Single Quarter Pound King	590	29	50
Whopper Burgers:			
Double Whopper	920	60	54
Impossible Whopper	630	34	62
Texas Double Whopper	1090	75	57
Triple with Cheese	1300	90	59
Whopper	670	41	54
Whopper with Bacon	750	49	55
Chicken Sandwiches:			
BK Royal Crispy:			
Bacon & Swiss	740	45	56
Crispy Chicken	600	33	54
Spicy Crispy Chicken	760	49	58
Chicken Jr.	440	27	39
Original Chicken	680	39	63
Chicken Nuggets: *Without Sauce*			
4 pieces	190	12	12
8 pieces	390	25	23
Dipping Sauces: BBQ	40	0	11
Buffalo	80	8	2
Ranch; Zesty Onion Ring, av.	145	15	2
Fish Sandwich,			
Big Fish	570	30	58
Platters: Pancake	235	7	42
with Sausage	415	23	42
Sides:			
Chicken Fries, 9 pieces	260	13	20
Classic Fries: Small	300	13	43
Medium	370	16	54
Mozzarella Sticks: 4 pieces	330	14	37
8pieces	660	29	73
Onion Rings: Medium	360	16	48
Large	520	24	70

Burger King® cont.. (Oct '23)

Breakfast:	C	F	Cb
Biscuits:			
Bacon, Egg & Cheese	450	30	33
Bacon, Sausage, Egg & Cheese	715	53	35
Egg & Cheese	410	27	33
Ham, Egg & Cheese	450	27	34
Sausage	430	30	30
Sausage, Egg & Cheese	590	43	33
Double	855	66	34
Burrito, Egg-Normous	830	46	69
Croissan'wich:			
Bacon, Egg & Cheese	410	25	31
Bacon, Sausage, Egg & Cheese	675	48	33
Egg & Cheese	370	22	31
Fully Loaded	715	49	34
Ham, Egg & Cheese	410	23	32
Sausage, Egg & Cheese	550	38	31
Double	885	66	33
Sides:			
French Toast Sticks with syrup:			
3 pieces	350	12	57
5 pieces	520	20	79
Hash Browns, small, 3 oz	290	19	29
Desserts:			
Chocolate Chip Cookies (2)	160	8	23
Hershey's Sundae Pie	310	18	32
Vanilla Soft Serve:			
Cone	200	5	33
Cup	180	5	28
Shakes:			
Chocolate	590	14	103
Chocolate Oreo	670	17	116
Classic Oreo	640	17	109
Strawberry	610	14	110
Vanilla	560	14	96
Beverages:			
Iced Coffee, Plain, medium	200	10	27
Fat Free Milk, glass	90	0	13
Simply Orange Juice, bottle	160	0	37
Sweetened Ice Tea, med., 29 fl.oz	160	0	49

Captain D's Seafood® (Oct '23)

From The Grill: *Without Sides, Rice, Hushpuppies or Breadstick*	C	F	Cb
Blackened Tilapia	210	7	2
Lemon Pepper White Fish Fillet	180	8	1
Shrimp Skewers (2)	210	6	3
White Fish & Shrimp Skewer	290	11	4
Wild Alaska Salmon	240	10	3
Variety Meals: *W/out Sides Or Hush Puppies*			
Butterfly Shrimp (15)	900	64	58
Deluxe Seafood Platter	1100	75	67
Fish & Shrimp	810	56	45
Supreme Sampler	1180	79	68
White Fish, Shrimp & Crab	940	64	52
Salads: *Without Dressing or Breadstick*			
Grilled Tilapia	320	13	10
Southern Style Breaded Chicken	470	28	32
Whats New: *W/o Sides, Rice, Hushpuppies or Breadstick*			
Cajun Catfish, 1 piece	510	37	20
Cajun Catfish & Shrimp Meal	750	54	35
Fried Oysters, 6 pieces	240	17	16
Seafood Gumbo, regular	190	7	21
Add-Ons: *Per Item/Serving*			
Baked Potato, plain, (1)	210	0	48
Loaded	400	15	49
Coleslaw	180	13	15
French Fries	330	22	28
Hush Puppy	80	4	9
Jalapeno Poppers	510	36	40
Mac & Cheese	170	8	18
Okra	320	20	31
Dessert, Cheesecake, no toppings	410	27	36

Caribou Coffee® (Oct '23)

Bakery:	C	F	Cb
Blueberry Muffin	410	22	52
Cinnamon Coffee Cake	530	23	81
Breakfast Sandwiches:			
Bacon, Egg & Cheese Bagel	610	28	60
Chicken Apple Sausage	440	21	38
Ham, Egg & Swiss Croissant	500	29	36
Lumberjack	740	36	67
Maple Waffle	480	26	42
Hot Beverages: *Per Medium*			
Berry White Mocha	600	32	66
Cappuccino	110	5	10
Chai Tea Latte	310	7	48
Chocolate	610	37	52
Crafted Press Coffee	170	9	15
Smoothie, Strawb. Ban. Yogurt, med.	360	0	85

For Complete Menu ~ See Calorieking.com

Carl's Jr.® (Oct '23)

California menu only. Please check instore for further nutritional information.	C	F	Cb
Charbroiled Burgers:			
Beyond Famous Star with Cheese	770	44	61
California Classic, Dble Cheeseburger	590	41	40
Guacamole Bacon Angus	970	65	55
Jalapeno: Angus	830	54	53
Double Cheeseburger	980	64	56
Original Angus	780	48	56
Super Star with Cheese	930	57	56
The Big Carl	930	58	56
Western Bacon Cheeseburger	780	36	77
Chicken Sandwiches:			
Charbroiled: BBQ Chicken	400	5	57
Chicken Club	650	30	53
Santa Fe Chicken	670	35	52
Hand Breaded: Bacon Swiss	780	42	61
Chicken	650	32	59
Chicken Stars: 6 pieces	270	15	19
9 pieces	410	23	29
Chicken Tenders, Hand Breaded:			
3 pieces, without sauce	260	13	13
5 pieces, without sauce	440	21	21
Breakfast:			
Biscuits: Bacon, Egg & Cheese	520	29	43
Monster Biscuit	830	56	47
Sausage, Egg & Cheese	640	42	44
Burger, Single	810	41	69
Burritos: Bacon, Egg & Cheese	620	35	37
Loaded Breakfast	650	36	50
Steak & Egg Burrito	530	26	41
Grilled Sandwiches: Bacon & Cheese	540	29	43
Ham & Cheese	490	24	43
Hash Rounds: Small	260	16	23
Medium	320	19	28
Large	450	27	40
Sides:			
Fried Zucchini, 5 oz	330	20	34
Jalapeno Poppers: 6 pieces	470	30	42
9 pieces	750	51	64
Natural Cut Fries: Small	300	15	39
Medium	420	21	55
Large	470	23	61
Onion Rings, 4.5 oz	560	30	66
Waffle Fries, 4.23 oz	380	25	36
Dessert: Choc. Chip Cookie	170	9	22
Chocolate Cake	290	11	46
Cinnamon Roll	520	16	89
Strawberry Swirl Cheesecake	320	17	35
Shakes: *With Ice Cream*			
Chocolate; Strawberry	690	35	85
Oreo Cookie	730	40	81
Vanilla	740	36	87

Carvel® (Oct '23)

Carvelanche:	C	F	Cb
M&M'S: Small, 12 oz	650	32	73
Regular, 16 oz	850	43	97
Large, 24 oz	1320	66	152
Classic Sundaes: *Per Small, 12 oz*			
Hot Caramel	620	27	79
Hot Fudge	620	32	72
Strawberry	530	26	61
Sundae Dashers: *Per Regular, 16 oz*			
Banana's Foster	1050	33	171
Fudge Brownie	1250	62	166
Mint Chocolate Chip	1080	56	144
Peanut Butter Cup	1850	110	174
Strawberry Shortcake	880	37	125
Ice Cream Scoops: *Per Medium*			
Butter Pecan	750	51	57
Chocolate	520	27	59
Mint Chcolate Chip	670	35	78
Peanut Butter Treasure	680	41	73
Thick Shakes: *Per 16 oz*			
Chocolate; Vanilla, av.	650	27	90
Coffee	720	27	58
Strawberry	590	27	73

Charley's Philly Steaks® (Oct '23)

Philly Cheessesteaks: *Per Regular with Toppings*	C	F	Cb
Bacon 3 Cheesesteak	850	43	58
Bacon Chipotle	830	41	56
Chicken Buffalo/Teriyaki, av.	735	30	62
Chicken California	800	40	56
Philly Cheesesteak	780	38	58
Chicken Wings: *Per Piece Without Sauce or Rubs*			
Boneless: Buffalo	110	7	7
Garlic Parmesan	160	12	8
Plain; Lemon Pepper	110	7	6
Sweet Teriyaki	140	7	13
Thai Chili	150	7	16
Classic: Plain	120	9	0
Bold BBQ/Thai Chili, average	160	9	9
Buffalo/Cajun Rub, average	130	9	1
Garlic Parmesan	180	14	1
Sweet Teriyaki	150	9	7
Fries: Original, regular	400	22	46
Gourmet: Cheese	550	30	62
Cheese & Bacon	680	41	63
Ultimate	790	54	61
Sides:			
Celery Sticks with Ranch Dip	210	21	3
Mozzarella Sticks	320	18	25
Breakfast: Bacon, Egg & Chse S'wich	490	26	36
Steak, Egg & Cheese Sandwich	520	25	36
Hashbrowns	280	18	27

For Complete Menu & Data ~ see CalorieKing.com

Cheesecake Factory® (Oct '23)

Cheesecake: *Per Slice*	C	F	Cb
Original	830	59	63
Godiva Chocolate	1400	105	110
Reese's P.B. Chocolate Cake	1510	95	154
White Chocolate Raspberry Truffle	1220	89	92
Appetizers: Avocado Eggrolls	930	48	111
Buffalo Blasts	1670	93	129
Chicken Pot Stickers	380	12	38
Fried Macaroni & Cheese	1310	96	70
Thai Lettuce Wraps w/ Satay. Chkn	850	27	105
Spicy Ahi Tempura Roll	770	51	45
Small Plates: Beets & Avoc. Salad	290	12	40
Chicken Taquitos	390	22	31
Crispy Fried Cheese	1080	75	50
Korean Fried Caulifl.	1150	71	113
Stuffed Mushrooms	510	42	19
Flatbread Pizza: Cheese	1000	50	86
Margherita	760	30	85
Pepperoni	1110	61	87
The Everything	1160	63	92
Glamburgers: *Without Sides*			
Americana Cheeseburger	1400	91	81
Bacon-Bacon Cheeseburger	1680	116	77
Classic Burger	1280	83	69
Impossible Burger	930	53	80
Macaroni & Cheese	1340	85	81
Mushroom	1460	100	73
Veggie	1340	83	124
Glamburger Sides: French Fries	530	23	76
Green Salad	130	12	5
Sweet Potato Fries	510	20	78
Fish & Seafood:			
Fish & Chips	1860	121	134
Shrimp Scampi	1260	76	105
Seared Ahi Tuna	990	38	121
Sandwiches: Chicken Parmesan	1960	125	99
Club	1290	68	112
Cuban	1200	73	64
Specialties: Baja Chicken Tacos	1230	50	125
Chicken Bellagio	2020	116	144
Chicken "Littles"	1990	106	160
Chicken Madeira	1300	73	72
Crispy Chicken Costoletta	1800	120	104
Factory Burrito Grande	1970	106	161
Grilled Fish Tacos	1040	42	121
Grilled Steak Tacos	1140	54	127
Spicy Cashew Chicken	1820	53	244
Thai Coconut-Lime Chicken	1960	118	156
Sides: Broccoli	260	18	15
French Fries	1060	46	152
Green Beans	140	10	10
Mac & Cheese	1550	109	92
Mashed Potatoes	450	25	49
Sauteed Spinach	650	67	10
Steamed White Rice	440	2	98
Sweet Potato Fries	1010	52	125

Chick-fil-A® (Oct '23)

Breakfast:	C	F	Cb
Biscuits: Bacon, Egg & Cheese	420	23	38
Chicken	460	23	45
Chicken, Egg & Cheese	550	28	48
Egg White Chicken Grill	300	8	31
Sausage, Egg & Cheese	620	42	38
Bowl, Hash Brown Scramble	470	30	19
Burrito, Hash Brown Scramble	700	40	51
Chick-n-Minis, 4 pieces	360	13	41
Hash Browns, 2.7 oz	270	18	23
Parfait, Greek Yogurt, fruit topping	270	9	36
Sandwiches: *Without Sauce*			
Chick-fil-A: Chicken	420	18	41
Deluxe	490	22	43
Grilled Chicken	390	12	44
Grilled Chicken Club	520	22	45
Spicy Deluxe	520	25	46
Chick-n-Strips, 3 count	310	14	16
Grilled Nuggets: 5 count	80	2	1
8 Count	130	3	1
Salads:			
Cobb: *With Avocado Lime Dressing*			
with Chick-n Strips	910	63	40
with Grilled Filet (warm)	700	51	25
Market: *With Zesty Apple Cider Vinaigrette*			
with Nuggets	690	40	51
without Chicken	440	29	40
Spicy Southwest: *With Creamy Salsa Dressing*			
with Grilled Nuggets	720	50	29
with Spicy Grilled Filet (cold)	690	49	29
Sauces: BBQ	45	0	11
Chick-fil-A	140	13	6
Honey Mustard Sauce	50	0	11
Sweet & Spicy Sriracha Sauce	45	0	11
Sides:			
Fruit Cup, medium	60	0	15
Chicken Noodle Soup, cup	170	4	25
Side Salad, w/ Avocado Lime Dressing and toppings	470	42	16
Mac & Cheese: Small	270	17	17
Medium	450	29	28
Waffle Potato Chips	220	13	25
Dessert:			
Chocolate Chunk Cookie	370	17	49
Chocolate Fudge Brownie	380	21	48
Milkshakes: *With Whipped Cream & Cherry*			
Chocolate, 14 oz	590	22	90
Cookies & Cream, 14.5 oz	630	26	90
Strawberry, 14.53 oz	570	19	93
Vanilla, 14.4 oz	580	23	82

Chili's® (Oct '23)

Starters: *As Served*	C	F	Cb
Bone In Wings:			
Bufffalo	890	65	3
House BBQ	860	55	18
Boneless Wings, Honey Chipotle	1190	57	125
Classic Chicken Nachos	1320	82	56
Fried Mozzarella	920	55	59
Quesadilla Bacon Ranch Chicken	1670	125	69
Quesadilla Brisket	1670	129	76
Southwestern Eggrolls	800	41	82
TX Cheese Fries, full order	1800	122	99
Baby Back Ribs: *Full Rack, without Sides*			
Dry Rub	1480	107	30
Honey Chipotle BBQ	1520	106	47
House BBQ	1440	107	21
Big Mouth Burgers: *Without Side Fries*			
Bacon Rancher	1710	123	48
Just Bacon	1020	69	47
Oldtimer with Cheese	850	53	46
Crispers,			
Honey Chipotle Crispy (4), w/o sides	1060	51	108
Guiltless Grill: *As Served*			
Ancho Salmon	630	32	41
Margarita Grilled Chkn	630	13	68
Sirloin (10 oz) with Grilled Avocado	510	26	13
Pasta, Ultimate Cajun Pasta	1310	62	109
Sandwiches: *Without Fries*			
Bacon Avocado Chicken	1150	62	74
Big Mouth Crispiest Chicken	1040	56	90
Buffalo Chicken Ranch	980	51	84
Sizzling Fajitas: *Without Toppings*			
Grilled: Chicken	1120	34	127
Steak	1220	44	130
Shrimp	950	30	126
Steaks: *Without Sides*			
Classic Ribeye	620	39	0
Classic Sirloin: 6 oz	250	12	1
10 oz	390	18	2
Sides: Asparagus	35	1	5
Black Beans	120	1	20
Coleslaw	230	20	13
Homestyle Fries	420	17	60
Loaded Mashed Potatoes	350	20	33
Roasted Street Corn	390	28	30
Steamed Broccoli	40	0	8
Sweet Corn on the Cob	180	6	29
Salads: *As Served*			
Quesadilla Explosion with Gr. Chkn	1170	78	68
Santa Fe Chicken with Crispers	910	60	44
Sweet Stuff:			
Cheesecake, slice	720	43	73
Molten Chocolate Cake	1170	59	155

Chipotle® (Oct '23)

Tortillas:	C	F	Cb
Burrito Size Flour Tortillas (1)	320	9	50
Tacos: Crispy Corn Tortilla	70	2	10
Soft Flour Tortilla	80	3	13
Meal Components:			
Barbacoa, 4 oz	170	7	2
Black/Pinto Beans, average, 4 oz	130	2	22
Cilantro Lime: Brown Rice, 4 oz	210	6	36
White Rice, 4 oz	210	4	40
Carnitas, 4 oz	210	12	0
Chicken, 4 oz	180	7	0
Fajita Vegetables, 2.5 oz	20	0	5
Guacamole, 3.5 oz	230	22	8
Monterey Jack, 1 oz	110	8	1
Romaine Lettuce	5	0	1
Sofritas, 4 oz	150	10	9
Steak, 4 oz	150	6	1
Condiments:			
Queso Blanco, 2 oz	120	9	4
Salsa: Chili Corn, 3.5 oz	80	2	16
Fresh Tomato	25	0	4
Green Tomatillo, 2 oz	15	0	4
Red Tomatillo, 2 oz	30	0	4
Sour Cream, 2 oz	110	9	2
Extras, Chips, 4 oz	540	25	73

Chuck E. Cheese® (Oct '23)

Appetizers & Sides:	C	F	Cb
Carrots, 4 oz	45	0	11
Cheesy Breadsticks	140	6	15
French Fries, 8 oz	420	13	67
Macaroni Salad, 4 oz	240	14	21
Mandarin Oranges, 4 oz	60	0	18
Rotini Pasta Salad, 4 oz	140	7	15
Specialty Pizzas: *Per Slice, 1⁄10 Medium Pizza*			
5 Meat	210	10	18
Supreme	190	9	19
Veggie	160	6	19
Traditional Wings: *Per 12 oz Wings with 2 oz Sauce*			
Small: With BBQ or Sweet Chili Sce	680	34	44
With Buffalo Sauce	600	37	16
Dessert: Chocolate Cake, 8", 1⁄12th	210	8	31
Giant Warm Cookie, 1⁄8th	200	9	28
Unicorn Churros (5)	485	25	62
Ice Cream: Big Bopper Sandwich	450	20	64
Brownie Batter Dip N Dots, large	320	15	40
Cookie N Cream Bar	230	11	32
Red, White & Blue Bomb Pop	80	0	21
Strawberry Shortcake Bar	190	9	26

Church's Chicken® (Oct '23)

Burgers & Sandwiches:	C	F	Cb
Cheeseburger	590	40	28
Cob Sandwich	810	55	50
Original Chicken Sandwich	650	35	53
Chicken: *Per Piece*			
Original: Breast, 1 piece	250	14	9
Leg, 1 piece	150	8	6
Thigh, 1 piece	360	27	12
Wing, 1 piece	290	18	8
Spicy: Breast, 1 piece	280	17	12
Leg, 1 piece	160	9	9
Thigh, 1 piece	380	25	21
Wing, 1 piece	350	20	19
Sides: *Per Regular Serving*			
Baked Macaroni & Cheese, 4.7 oz	210	12	19
Cole Slaw, 4.2 oz	170	11	16
French Fries, 2.6 oz	210	9	29
Honey Butter Biscuit, 2.2 oz	230	15	25
Jalapeno Cheese Bombers (4)	220	11	24
Mashed Potatoes & Gravy, 4.5 oz	110	1	24
Okra, 3.4 oz	260	15	30
Sauces: Honey BBQ, pkt	45	0	11
Creamy Jalapeno, pkt	120	13	2
Honey Mustard/Ranch, av., pkt	140	14	3
Dessert, Apple Pie	270	13	37

Cici's Pizza® (Oct '23)

Pizza:	C	F	Cb
Regular Crust: *Per Slice, 1⁄10 of Large 14" Pizza*			
Alfredo; Spinach Alfredo, average	170	5	26
Pepperoni	200	7	26
Flatbread: Chicken Bacon Club	120	8	6
Pepperoni	100	6	6
Spinach Alfredo	70	4	6
Stuffed Crust, Cheese	270	10	32
Bone In Wings: BBQ (1)	85	6	2
Garlic Parmesan (1)	130	11	1
Mild Buffalo (1)	105	9	1
Sides: Chicken Noodle Soup, 8 fl.oz	135	3	16
Garlic Cheesy Bread, 1slice	205	10	24
Pasta	255	4	48
Dessert: Brownie, 1 square	140	6	21
Apple/Barvarian Pizza, 1 slice	165	3	30

Cinnabon® (Oct '23)

	C	F	Cb
Cinnabon Classic Roll (1)	880	37	129
MiniBon Roll (1)	350	15	52
Cheese Roll Paninis: Grilled Cheese	480	24	46
Black Forest Ham	540	25	48
Smoked Turkey Club	530	24	49
Chillata: *Per 16 fl.oz*			
Chocolate Mocha	380	13	61
Oreo Cookies & Cream	710	27	109
Strawberries & Cream	530	18	86

Claim Jumper® (Oct '23)

Appetizers: As Served	C	F	Cb
Beef Sliders with Cheese	740	35	67
Chips & Salsa	540	10	90
Spinach & Artichoke Dip, share	1735	64	233
Burgers: *Without Sides*			
Bacon & Mac	950	48	89
Classic Hamburger	750	40	60
Impossible Burger	1230	75	91
Widow Maker Burger	1565	89	126
Meals: *As Per Menu Description*			
Classics: After The Gold Rush	890	47	47
Country Fried Steak	1175	50	116
Fish & Chips	1115	37	148
Meatloaf & Mashed Potatoes	1180	73	83
Combo Plates: Steak & Shrimp	770	52	17
Tri-Tip Prospector	765	42	9
Pasta: Black Tie Chkn	1895	97	161
Shrimp Fresca	2005	143	110
Seafood: Blackened Salmon	405	26	3
Coconut Shrimp	1305	36	202
Grilled Shrimp	550	22	53
Wood Fired Pizza, Classic Crust: *Per Whole Pizza*			
BBQ Chicken, 8 slices	1960	80	230
Sausage & Pepperoni, 8 slices	2010	100	190
Sides: Baked Potato with Butter	635	27	82
Brussels Sprouts	190	14	11
Charbroiled Asparagus	235	19	7
Chili French Fries	580	35	44
Loaded French Fries	550	35	39
Mac & Cheese	460	25	40
Mashed Potatoes	270	16	28
Roasted Veggies	55	3	6
Sweets: Chocolate Motherlode Cake	3415	158	459
Raspberry Cream Cheese Pie	1570	97	147

Cold Stone Creamery® (Oct '23)

Ice Cream:	C	F	Cb
Amaretto: Like it	340	21	36
Love it	550	33	57
Gotta Have it	820	49	85
Caramel Chocolate Cheeecake:			
Like It	340	19	39
Love It	550	31	63
Gotta Have It	820	46	94
Cheesecake: Like It	340	19	40
Love It	540	31	63
Gotta Have It	810	47	95
Chocolate: Like it	330	20	34
Love it	520	31	54
Gotta have it	780	47	81

Cold Stone Creamery® cont...(Oct '23)

Sorbet:	C	F	Cb
Strawberry Mango Banana:			
Like it, 5 oz	210	0	54
Love it, 8 oz	340	0	87
Gotta have it, 12 oz	510	0	130
Shakes: *Per 20 oz With Whipped Topping*			
Cake Batter 'n Shake	1440	76	176
Oh Fudge; Very Vanilla, average	1320	76	149
Savory Strawberry	1200	71	133
Signature Creations:			
Berry Berry Berry Good: Like It	380	21	47
Love It	580	33	69
Gotta Have It	850	31	97
Coffee Lovers: Like It	480	29	50
Love It	790	48	85
Gotta Have It	1060	34	114
Cookies Make Everything Batter:			
Like It	520	28	65
Love It	840	44	108
Gotta Have It	1130	59	143
Sundaes: Banana Split Decision	650	37	77
Who You Callin' Shortcake	560	31	68

Cousins Subs® (Oct '23)

Subs: *Per 7.5", Standard Toppings*	C	F	Cb
Grilled To Order:			
Chkn Bacon Cheddar	580	21	50
Chicken Cheese Steak	530	16	50
Double Steak Cheese Steak	790	28	52
Classics:			
Club, with Mayo	670	32	54
Italian Special, with Oil	830	51	51
Tuna with Mayo	650	36	51
Deli Fresh:			
Ham & Provolone, with Mayo	630	32	52
Roast Beef & Cheddar, with Mayo	740	37	52
Turkey Breast with Mayo	550	25	53
Cheese Curds: Regular, 5 oz	680	56	13
Large, 10 oz	1380	113	26
French Fries:			
Regular, 4.5 oz	240	12	29
Large, 9 oz	470	24	57
Soup: *Per Cup*			
Broccoli Cheese	150	9	12
Chicken Noodle	100	2	15
Chicken & Wild Rice	160	9	17

For Complete Nutritional Data ~ see CalorieKing.com

Culver's® (Oct '23)

ButterBurgers:	C	F	Cb
Original: Single	390	17	38
Double	560	30	38
Triple	730	43	38
Bacon Deluxe: Single	610	38	40
Double	850	56	41
Triple	1090	76	42
Cheese: Single	460	23	39
Double	700	42	40
Culver's Deluxe: Single	570	34	41
Double	810	53	42
Triple	1050	72	43
Mushroom & Swiss, Single	530	28	41
Sourdough Melt, Single	490	25	42
Wisconsin Swiss Melt, Single	470	24	39
Homestyle Favorites:			
Beef Pot Roast Dinner	490	16	46
Beef Pot Roast Sandwich	410	13	40
Chopped Steak Dinner	600	36	32
Grilled Reuben Melt	660	38	43
Pork Loin Sandwich	630	25	72
Sides:			
Classic: Coleslaw, medium	200	16	15
Mshd Pot. & Gravy, med.	130	1	25
Steamed Broccoli	40	0	7
Premium, Onion Rings, medium	400	22	44
Signature: Chili Cheddar Fries	690	32	80
George's Chili	300	13	26
Fries, Crinkle Cut, medium	360	14	53
Seafood Dinner: *With Dinner Role, Butter & Menu Set Sauce*			
Butterfly Jumbo Shrimp, 6 pieces	380	18	42
North Atlantic Cod, Fried, 2 pieces	920	68	42
Soup: Broccoli Cheese	220	12	17
Chicken Noodle	100	2	15
Potato with Bacon	240	10	28
Salads: *Without Dressing*			
Chicken Cashew with Gilled Chicken	450	24	13
Cranberry Bacon Bleu, with Grilled Chicken	360	14	14
Garden Fresco with Grilled Chicken	350	14	15
Strawberry Fields with Gr. Chicken	390	22	9
Dressings: Bleu Cheese	200	21	2
Buttermilk Ranch	180	19	2
Country French	190	15	13
Honey Mustard	130	6	20
Raspberry Vinaigrette	50	0	12
Kid's Meals:			
Corn Dog	240	14	23
Grilled Cheese Sourdough Sandwich	360	17	39
Original Chicken Tenders, 2 pieces	270	12	21

Culver's® cont... (Oct '23)

Concrete Mixers: *No Toppings*	C	F	Cb
Chocolate & PB Cups, med.	980	51	116
Vanilla, with Oreo, medium	950	53	105
Sundaes: *Per 2 Scoops*			
Banana Split	1080	61	119
Caramel Cashew	1000	52	121
Turtle	1040	61	111
Shakes: Chocolate, medium	850	38	114
Mint, medium	840	38	114
Peanut Butter, medium	1040	74	78
Strawberry, medium	700	38	78

D'Angelo® (Oct '23)

Deli Sandwiches: *Per Medium*	C	F	Cb
Italian Sub Bread	350	4	65
Add Chicken Salad	700	62	3
Add Ham & Cheese	300	24	3
Add Tuna Salad	640	64	3
Wraps: *Per Medium*			
Tortilla Wrap Only	250	6	42
Add Buffalo Chicken	490	40	13
Add Chicken Caesar	500	38	14
Add Greek	390	31	17
Fresh Salads: *With Dressing, without Pokket*			
Entree: Caesar	490	39	24
Greek	520	45	19
Grilled Topped:			
Chicken Cobb	810	59	25
Steak Cobb	880	65	25
Steak Greek	840	68	20
Soup: *Per Bowl*			
Beef Stew	330	12	34
Broccoli & Cheddar	370	28	18
Main Lobster Bisque	540	43	24
New England Clam Chowder	480	27	46

For Complete Menu & Data ~ see CalorieKing.com

Dairy Queen® (Oct '23)

Signature Stackburgers:	C	F	Cb
Backyard Bacon Ranch, double	820	51	53
Bacon Two Cheese Deluxe, double	720	47	39
FlameThrower, double	720	49	37
Loaded A.1. Steakhouse Double	820	51	52
Original Cheeseburger, single	370	18	37
Chicken Strips:			
3 Pieces	430	20	41
Basket: 4 Pieces	1020	48	111
6 Pieces	1300	61	139
Sandwiches:			
Crispy Chicken	550	26	62
Spicy Chicken	530	23	63

Dairy Queen® cont... (Oct '23)

Hot Dogs:	C	F	Cb
Bacon Cheese	420	26	27
Cheese Dog	390	24	27
Chili Dog	360	22	27
Chili Cheese Dog	420	26	28
Classic Hot Dog	330	19	25
Salads: *Without Dressing*			
Crispy Chicken Strips Bowl	430	22	35
Rotisserie Style Chicken Bites Bowl	310	15	8
Dressing:			
Fat Free Italian	25	0	4
Honey Mustard	130	9	12
Light Italian	15	1	2
French Fries: Regular	280	13	36
Large	450	21	59
Sides:			
Cheese Curds: Regular	500	34	26
Large	1000	67	52
Onion Ring: Regular	290	13	39
Large	450	20	60
Pretzel Sticks with Zesty Queso	330	9	52
Desserts: *Per Medium*			
Blizzard Treats:			
Choco Brownie Xtreme	810	36	111
Choc. Chip Cookie Dough	1030	41	151
M&M's	800	27	124
Oreo Cookie	790	31	117
Reese's P'nut Butter Cup	750	31	102
Turtle Pecan Cluster	1020	52	123
Curl On Top Treats:			
Banana Split	520	14	94
Brownie & Oreo Cupfection	720	23	122
Peanut Buster Parfait	710	31	95
Triple Chocolate Brownie	540	25	74
Dipped Cone, Chocolate	460	22	58
DQ Sundaes: Caramel	430	11	73
Hot Fudge	430	15	66
Strawberry	340	10	56
MooLatte: Caramel	620	18	103
Mocha	620	23	94
Vanilla	560	17	93
Shakes: Caramel	750	25	115
Chocolate	710	23	110
Strawberry	630	23	92
Vanilla	660	23	97
Treatzza Pizza: Choco Brownie, slice	190	10	26
Reese's Peanut Butter Cup, slice	200	10	24

Daphne's Greek Cafe® (Oct '23)

Califonia Menu Only. Check Instore for Latest Information

Starters:	C	F	Cb
Fire Feta & Warm Pita	340	17	39
Hummus & Warm Pita	320	12	47
Classic Pita Sandwiches: *Without Tzatziki Sauce*			
with Chicken	410	16	41
with Crispy Shrimp	410	17	48
with Falafel	640	17	96
with Gyro	680	45	49
Plates: *Without Pita or Tzatziki Sauce*			
Cali-Greek Bowls: Crispy Shrimp	930	38	117
Falafel	1160	39	165
Grilled Chicken	930	37	109
Grilled Shrimp	1060	46	91
Mediterranean Veggie	1300	56	161
Surf & Turf	690	25	85
Classic Greek Salads: *W/ Dressing, w/o Pita & Sauce*			
Crispy Shrimp	440	31	25
Falafel	670	31	74
Grilled Chicken	440	30	18
Add, Pita & Tzatziki	135	3	21
Sides: Cucumber-Tomato Salad	120	11	5
Fire Roasted Vegetables	70	3	12
French Fries	440	22	55
Seasoned Rice	60	8	68
Small Greek Salad	140	12	7

Davanni's® (Oct '23)

Hot Hoagies: *Per Half, with 6" White Bun & Standard Toppings*	C	F	Cb
Chicken & Bacon, w/ Honey Mustard	505	22	46
Chicken Breast	510	28	40
Club	495	27	40
Ham	460	25	39
Meatball	565	33	49
Roast Beef	470	25	39
Tuna Melt	645	44	42
Turkey Bacon Chipotle	565	33	39
Pasta: *As Served, with Garlic Toast*			
Chicken Florentine, half portion	610	28	56
Lasagna, half portion	625	43	37
Calzones:			
BBQ Chicken w/ Bacon	790	34	79
Veggie	810	43	76
Works	910	53	76
Pizzas: *Per ⅛ Medium Pizza, with Red Sauce*			
Five Meat: Thin Crust	255	13	19
Traditional Crust	305	13	30
Gluten Free Crust	215	12	16
Veggie: Thin Crust	220	10	19
Traditional Crust	275	10	30
Works: Thin Crust	265	14	19
Traditional Crust	315	15	30

Del Taco® (Oct '23)

Breakfast:	C	F	Cb
Burritos: Bacon	520	26	36
Carne Asada	450	19	38
Egg & Cheese	380	16	35
Shredded Pork Carnitas	500	26	36
Donut Bites (4)	240	16	22
Hash Brown Sticks, 5 pieces	230	17	18
Rollers: Bacon	290	14	24
Egg & Cheese	250	11	24
Wraps: Bacon	400	23	32
Carne Asada Steak	400	21	34
Egg & Cheese	330	17	32
Burgers: *Without Fries*			
Bacon Double Del Cheeseburger	760	51	35
Del Cheeseburger	470	28	34
Double Del Chseburger	690	47	35
Burritos:			
Bean & Cheese, red	460	10	68
8-Layer Veggie	520	17	70
Classic Grilled Chicken	520	32	39
Del Beef	470	22	39
Del Combo	470	16	53
Chicken Cheddar Rollers: Chipotle	280	12	30
Original	250	9	30
Ranch	270	12	30
Epic Cali Bacon: Carne Asada	1050	60	73
Grilled Chicken	1020	60	72
Epic Fresh Guacamole:			
Carne Asada	750	25	89
Grilled Chicken	720	25	87
Epic Loaded Queso: Carne Asada	890	44	75
Grilled Chicken	860	45	73
Crunchtada, Tostada	330	14	41
Fries: Carne Asada Steak	760	56	45
Chilli Cheddar	570	35	42
Deluxe Chili Cheddar	610	37	44
Crinkle Cut Fries:			
Small, 3 oz	160	10	17
Medium, 6 oz	320	19	34
Macho, 7.7 oz	410	25	43
Queso Loaded	660	44	46
Nachos & Chips:			
Chips & Queso Dip, regular, 8 oz	640	40	59
Queso Loaded Nachos: *Per Regular*			
Beef	1030	54	99
Carne Asada Steak	970	47	99
Grilled Chicken	950	47	98
Quesadillas: Cheddar	480	27	35
Carne Asada; Chicken Cheddar, av.	545	30	37

Del Taco® cont... (Oct '23)

Tacos:	C	F	Cb
Beer Battered Crispy Fish	200	11	19
Chicken Del Carbon	110	4	13
Chipotle Crispy Chicken	240	13	18
Habero Crispy Chicken	240	14	18
Ranch Crispy Chicken	230	13	18
Shredded Pork: Del Carbon	150	4	12
Guac'd Up	170	9	13
Taco Salads: *With Fresh Guacamole*			
Carne Asada Steak	440	26	23
Grilled Chicken	420	26	22
Seasoned Beef	510	24	23
Desserts:			
Caramel Cheesecake Bites (2)	410	23	48
Mini Cinnamon Churros (2)	200	10	25
Shakes:			
Regular: Chocolate	550	9	102
Strawberry	520	9	96
Vanilla	480	9	85
Mini: Chocolate; Strawberry, average	265	5	49
Vanilla	240	5	40

Denny's® (Oct '23)

Signature Breakfast: *With Hash Browns Unless indicated*	C	F	Cb
Country Fried Steak, with Gravy & White Toast	810	43	82
Moons Over My Hammy	1040	54	90
Santa Fe Sizzlin' Skillet, without Hash Browns or Egg	770	58	38
T'Bone Steak, with White Toast	910	49	55
The Grand Slamwich	1300	79	94
3 Egg Omelettes: *With Hash Browns & White Toast*			
Loaded Veggie, 19 oz	920	56	63
Mile High Denver, 19 oz	1090	67	69
Ultimate, 21 oz	1140	77	63
Pancakes: *Two Pancakes Without Extras*			
Choconana	830	25	149
Cinnamon Roll w/ Cream Cheese	1100	26	207
Double Berry Banana	490	7	97
Hearty 9 Grain	410	11	68
Maple Flavored Syrup, 2 fl.oz	220	0	54
Slams: *With Hash Browns Unless Indicated*			
All American with White Toast	1170	80	57
Fit Slamm as per menu description	450	12	59
French Toast w/o Eggs or H. Browns	800	52	52
Lumberjack with White Toast without Eggs	1230	56	135

Denny's® cont... (Oct '23)

Breakfast Extras:	C	F	Cb
Bacon Strips (2)	100	8	1
Egg: Boiled (2)	130	8	1
Fried (20	190	16	1
Scrambled (2)	220	17	1
Whites (2)	80	1	1
English Muffin without Margarine	140	1	29
Grilled Ham Slice, 3 oz	120	4	7
Hash Browns, 5 oz	180	8	24
Pancakes, Buttermilk (2), w/ Marg.	450	11	77
Sausage Links (2)	160	15	0
Turkey Bacon Strips (2)	70	4	1
White Toast with Margarine, 2 slices	240	10	31
Starters: *Without Dipping Sauce*			
BBQ Boneless Chicken Wings, 8 oz	740	36	71
Premium Chicken Tenders (5)	680	40	38
Samplers:			
Beer Battered Onion Rings, 5 oz	400	27	35
Mozzarella Cheese Sticks, 8 oz	360	15	35
Zesty Nachos (serves 4), 25 oz	1660	106	170
Condiments:			
BBQ Sauce, 1.5 oz	90	0	23
Bourbon Sauce, 1 oz	110	0	26
Brown Gravy, 1 oz	10	0	2
Buffalo Sauce, 1.5 oz	110	12	1
Country Gravy, 1 fl.oz	20	10	2
Pico de Gallo, 2 oz	15	0	3
Sour Cream, 1 oz	45	4	1
Tomato Sauce, 1.5 oz	25	1	3
Whipped Margarine, 0.5 oz	40	5	0
Burgers: *Without Sides*			
Bacon Avocado Cheeseburger, 15 oz	1020	69	54
Double, 20 oz	1420	99	54
Bourbon Bacon, 15 oz	880	50	62
Double, 20 oz	1290	80	62
Flamin' 5 Pepper, 15 oz	1000	66	53
Double, 20 oz	1400	97	53
Slamburger, without egg, 11 oz	840	47	58
Double, without egg, 16 oz	1240	77	59
Dinners: *Without Sides or Sauce*			
Bourbon Chicken Sizzlin Skillet	910	43	71
Cntry Fried Stk w/ Gravy & Din. Bread	960	56	78
Crazy Spicy Sizzlin' Skillet, w/out Egg	1040	69	48
Mac 'N Sizzlin Skillet	990	60	110
Oven Baked Lasagna w/ Dinn. Bread	1130	51	110
Plate Likin' Fried Chkn w/ Dinn. Bread	1070	62	68
Premium Chkn Tenders & Dinner Bread	860	47	63
Sirloin Steak with Dinner Bread	530	25	27
T-Bone Steak with Dinner Bread	680	38	26
Wild Alask. Salmon With Dinner Bread	540	31	27

Denny's® cont... (Oct '23)

Melts & Handhelds: W/out Sides	C	F	Cb
Cali Club Sandwich	890	55	59
Nashville Hot Chkn Melt	1250	76	95
Slow Cooker Meaty Melt	1060	60	67
The Super Bird	760	33	69
A La Carte/Dinner Sides:			
Beer Battered Onion Rings	400	27	35
Fresh Vegetable Medley	70	5	6
Garden Salad, without dressing	170	9	16
Herb Glazed Corn	300	18	30
Red Rustic Mashed Potatoes	250	11	32
Red Skinned Potatoes	250	13	30
Seasoned Fries	490	26	57
Seasonal Fruit	100	0	25
Wavy-Cut Fries	400	22	46
Whole Grain Rice	240	3	48
55 & Over: *Without Extras*			
B'fast, Scrambled Eggs & Cheddar	1010	58	80
Grilled Cheese Sandwich	550	26	66
Omelette w/ H Browns & Toast	900	57	60
Salads: *Without Dressing*			
Cobb	480	34	23
House Salad:			
without Meat	190	9	19
with Chicken Tenders (3)	600	33	42
with Grilled Chicken	390	18	19
with Wild Alaska Salmon	500	28	21
Dressings: *Per 1.5 fl.oz*			
Balsamic Vinaigrette	60	2	11
Blue Cheese	150	16	2
Honey Mustard	190	15	12
Fat Free Italian	20	0	4
Ranch	200	21	1
Thousand Island	180	16	7
Desserts: *As Served*			
Lava Cookie Skillet, 9 oz	820	40	108
New York Style Cheesecake, plain	490	32	42
Beverages:			
Chocolate Milk, reduced fat, 15 fl.oz	290	5	46
Hot Chocolate, 8 fl.oz	190	3	37
Lemonade, 12 fl.oz	150	0	40
Mango Lemonade, 15 fl.oz	210	0	57
Orange Juice, 15 fl.oz	210	0	51
Milk Shakes:			
Chocolate, 16 fl.oz	870	43	111
Oreo, 17 fl.oz	1050	56	125
Strawberry, 17 fl.oz	780	34	114
Vanilla, 16 fl.oz	800	43	97
Smoothie, Mango, 15 fl.oz	340	0	86

Dippin' Dots® (Oct '23)

Ice Cream: Per ⅔ Cup	C	F	Cb
Birthday Cake, 3.4 oz	190	10	24
Choc. Chip Cookie Dough, 3.5 oz	230	10	31
Chocolate, 3 oz	190	9	25
Cookies 'N Cream, 3.17 oz	210	10	26
Cotton Candy, 3 oz	170	9	20
Ultimate Brownie Batter, 3.77 oz	220	10	30
***Yogurt:** Per 2.54 oz Packet*			
Banana Split	90	1	18
Cookie Dough;Strawb. Cheesecake, av.	110	2	23

Donatos Pizza® (Oct '23)

***Pizzas:** Per Slice*	C	F	Cb
Cauliflower Crust, 10":			
Spinach Mozzarella	80	4	6
Other varieties, average	70	4	7
Hand Tossed Signature Pizzas: *Per Slice of 14" Pizza*			
Chicken Spinach Mozzarella	330	15	31
Founder's Favorite	330	14	33
Mariachi Beef	300	12	33
Mariachi Chicken	290	11	33
The Works	320	13	34
Thick Crust Signature Pizzas: *Per Slice of 14" Pizza*			
Chicken Spinach Mozzarella	150	7	15
Double Bacon Pepperoni	190	9	16
Founders Favorite	160	7	16
Margherita	160	8	15
Serious Meat, Ground Beef	190	9	16
The Works	170	8	17
Oven Baked Subs:			
Big Don Italian with Marinara Sauce	600	24	61
Chicken Bacon Ranch	740	34	59
Fresh Vegy	490	18	61
Ham & Smoked Prov.	560	20	65
Meatball	850	37	76
***Salad:** Entree Size, with Menu Set Dressing*			
Chicken Bacon Ranch	590	45	12
Chicken Caprese	390	26	17
Italian Chef	500	42	13
Side: Caprese	230	19	11
Italian	330	31	7
***Wings:** Per 6 pieces, without Dipping Sauce*			
Boneless:			
Mild/Hot Sauce, average	345	15	30
BBQ Sauce	380	12	45
Dessert: Cinnamon Bread, ¼ bread	260	8	41
Fudge Brownie (1)	360	21	45
Triple Chocolate Chunk Cookie (1)	310	15	35

For Complete Nutritional Data ~ see CalorieKing.com

Domino's® (Oct '23)

With Regular Cheese Base	C	F	Cb
***12" Hand Tossed:** Per Slice, ⅛ Pizza, with Honey BBQ Sauce Unless Indicated*			
Bacon, Beef, & Italian Sausage	290	15	27
Beef, Green Peppers, Onions, & Mshrm	210	8	27
Chicken, Black Olives, Green Peppers, Mshrm &Tomatoes, Marinara Sauce	200	7	25
Ham & Pineapple, no sauce	190	7	23
Italian Sausage & Pepperoni	250	12	26
Italian Sausage, Beef & Pepperoni	280	14	26
Pepperoni & Salami	240	10	26
***14" Brooklyn:** Per Slice, ⅙ Pizza, with Hearty Marinara Sauce Unless Indicated*			
Beef, Green Pepp., Onions & Mshrm	260	11	29
Chicken, Black Olives, Green Peppers, Onions, Mushrooms, Tomatoes	290	12	30
Ham & Pineapple, no sauce	260	11	27
Italian Sausage	350	19	27
Pepperoni, no sauce	290	15	24
Pepperoni & Italian Sausage, no sauce	340	20	24
***14" Thin Crust:** Per Slice, ⅛ Pizza, with Garlic Parmesan White Sauce Unless Indicated*			
Bacon, Beef & Italian Sausage	320	24	15
Beef, Green Pepp., Onions & Mshrm	260	18	16
Chkn, Black Olives, Green Peppers, Onions, Mushrooms & Tomatoes	260	17	17
Ham & Pineapple, no sauce	190	9	17
Italian Sausage, Marinara Sce	250	16	17
Pepperoni, no sauce	210	12	15
Pepperoni & Italian Sausage	320	24	15
***12" Specialty Handmade Pan:** Per Slice, ⅛ Pizza*			
Cali Chicken Bacon Ranch	380	22	29
Deluxe	320	17	30
Memphis BBQ Chicken	330	16	34
Spinach & Feta	310	16	29
***12" Specialty Hand-Tossed:** Per Slice, ⅛ Pizza*			
Deluxe	240	12	24
ExtravaganZZa	270	14	25
MeatZZa	260	13	24
Philly Cheeese Steak	230	10	24
Ultimate Pepperoni	260	13	24
***14" Specialty Thin Crust:** Per Slice, ⅛ Pizza*			
Cali Chicken Bacon Ranch	330	23	17
Deluxe	260	16	18
Honolulu Hawaiian	250	14	19
Memphis BBQ Chicken	270	14	22
Wisconsin 6 Cheese	250	15	18

Domino's® cont... (Oct '23)

Chicken Wings: Without Sauce	C	F	Cb
Garlic Parmesan, 4 wings	390	34	10
Honey BBQ, 4 wings	310	20	22
Chicken Dipping Cups:			
Blue Cheese, 1.25 oz	200	21	2
Honey BBQ, 1.25 oz	70	0	17
Hot Buffalo, 1.25 oz	15	1	1
Ranch, 1.5 oz	220	24	2
Sweet Mango Habanero, 1.25 oz	70	0	17
BreadBowl Pasta: *Per ½ Bowl*			
Chicken Alfredo, 10.5 oz	690	25	92
Chicken Carbonara, 11.6 oz	730	28	93
Italian Sausage Marinara, 11.85 oz	740	28	96
Pasta Primavera, 11 oz	660	23	92
Oven Baked Sandwiches: *Per Sandwich*			
Buffalo Chicken	860	42	78
Chicken Bacon Ranch	900	44	74
Chicken Parmesan	800	30	76
Italian	820	38	74
Mediterranean Veggie	720	30	78
Philly Cheese Steak	760	30	76
Sweet & Spicy Chicken Habanero	780	28	88
Pasta In Dish: Chicken Alfredo, 11.5 oz	600	29	60
Chicken Carbonara, 13 oz	690	34	63
Italian Sausage Marinara, 13.5 oz	700	36	68
Pasta Primavera, 11.9 oz	530	26	62
Salads: *Without Dressing*			
Chicken Caesar	220	8	14
Classic Garden	80	4	8
Salad Dressings: *Per 1.5 oz Package*			
Caesar Dressing	230	25	1
Italian	160	17	4
Light Balsamic Dressing	100	8	5
Ranch Dressing	220	24	2
Bread Side Items:			
Garlic Bread Twists, 2 pcs	220	11	27
Jalap. Bacon Stuffed Cheesy Bread (1)	170	8	17
Parmesan Bread Bites, 4 pieces	220	10	27
Spin. & Fetta Stuffed Cheesy Bread, 1 piece	160	7	17
Stuffed Cheesy Bread, 1 piece	150	7	16
Bread Dipping Sauces: *Per Container*			
Garlic, 1 oz cup	250	28	0
Marinara, 2 oz cup	30	0	6
Dessert: Choc. Lava Crunch Cake, 3 oz	350	17	47
Marbled Cookie Brownie, 1.5 oz	200	10	26
Sweet Icing, Dipping Cup, 2.25 oz	220	4	52

Dunkin'® (Oct '23)

Bagels: *Per Bagel*	C	F	Cb
Plain	300	1	64
Cinnamon Raisin	320	1	67
Everything	340	3	67
Multigrain	380	8	63
Sesame Seed	350	5	64
White Cheddar Twist	390	8	64
Donuts: Apple 'n Spice	230	10	31
Apple Crumb	290	11	44
Bavarian Kreme	240	11	31
Bismark	480	22	63
Boston Kreme	270	11	39
Butternut	430	21	57
Chocolate Butternut	450	24	57
Chocolate Dipped French Cruller	280	15	33
Chocolate Frosted Cake	360	20	41
Chocolate Headlight	310	14	41
Chocolate Long John	320	15	41
Cinnamon	330	20	34
Coconut; Coffee Roll, average	400	20	49
Double Chocolate	380	23	41
French Cruller	230	14	21
Glazed	240	11	33
Glazed Chocolate	370	23	41
Glazed Jelly	280	10	44
Jelly	250	10	36
Lemon	230	10	31
Maple Creme	290	14	38
Maple Frosted	260	11	35
Maple Vanilla Creme	330	15	45
Old Fashioned	310	19	30
Peanut	470	27	50
Plain Stick	420	30	36
Powdered	330	20	34
Strawberry Frosted	260	11	35
Sugared	210	11	24
Toasted Coconut	430	22	52
Vanilla Creme	300	15	37
Vanilla Long John	320	15	42
Muffins: Blueberry	460	15	77
Chocolate Chip	550	21	85
Coffee Cake	590	24	88
Corn	460	16	73
Munchkins: Cinnamon	60	4	6
Glazed	60	3	7
Glazed Chocolate	60	4	8
Jelly	60	3	8
Old Fashioned	50	3	6
Powdered	60	4	7
Other Bakery Items: Eclair	370	16	50
English Muffin	190	2	35
Plain Croissant	340	19	37

..continued next page

Dunkin'® cont... (Oct '23)

Sandwiches:	C	F	Cb
Plain Bagel Sandwiches:			
Bacon, Egg & Cheese	520	18	67
Egg & Cheese	460	13	66
Sausage, Egg & Cheese	680	34	68
Croissants: Bacon, Egg & Cheese	560	36	41
Egg & Cheese	500	31	40
Sausage, Egg & Cheese	720	52	42
English Muffin Sandwiches:			
Bacon, Egg & Cheese	400	19	39
Sausage, Egg & Cheese	560	35	40
Sourdough Breakfast Sandwich	650	32	58
Wake-Up Wraps: Egg & Cheese	180	10	14
Bacon, Egg & Cheese	220	13	15
Turkey Sausage	240	15	15
Hash Browns, 6 pieces	110	6	13
Hot Beverages:			
Original Chocolate: Small	220	7	40
Medium	330	10	59
Large	460	14	82
Iced Drinks: *Per Medium*			
Butter Pecan Swirl Iced Cappuccino:			
with Skim Milk	230	0	48
with Whole Milk	280	6	47
Butter Pecan Swirl Iced Latte:			
with Skim Milk	260	0	52
with Whole Milk	330	9	52
Butter Pecan Swirl Iced Macchiato:			
with Skim Milk	230	0	48
with Whole Milk	280	6	48
Frozen Drinks: *Per Medium*			
Caramel Swirl Frozen Coffee:			
with Skim Milk	650	5	142
with Whole Milk	680	9	141
Frozen Chocolate,			
French Vanilla Swirl	700	14	135
Frozen Matcha Latte: Skim milk	360	0	83
Whole milk	390	5	83

Eat 'N Park® (Oct '23)

Breakfast: *Without Extras*	C	F	Cb
Bananas Foster French Toast, 2 sl.	440	6	88
Country Fried Steak & Eggs	690	36	51
Ham Steak & Eggs	410	24	3
Omelettes:			
Ham & Cheese	660	47	6
Mushroom & Swiss	490	25	5
Pancakes: *With Whipped Topping*			
Bananas Foster (2) with Sauce	660	13	129
Blueberry (2)	460	12	78
Chocolate Chip (2)	720	29	110
Scramblers:			
All American with Bacon & Cheese	580	20	58
All American with Sausage & Chse	740	42	58
Appetizers:			
Fresh Potato Chip Basket	620	40	63
Fried Cheese Sticks	590	35	41
Fried Ravioli	410	17	52
Loaded Tater Tots	690	43	75
Burgers: *Without Sides*			
Bacon Cheeseburger	810	51	37
Eat 'N Park Beyond	850	60	45
Mushroom & Onion	790	48	41
Superburgers: Black Angus	1100	71	39
Original	670	42	37
Sandwiches: *Without Sides*			
Bacon Grilled Cheese	600	41	33
Chargrilled Chicken	470	16	41
Classic Grilled Cheese	530	36	33
Crispy Chicken Bacon Club	1090	67	63
Philly Cheesesteak	800	42	50
Shredded Pot Roast	540	31	28
Turkey Club	850	46	48
Whale of a Cod Fish	930	35	96
Dinners: *Without Sides or Sauces Unless Indicated*			
Baked Chicken Parmigiana,			
with Marinara Sauce	920	41	84
Baked Cod, 1 fillet	220	12	3
Breaded Shrimp (6) w/ Cocktail Sce	430	18	39
Chicken Bruschetta, 1 breast	500	27	27
Chicken Tenders, 4 pieces	630	31	33
Country Fried Steak & Gravy	490	20	50
Nantucket Cod & Stuffing, 1 piece	400	28	10
Spaghetti Marinara	680	8	130
Whale & Mac	1080	52	83
Whale of a Cod with Hogie	930	35	96

Eat 'N Park® cont... (Oct '23)

Salads:	C	F	Cb
Chicken & Strawberry: *W/- Poppy & Sesame Seed Dressing*			
Grilled Chicken	510	25	35
Herb Crusted Chicken	700	44	40
Chicken Bacon Ranch, w/ Ranch Dr.	930	64	24
Sides: Baked Potato	190	0	44
Broccoli	40	0	8
Carrots	40	1	9
Coleslaw	120	8	12
French Fries	380	24	37
Mac'n Cheese	450	22	44
Mashed Potatoes	110	6	13
Tater Tots	250	14	30
Soup Bowls: *Per Bowl*			
Chicken Noodle	270	8	34
Clam Chowder	420	18	48
Cream of Broccoli	300	12	39
Cream of Potato	310	14	39
Desserts: *Per Slice, without Whipped Cream*			
Pies: Apple Pie	390	14	65
Bananas Foster Creme Pie	560	29	74
Chocolate Cream Pie	510	28	58
Dutch Apple Pie	410	16	65
Peach	380	15	57

Edo Japan® (Oct '23)

	C	F	Cb
Chop Chop Bowls: *Without Teriyaki Top Sauce*			
Beef	680	21	80
Chicken	565	9	80
Chicken & Beef	620	15	80
Tempura Shrimp	600	17	92
Veggie	390	3	77
Noodle Meals: *W/ Asian Veggies, w/out Teriyaki Top Sauce*			
Noodleful: Beef	795	37	72
Chicken	680	25	72
Shrimp	625	22	71
Veggie	550	20	79
Yakisoba: Beef	615	23	61
Chicken	505	11	62
Chicken & Beef	560	17	62
Rice Meals: *With Asian Veggies, w/out Teriyaki Top Sauce*			
Beef & Shrimp	825	34	80
Chicken & Beef	570	12	76
Chicken & Shrimp	715	22	80
Fresh Grilled Vegetables	445	1	96
Hawaiian Chicken	505	6	75
Sizzling Shrimp	470	4	78
Teriyaki Salmon	540	8	79
Sushi: *Per 4 Rolls without Sauce*			
Beef	165	5	23
California Rolls	170	4	27
Dynamite Rolls	180	6	26
Salmon	145	2	22

Einstein Bros® (Oct '23)

Bagels: *For Nutritional Information on Menu Items at Licensed Locations ~ see In Store*	C	F	Cb
Classic: Ancient Grain	290	5	50
Cranberry	310	4	59
Everything	280	1	57
Onion	280	1	58
Plain	270	1	56
Poppy Seed	280	2	56
Sesame Seed	290	2	56
Gourmet: Apple Cinnamon	420	7	78
Cheesy Hash Brown	400	12	60
Green Chili	390	12	54
Spinach Florentine	370	12	53
Signature: Asiago Cheese	300	4	54
Blueberry	280	1	60
Chocolate Chip	280	3	56
Cinnamon Sugar	300	2	61
French Toast	380	7	70
Signature Lunch Sandwiches:			
Avocado Veg Out on Sesame, 9.1 oz	410	11	66
Ham & Swiss on Plain Bagel, 10.4 oz	540	20	63
Nova Loxon Plain Bagel, 8.7 oz	520	8	61
Tasty Turkey on Asiago Bagel, 11.6 oz	510	15	67
Turkey & Chedd. on Plain Bagel, 10.4 oz	540	19	64
Cream Cheese: *Per 1.2 oz Schmear*			
Plain	120	12	2
Onion and Chive	110	10	4
Reduced Fat:			
Garden Veggie	100	9	5
Honey Almond; Strawberry, av.	120	8	10
Jalapeno Salsa	100	9	5
Classic One Egg Sandwiches: *On Plain Bagel*			
Applewood Bacon & Cheddar	450	16	58
Ham & Swiss	450	12	59
Turkey Sausage & Cheddar	490	17	57
Signature Egg Sandwiches:			
All-Nighter, on Cheesy Hash Brown Bagel	900	58	65
Bacon, Avoc., Tomato on Plain Bgl	400	17	47
F'house on Cheesy H.Brown Bagel	680	32	64
Sides, Twice Baked Hash Brown	170	11	11
Desserts, Blueberry Muffin	440	25	48

El Pollo Loco® (Oct '23)

Bowl:	C	F	Cb
Original	580	10	83
Double Chicken	930	33	87
Grand Avocado Chicken	790	27	90
Shredded Chicken & Cheese	590	14	84
Street Corn Chicken	600	11	84
Burritos:			
Chicken Avocado	920	47	68
Chipotle Chicken Avocado	920	40	81
Classic Chicken Burrito	480	13	66
Original BRC	410	11	63
Fire-Grilled Combos:			
Chicken Tacos Al Carbon	510	15	46
Classic Chicken Burrito	480	13	66
Original Pollo Bowl	580	10	83
Shredded Chkn Quesadilla	500	24	40
Fit Menu:			
Double Chicken Avocado Salad	430	20	13
The World's First Keto Burrito	510	29	30
Extras:			
Chicken Taco Al Carbon	170	5	17
Chips & Guacamole:			
5.9 oz	490	32	49
11.8 oz	990	63	98
Fried Tortilla Chips, 5 oz	760	44	83
Tortilla Soup: Small	250	9	19
Large	450	17	34
Street Tacos:			
Chicken Avocado	340	19	18
Chicken Taco Al Carbon	170	5	17
Tostada Salads: Classic	830	39	79
Double Chicken	990	46	82
Sides:			
Broccoli, small, 3 oz	30	0	6
Coleslaw, small, 4 oz	130	10	9
Corn, small, 5 oz	160	5	24
Loco Side Salad, small	160	14	8
Macaroni & Cheese: Small, 6 oz	310	19	24
Large, 15 oz	770	48	60
Mashed Potatoes & Gravy:			
Small, 6 oz	105	1	21
Large, 17 oz	340	5	69
Pinto Beans, small, 6 oz	140	1	25
Rice: Small, 4.5 oz	160	2	33
Large, 10.75 oz	380	4	78
Condiments:			
Creamy Cilantro Dressing, 3 oz	310	33	2
Ranch Dressing, 1.5 oz	190	21	2
Salsa: Avocado, 1.3 oz	30	3	2
House; Pico de Gallo, Roja, 1.3 oz	10	0	2
Sour Cream, 1.3 oz	80	7	1

Fatburger® (Oct '23)

Burgers: *Without Extras*	C	F	Cb
Fatburger: Baby Fat	400	21	37
Original	590	31	46
Kingburger	850	41	69
Double	1270	69	69
Triple	1685	97	69
Impossible Burger	525	13	54
Thousand Island	770	47	46
Turkeyburger	480	21	50
Veggieburger	510	20	60
Western BBQ	780	38	66
Hot Dogs: *Without Extras*			
Chili Cheese	480	27	35
Regular Hot Dog	320	15	32
Sandwiches: *Without Extras*			
Bacon & Egg	350	16	37
Chicken: Crispy	660	16	91
Grilled	430	14	42
Sausage & Egg	780	53	47
Spicy Chicken	520	21	58
Fries: Fat Fries	380	18	47
with Chili & Cheese	590	33	53
Skinny Fries	390	15	58
with Chili Cheese	600	30	64
Sweet Potato	480	24	66
Sides: Chili Cup	200	11	10
with Cheese & Onions	320	20	12
Onion Rings	540	29	64
Shakes: Chocolate	910	45	115
Maui Banana	940	44	126
Strawberry	880	44	111
Vegan Strawberry/Vanilla, av	540	24	81

For Complete Nutritional Data ~ see CalorieKing.com

Fazoli's® (Oct '23)

Fan Favorites: *Per Serving*	C	F	Cb
Fettuccine Alfredo	700	26	102
Penne Creamy Basil	830	40	102
Ravioli Meat Sauce	530	21	59
Spaghetti with Meatballs	730	22	110
Specialty Pastas:			
Chicken Carbonara	1050	48	107
Loaded Fettuccini Alfredo	1000	43	105
Breadsticks, (2)	250	11	31

Fazoli's® cont... (Oct '23)

Samplers: Per Serving	C	F	Cb
Classic	790	25	119
Oven Baked	940	37	120
Ultimate	1010	28	161
Signature Bakes:			
Chicken Broccoli Penne	1070	60	84
Loaded Baked Spaghetti	1070	53	100
Spicy Baked Ziti with Chicken	790	32	78
Subs:			
Club	750	42	54
Meatball	1070	67	74
Salads:			
Crispy Chkn Bacon Ranch w/ Ranch	770	62	32
House Side without Dressing	110	7	7

For Complete Nutritional Data ~ see CalorieKing.com

Firehouse Subs® (Oct '23)

Hot Subs: Per Medium White Sub, with Standard Toppings	C	F	Cb
Cajun Chicken	710	35	54
Club on a Sub	760	40	64
Engineer	700	35	61
Hook & Ladder	710	36	64
Italian	930	57	66
Jamaican Jerk Turky	720	36	68
Meatball	830	51	59
Steak & Cheese	840	51	56
Sides, 5 Cheese Mac & Cheese	380	20	33
Under 500 Calorie Salads:			
Firehouse Chopped: *Without Dressing*			
with Grilled Chicken	380	10	14
with Ham	290	9	27
with Turkey	220	7	15
Italian, with Grilled Chicken	410	22	14

Five Guys® (Oct '23)

	C	F	Cb
Bun, 2.7 oz	240	9	39
Meat Choices:			
Bacon, 2 pieces	70	6	0
Hamburger Patty	300	17	0
Hot Dog	280	26	1
Veggie Toppings: Cheese Slice	70	6	1
Green Peppers, 0.9 oz	3	0	1
Grilled Mushrooms, 0.75 oz	6	0	1
Jalapeno Peppers, 0.4 oz	3	0	1
Lettuce, 1 oz	3	0	1
Onions/Grilled, 1 oz	10	0	2
Pickles, 1 oz	4	0	1
Relish, 0.5 oz	15	0	4
Tomatoes, 1.83 oz	8	0	2

Five Guys® cont... (Oct '23)

Sauces:	C	F	Cb
A.1 Original, 0.6 oz	15	0	3
BBQ, 1 oz	60	0	15
Ketchup, 0.6 oz	30	0	5
Mayo, 0.5 oz	110	11	0
Fries: Little, 8 oz	525	23	72
Regular, 14.5 oz	955	41	131
Large, 20 oz	1315	57	181

Flame Broiler® (Oct '23)

Bowls: Regular Single Protein with White Rice, without Toppings or Cooking Sauce	C	F	Cb
Beef, marinated	700	10	103
Chicken	650	12	85
Tofu	620	13	89
Plates: *Regular Single Portion with White Rice, without Toppings or Sauce*			
Beef, marinated	780	14	111
Chicken	770	17	86
Rib (beef), marinated	920	34	93

Freshens® (Oct '23)

	C	F	Cb
Crepes: Chicken Bacon Ranch	610	40	28
Denver, with Bacon	540	29	30
Egg White Florentine	310	9	27
Fresh Tomato, Chse & Basil	380	10	38
Nashville Hot	520	28	38
Nutella & Strawberry	390	15	54
Rice Bowls: Baja Queso	680	33	74
Buffalo Chicken	600	23	70
KC BBQ	610	11	97
Meatless Mexican	730	29	91
Mexican	710	29	83
Power Protein	810	30	94
Salads: Buffalo Chkn	480	27	29
Gr. Chicken Caesar	520	37	26
Roadhouse BBQ Chkn	420	17	42
Strawberry & Kale	490	15	56
Smoothies: *100% Juice*			
Blended Fruit Classics: *Per 20 fl.oz*			
Bangin' Berry	330	0	80
Caribbean Craze; Wild Strawberry	300	0	73
Goin' Green	280	1	70
Maui Mango	390	0	97
Orange Sunrise	330	3	73
Peanut Butter Protein	480	12	69
Super C Immune Support	340	3	75
Tropical Therapy	430	11	79

For Complete Nutritional Data ~ see CalorieKing.com

Godfather's Pizza® (Oct '23)

Golden Crust Pizza: Per Slice	C	F	Cb
Cheese: Medium, ⅛ pizza	210	8	25
Large, 1/10 pizza	230	10	27
Classic Combo: Medium, ⅛ pizza	270	13	27
Large, 1/10 pizza	310	15	30
Super Combo:			
Medium, ⅛ pizza	310	15	28
Large, 1/10 pizza	350	18	30
Original Crust Pizza:			
BLT: Individual, ⅙ pizza	170	7	18
Small, ⅙ pizza	290	14	29
Medium, ⅛ pizza	320	15	32
Jumbo, 1/12 pizza	430	21	42
Buffalo Chicken: Individ., ⅙ pizza	150	6	18
Small, ⅙ pizza	250	9	29
Medium, ⅛ pizza	270	9	32
Jumbo, 1/12 pizza	370	14	41
Taco Pie: Individual, ⅙ pizza	170	7	19
Small, ⅙ pizza	300	12	32
Medium, ⅛ pizza	330	14	35
Jumbo, 1/12 pizza	460	20	45
Thin Crust Pizza:			
BBQ Chicken: Medium, ⅛ pizza	200	8	20
Large, 1/10 pizza	240	10	24
Pepperoni: Medium, ⅛ pizza	200	11	15
Large, 1/10 pizza	230	13	18
The Don: Medium, ⅛ pizza	250	14	16
Large, 1/10 pizza	290	17	19
Sides: Baked Beans, 4 oz	120	1	25
Biscuit, 1 oz	100	3	11
Cheesy Potatoes, 4 oz	310	19	30
Coleslaw, 4 oz	200	17	12
Gravy, 2 oz	30	1	4
Green Beans, 4 oz	140	10	8
Mshd Potatoes, 4 oz	100	3	17
Potato Wedges, 4 oz	180	7	27

Gold Star Chili® (Oct '23)

Burgers: Per Single	C	F	Cb
Bacon Cheeseburger	870	58	46
Chili	680	39	50
Hamburger	560	33	44
Coneys, Original Chili: Plain	210	11	21
Cheese, plain	300	18	21
Chili Cheese Sandwich, plain	250	14	20
Ways, Origninal Chili:			
Regular: 3-Way	760	41	56
5-Way	850	41	74
Chili Spaghetti	240	1	48
Double Deckers: *With White Bread*			
Ham & Bacon	1080	80	46
Ham & Turkey	760	46	46
Turkey & Bacon	1070	78	46

Gold Star Chili® cont...(Oct '23)

Salads: Full Salad, without Dressing	C	F	Cb
BBQ Chicken	490	24	36
Harvest Pecan Chkn	340	16	25
Fries: French, regular	460	19	67
Chili	490	22	63
Chili Cheese	840	51	64
Garlic Parmesan	870	62	71
Vegetarian Chili	540	24	71

Golden Corral® (Oct '23)

Breakfast: Per ½ Cup	C	F	Cb
Corned Beef Hash	230	15	14
Hashbrown Casserole	100	4	14
Scrambled Eggs	180	14	2
Beef: Asian, 3 oz	110	4	10
BBQ, 3 oz	120	5	0
Enchiladas, each	200	12	11
Smoked Beef Short Ribs, 3 oz	340	27	0
Smothered Chopped Steak, 5.9 oz	290	18	4
Chicken: Buffalo Chicken S'wich	200	9	21
Chicken & Noodle Dumplings, 1 cup	210	7	25
Orange Chicken, 1 cup	360	14	35
Smoked White Meat Chicken, 3 oz	150	6	0
Fish: Baked, 3 oz	150	8	1
Fried Catfish, 3 oz	180	10	12
Pork: Baby Back Ribs, 3 oz	190	13	3
Sweet & Sour, 6 oz	220	11	18
Sides: BBQ Baked Beans, ½ cup	160	1	35
Creamed Spinach, ½ cup	170	12	10
Fries, Seasoned Wedges (10)	190	12	21
Fried Okra (10)	110	7	10
Mac & Cheese, ½ c.	180	10	19
Mshd Potatoes, ½ c.	200	15	16
Rice Pilaf, ½ cup	130	5	18
Salad Buffet: *Per ½ Cup Unless Indicated*			
Caesar, without dressing, 1 cup	110	8	8
Chicken	250	22	3
Coleslaw	80	6	7
Macaroni	280	11	41
Marinated Vegetable	35	2	3
Potato	230	18	14
Romaine Lettuce, 1 cup	10	0	2
Seafood	110	6	8
Spinach, 1 cup	15	0	2
Strawberry Spinach, 1 cup	40	3	5
Tuna	190	12	4

Great American Bagel Co® (Oct '23)

Bagels:	C	F	Cb
Asiago Cheese	520	16	72
Cheddar Herb	390	8	66
Cinnamon Raisin	380	4	76
Jalapeno Cheddar	370	7	63
Plain	360	4	71
Spinach Tomazzo	640	20	86
Tomazzo	520	13	77
Cream Cheese Filling: *Per 1 oz*			
Plain	100	10	1
Strawberry; Vegetable, average	90	8	4
Paninis: *With Set Menu Ingredients On Regular Baguette*			
Chicken Pesto	770	35	70
Ham & Swiss	600	26	58
Philly Beef	920	40	92
Turkey Club	680	29	67
Sandwiches: Asiago Omelet	720	29	80
BLT	550	17	72
Chicken Parmigiana	740	22	81
Ham	460	9	71
Roast Beef	465	9	71
Turkey	435	5	72
Pastries:			
Cookies: Chocolate Chunk, 4 oz	110	4	19
Oatmeal Raisin, 4 oz	120	5	18
Muffins: Banana Nut, 4.25 oz	430	18	61
Blueberry, 4.25 oz	430	16	64

The Great Steak® (Oct '23)

Breakfast:	C	F	Cb
Potatoes: Original	300	16	35
Deluxe	330	17	41
Sandwiches: Bacon, Egg & Cheese	550	31	38
Ham, Egg & Cheese	530	27	41
Sausage, Egg & Cheese	660	42	38
Steak, Egg & Cheese Sandwich	540	27	38
Cheesesteaks:			
Regular 7": Bacon Cheddar	590	23	55
Chicagoland	610	24	59
Great Steak	790	45	55
Original Philly	510	17	55
Super Steak	800	45	57
Large: Bacon Cheddar	1000	38	91
Chicagoland	1050	41	97
Great Steak	1360	79	92

The Great Steak® cont... (Oct '23)

Chicken Philly Sandwiches:	C	F	Cb
Regular: Original	570	21	56
Buffalo Chicken	750	38	61
Teriyaki Chicken	820	44	68
Ultimate Chicken	800	44	60
Grilled Sandwiches:			
Regular:			
Chicken Bacon Ranch	820	44	60
Veggie Delight	490	19	61
Large:			
Chicken Bacon Ranch	1430	78	101
Veggie Delight	770	28	103
Baked Potatoes:			
Bacon & Cheese	440	23	36
Broccoli & Cheese	250	6	45
Sour Cream & Chives	250	10	38
The Great Potato: Chicken	460	19	49
Ham	450	19	52
King	540	32	38
Steak	470	20	46
Turkey	430	17	48
Burgers: Bacon Cheeseburger	1050	72	45
Philly Cheeseburger	780	48	44
Fries:			
Bacon Ranch: Regular	650	42	51
Large	1520	91	139
Cheese: Regular	410	21	51
Large	1040	48	140
Chili Cheese: Regular	490	23	62
Large	1220	53	163
Great Fry: Regular	370	18	48
Large	930	40	132
King Fry, regular	480	27	52
Philly, large	1090	48	131
Great Salads: *Without Dressing*			
Grilled Chicken	370	22	16
Grilled Ham	360	22	19
Steak	390	23	17
Turkey	350	20	19
Salad Dressings: Mayo, reg., 1 oz	200	22	0
Ranch, 1 oz	150	16	2
Thousand Island, 1 oz	130	12	4
Sauce: BBQ, 1 oz	50	0	12
Buffalo, 1 oz	10	0	1
Honey Mustard, 1 oz	40	1	7
Teriyaki, 1 oz	25	0	3

Haagen-Dazs® (Oct '23)

Classic Flavors: Per ⅔ Cup	C	F	Cb
Bourbon Praline Pecan	360	20	40
Bourbon Van. Bean Truffle	340	20	36
Butter Pecan	370	28	26
Caramel Cone	400	25	38
Cherry Vanilla	290	18	29
Chocolate	330	21	28
Chocolate Chip Cookie Dough	380	22	41
Chocolate Chocolate Chip	380	24	34
Chocolate Peanut Butter	440	29	36
Coffee	300	21	25
Coffee Chip	340	22	30
Coffee Chocolate Brownie	360	20	38
Cookies & Cream	320	20	29
Creamy Mango	330	17	40
Double Belgian Chocolate Chip	420	27	39
Dulce de Leche	350	20	36
Honey Salted Caramel Almond	350	22	33
Irish Cream Brownie	340	20	36
Matcha Green Tea	310	21	25
Peppermint Bark	360	20	40
Pineapple Coconut	290	16	32
Pistachio	340	23	27
Rocky Road	370	21	37
Rum Raisin	320	20	29
Strawberry	310	19	29
Triple Chocolate Fudge Cookie	360	20	40
Vanilla	320	21	26
Vanilla Bean	340	21	32
Vanilla Chocolate Chip	370	24	33
Vanilla Swiss Almond	370	25	30
White Chocolate Raspberry Truffle	360	20	41
***City Sweets Collection:** Per ⅔ Cup*			
Black & White Cookie	410	24	42
Chocolate Peanut Butter Pretzel	450	30	38
Coffee Chocolate Brownie	360	20	38
Dulce De Leche Churro	390	23	41
Summer Berry Cake Pop	320	20	31

Ice Cream Bars/Cones ~ See Page 109

Hardee's® (Oct '23)

Charbroiled Burgers:	C	F	Cb
Famous Star with Cheese	660	37	55
Super Star w/ Cheese	920	56	59
The Big Hardee	920	58	55
Western Bacon Cheeseburger	810	38	80
Cheeseburgers: Big	540	23	56
Double	530	26	56
Thickburgers: Original, ⅓ lb	820	51	56
Bacon Cheese, ⅓ lb	790	49	54
Frisco, ⅓ lb	760	50	43
Monster Double, ⅔ lb	1400	97	53
Mushroom 'N' Swiss, ⅓ lb	620	33	52
Original Beyond Meat	780	46	61
Double	1110	70	66
***All Star Meals:** Per Set Menu, without Dipping Sauce*			
Double Cheeseburger:			
w/ Spicy Chicken S'wich	1280	71	131
w/ Jumbo Hot Dog	1160	64	111
Sandwiches:			
Beef: Big Roast Beef	500	22	49
Monster Roast Beef	870	33	52
Big Hot Ham 'N' Cheese	530	20	51
Chicken: Big Chicken Fillet	590	29	61
Charbroiled Chicken Club	650	29	53
***Chicken Tenders:** Without Sauce*			
Hand Breaded:			
3 pieces, 4.5 oz	260	13	13
5 pieces, 7.5 oz	440	21	21
Boxes: 10 Pieces	880	42	42
15 Pieces	1320	63	63
20 Pieces	1760	84	84
Chili Dog, Jumbo	390	26	23
Natural Cut Fries:			
Kid's, 3 oz	240	12	31
Small, 3.7 oz	300	15	39
Medium, 5.9 oz	420	21	55
Large, 6.5 oz	460	22	59
Sides:			
Beer Battered Onion Rings	670	35	77
Crispy Curls:			
Small, 4.1 oz	310	15	39
Medium, 5.36 oz	420	21	53
Large, 6.5 oz	460	23	58
Side Salad	120	7	7

Hardee's® cont... (Oct '23)

Breakfast:	C	F	Cb
Bowls:			
Loaded Hash Round	510	36	30
Low Carb	760	68	0
Burritos: Beyond Sausage	730	41	51
Loaded	580	30	46
Southwest Omelet	690	41	44
Made From Scratch Biscuits:			
Bacon, Egg & Cheese	620	40	44
Beyond Sausage	480	26	44
with Egg	600	35	47
Biscuit 'N' Gravy	600	38	54
Chicken Fillet	660	43	50
Country Ham	510	32	42
Country Fried Steak	650	44	49
Loaded Omelet	630	41	46
Monster	890	63	45
Pork Chop 'N' Gravy	550	34	48
Sausage	630	45	42
with Egg	700	50	44
Smoked Sausage, Egg & Cheese	700	48	45
Platters: With Bacon	1050	68	76
With Chicken Fillet	980	58	63
With Country Ham	990	61	75
With Country Steak	970	60	62
With Pork Chop	990	56	66
With Sausage	1150	79	76
Sandwich, Frisco Breakfast	430	19	42
Sunrise Croissant: Bacon	420	26	29
Ham	390	23	29
Sausage	550	40	30
Breakfast Sides:			
Hash Rounds: Small, 2.9 oz	240	14	21
Medium, 4.2 oz	370	22	33
Large, 5.8 oz	490	29	43
Starpals Kids Meals: *Without Drink*			
Cheeseburger	530	22	55
Hamburger	480	18	54
Hot Dog	650	38	60
Desserts:			
Apple Turnover, w/out Cinnamon Sugar	270	13	35
Chocolate Chip Cookie, 1.5 oz	200	10	26
Ice Cream Shakes: *Per 14 oz*			
Hand Scooped: Chocolate	690	36	84
Strawberry	690	35	83
Vanilla	700	35	86

Hissho Sushi® (Oct '23)

Natural Food Store Menu Items	C	F	Cb
Maki Sushi Rolls: *Per Package*			
California, 11.5 oz	330	7	60
Dazzling Dragon, 13 oz	510	22	52
Krispy Krab, 9.8 oz	410	19	53
Living Color, 10.6 oz	340	11	40
Philadelphia, 11.4 oz	470	20	62
Rising Sun, 13.4 oz	680	40	50
Southern Charm, 9.8 oz	390	19	46
Spicy California, 13 oz	440	16	66
Spicy Salmon, 12 oz	420	15	53
Spicy Tuna, 12 oz	390	9	53
Sriracha Party, 10 oz	380	11	50
Tempura Shrimp, 12.87 oz	520	23	70
TNT, 10.3 oz	440	19	42
Veggie, 12 oz	320	7	60
Wasabi Crunch, 9.45 oz	290	9	43

Hot Dog on a Stick® (Oct '23)

Menu Items:	C	F	Cb
On A Stick: American Cheese	260	16	20
Beef Hot Dog	330	21	25
Pepper Jack Cheese	260	15	22
Turkey Hot Dog	240	5	27
Veggie Dog	200	6	26
Fish & Zucchini Platter	470	15	53
Fish Platter with Tartar Sauce	320	14	27
Zucchini Platter with Ranch Sauce	420	23	45
Condiments: Ketchup, 0.5 oz	10	0	3
Mayo, 0.5 oz	80	9	0
Sweet Relish, 0.3 oz	10	0	3
Yellow Mustard, 0.2 oz	5	0	1
French Fries: Small, 7.2 oz	500	29	57
Regular, 14.4 oz	1000	59	113
Funnel Cake Sticks:			
with Chocolate Sauce, 3.4 oz	300	6	48
with Powdered Sugar, 2.6 oz	210	5	26
with Raspberry Sauce, 3.4 oz	270	5	40
Beverages: *Per Regular Size, 16 fl.oz*			
Lemonade:			
Original	150	0	38
Cherry	210	0	52
Lime	230	0	57

Hungry Howie's Pizza® (Oct '23)

Pasta: Per Regular	C	F	Cb
Baked:			
Orig.; Pasta & Mushrms	450	12	64
Pasta & Meatballs	780	36	70
Chicken Parmesan	740	29	81
Specialty Pizza: *12" Pizza, Per ⅛ Slice*			
Bacon Cheddar Cheeseburger	270	13	25
BBQ Chicken	230	8	29
Buffalo Chicken	210	8	24
Howie Special	210	7	26
Meat Eaters	250	11	25
Works	250	11	26
Veggie	200	6	28
Spicy Chicken Tenders, each	130	7	9
Subs: *Per ½ of Large Sub, with Set Menu Toppings*			
Deluxe Combo	540	20	60
Ham & Cheese	590	23	62
Italian	620	27	62
Steak & Cheese	650	29	62
Veggie	580	24	69
Salads: *Regular Size, without Dressing*			
Antipasto	400	26	14
Chicken Asiago; Chicken Caesar, av.	230	9	15
Garden	90	3	14
Greek	230	11	18
Grilled Chicken	360	19	15
Spicy Chicken	640	36	39
Dressings: *Per Packet*			
Caesar	180	18	2
Greek	220	24	1
Ranch; Thousand Island, average	205	22	4

In-N-Out Burger® (Oct '23)

Burgers:	C	F	Cb
Hamburger: with Onion	390	19	39
w/ Mstrd & Ketchup, w/out Spread	310	10	41
Protein Style with Lettuce Wrap, without Bun	240	17	11
Cheeseburger: with Onion	480	27	39
w/ Mstrd & Ketchup, w/out Spread	400	18	41
Protein Style with Lettuce Wrap, without Bun, with Lettuce	330	25	11
Double Double: with Onion	670	41	39
w/ Mstrd & Ketchup, w/out Spread	590	32	41
Protein Style with Lettuce Wrap, without Bun	520	39	11
French Fries, 4.5 oz	370	15	52
Hot Cocoa: 8 fl.oz	130	3	26
with Marshmallows, 8 fl.oz	150	3	32
Shakes: *Per 15 fl.oz*			
Chocolate	580	39	95
Strawberry	590	24	114
Vanilla	570	30	65

IHOP® (Oct '23)

Crepes: With Menu Set Toppings	C	F	Cb
Fresh Berry	540	22	71
Lemon Ricotta Blueberry	540	24	68
Pancakes: *With Menu Set Toppings*			
Orig. Buttermilk with Wh. Butter (3)	450	18	59
Chocolate Chip w/- Wh. Topping (4)	770	25	123
Cinn-a-Stack w/- Wh. Topping (4)	870	29	136
French Toast: *With Menu Set Toppings*			
Lemon Ricotta Blueberry	950	39	125
Strawberry Banana	960	34	144
Waffles, Belgian w/- Wh. Butter	570	33	60
Omelettes: *As Served, without Extra Side Choices*			
Big Steak	1040	69	39
Chicken Fajita	900	58	21
Colorado	1270	100	18
Spicy Poblano	1090	88	23
Spinach & Mushroom	950	78	20
Breakfast Sides: Cripsy Potatoes	280	13	37
Hash Browns	220	14	20
Seasoned Fresh Fruit	50	0	14
Burgers: *With American Cheese, w/out Sides or Add Ons*			
Big Brunch: With Beef	1050	68	63
With Crispy Chicken	890	53	61
Cowboy BBQ: With Beef	1050	65	80
With Grilled Chicken	920	44	80
Jalapeno Kick: With Beef	1080	83	46
With Crispy Chicken	1050	72	62
The Classic: With Beef	780	53	45
With Crispy Chicken	750	42	62
With Grilled Chicken	630	32	45
Melts: *Without Add Ons, Sides*			
Buffalo Chicken	1250	76	88
Cali Roasted Turkey	1130	72	63
Philly Cheese Steak Stacker	820	47	55
Entrees: *Without Sides, Gravy or Bread*			
Buttermilk Crispy Chicken	550	27	36
Pot Roast	360	20	11
Salisbury Steak	680	56	11
Sirloin Steak Tips	510	31	21
Entree Sides: Brocc.w/-Garlic Butter	90	7	5
Garlic Bread	150	8	15
House Salad without Dressing	140	9	7
Loaded Mashed Potatoes	410	27	31
Mac & CHeese	350	20	32
Onion Rings	570	31	65
Red Skin Mshd Potatoes	240	13	30
Seasoned Fries	320	15	42
55+ Sandwiches: *Without Sides*			
BLT on White Bread	390	25	27
Roasted Turkey on Multigrain Bread	770	42	55

IHOP® cont... (Oct '23)

Bowls: Without Side Options	C	F	Cb
New Mexico Chicken	860	46	67
Southwest Chicken	1080	77	42
Spicy Shredded Beef	800	41	65
Spicy Shredded Beef	890	42	83
The Classic: With Bacon	850	63	30
With Pork Sausage	900	71	29
Burritos:			
New Mexico Chicken	1160	53	118
Southwest Chicken	1380	84	92
Spicy Shredded Beef	1100	49	115
The Classic with Bacon	1150	71	80

Jack in the Box® (Oct '23)

Sandwiches & Burgers:	C	F	Cb
Bacon Swiss Buttery Jack	810	53	48
Bacon Ultimate Cheeseburger	930	65	32
Cheeseburger	370	21	30
Classic Buttery Jack	790	51	51
Double Jack	830	58	33
Jumbo Jack	520	33	32
Jumbo Jack Cheeseburger	600	40	33
Sourdough Jack	700	45	39
Ultimate Cheeseburger	840	59	31
Chicken & Fish Sandwiches:			
Chicken Fajita Pita with Salsa	330	9	35
Chicken	510	32	40
Fish	450	23	47
H'style Ranch Chicken Club	700	36	60
Jack's Spicy Chicken	620	34	50
The Cluck Chicken	670	36	60
Chicken: Crispy Strips, 4 pieces	620	31	42
Nuggets, 5 pieces	240	17	13
Teriyaki Bowl	630	6	109
Breakfast:			
Biscuit: Bacon, Egg & Cheese	410	25	26
Sausage, Egg & Cheese	530	38	27
Breakfast Jack: Bacon	380	21	30
Ham	350	18	30
Sausage	500	34	30
Burrito: *With Salsa*			
Meat Lovers	810	51	50
Grand Sausage	1070	72	70
Croissants: Sausage	480	33	28
Supreme	370	21	28
Mini Pancakes (8), without syrup	140	2	28
Sandwiches: Extreme Sausage	650	49	29
Grilled Sourdough Swiss	580	34	36
Loaded	710	47	36
Ultimate	520	31	30

Jack in the Box® cont... (Oct '23)

Munchie Meals: Includes 2 Tacos, Halfsie Fries & 20 fl.oz Coke	C	F	Cb
Chick-N-Tater Melt	1940	103	215
Spicy Nacho Chicken S'wich	1880	89	227
Srircha Curly Fry Burger	1720	87	196
Stacked Gr. Cheese Burger	1870	92	211
Snacks & Sides:			
Bacon Cheddar Friess	580	34	54
Egg Roll (1)	210	12	20
French Fries: Small	300	14	40
Medium	430	20	58
Large	550	25	75
Panko Onion Rings (8)	440	24	52
Seasoned Curly Fries: Small	280	16	30
Medium	430	25	46
Large	480	28	52
Stuffed Jalapenos: 3 Pieces	220	12	21
7 Pieces	510	29	49
Salads: *Without Dressing or Toppings/Croutons*			
Chicken Club: Crispy Chicken Strips	540	31	29
Grilled Chicken	220	8	13
Side Salad	20	0	4
Southwest Chicken:			
Crispy Chicken Strips	530	26	45
Grilled Chicken	340	14	28
Croutons	70	3	9
Dressing: Creamy S'thwest, 1.75 oz	190	19	3
Ranch, 1.75 oz	250	25	5
Low Fat Balsamic Vinaigrette, 1.5 oz	25	2	3
Desserts: Mini Churros (5)	350	18	42
Choc. Overload Cake	300	7	57
NY Style Cheesecake	310	17	32
Ice Cream Shakes: *16 fl.oz, with Whipped Topping*			
Chocolate	680	23	107
Oreo Cookie	690	28	100
Strawberry	650	23	100
Vanilla	580	23	83

For Complete Nutritional Data ~ see Calorieking.com

Jack's® (Oct '23)

Burgers & Sandwiches:	C	F	Cb
Big Bacon	800	57	36
Big Jack	720	47	43
Cheeseburger	440	23	38
Double Cheeseburger	775	50	42
Hamburger	400	19	38
Fried Chicken: Breast	670	36	37
Drumstick	200	11	12
French Fries, large	380	23	39
Sides: Coleslaw, 4 oz	210	18	13
Mashed Potatoes, 4 oz	140	4	26
Breakfast: Hash Browns, regular	360	25	31
Bacon, Egg & Cheese Biscuit	520	36	32
Big Breakfast Sausage Sandwich	830	60	44

Jamba Juice® (Oct '23)

Freshly Squeezed Juice: *Medium*	C	F	Cb
Orange Carrot Twist	280	2	64
Purely Carrot	250	2	62
Purely Orange	310	2	71
Veggie Vitality	230	1	52
Smoothies: *Per Medium,, without Boosts or Add Ins*			
Classic:			
Aloha Pineapple	360	2	81
Caribbean Passion	330	2	80
Mango-A-Go-Go	390	2	96
Orange Dream Machine	420	2	91
PB Chocolate Love	670	25	99
Peanut Butter Moo'd	730	20	120
Razzamatazz	350	2	84
Strawberry Surf Rider	330	2	80
Strawberries Wild	320	0	77
Watermelon Breeze	410	2	98
Plant-Based: Apple 'n Greens	320	1	76
Greens 'n Ginger	290	1	70
Mega Mango	280	1	74
Peach Perfection	310	1	76
Pomegranate Paradise	320	1	79
Smooth Talkin' Mango	380	9	75
Strawberry Whirl	290	1	49
Vanilla Blue Sky	280	5	59
Super Blends:			
Acai Super-Antioxidant	430	6	88
PB & Banana Soy Protein	530	23	57
PB & Banana Whey Protein	650	25	71
Soy Protein Berry Workout	390	1	76
Tasty Bites:			
Baked Goods: *Per Item*			
Belgian Waffle	310	15	39
Cheddar Tomato Twist	250	6	41
Savory Pretzel	420	11	69
Sweet Pretzel	390	5	78
Breakfast Handwiches:			
Classic Sausage, Egg & Cheese	320	23	14
Impossible	220	12	16
Oatmeal, plain	170	3	31
Spring Veggie Egg Bake	200	14	8
Energy Bowls: *Per 16 fl.oz without Add-Ons*			
Acai Primo	520	11	103
Chunky Strawberry	610	18	96
Dragon Fruit Delight	500	8	105
Vanilla Blue Sky	320	9	60

Jersey Mike's Subs® (Oct '23)

Cold Subs: *Per Regular, on White Roll, with Standard Menu Components*	C	F	Cb
#1 BLT, with Mayo	750	47	59
#2 Jersey Shore Favorite	800	44	63
#3 Ham & Provolone	790	44	62
#5 Super Sub	810	44	65
#6 Roast Beef & Provolone	890	46	60
#7 Turkey & Provolone	790	41	61
#8 Club Sub with Mayonnaise	1130	77	63
#9 Club Supreme w/ Mayonnaise	1150	76	62
#10 Tuna	1030	74	62
#13 Original Italian	930	54	66
#14 Veggie	910	58	63
Hot Subs: *Per Reg., on White Roll, with Standard Menu Components*			
#16 Mike's Chicken Philly			
#17: Mike's Philly	650	22	65
#20 Grilled Pastrami Reuben	700	30	67
#42 Chipotle Chicken Cheese Steak	940	54	66
#43 Chipotle Cheese Steak	1000	62	67
#55 Big Kahuna Chkn Cheese Steak	700	27	67
#56 Big Kahuna Cheese Steak	770	35	67
French Fries: 5 oz	310	19	34
6 oz	370	23	41
Salads: *Without Dressing*			
Grilled Chicken	800	25	51
Tossed	180	2	39
Mini Breakfast Subs: *On White Bread, w/ Standard Menu Components, without Ketchup*			
#2: Bacon, Egg & Cheese	510	27	38
#3: Sausage, Egg & Cheese	880	64	38
#4: Ham, Egg & Cheese	490	23	39
#5: Steak, Egg & Cheese	540	23	38
Kid's: *On White Bun, with Standard Menu Components without Condiments*			
Ham Sub	220	6	30
Salami Sub	250	10	30
Turkey Sub	230	5	30
Desserts:			
Brownie, regular	500	28	63
Choc. Chip Cookie, mini	180	9	26
Tastykake: Butterscotch Krimpet (2)	220	7	39
Chocolate Kandy Cake (2)	190	10	20
Cream Filled Buttercream Cupcake (2)	270	10	43

Jimmy John's® (Oct '23)

Original Subs: (8") Figures Based on French Bread w/ Standard Menu Board Toppings	C	F	Cb
#1. Pepe	600	29	50
#2. Big John	500	21	47
#3. Totally Tuna	500	22	51
#4. Turkey Tom	480	19	48
#5. Vito	580	27	51
#6. Veggie	670	39	50
JJBLT	590	32	47
Favorite Subs : (8") Figures Based on French Bread. with Standard Menu Board Toppings			
#7. Spicy East Coast Italian	850	49	53
#8. Billy Club	810	33	73
#9. Italian Night Club	930	46	77
#10. Hunter's Club	830	34	70
#11. Country Club	780	31	74
#12. Beach Club	860	40	74
#13. Jimmy Cubano	720	38	47
#14. Bootlegger Club	680	23	71
#15. Club Tuna	850	42	75
#16. Club Lulu	690	26	71
#17. Ultimate Porker	690	28	72
***Plain Slims:** Figures Based on French Bread without Toppings, Dressing or Mayo*			
Slim 1. Ham & Provolone Cheese	540	13	69
Slim 2. Roast Beef	440	5	66
Slim 3. Tuna Salad	600	23	70
Slim 4 .Turkey Breast	420	3	68
Slim 5. Salami Capicola & Cheese	630	23	69
Slim 6. Double Provolone	590	21	68
Sides:			
Brownie, Fudge Chocolate	350	19	46
Cookies: Chocolate Chip, 3 oz	410	19	56
Oatmeal Raisin, 3 oz	370	13	57
Jimmy Chips: Average	290	17	33
Thinny	260	11	39
Jumbo Kosher Dill Pickle, 6.9 oz	20	0	3

Johnny Rockets® (Oct '23)

Starters:	C	F	Cb
Chili Bowl	620	50	20
Fries: Plain	330	10	50
Bacon Cheese	630	30	60
Cheese	540	30	60
Chili Cheese	820	50	70
Onion Rings	630	30	80
Tots: Plain	740	50	70
Bacon Cheese	1050	70	80
Cheese	960	70	80
Chili Cheese	1230	90	90

Johnny Rockets® cont... (Oct '23)

***Burgers:** Per Regular Size Bun*	C	F	Cb
Bacon Cheddar:			
Beef Burger	780	50	40
Boca Veggie Burger	680	40	50
Grilled Chicken	720	40	40
Original: Beef Burger	680	40	40
Gardein	640	40	70
Rocket: Beef Burger	690	40	40
Boca Veggie Burger	590	30	50
Turkey	810	60	40
Smokehouse: Beef Burger	800	40	70
Boca Veggie Burger	710	30	80
Gardein Burger	760	40	90
Spicy Houston:			
Beef Burger	640	40	40
Grilled Chicken	580	30	40
Turkey	770	50	40
Chicken, Tenders, BBQ Sauce	670	20	90
Hot Dogs:			
Rocket Dog	480	30	40
Rocket Chili Dog	670	50	40
Philly Cheese Steak, Beef	780	40	60
Melts:			
BBQ Chicken	940	30	100
Tuna on Sourdough	650	40	50
***Sandwiches:** On Sourdough, without Substitutions*			
BLT	690	50	50
Fried Chicken Club	910	50	70
Grilled Chicken Club	800	40	50
Grilled Cheddar Cheese	600	40	50
Sourdough Burger Melt	680	40	50
***Salads:** Without Dressing*			
Crispy Chicken Club	420	20	20
Grilled Chicken Club	400	20	10
Garden Salad	150	10	10
***Breakfast:** Standard, without Subsititutions*			
French Toast: 2 slices	620	10	100
3 slices	800	20	130
Pancakes: B'milk (2) w/ Sausage	1020	50	110
Buttermilk (2), with Bacon	700	20	110
Scramblers: Bacon Denver	1130	60	80
Biscuits, Sausage & Gravy	2010	130	120
Cheesy Bacon Lovers	1170	70	80
***Shakes:** Without Malt*			
Banana	830	40	90
Chocolate Baana	910	40	110
Hershey's Chocolate	920	40	110
Oreo Cookies & Cream	1020	50	120
Peanut Butter Banana	1050	60	100

For Complete Menu & Data ~ see CalorieKing.com

KFC® (Oct '23)

Chicken On The Bone: Per Piece	C	F	Cb
Original Recipe:			
Breast, 6 oz	390	21	11
Drumstick, 1.87 oz	130	8	4
Thigh, 3.7 oz	280	19	8
Whole Wing, 1.5 oz	130	8	3
Extra Crispy:			
Breast, 6.3 oz	530	35	18
Drumstick, 1.9 oz	170	12	5
Thigh, 3.5 oz	330	23	9
Whole Wing, 1.7 oz	170	13	5
Kentucky Grilled:			
Breast, 4.6 oz	210	7	0
Drumstick, 1.4 oz	80	4	0
Thigh, 2.5 oz	150	9	0
Whole Wing, 1 oz	70	3	0
Spicy Crispy:			
Breast, 5.2 oz	350	20	11
Drumstick, 1.6 oz	130	8	5
Thigh, 2.8 oz	270	20	10
Whole Wing, 1.2 oz	120	8	5
Chicken			
Extra Crispy Tenders, each	140	7	8
Fried Nuggets, each	35	2	1
Nashville Hot Spicy Crispy:			
Breast	540	40	14
Drumstick	190	14	6
Thigh	390	32	12
Whole Wing	180	15	5
Famous Bowls & Pot Pie:			
Chicken Pot Pie, 14 oz	720	41	60
Famous Bowl, regular	590	23	67
***Salads:** W/out Dressing or Croutons*			
Caesar side	40	2	2
House Side Salad	15	0	3
Salad Dressings & Croutons:			
ButtermilkDressing	160	17	1
Creamy Parmesan Caesar	260	26	4
Light Italian Dressing	15	1	2
Original Fat Free Ranch	35	0	8
Parmesan Garlic Croutons	60	3	8

KFC® cont... (Oct '23)

Condiments:	C	F	Cb
Colonel's ButterySpread	35	4	0
Grape Jelly	35	0	9
Lemon Juice Packet	5	0	1
Strawberry Jam	35	0	9
Dipping Sauces:			
Per 0.9 oz Container			
BBQ Dipping Sauce Cup	45	0	11
Colonel's Buttery Spread	35	4	0
Honey Musard Dipping Sauce	110	9	6
Honey Sauce; Ketchup	30	0	8
KFC Dipping Sauce Cup	90	8	5
Ranch Dipping Sauce Cup	130	14	2
Sandwiches:			
Chicken Littles,			
Extra Crispy Tender	300	15	27
Classic Chicken	650	35	49
Crispy Twister	630	34	53
Spicy Chicken	620	33	49
***Homestyle Sides:** Per Individual Portion*			
BBQ Baked Beans, 4.25 oz	190	1	34
Biscuit	180	8	22
Coleslaw, 4.2 oz	170	12	14
Corn on the Cob, 2.5 oz	70	1	17
Green Beans	25	0	5
Mac. & Cheese, 4.8 oz	140	6	17
Mashed Potatoes, 4.2 oz	110	4	17
Mashed Potatoes with Gravy, 5 oz	130	5	20
Potato Salad	340	28	19
Sweet Kernel Corn, 2.75 oz	70	1	16
Kids, Fried Chicken Nuggets (5)	170	8	7
Desserts:			
Apple Turnover, 2.9 oz	230	10	32
Cafe Valley: Choc. Chip Cake, 1 slice	300	15	39
Mini Choc. Chip Cake (1)	300	12	49
Lemon Cake, 1 slice	220	10	30
Mini Lemon Cake	300	13	43

Krispy Kreme® (Oct '23)

Doughnuts:	C	F	Cb
Cake Batter	350	18	45
Chocolate Iced: Custard Filled	360	15	37
Glazed	240	11	33
With Sprinkles	260	11	36
Kreme Filling	350	19	41
Glazed: Blueberry Cake	300	15	40
Cinnamon Roll	280	11	42
Lemon Filled	290	15	37
Raspberry Filled	300	15	38
Original	190	11	22
Strawberry Iced with Sprinkles	260	12	36
Holes, Original Glazed (1)	45	3	5
Mini Doughnuts:			
Glazed: Chocolate Iced	120	5	19
With Sprinkles	130	5	20
Original	90	5	11
Strawberry Iced with Sprinkles	130	5	20
Hot Beverages:			
Chocolate: 12 fl.oz	410	12	63
16 fl.oz	490	14	76
20 fl.oz	610	17	99
Cappuccino: 12 fl.oz	120	4	12
16 fl.oz	150	5	15
20 fl.oz	190	7	20
Latte with Whipped Cream: *Per 16 fl.oz*			
Caramel Mocha Specialty	350	10	50
Caramel Specialty	450	11	73
Mocha Specialty	400	11	62
Frozen Lattes: *Per 16 fl.oz with Whipped Cream*			
Caramel Specialty	420	17	62
Caramel Mocha Specialty	410	17	60
Original Glazed Specialty	330	10	56
Frozen Lemonade Chiller, 16 fl.oz	280	0	73
Iced: *Per 16 fl.oz with Whipped Cream,*			
Caramel Specialty Latte	400	11	67
Caramel Mocha Specialty	300	11	44
Mocha Specialty	340	11	54

For Complete Menu & Data ~ See CalorieKing.com

Krystal® (Oct '23)

Krystals:	C	F	Cb
Bacon Cheese	210	12	15
Original	150	7	14
with Cheese	170	9	14
Double	250	14	22
with Cheese	300	18	22
Chik, regular/spicy	400	25	29
Pups: Chili Cheese Pup	250	15	19
Classic	200	10	20
Fries:			
Chili Cheese	620	40	49
French Fries: Small	220	14	21
Medium	300	19	29
Large	440	28	42
Junkyard: Fries	790	57	50
Tots	830	64	45
Tots: Small	260	19	20
Medium	330	24	25
Large	480	35	37
Chili Cheese	670	47	44
Sauces:			
Honey Mustard; Ranch, average	130	12	2
Sweet & Sour/Baby Rays BBQ, av.	50	0	13
Wings, (10)	1030	83	30
Breakfast:			
3 Egg Plates:			
Biscuit, Bacon & Grits	740	37	74
Biscuit, Sausage & Tots	1050	75	64
Biscuits: Bacon, Egg & Cheese	430	28	31
Chik	530	32	45
Sausage, Egg & Cheese	650	51	30
Scramblers:			
Original: with Bacon	330	21	17
with Sausage	520	41	16
Low-Carb Scramblers:			
with Bacon	500	36	3
with Sausage	880	76	1
Sunriser	450	35	18
Sides: Grits, bowl	180	4	35
Tots, small	260	19	20
Dessert, Apple Turnover	370	26	33
Hand-Spun Shakes: *Regular*			
Chocolate	580	15	102
Oreo	580	19	89
Strawberry	480	14	79
Vanilla	440	14	68

For Complete Menu & Data ~ see CalorieKing.com

LaRosa's Pizzeria® (Oct '23)

Classic Specialty Pizzas:	C	F	Cb
Hand Tossed: *Per Slice, 1/8 of 12" Medium Pizza*			
Chicken Bacon Ranch	330	18	29
Double Pepperoni	290	13	30
Hawaiian	280	11	33
Zesty BBQ Chicken	290	10	34
Traditional: *Per Slice, 1/12 of 14" Large Pizza*			
Chicken Bacon Ranch	290	18	18
Double Pepperoni	230	13	19
Hawaiian	240	11	21
Zesty BBQ Chicken	240	11	23
Deluxe Pizzas:			
Hand Tossed: *Per Slice, 1/8 of 14" Large Pizza*			
Buddy	490	24	47
Meat	560	30	46
Original	490	23	47
Veggie	370	12	48
Pan: *Per Slice, 1/8 of 14" Large Pizza*			
Buddy	510	26	47
Meat	580	31	46
Original	500	25	47
Veggie	380	13	48
Hoagies: *With White Bun & Provolone Cheese*			
Baked Meatball & Pasta Sauce	810	36	89
Fried Cod, w/ Tartar Sce & Provolone	820	28	99
Steak w/ Tomato, Onion & Mayo	880	48	71
Pasta Entrees: *Without Bread, Soup or Salad*			
Lasagna, with Meat Sauce	1040	62	77
Ravioli: Cheese, with Pasta Sauce	750	29	89
Meat, with Pasta Sauce	730	26	89
Spaghetti, 3 Meatballs & Pasta Sce	1010	32	146
Ziti, Chicken Alfredo	890	27	112
Salad : *Entree, without Dressing or Breadstick*			
Antipasto for One	370	26	14
Crispy Chicken	500	27	36
Grilled Chicken	280	11	11
JoJo BLT	160	11	9
Tossed Garden	160	9	11
Salad Dressings: *Per 2 oz Cup*			
Blue Cheese	280	30	2
Honey French	250	19	18
Italian	320	34	4
Soup: *With 2 Packets Saltine Crackers*			
Baked Onion	220	9	29
Minestrone	120	2	24

LaRosa's Pizzeria® cont... (Oct '23)

Appetizers:	C	F	Cb
Cheesy Flatbread, w/ Pizza Sauce	1480	88	117
Fried Mozz. Chse Stick w/ Pizza Sce	640	35	46
Garlic Fries, w/ Ranch Dressing	920	65	76
Rondos:			
Pepperoni, with Pizza Sauce	1410	84	115
Spinach, with Pizza Sauce	1290	71	114
Traditional Wings with Sauce: *Without Sauce Cup*			
BBQ (5)	400	23	19
Diablo (5)	470	31	17
Garlic-Romano (5)	610	51	9

La Salsa Fresh Mexican® (Oct '23)

Breakfast:	C	F	Cb
Burritos: Chicken	660	30	56
Steak	700	36	55
Huevos Ranchero Platter:			
Chicken	500	14	59
Chorizo	610	27	61
Steak	550	20	58
Taco	200	10	14
Burritos: *Without Chips*			
Black Beans & Cheese:	720	37	62
with Carnitas	820	41	62
with Grilled Chicken	810	40	63
California Steak, w/ Black Beans	830	39	81
Grande, Black Beans:			
with Carnitas/Chicken, average	750	31	79
with Steak	810	38	80
Pinto Beans & Cheese: no meat	810	37	79
with Carnitas	910	42	79
with Steak	970	49	80
Overstuffed Burrito:			
with Carnitas	860	35	56
with Grilled Chicken	860	32	59
with Steak	980	49	58
Platters:			
Enchiladas:			
Pinto Beans: Carnitas; Chicken, av.	985	53	59
Cheese	850	49	58
Steak	1070	63	59
Taquitos & Quesadillas:			
Pinto Beans: Carnitas; Chicken, av.	1600	76	134
Cheese	1470	72	129
Steak	1660	84	134
Three Pepper Fajita Flour Tortilla:			
Black Beans: Carnitas	700	29	55
Chicken	690	27	58
Steak	820	44	57
Tacos: *Without Chips*			
Baja Grilled Fish	260	12	23
Baja Shrimp	250	9	23
Guadalajara Carnitas	300	17	22

La Salsa Fresh Mex® cont... (Oct '23)

Favorites: Without Chips	C	F	Cb
Classic Quesadillas: Carnitas	980	58	59
Cheese	880	54	59
Chicken	980	57	60
Steak	1040	65	60
Fire Roasted Bowls:			
Black Beans: Carnitas	510	18	54
Chicken	500	16	55
Steak	570	25	55
Nachos:			
Black Beans: with Carnitas	1150	56	93
with Chicken	1150	54	95
with Steak	1210	63	94
Pinto Beans:			
with Carnitas	1190	56	101
with Chicken	1170	54	98
with Steak	1230	63	98
Stuffed Fajita Quesadilla:			
Carnitas	930	49	59
Cheese	830	45	59
Chicken	930	48	60
Steak	990	57	60

Little Caesars® (Oct '23)

Large 14" Pizza: Per ⅛ Pizza	C	F	Cb
Classic: Beef, seasoned	275	11	32
Cheese	245	8	31
Italian Sausage	285	11	32
Pepperoni	290	12	31
Detroit Style Specialty Deep Dish:			
3 Meat Treat; 5 Meat Treat, av.	435	22	40
Hula Hawaiian	335	11	43
Ultimate Supreme	380	16	42
Veggie	340	12	42
***Caesar Wings:** Per 8 Wing*			
BBQ	620	35	32
Buffalo	510	35	3
Garlic Parmesan	670	51	5
Oven Roasted	510	35	3
***Caesar Dips:** Per 1.5 oz Container*			
Buffalo Ranch	230	23	4
Butter Garlic Flavor	370	42	0
Cheezy Jalapeno	210	21	3
Ranch	230	23	4
Bread: Crazy Bread, 1 stick	100	3	16
Italian Cheese Bread	135	6	14
Crazy Sauce, 1 cup	30	0	7

Long John Silver's® (Oct '23)

Sandwiches:	C	F	Cb
Baja Fish	410	21	40
Fish	400	16	44
***Seafood:** Without Sides*			
Baked Cod, 1 piece, 6 oz	160	1	1
Battered Alaskan Cod, 1 piece, 3 oz	190	11	9
Breaded Clam Strips	340	20	35
Lobster Stuffed Crab Cake (1), 2.2 oz	280	15	26
Popcorn Shrimp, 3 oz	210	9	24
Grilled:			
Rice Bowls: Seasoned Salmon	360	8	45
Seasoned Shrimp	360	8	47
Southwest Salmon	420	15	45
Southwest Shrimp	420	16	48
Sweet Chili Salmon	370	9	48
Sweet Chili Shrimp	390	11	51
Tacos: Baja Salmon (1)	210	9	23
Seasoned Shrimp (1)	180	5	23
Southwest Salmon (1)	220	9	23
Sauces & Condiments:			
Dipping Sauces: BBQ, 1 oz	40	0	10
Cocktail; Marinara, av.	20	0	4
Sweet & Sour 1 oz	45	0	12
Other Sauces & Condiments:			
Honey Mustard, 0.4 oz packet	60	6	2
Ketchup, 1oz pouch	30	0	8
Louisiana Hot Sauce, 1 tsp	0	0	0
Tartar Sauce, 0.5 oz packet	40	4	3
Sides: Baked Potato, 12 oz	295	0	67
Battered Onion Rings, 4 oz	480	35	39
Breaded Mozzarella Sticks (3)	370	23	24
Broccoli Cheese Bites, 5 pieces	310	24	18
Broccoli Cheese Soup, 1 bowl, 7.4 oz	220	18	8
Clam Chowder, 1 bowl, 8 oz	230	16	16
Cole Slaw, 4 oz	170	11	18
Corn Kernels, 4 oz	160	8	19
Crumblies, 1 oz	170	12	13
Green Beans, 4 oz	25	0	4
Hushpuppies, 2 pcs	150	7	19
Jalapeno Peppers (1)	15	0	2
Macaroni & Cheese, 4 oz	150	6	19
Rice, 5 oz	180	1	37
Fries, 3.7 oz	350	17	44
Dessert: Choc. Chip Cookie (1)	190	11	22
Chocolate Cream Pie, 1 slice	280	17	28
Strawberry Swirl Cheesecake, 1 sl.	320	17	35

For Complete Menu & Data ~ see CalorieKing.com

Macaroni Grill® (Oct '23)

Antipasti: As Served	C	F	Cb
Calamari Fritti	760	55	33
Caprese Salad	510	44	15
Crispy Brussels Sprouts	370	25	37
Crispy Fresh Mozzarella	820	79	17
Mac & Cheese Bites	920	70	44
Spinach & Artichoke Dip	1100	61	109
Stuffed Mushrooms	510	38	20
Land & Sea: *With Menu Set Sides*			
Braised Lamb Shank	1350	101	29
Chicken Marsala	790	32	61
Chicken Scaloppine	1240	76	83
Grilled Salmon	930	45	82
Shrimp Portofino	1200	78	93
Steak & Potatoes & Rosemary Butter	1250	94	34
Pasta: Butternut Tortellaci	980	66	63
Fettuccine Alfredo	1140	56	114
with Chicken	1370	72	117
with Shrimp	1310	71	115
Mama's Trio	2110	129	140
Mushroom Ravioli	930	66	53
Pasa Milano	1040	39	123
Penne Rustica	1060	52	82
Seafood Ravioli	920	74	36
Truffle Mac & Cheese	1060	89	24
Sandwiches: *Boxed Lunch*			
Chicken Parmesan	1490	79	144
Italian Pesto Caprese	1470	92	132
Meatball	1670	92	142
Sides:			
Broccolini	100	7	7
Buttermilk Mashed Potatoes	480	40	21
Crispy Brussels Sprouts	190	13	18
Grilled Asparagus	150	14	3
Parmesan Fries	610	32	74
Rosemary Peasant Bread	480	6	89
Sauteed Spinach	220	18	7
Spinach & Sundried Tomato Pasta	530	24	71
Kids:			
Chicken Strips w/- Broccolini & Fries	860	45	67
Fettuccine Alfredo	470	24	42
Macaroni & Cheese	540	31	44
Spaghetti, with Pomodoro Sauce	290	8	43

Macaroni Grill® cont... (Oct '23)

Salads: With Menu Set Dressing	C	F	Cb
Bibb & Bleu: with Salmon	830	57	14
with Shrimp	590	43	18
Italian Chopped	490	34	20
Parmesan Crusted Chicken	1080	48	100
Rosa's Signature Caesar	470	41	14
with Chicken	630	41	15
with Salmon	990	77	18
Dessert: Decadent Choc. Cake	1090	88	79
Chocolate Chip Cookie	300	13	45
NY Style Cheesecake	690	41	70
Romano's Cannoli	640	32	69
Tiramisu	600	39	54

Manhattan Bagel® (Oct '23)

Bagels: Per Bagel	C	F	Cb
Blueberry	310	1	67
Cheddar	300	1	60
Chocolate Chip	290	3	58
Cinnamon Raisin	310	1	63
Everything	330	3	62
Plain; Salt, average	305	1	64
Gourmet: Asiago	340	4	60
California Power	310	4	59
Cheesy Hash Brown	390	11	59
Cream Cheese: *Per 1.2 oz*			
Plain	120	12	2
Onion & Chive	110	10	4
Reduced Fat: Honey Almond	120	9	10
Strawberry	120	9	9
Sandwiches:			
Deli:			
BLT on Multigrain Bread	510	34	34
Chicken Salad Croissant	650	44	45
Ham & Swiss on Sesame Bagel	580	17	67
Nova Lox	690	34	71
Turkey & Cheddar	610	39	37
Signature Lunch Sandwiches:			
Avocado Veg Out	470	14	74
Ellis Isl. Hot Pastrami	560	15	67
Manhattan Cheesesteak	660	30	59
Soup, Chicken Noodle, 8 fl.oz	110	4	12
Breakfast Sandwiches:			
Plain Bagel: Cheese	490	15	65
Bacon & Cheese	540	19	66
Pork Roll & Cheese	720	33	67
Croissant: Bacon & Cheese	650	41	44
Ham & CHeese	650	39	45
Sausage & Cheese	830	60	44

Marie Callender's® (Oct '23)

Appetizers: As Served	C	F	Cb
Crispy Chicken Tenders, 12.9 oz	870	47	72
Crispy Green Beans, 10.5 oz	810	52	75
Mozzarella Sticks, 8.6 oz	690	42	46
Onion Rings	1150	63	129
***Burgers and Sandwiches:** With Fries*			
Original Burger	1290	87	84
Albacore Tuna Melt	1430	92	99
Callender's Cheeseburger	1450	99	85
Frisco Chicken Breast	1290	81	95
Meatloaf on Parm. Sourdough	1250	78	96
Roasted Turkey Croissant Club	1450	97	95
Main Meals:			
Comfort Classics: *With Menu Set Sides & Sauces*			
Braised & Slow Rstd Pot Roast	740	39	39
Chicken & Broccoli Fettuccine	1090	49	98
Crispy Fish & Shrimp Platter	1700	97	143
Home-Style Beef Stroganoff	850	30	99
Home-Style Meatloaf Dinner	610	35	34
Honey Ginger Glazed Salmon	570	30	29
Roasted Turkey Dinner	730	36	65
Shrimp & Chicken Carbonara	1140	50	93
Pies, Chicken Pot Pie, w/out sides	1140	79	70
Savory Skillets: *With Herb Rice & Set Sauces*			
Kickin' Chicken Bacon Broccoli	720	37	40
Spicy Beef & Chicken	790	54	27
Thai Shrimp	730	43	52
Salads:			
Cobb without Dressing	570	31	15
Combo Caesar with Caesar Dressing	240	18	9
Honey Mstd Chkn Crunch w/ dressing	950	61	54
Trad. Caesar w/ Caesar Dressing	490	35	28
Sides: Almond Coleslaw	250	21	14
Cornbread, w/ Honey Spread	340	21	33
French Fries, 4 oz	380	20	45
House Dinner Salad without dressing	160	8	15
Loaded Mashed Potatoes, 6.2 oz	340	23	23
Macaroni & Cheese, 6.4 oz	230	9	26
Tater Tots, 5 oz	330	20	33
***Soups:** Per Bowl*			
Chicken Tortilla	230	10	26
Clam Chowder	270	13	22
Hearty Vegetable	90	3	13
Potato Cheese	590	40	49
***Breakfast:** With Menu Set Items*			
Classics: Croissant Sandwich	1100	70	76
Calif. Eggs Benedict	830	53	66
Triple Egg Dare Ya	1380	71	132

Marie Callender's® cont... (Oct '23)

Breakfast (Cont.):	C	F	Cb
Griddle Greats: *As Served*			
Banana Crm Pie P'cakes w/Wh. Crm	800	28	118
Belgian Waffles	600	19	99
Buttermilk Pancakes (3)	670	28	92
Old Fashioned French Toast	830	31	123
Omelets, w/out Tater Tots: BTA	1210	66	103
Oh My	1340	74	98
Veggie	570	37	23
Quiche: *As Served*			
Bacon; Veggie, average, 1 slice	990	79	44
Ham, 1 slice	1030	81	40
***Desserts:** Per Slice Unless Indicated*			
NY Style Cheesecake, slice	740	52	58
Pies: Cream Cheese	620	38	63
Banana Cream, with Meringue	510	24	66
Kahlua Cream Cheese	670	36	76

Max & Erma's® (Oct '23)

Shareables: As Served	C	F	Cb
Chicken Fajita Quesadillas	1250	78	80
Knock Out Nachos	1570	100	116
Loaded Tots	1230	90	71
Potato Skins	1970	95	231
Wings with Blue Cheese Dressing:			
Cherry Cola BBQ	1990	120	95
Sweet Chili	1830	120	53
***Burgers & Sanwiches:** Without Fries*			
BBQ Pulled Pork Sandwich	760	33	71
Big Ol' Buffalo Chicken Sandwich	1370	71	144
Bodalicious Bacon Burger	1230	83	59
Cola BBQ Bacon Burger	1510	99	94
Garbage Burger, 6 oz	1680	126	61
Irish Boss Burger	1410	96	67
Sauteed Mushrm & Swiss Burger	1200	85	53
Tortilla Burger	1270	84	62
Turkey Avocado Swiss Burger	830	55	35
***Salads:** Entrée Size, with Dressing, without Breadstick*			
3rd Street	1160	100	41
Grilled Chicken Santa Fe	1090	83	46
Mediterranean Salmon	610	42	16
Village	410	39	13
Garlic Breadstick	160	6	23
Sides: Baked Potato, plain	220	0	51
Creamy Coleslaw	160	12	14
Fresh Fruit Salad	100	0	25
Mashed Potatoes	270	14	32
Seasoned Fries	360	17	49
Steamed Broccoli	30	1	6
Tater Tot	320	19	33
Dessert: Banana Cream Pie	790	37	107
Chocolate Cake a la Mode	1600	82	206

McAlister's Deli® (Oct '23)

Sandwiches: *W/- Menu Set Ingredients Without Sides*	C	F	Cb
Black Angus Club On Wheat Bread	940	51	75
French Dip on 6" Baguete	660	30	45
Grilled Chicken Club on Wheat Bread	890	41	79
Harvest Chicken Salad on Croissant	690	44	53
McAlister's Club n Wheat Bread	870	42	80
Reuben on Marbled Rye Bread990	50	80	
Sweet Chipotle Chicken on Ciabatta	700	19	83
Giant Spuds: Bl. Angus Roast Beef	1020	31	134
Chipotle Chicken & Bacon	1200	46	139
Spud Max	1070	40	135
Sides: Mac & Cheese	220	12	20
Potato Salad	230	14	20
Steamed Broccoli	100	8	6
Tomato & Cucumber Salad	70	4	6

Mellow Mushroom® (Oct '23)

Burgers:	C	F	Cb
Mel's Classic	900	52	59
Pizzaiola	1400	93	65
Ritz Burger	1150	75	62
Hoagies, Whole: *With French Hoagie*			
Chicken & Cheese	1360	78	94
Italian	1290	78	88
Meatball	810	29	93
Steak & Cheese	1600	107	89
Munchies: Bruschetta	330	24	24
Magic M'shrm Soup	350	24	15
Meatball Trio	360	24	11
Spinach & Artichoke Dip	760	44	67
Wings: *Without Extras*			
Hot(10)	580	33	32
Sweet Thai Chili (10)	780	33	60
Pizzas: *With Baked Crust, Per Medium Slice*			
Buffalo Chicken	510	31	46
Funky Q Chicken	440	20	51
Kosmic Karma	421	22	48
Salads: *Per Regular Size*			
Caesar, with Caesar Dressing	830	75	19
Greek, without Dressing	280	17	17
Dressing, Balsamic Vinaigrette, 1 oz	90	8	5
Desserts: *With Whipped Cream*			
Time For A Sundae:			
with a Brownie	800	48	85
with PB Cookie	970	56	104
with Sugar Cookie	1020	57	114
with Triple Chocolate Chunk Cookie	990	53	122

McDonald's® (Oct '23)

Beef Burgers:	C	F	Cb
Big Mac	590	34	46
Cheeseburger: Regular	300	13	32
Double	450	24	34
Double Quarter Pounder, w/ Cheese	740	42	43
Hamburger	250	9	31
McDouble	400	20	33
Quarter Pounder: with Cheese	520	26	42
with Cheese Deluxe	630	37	44
with Cheese & Bacon	630	35	43
Chicken Sandwiches:			
Deluxe McCrispy	530	26	48
Filet-O-Fish, regular bun	390	19	39
McChicken	400	21	39
McCrispy	470	20	46
Spicy McCrispy	530	26	48
Spicy Deluxe McCrispy	530	26	49
Chicken McNuggets:			
4 pieces	170	10	10
6 pieces	250	15	15
10 pieces	410	24	26
Sauces: *Per Packet*			
Creamy Ranch	110	12	1
Honey Mustard	60	4	6
Mayonnaise	90	10	0
Mustard	0	0	0
Spicy Buffalo	30	3	1
Sweet 'N Sour; Honey, average	50	0	12
Tangy BBQ	45	0	11
Happy Meals: *Includes Small Fries, Milk Jug & Apple Slices*			
Chicken McNuggets Meal:			
with 4 nuggets	515	23	57
with 6 nuggets	595	28	62
Hamburger	475	16	62
Meals: *Includes Small Black Coffee & Hash Browns*			
Biscuit: Bacon, Egg & Cheese	605	34	58
Sausage, Egg & Cheese	675	43	57
McGriddle: Bacon, Egg &Cheese	575	29	63
Sausage, Egg & Cheese	695	41	63
McMuffin: Egg	455	21	49
Sausage, Egg & Cheese	625	39	49
French Fries: Kids, 1.3 oz	110	5	15
Small, 2.6 oz	230	11	31
Medium, 3.9 oz	320	15	43
Large, 5.9 oz	480	23	65
Ketchup, packet	10	0	2

McDonald's® cont... (Oct '23)

Breakfast:	C	F	Cb
Big Breakfast	760	48	57
with Hotcakes	1340	63	158
Biscuits: Bacon, Egg & Cheese	460	26	39
Sausage	460	30	37
Sausage with Egg	530	35	38
Fruit & Maple Oatmeal, with Apples, Cranberries & Light Cream	320	5	64
Hash Brown, 2 oz	140	8	18
Hotcakes: with Syrup	580	15	101
with Sausage & Syrup	770	33	102
McGriddles: Sausage	430	24	41
Sausage, Egg & Cheese	550	33	44
McMuffin: Egg	310	13	30
Sausage & Egg	480	31	30
Snacks, Apple Slices, pkt	15	0	4
McFlurry's:			
M&M's Candy, regular	640	21	96
Oreo Cookies, regular	510	16	80
Shakes:			
Chocolate: Small	520	14	85
Medium	650	17	107
Large	800	20	134
Strawberry: Small	470	13	77
Medium	600	16	99
Large	850	21	143
Vanilla: Small	480	13	80
Medium	570	15	97
Large	780	19	133
Sundaes:			
Hot Caramel	330	7	58
Hot Fudge	330	10	51
Vanilla Cone	200	5	33
Beverages:			
Milk: 1% Low Fat Milk Jug	100	2	12
Low Fat, Red. Sugar Choc Milk Jug	130	3	18
Orange Juice: Small	150	0	36
Medium	190	0	45
Large	270	0	65
Sweet Tea, Iced: Small	100	0	26
Medium	130	0	31
Large	170	0	43
McCafe Bakery:			
Baked Apple Pie	230	11	33
Chocolate Chip Cookie	170	8	22

McDonald's® cont... (Oct '23)

McCafe Beverages:	C	F	Cb
Cappuccino: *With Whole Milk*			
Regular: Small, 16 fl.oz	110	5	10
Medium, 22 fl.oz	160	7	14
Large	200	10	18
Caramel: Small	210	5	35
Medium	260	6	44
Large	340	8	55
French Vanilla: Small	210	5	37
Medium	260	6	47
Large	340	8	58
Frappes: *With Whipped Cream & Drizzle*			
Caramel, medium	490	20	70
Mocha, medium	490	20	72
Iced Coffee: *With Standard ingredients*			
Regular: Small, 16 fl.oz	140	5	24
Medium, 22 fl.oz	190	6	32
Large, 30 fl.oz	260	9	45
Caramel: Small, 16 fl.oz	140	5	23
Medium, 22 fl.oz	190	7	31
Large, 30 fl.oz	270	9	46
Iced Mocha: *With Whole Milk, Whipped Cream & Drizzle*			
Small	280	10	39
Medium	320	11	48
Large	450	15	69
Lattes: *With Whole Milk*			
Regular: Small	140	8	12
Medium	190	10	15
Large	250	13	20
Caramel: Small	250	7	39
Medium	320	8	50
Large	390	11	60
French Vanilla: Small	250	6	39
Medium	310	8	50
Large	390	11	60
Iced Regular: Small	90	5	7
Medium	120	6	10
Large	170	8	15
Macchiato: *With Whole Milk*			
Hot Caramel: Small	260	6	41
Medium	320	8	51
Large	400	10	62
Iced Caramel: Small	200	5	33
Medium	240	6	41
Large	360	9	59
Smoothie: *With Standard ingredients*			
Mango Pineapple, medium	250	1	57
Strawberry Banana, medium	240	1	55

Mimi's Cafe® (Oct '23)

Bakery:	C	F	Cb
Just Baked Croissants: All Butter	360	20	38
Almond	370	20	40
Just Baked Muffins: Blueb. Crumble	590	30	74
Buttermilk Spice	575	21	85
Carrot Raisin Nut	520	27	64
Chocolate Chip	865	44	105
Breakfast: *Without Potatoes*			
Benedicts: Eggs, Original	645	39	34
Corned Beef Hash	730	44	46
Smoked Salmon	605	39	33
Add Roasted Potatoes	150	5	23
French Toast Items: *Without Side Options*			
Brioche	595	23	74
Cinnamon Roll	715	29	95
Griddlecakes: *With Eggs, Any Style*			
Berry	1030	38	135
Buttermilk	1025	44	120
3 Egg Omelets: *With Roasted Potatoes*			
Bacon Avocado	920	65	30
Hickory-Smoked Ham & Cheese	675	45	27
Mushroom Bacon & Brie	775	56	28
Smoked Salmon	555	35	24
Malted Berry Waffles:			
with Eggs any style	585	28	61
with Pork Sausage	790	49	61
Lunch & Dinner: *Without Side Choices*			
Burgers: Brioche Cheeseburger	775	41	56
Hickory Bacon Cheddar	945	50	68
Mushroom & Brie	890	51	51
The French Quarter	1285	90	48
Sandwiches: Croque Monsieur	835	42	62
French Dip	585	14	70
Grilled Chicken Pesto Baguette	920	47	56
Roasted Chicken Croque Monsieur	1090	64	57
Turkey Hummus	560	25	54
West Coast Reuben	1335	72	99
Entrees:			
Beer Battered Fish & Fries	1185	78	79
Coastal Shrimp Pasta	1035	53	99
French Pot Roast	515	32	22
Mimi's Meatloaf	445	25	15
Slow Roasted Turkey	700	29	69
Sides: Broccoli	115	9	5
Coleslaw	250	23	7
French Fries	125	3	22
Garlic Spinach	70	4	4
Mashed Potatoes	130	4	21
Potatoes au Gratin	490	32	32
Roasted Potatoes	150	5	23

Mr. Goodcents® (Oct '23)

Cold Subs:	C	F	Cb
Per 8" White Bread Sub with Standard Toppings			
Bologna	760	45	64
Centsable	660	33	64
Garden Veggie without Cheese	480	19	67
Goodcents Original	730	43	62
Oven Roasted Chicken Breast	540	19	58
Penny Club	530	19	59
Pepperoni	990	81	56
Tuna Salad	690	37	64
Toasted Sub: *Per 8" Wheat Bread Sub with Standard Toppings*			
Chicken Bacon Ranch	660	27	57
Chipotle Cheesesteak	630	28	65
Meatball	790	35	66
Pasta To Go: Chicken Alfredo	700	34	62
Chicken Tortellini	680	33	57
Pasta with Meatballs	690	25	78
Soup: *Per 16 fl.oz Bowl*			
Broccoli Cheese	390	26	28
Chicken Homestyle Noodle	160	5	22

Mr. Hero® (Oct '23)

7" Subs & Burgers: *Per Medium*	C	F	Cb
Burgers:			
Cheeseburger	1110	76	67
Romanburger	1235	87	69
Romanburger BTE	1535	111	73
Chicken Subs:			
Chicken Bacon Ranch	890	43	66
Chicken Philly	770	32	69
Deli Subs:			
Italiano	920	46	87
Original Italian	830	44	77
Tuna 'N Cheese	1030	82	68
Turkey	490	4	75
Steak Subs:			
Sicilian Parm	1075	70	61
Zesty Bacon & Swiss	1010	62	60
Sides: *Per Regular Size*			
Mozzarella Sticks	505	33	37
Onion Petals	545	36	52
Potato Waffers	360	27	29
Kids: Cheeseburger	260	14	20
Nuggets	275	19	11
Desserts:			
Choc.Chip Brownie	500	28	63
Funnel Cake Fries, Regular, with Caramel Sauce	285	6	57

Mrs Fields Cookies® (Oct '23)

Brownie Bites: Per 3 Bites	C	F	Cb
Butterscotch Blondie	200	8	29
Double Fudge	200	10	27
Toffee Fudge	200	11	26
***Bite Size Nibbler Cookies:** Per 3 Cookies*			
Cinnamon Sugar	180	8	25
Debra's Special	160	7	22
Semi-Sweet Chocolate	170	8	23
Triple Chocolate	160	8	22
White Chunk Macadamia	180	9	22
Cake, Chocolate Chip, 3 oz	350	17	45
***Cookies:** Per Cookie*			
Cinnamon Sugar	210	8	31
Frosted	270	11	39
Cut Out	280	11	44
Debra's Special	200	9	27
Oatmeal, Raisins & Walnuts	200	9	27
Semi-Sweet Chocolate	210	10	29
Triple Chocolate	210	10	28
White Chunk Macadamia	230	12	28
Muffins: Blueberry	190	9	24
Chocolate Chip	200	10	26

For Complete Nutritional Data ~ see CalorieKing.com

My Favorite Muffin® (Oct '23)

Muffins: Per Large Muffin	C	F	Cb
Blueberry	590	28	78
Boston Cream Pie	740	33	105
Chocolate Chip	790	39	100
Carrot Cake	850	42	112
Deep Dish Apple Pie	560	22	85
Lemon Poppy Seed	670	32	90
New York Almond Cheesecake	690	41	74
Pumpkin Spice	600	26	86
Strawberry Cheesecake	580	31	67

Nathan's Famous® (Oct '23)

Burgers: Single, Without Sides	C	F	Cb
Hell's Kitchen	790	53	39
Manhattan	750	51	44
NY Attitude on Everythin Bun	940	66	49
Cheesesteak, Original Philly	580	23	62
***Hand Dipped Chicken Sandwiches:** Per Single*			
Buffalo Chickn: Fried	750	48	54
Grilled	510	28	40
Chicken Club: Fried	850	57	53
Grilled	610	38	38
Hell's Kitchen: Fried	770	47	52
Grilled	530	27	37
Southern: Fried	670	40	50
Grilled	430	20	35

Nathan's Famous® cont... (June -23)

Hot Dogs: With Natural Casings	C	F	Cb
Original, 3.5 oz	270	16	22
Chili, 5.5 oz	390	26	28
Chili Cheese, 6.5 oz	430	28	21
Hot Dog Nuggets, 6 pieces, 3.5 oz	410	25	36
***Fries:** Per Regular Size*			
Bacon Cheese	680	51	41
Bacon Ranch	900	76	39
Cheese	570	43	41
Chili Cheese	690	52	46
Original Crinkle Cut	520	39	36
Onion Rings:			
Beer Battered, ½ lb	530	28	62
Hand Dipped, ½ pound	350	22	37

New York Fries® ~ *See CalorieKing.com*

Ninety Nine® (Oct '23)

Standout Starters: As Served	C	F	Cb
Boneless Wings, without sauce	930	33	89
Mozzarella Moons	850	50	65
Seafood Stufffies	770	59	47
***Burgers:** Without Sides*			
Bacon & Cheese	820	40	57
Cheeseburger	700	31	57
Plain Burger	640	25	57
Vermont Cheddar	910	46	63
***Sandwiches::** Without Sides*			
Honey BBQ Chicken Wrap	910	33	108
Spicy Crispy Chicken Sandwich	880	37	92
***Entrees:** Without Sides Unless Noted*			
Broiled Sirloin Tips, smothered	620	44	0
Cntry Fried Chkn, Mashed Pot & Bisc.	1270	57	144
Fish & Chips with Fries & Coleslaw	1790	113	134
Seafood Trio	690	37	41
Top Sirloin Steak, 8 oz	310	13	0
Sides: Broccoli Florets	50	1	9
Coleslaw	290	23	19
Corn	240	8	44
French Fries, 16 oz	1040	64	107
Rice Pilaf	310	8	55
Russet Mashed Potatoes	240	11	30
Desserts: Ban. Coconut Petite Treat	300	17	33
Towering Midnight Fudge Cake	1680	82	217

Noodles & Company® (Oct '23)

Asian Noodles: Per Reguar Size	C	F	Cb
Japanese Pan Noodles	640	12	114
Pad Thai	1040	42	143
Spicy Korean Beef Noodles	890	34	114
Bowls: *Per Regular*			
Paleo Friendly:			
Zucc. with Rstd Garlic Cream Sauce	400	30	20
Zucchini Rosa with Grilled Chicken	450	23	24
Vegetarian: Jap. Pan Noodles w/ Tofu	870	26	120
Zucchini Scampi	350	23	25
Classic Noodles: *Regular Size*			
Alfredo MontAmore Parm Crusted Ckn.	1630	104	117
Buttered Noodles	760	35	98
Penne Rosa with Parm	730	25	104
Pesto Cavatappi with Parm	740	31	96
Spaghetti & Meatballs	980	48	102
Macs: *Per Regular Size*			
BBQ Chicken	1190	44	129
Buffalo Chicken	1100	39	128
Gluten Sensitive Pipette Mac	850	34	105
Wisconsin Mac & Cheese	980	38	119
Zoodles: *Per Regular*			
Zucchini Pesto Crm w/ Grilled Chicken	500	30	22
Zucchini Roasted Garlic Cream Sauce	400	30	20
Zucchini with Grilled Chicken	450	23	24
Salads: *Per Regular with Dressing*			
Backyard BBQ	470	27	24
Grilled Chicken Caesar	610	45	17
The Med with Chicken	430	17	32
Soup, Chicken Noodle, regular	360	10	41

O'Charley's® (Oct '23)

Appetizers: As Served	C	F	Cb
Chipotle Chicken Tenders	1160	40	107
Loaded Potato Skins	1400	109	44
Meatball Costini	980	47	93
Shrimp Stuffed Crab	890	65	57
Spicy Jack Cheese Wedges (7)	720	48	44
Top Shelf Combo Platter	1880	132	74
Burgers: *Without Sides*			
Bacon Cheddar	1000	68	49
Classic Cheeseburger	930	61	47
Chicken & Pasta: *Without Sides*			
Balsamic Glazed Chicken	560	41	16
Bayou Shrimp Pasta	1060	56	100
Chicken Tenders & Fries	1410	85	74
Chicken Tender Dinner:			
Buffalo	1070	64	31
Chipotle	1040	40	77
Country Style Tenders	960	47	50

O'Charley's® cont... (Oct '23)

Classic Combos: Without Sides	C	F	Cb
BBQ Pork Chip & Baby Back Ribs	1490	77	65
BBQ Ribs & Chicken Tenders	950	37	84
Steak, 6 oz & Baby Back Ribs	890	49	48
Steak & Chicken Tenders, 6 oz	1030	67	26
Steak & Gr. Atlantic Salmon, 6 oz	750	33	5
Steak & Half Rack Baby Back Ribs	890	49	48
Steak, Ribs & Chops: *Without Sides*			
Baby Back Ribs, regular	1220	62	95
Steak:			
Filet Mignon, w/ Garlic Butter	580	47	1
Grilled Top Sirloin, 6 oz	270	18	0
Louisiana Sirloin	600	43	3
Pork Chop, Bone In	1070	66	12
Ribeye, Bone In, 14 oz	1060	85	1
Sandwiches: *Without Sides Unless Indicated*			
Buffalo Chicken with Fries	1400	89	104
Chicken with Fries	1360	85	100
Chicken Bacon Ranch	1140	62	81
Club	950	85	91
Seafoodl Favorites: *Without Sides Unless Indicated*			
Bayou Salmon, 9 oz	1130	74	41
Grilled Blackened Atl. Salmon, 9 oz	500	31	3
Hand Battered Fish & Chips	1420	92	85
Hand Breaded Catfish, w/ Fries & Slaw	1720	124	103
Seafood Platter	1950	121	141
Sides: Baked Potato (1)	200	1	50
Broccoli, 5 oz	110	8	6
Coleslaw	200	15	12
French Fries, 6 oz	400	24	40
Grilled Asparagus	60	5	3
Loaded Baked Potato, 1 portion	490	27	53
Mac & Cheese	450	22	47
Seasoned Rice Pilaf, 1 portion	160	4	27
Smashed Potatoes	350	16	44
Salads: *Per Full Salad with Dressing*			
California Chicken	1020	67	71
California Salmon	1210	83	68
Southern Fried Chicken	1550	110	48
Southern Pecan Chicken Tender	1550	106	95
Signature Soup: *Per Bowl*			
Chicken Tortilla	170	7	18
Loaded Potato	360	24	29
Desserts: *Per slice*			
Blackberry Cobbler, Double Scoop	1010	28	191
Brownie Lover's Brownie	1650	77	227
Peach Cobbler, Double Scoop	1010	31	181
Ooey Gooey Caramel Pie	640	39	76
Strawberry Cheeesecake	710	46	71
Tiramisu	570	36	57

Old Spaghetti Factory® (Oct '23)

Appetizers: As Served	C	F	Cb
Spinach & Artichoke Dip	640	46	44
Sicilian Garlic Chse Bread	1220	78	97
with Bacon	1450	95	97
Entrées, Lunch/Dinner:			
Classics:			
Italian Sausage with Meat Sauce	980	38	109
Sicilian Meatballs	1040	36	115
Spaghetti: with Marinara Sauce	570	7	106
with Rich Meat Sauce	650	11	108
with White Clam Sauce	790	29	107
Founder's Favorites:			
Baked Lasagna, 17.6 oz	820	45	61
Garlic Mizithra, 17 oz	1360	85	102
Tenderloin w/ Mizithra & Brocc.	1260	87	59
Manager Favorites:			
Marinara: Clam, 15 oz	690	18	107
Meat, 15 oz	600	8	108
Mushroom, 16.5 oz	610	10	109
Signature Pasta:			
Angel Hair Pomodoro, 16.6 oz	570	8	98
Fettuccine Alfredo, 13.3 oz	1090	72	91
Spinach & Cheese Ravioli, 11 oz	470	16	63
Specialty Selections:			
Crab Ravioli	810	45	73
Spaghetti Vesuvius	860	29	112
Dessert, Tiramisu, 4.5 oz	295	14	43

Olive Garden® (Oct '23)

Appetizers:	C	F	Cb
Calamari	670	42	48
Fried Mozzarella	800	49	57
Marinara Sauce	35	2	4
Lasagna Fritta	1130	76	75
Lunch Entrees: Fettuccine Alfredo	650	45	47
Chicken Parmigiana	630	29	61
Eggplant Parmigiana	660	32	75
Lasagna Classico	500	30	33
Shrimp Scampi	480	19	53
Dinner Entrees:			
Chicken & Shrimp Carbonara	1390	94	75
Five Cheese Ziti al Forno	1170	69	98
Grilled Chicken Alfredo	1570	95	96
Sides: French Fries	290	14	37
Seasoned Parmesan Garlic Broccoli	150	13	8
Desserts: Black Tie Mousse Cake	750	50	76
Choc. Brownie Lasagna	910	52	144
Strawb. Cream Cake	540	26	69
Tiramisu	470	27	54
Warm Italian Donuts without sauce	810	28	119

On the Border® (Oct '23)

Starters: As Served	C	F	Cb
Border Sampler	2160	147	120
Quesadillas:			
Fajita Chicken	1210	86	60
Fajita Steak	1270	93	59
Stacked Nachos with Seasoned Beef	2050	128	145
Bowls: *As Served*			
Grilled: Chicken	670	20	91
Portobello	580	15	94
Shrimp	670	24	91
Classic Burritos: *Without Beans, Rice or Sauce*			
Seasoned Ground Beef	850	44	56
Shredded Chicken Tinga	730	33	52
Chimichangas: *Without Beans, Rice or Sauce*			
Seasoned Ground Beef	970	57	56
Shredded Chicken Tinga	850	47	52
Salads: *W/out Dressing*			
Fajita: Chicken	410	21	27
Steak	490	31	26
Grande Taco Salad:			
Seasoned Ground Beef	730	48	41
Shredded Chicken Tinga	630	40	38
Dressings: Ranch	230	24	2
Smoked Jalapeno Vinaigrette	120	10	9
Tacos: *Without Beans or Rice*			
Dos XX Fish Taco w/ Red Chili Sce	400	25	31
Shredded Chicken Tinga, Crispy	200	10	15
Sides: Black Beans	210	2	36
Cilantro Lime Rice	180	2	37
Corn Tortilla (1)	60	1	12
Mexican Rice	220	5	39
Refried Beans	220	7	30
Sauteed Vegetables	90	7	7

For Complete Nutritional Data ~ see CalorieKing.com

Orange Julius® (Oct '23)

Julius Originals: Per Medium Size	C	F	Cb
Mango Pineapple	320	0	78
Orange Julius	260	0	65
Pina Colada	540	7	117
Strawberry Banana	460	7	99
Premium Fruit Smoothies: *Per Medium Size*			
Mango Pineapple	340	0	80
Pomegranate Berry Blast	380	0	89
Strawberry Banana	360	0	85
Strawberry Watermelon Sensation	340	1	80
Light Smoothies: *Per Medium Size*			
Berry Pomegranate Twilight	210	0	51
Tripleberry	210	0	51
Boost, Banana, Small drink	30	0	7

Outback Steakhouse® (Oct '23)

Aussie-Tizers: *Per Regular Size, with Selected Dressing/Sauce*	C	F	Cb
Aussie Cheese Fries	2620	182	153
Bloomin' Onion	1620	126	107
Kookaburra Wings, 10 count:			
Hot	2170	175	53
Medium,	1740	130	52
Mild, 10 count	1780	125	72
Seared Peppered Ahi, large	440	17	30
Steakhouse Mac & Cheese Bites	660	43	36
Three Cheese Steak Dip	2050	119	179
Burgers/Sandwiches: *Without Sides*			
Bloomin' Fried Chicken Sandwich	700	34	62
Outback Burger with Aerican Cheese	810	50	50
Prime Rib Sandwich	1330	101	51
The Bloomin' Burger	1140	80	65
Chicken & Ribs:			
Alice Springs Chicken	780	47	14
Drover's Rib & Chicken Platter	1190	54	63
Grilled Chickn On The Barbie, 8 oz,	410	9	22
Hand Breaded Chkn Tenders w/ Fries	1000	59	67
Queensland Chicken & Shrimp Pasta	1360	49	135
Signature Steaks: *Without Sides*			
Melbourne Porterhouse, 22oz	660	34	1
Outback Centre Cut Sirloin: 6 oz	370	20	1
8 oz	450	23	1
Ribeye, 12 oz	900	72	1
Victoria's Filet Mignon, 6 oz	690	36	1
Straight From The Sea: *Without Sides*			
Grilled Shrimp on the Barbie	550	35	3
Lobster Tails	490	25	0
Grilled Salmon with Remoulade	550	39	1
Toowoomba Samon	760	53	7
Big Bowl Salads:			
Aussie Cobb: *Without Dressing*			
with Crispy Chicken	940	54	62
with Grilled Chicken	680	34	29
Steakhouse, with dressing	1170	80	46
Side Salads: *With Dressing*			
Caesar	260	20	14
House: Base Salad	180	10	16
add Blue Cheese Vinaigrette	150	16	1
add Caesar Dressing	220	23	2
add Honey Mustard	220	19	12
add Mustard Vinaigrette	230	24	4
add Ranch Dressing	200	21	1

Outback Steakhouse® cont...(Oct '23)

Soups: *Per Cup*	C	F	Cb
Baked Potato	250	18	17
Cream of Broccoli	160	12	10
Creamy Onion	220	18	11
Sides: Aussie Fries	500	23	67
Broccoli	130	10	8
Creamed Spinach	570	45	23
Fresh Seasonal Mixed Veggies	70	2	13
Grilled Asparagus	40	2	5
Homestyle Mashed Potatoes	230	11	28
Loaded Baked Potato	340	14	47
Loaded Sweet Potato	250	7	45
Seasoned Rice	320	6	57
Steakhouse Mac & Cheese	720	37	74
Sweet Potato, with everything	410	11	72
Kid's Menu:			
Boomerang Cheeseburger	610	37	41
Grillded Cheese -A-Roo	580	35	50
Grilled Chcken On The Barbie	170	4	0
Mac-A-Roo 'N Cheese	550	19	73
Desserts: *Per Whole Dish*			
Choc. Thunder From Down Under	800	53	79
Salted Caramel Cookie Skillet	910	40	129
Tim Tam Brownie Cake	1500	85	174
Triple Layer Carrot Cake	1070	61	131

For Complete Menu & Data ~ see CalorieKing.com

Panda Express® (Oct '23)

Appetizers:	C	F	Cb
Chicken Egg Roll (1)	200	10	20
Cream Cheese Rangoon (3)	190	8	24
Veggie Spring Rolls (2	240	14	24
Entrées:			
Beef: Beijing Beef	480	27	46
Black Pepper Angus Steak	210	10	13
Broccoli Beef	150	7	13
Chicken:			
Black Pepper Chicken	280	19	15
Breast: Honey Sesame	340	15	35
String Bean	210	12	13
Sweet & Sour	300	12	40
SweetFire	360	15	40
Kung Pao Chicken	290	19	14
Teriyaki Chicken	340	13	14

Panda Express® cont... (Oct '23)

Entrees (Cont):	C	F	Cb
Fish, Steamed Ginger	200	12	8
Shrimp: Golden Treasure	360	18	35
Honey Walnut	360	24	27
Wok Fired	190	5	19
Vegetables: Eggplant Tofu	340	24	23
Super Greens	45	2	5
Sides:			
Chow Mein	510	20	80
Fried Rice	520	16	85
Stamed Brown Rice	420	4	86
Steamed White Rice	380	0	87
Super Greens	90	3	10
Dessert: Choc Chip Chunk Cookie	160	7	25
Fortune Cookies, 0.18 oz	20	0	5

Panera Bread® (Oct '23)

Bagels:	C	F	Cb
Asiago Cheese	320	5	56
Cinnamon Crunch	420	7	84
Breakfast Sandwiches:			
Avocado, Egg White, Cheese & Spinach, on Flat Sprouted Grain Bagel	350	14	39
Bacon, Scr. Egg & Cheese on Artisan Ciab.	440	21	40
Bacon, Scramb. Egg & Chse on Brioche	450	26	33
Ssg, Scramb. Egg & Cheese on Brioche	590	40	33
Sandwiches: *Per Full Sandwich*			
Bacon Turkey Bravo on Tomato Basil	1000	41	104
Classic Grilled Cheese on White Miche	880	51	68
Mediterranean Veggie on Tomato Basil	640	14	106
Roasted Turkey & Avocado BLT, on Country Rustic Sourdough	940	53	73
Tuna Salad on Black Pepper Focaccia	710	31	80
Entree:			
Bowls, Baja with Chicken	660	31	71
Flatbread Pizza, Cheese	920	41	95
Mac & Cheese:			
Small, 1 cup	480	32	34
Large, 2 cups	960	64	67
Salads: *Full Size, with Dressing, without Bread*			
Asian Sesame w/ Chicken	410	22	26
Chicken Caesar	440	27	20
Fuji Apple w/ Chicken	560	34	38
Greek	410	35	17
Stawberry Poppyseed	240	12	34

Panera Bread® cont... (Oct '23)

Soups: *Per Cup, without Bread*	C	F	Cb
Bistro French Onion	180	7	21
Broccoli Cheddar	230	15	16
Cream of Chkn & Wild Rice	180	10	18
Homestyle Chicken Noodle	60	1	8
Ten Vegetables	60	1	10
Vegetarian Creamy Tomato	240	14	24
Pastries & Sweets:			
Bear Claw	500	23	65
Chocolate Croissant	410	21	49
Brownie	470	18	69
Cookie: Kitchen Sink	820	44	99
Lemon Drop Favored	440	20	60
Muffin: Blueberry	510	18	79
Chocolate Chip	670	26	101

Papa Gino's® (Aug '22)

Burgers: *Without Fries*	C	F	Cb
Cheeseburger	550	31	37
Classic Burger	690	44	42
Double Cheeseburger	830	49	37
Hamburger	520	28	36
Entree Pasta:			
Penne	580	6	118
Penne Alfredo	730	23	112
Spaghetti Alfredo	650	22	95
Pizzas:			
Thin Crust: *Per Slice, ⅛ Large Pizza*			
Boss BBQ Chicken	310	11	39
Cheese	230	7	32
Crispy Buffalo, w/ Blue Cheese	370	18	36
Meat Combo	390	16	44
Pepperoni	280	11	32
Super Veggie	250	8	35
Works	310	13	33
Subs: *Per Small Sub*			
BLT	720	43	60
Chicken Parm	1000	37	109
Crispy chicken	960	48	95
Italian	890	48	68
Meatball Parmesan	1110	68	80
Tuna	820	51	58
Turkey	450	6	52
Turkey Club	740	35	62
Salads: *Without Breadstick*			
Caesar, with Caesar Dressing	190	10	18
Garden with Croutons, w/o Dressing	190	8	27
Breadstick, Cheese w/ Marinara (1)	230	8	30
French Fries, 10.23oz	450	19	67
Dressings: Blue Cheese, 1.7 fl.oz	270	28	3
Greek, 1.5 fl.oz	210	24	1
Ranch, 1.5 fl.oz	150	15	2

Papa John's® (Oct '23)

Pizzas:	C	F	Cb
Original Crust (14"): *Per 1/8 of Large 14" Pizza*			
BBQ Chicken & Bacon	340	11	45
Cheese	290	10	38
Extra Cheesy Alfredo	320	13	37
Fiery Buffalo Chicken	330	12	38
Garden Fresh	280	9	39
Meatball Pepperoni	360	15	38
Pepperoni Sausage & Six Cheese	390	20	36
Philly Cheesesteak	330	12	38
The Meats	380	17	38
The Works	340	14	39
Papadias: Italian	940	53	76
Meatball Pepperoni	940	49	79
Philly Cheesesteak	810	35	80
Wings: *Per 8 Wings, with Dipping Sauce*			
BBQ	880	57	20
Honey Chipotle	900	57	27
Spicy Buffalo	840	58	8
Sides:			
Bacon Cheesesticks, 10"	110	5	11
Chicken Poppers: 5 Poppers	270	10	21
10 Poppers	530	21	42
Breadsticks:			
Regular, 1 X 12"	130	2	24
Cheesesticks, 1 X 10"	90	4	10
Garlic Parmesan, 1 X 12"	160	5	24
Garlic Knots, each	110	5	14
Desserts: Chocolate Chip Cookie	190	9	26
Double Chocolate Chip Brownie	240	12	34

Papa Murphy's® (Oct '23)

Pizzas:	C	F	Cb
Original Crust: *Per 1/8 of Family Size Pizza*			
BBQ Chicken	330	13	36
Chicken Garlic	310	14	29
Cowboy	360	18	31
Garden Veggie	260	10	31
Gourmet Vegetarian	300	14	30
Hawaiian	270	9	32
Murphy's Combo	340	17	31
Papa's Favorite	340	17	31
Pepperoni	290	13	29
Rancher	310	14	30
Thai Chicken	330	12	39
Stuffed Pizzas: *Per 1/16 of Family Size Pizza*			
5 Meat	440	18	49
Big Murphy	440	18	50
Chicago Style	440	18	49
Chicken and Bacon	420	16	49

Papa Murphy's® cont... (Oct '23)

Salads: *Per Whole Salad, without Dressing or Croutons*	C	F	Cb
Caesar	100	5	7
Club	270	16	12
Garden	190	11	13
Italian	270	19	11
Mediterranean	320	17	23
Desserts:			
Choc. Chip Cookie, 2 oz slice	170	11	34
Cinnamon Wheel, 3 oz	260	7	44
S'mores Dessert Bar	130	7	25

Pei Wei Asian Diner® (Oct '23)

Shareables: *Without Sauce*	C	F	Cb
Crab Wonton (1)	120	6	12
Chicken Dumpling	30	1	4
Trad'nl Edamame	250	11	20
Vegetable Spring Rolls (1)	110	5	16
Entrees: *Per Regular Size*			
Classic: Beef & Broccoli	730	38	50
Honey Seared Chicken	800	34	80
Mongolian Steak	710	38	45
Orange Chicken	720	23	81
Kung Pao Shrimp	780	38	80
Pei Wei Original Shrimp	720	30	89
Spicy Korean BBQ Steak	700	42	38
Teriyaki Tofu	570	15	95
Thai C'nut Curry Chkn	770	48	45
Rice & Noodle Entrees:			
Chicken Fried Rice	1050	32	157
Chicken Lo Mein	1040	34	128
Chicken Pad Thai	1360	43	168
Dan Dan Chicken Noodles	1070	40	126
Spicy Drunken Noodles	1070	26	144
Salad Bowl,			
Asian Chopped Chkn w/out Drssng	400	16	34
Sides: *Per Regular*			
Brown Rice	350	3	73
Fried Rice	680	21	102
White Rice	400	0	90
Soup, Thai Wonton, bowl	230	11	29
Dessert:			
Fudge Brownie	430	22	57
Thai Donuts	280	10	43

Pepe's Mexican® ~ see CalorieKing.com

Perkins® (Oct '23)

Breakfast: W/out Side or Extras	C	F	Cb
Classic: Country Fried Steak & Eggs	770	47	47
Hearty Man's Combo	800	69	11
Magnificent Seven	720	39	68
Eggs Benedict Classic	660	31	61
Omelets: Everything	550	40	14
Farmer's	660	54	8
Granny's Country	640	41	34
Griddle Greats: Belgian Waffle	410	21	49
Blueberry Pancakes (3)	520	21	73
Buttermilk Pancakes (3)	490	21	66
Platters: Belgian Waffle	570	33	51
French Toast	570	27	53
Potato Pancake	650	42	48
Syrups & Toppings:			
Apricot Syrup, 2 oz	120	0	30
Glazed Blueberries, 6 oz	200	0	51
Glazed Strawberries, 6 oz	140	0	36
Pancake/Twinberry Syrup, 2 oz, av.	130	0	33
Sugar Free Pancake Syrup, 2 oz (contains sugar alcohol)	20	0	6
Side Choices: Bacon, 4 slices	140	12	0
Blueberry Muffin, with margarine	600	27	81
Breakfast Potatoes, 5 oz	280	17	30
Eggs Beaters, 2	80	4	2
English Muffin, with butter	180	6	28
Fresh Cut Fruit, 4 oz	70	0	19
Ham, sliced, 3.4 oz	140	5	4
Hash Browns, 4.3 oz	210	13	22
Oatmeal, with butter blend, 2% Milk & Brown Sugar	340	9	57
Sausage Patties (2)	380	38	1
Smoked Sausage, 4.1 oz	380	34	8
Sticky Bun, with marg.	740	36	98
Tot's,7 oz	470	28	47
Turkey Bacon, 4 slices	100	6	0
White Toast (2), with margarine	260	11	34
Whole Wheat Toast (2), with marg.	260	8	38
***Burgers:** Without Sides*			
BBQ Tangler	1190	73	82
Big BLT on Brioche Bun	630	43	42
Classic: Burger	710	40	48
Cheeseburger	870	54	48
***Melts:** Without Sides*			
Chicken Strips on Sourdough	1190	70	88
Country Club Melt on Sourdough	940	52	64
Patty Melt on Rye	1070	69	61
Pot Roast on Sourdough	880	49	63
Reuben Melt on Brioche Bun	1070	69	56

Perkins® cont... (Oct '23)

Lunch & Dinners:	C	F	Cb
Comfort Classics Dinner: *Without Sides*			
Chicken Strips	800	43	59
Country Fried Steak	600	34	45
Grilled Garlic Tilapia & Shrimp	580	24	57
Grilled Salmon	430	29	2
Turkey & Dressing, w/- Cranb. Sce	400	17	21
Comfort Classics Lunch: *Without Sides Unless Indicated*			
Fish 'n Chips, with Garden Salad and Tartar Sauce	1380	88	108
Grilled Cajun Tilapia & Shrimp	490	14	57
Mini Chicken Pot Pie	690	43	50
Supper Skillets:			
Hibachi Fried Chicken	780	29	103
Hibachi Grilled Shrimp	610	20	85
Steak & Pepper with B'fast Pot.	820	45	58
Dinner Sides: Applesauce	40	0	9
Baked Potato with Lt. Sour Cream	250	7	42
Buttered Corn	120	4	17
French Fries	570	36	56
Green Beans & Bacon	45	3	4
Herb Rice Pilaf	270	6	50
H'style Seasoned Potato	210	3	40
Macaroni & Cheese	340	18	32
Mashed Potatoes & Gravy	210	5	35
Potato Pancakes (2)	280	17	27
Sauteed Spinach	70	4	4
Tater Tots	470	28	47
***Soups:** Per Bowl, Includes Crackers*			
Chicken Noodle	260	6	37
Loaded Potato; Tomato Basil	460	26	46
***Salads:** With Set Dressing Unless Indicated*			
Honey Mustad Chicken Crunch	980	63	63
Southwest Avocado Chhicken	820	50	61
***55 Plus Lunch/Dinner:** Without Sides*			
Cheeseburger	640	34	41
Pork Chop Dinner	560	32	8
Pot Roast Dinner	530	27	17
***Dessert:** As Served*			
Muffins: *Includes Whipped Margarine Blend*			
Apple Cinnamon	580	27	76
Banana Nut	740	41	85
Blueberry	600	27	81
Pies: *Per Slice*			
Banana Cream Pie with Wh. Crm	650	43	62
Caramel Apple, 7.2 oz	500	22	68
Cherry	580	27	75
Chocolate French Silk w/ Wh. Crm.	730	52	63
Southern Pecan, 5.5 oz	670	33	86
Wildberry, no sugar added, 7 oz	470	27	50

Peter Piper Pizza® (Oct '23)

Signature Pizzas:	C	F	Cb
Original Crust: *Per ⅛ of Large 14" Pizza*			
5 Meat Supreme	360	15	39
California Veggie	290	9	41
Cheese	320	11	39
Chicago Classic	330	13	40
Hearty Hawaiian	310	9	41
New York 3 Cheese with Pepperoni	390	18	39
Spinach Chkn Alfredo	350	15	37
The Werx	310	11	40
Veggie Harvest	300	9	42
Original Crust: *Per 1/12 of Extra Large 16" Pizza*			
5 Meat Supreme	350	16	34
California Veggie	250	8	35
Cheese	280	10	34
Chicago Classic	300	12	35
Hearty Hawaiian	270	8	36
New York 3 Cheese w/ Pepperoni	350	16	34
Pizza Mexicana	340	15	34
Spinach Chicken Alfredo	310	14	32
The Werx	290	11	34
Veggie Harvest	260	8	36
Pasta: *With Breadsticks*			
Mac & Pepperoni	1670	91	168
Meaty Ziti	1240	78	79
Spinach Alfredo	1640	89	153
Salads: *Small Size, without Dressing*			
Caesar, with Croutons	320	14	35
Chopped Italian	260	19	10
Wings & More: *Without Sides*			
Cheddar Bacon Roll (1)	350	18	34
French Fries	510	32	53
Garlic Chse Bread, 3.25 oz	390	17	45
Handmade Breadsticks, with Marinara Sauce (6)	1190	31	199
Loaded Tots	1280	102	70
Bone In Wings: *Without Sauce or Sides Unless Indicated*			
Plain (10)	1160	97	0
Louisiana Honey Hot with Ranch	1590	134	28
Boneless: 10 oz	880	58	47
Mango Havanero, with Ranch, 10 oz	1510	95	123
Sweet BBQ,	1130	58	110
Dipping Sauces:			
BBQ	240	0	60
Buffalo	120	9	6
Ranch	320	36	2
Sweet Chili	200	0	46
Xtra Hot Buffalo	90	6	5
Dessert:			
Cinnamon Crunch, small slice	380	9	69
Vanilla Soft Serve: Cone	200	6	35
Cup	180	6	31

P.F. Chang's® (Oct '23)

Shareables/Sides: *Per Single Serve*	C	F	Cb
Chang's BBQ Pork Spare Ribs (6)	430	14	17
Chang's Chicken Lettuce Wraps	330	13	33
Chang's Vegetarian Lettuce Wraps	260	14	23
Crispy Green Beans	500	39	35
Dynamite Shrimp	290	21	20
Edamame with Kosher Salt	200	8	12
Kung Pao Brussels Sprouts	370	21	43
Entrées:			
Beef: *Per Serving For One Without Sides*			
Beef with Broccoli	330	15	24
Mongolian Beef	380	19	21
Pepper Steak	300	15	15
Chicken: *Per Serving For One Without Sides*			
Chang's Spicy	570	29	49
Crispy Honey Chkn	570	31	44
Ginger Chicken with Broccoli	250	7	18
Kung Pao	520	34	15
Sesame Chicken	490	24	30
Sweet & Sour Chicken	440	21	44
Seafood: *Per Serving For One Without Sides*			
Crispy Honey Shrimp	510	28	40
Kung Pao Shrimp	510	35	27
Miso Glazed Salmon	320	18	14
Oolong Chilean Sea Bass	280	18	15
Salt & Pepper Prawns	460	34	22
Shrimp with Lobster Sauce	210	11	6
Other Entrees:			
Fire Braised Short Ribs	770	50	51
Ma Po Tofu	490	31	33
Stir Fried Egg Plant	280	18	29
Noodles & Rice: *Per Serving for One*			
Fried Rice: Combo	530	14	77
with Beef	1540	15	78
with Chicken	420	10	76
with Pork	550	15	76
with Shrimp	460	8	76
Lo Mein: Beef	450	14	59
Chicken	330	9	57
Combo	420	12	58
Pork	440	13	57
Shrimp	380	9	58
Vegetables	360	7	63
Pad Thai: Chicken	670	18	95
Combo	650	19	93
Shrimp	630	18	93

P.F. Chang's® cont... (Oct '23)

Noodles & Rice (cont):	C	F	Cb
Korean Glass Noodles	370	12	60
Singapore Street Noodles	610	7	112
Lunch Bowls: *Without Rice*			
Beef & Brocoli	390	17	34
Crispy Honey Chicken	840	42	71
Mongolian Beef	460	24	26
Spicy Chicken	810	44	58
Sides: Brown Rice, 6 oz	190	0	40
Fried Rice	500	15	76
Noodles	570	13	96
White Rice, 6 oz	220	0	49
Sushi: California Roll	390	16	53
Kung Pao Dragon Roll	510	23	60
Shrimp Tempura Roll	580	25	69
Spicy Tuna Roll	300	6	43
Salad: Asian Caesar	210	15	11
Mandarin Crunch	370	23	38
Add: Chicken	140	7	1
Salmon	160	13	0
Soup: Egg Drop, bowl	240	6	36
Hot & Sour, bowl	420	12	54
Wonton, bowl	780	21	84
Dessert: *Per Serving*			
Banana Spring Roll	470	17	75
Chang's Apple Crunch	460	21	62
Chocolate Souffle	400	25	42
New York Style Cheese Cake	480	31	42
The Great Wall of Chocolate	970	40	154

Pita Pit® ~ *See CalorieKing.com*

Pizza Hut® (Oct '23)

All Pizzas are with Standard Ingredients & Sauce

Hand-Tossed Style: *Per ⅛ of Medium 12" Pizza*	C	F	Cb
Buffalo Chicken	190	6	24
Cheese	210	7	26
Meat Lover's	280	15	26
Pepperoni	220	9	25
Pepperoni Lover's	260	12	26
Supreme	230	10	26
Veggie Lover's	190	6	27
Original Pan: *Per ⅛ of Medium 12" Pizza*			
Backyard BBQ Chicken	260	9	33
Cheese	240	10	28
Meat Lover's	310	17	28
Pepperoni	250	11	28
Pepperoni Lover's	290	15	28
Supreme	260	12	28
Veggie Lover's	230	9	29

Pizza Hut® cont..(Oct '23)

Personal Pan: *Per ¼ of 6" Pizza, with Standard Ingredients & Sauce*	C	F	Cb
Backyard BBQ Chicken	180	6	25
Meat Lover's	190	9	17
Pepperoni	150	7	17
Pepperoni Lover's	180	9	18
Supreme	160	7	18
Veggie Lover's	140	5	18
Rectangle Slices: *Per Slice, ⅛ of Pizza*			
Backyard BBQ Chicken	260	9	34
Buffalo Chicken	220	8	28
Cheese	240	9	29
Pepperoni	250	11	29
Supreme	270	12	30
Veggie Lovers	230	8	30
Thin 'n Crispy: *Per ⅛ of Medium 12" Pizza*			
Backyard BBQ Chicken	210	7	27
Buffalo chicken	170	5	21
Cheese	180	7	22
Cheesesteak	210	9	21
Hawaiian Chicken	190	6	24
Pepperoni Lover's	250	13	22
Supreme	220	10	23
Veggie Lover's	170	5	24
Pastas, Tuscani:			
Chicken Alfredo, 9.9 oz	930	49	85
Italian Meats 9.6 oz	860	37	97
Sides:			
Saucy Wings: BBQ (1)	60	4	2
Buffalo (1)	60	4	1
Breadstick (1), without sauce	140	5	19
Cheese Stick without sauce	150	5	20
Garlic Bread, 1 piece	190	6	29
with Cheese	210	13	16
Salad: *Without Dressing*			
BLT	290	16	29
Chicken Caesar	410	21	30
Chicken Garden	420	19	39
Crispy Chicken Caesar	830	53	60
Zesty Italian	390	23	33
Dressing: Blue Cheese, entree size	450	48	3
Creamy Caesar, entree size	360	37	5
French, entree size	330	23	29
Light Italian Vinaigrette, entree size	150	11	11
Desserts: Fried Apple Pie, no sauce	170	9	22
Triple Choc. Brownie, ⅑ square	230	10	34
Ultimate Chocolate Chip Cookie	190	9	26

Pizza Ranch® (Oct '23)

Specialty Pizza:	C	F	Cb
Original Crust: *Per Slice, 1/10 of Medium Pizza*			
Bacon Cheeseburger	180	7	20
BBQ Chicken	170	5	22
Bronco	200	8	19
Buffalo Chicken	180	8	18
Chicken Bacon Ranch	220	11	18
Macaroni 'N' Cheese	220	10	23
Prairie (Veggie)	170	5	20
Stampede	200	7	20
Sweet Swine	170	6	20
Texan Taco	180	7	21
Thin Crust: *Per 1/10 Slice of Medium Pizza*			
BBQ Chicken	110	5	11
Bronco	140	8	9
Mac 'N' Cheese	160	9	12
Ranch Wraps: *Without Sides*			
BBQ Chicken	930	29	118
Caesar Chicken	1030	61	68
Chicken Bacon	1260	83	68
Sides: *Single Serving*			
Coleslaw	280	23	18
Corn	180	1	38
Mashed Potatoes & Gravy	250	7	39
Ranch Potato Wedges (6)	620	34	68
Salads: *Without Dressing*			
Chef	430	17	14
Chicken Fiesta	180	7	9
Garden	90	5	7
Taco	620	33	51

For Complete Menu & Data ~ see CalorieKing.com

Pollo Tropical® ~ *See CalorieKing.com*

Popeye's® (Oct '23)

Chicken: *Hand Battered, Breaded & Fried*	C	F	Cb
Ghost Pepper Wings:			
6 Pieces	670	46	21
12 Pieces	1350	91	43
Nuggets: 8 Pieces	425	24	39
12 Pieces	570	36	28
Tenders: 3 Pieces	460	20	35
5 Pieces	770	33	58
Combo Meals: *W/ Regular Cajun Fries & Small Coca Cola*			
#1. Classic Chicken Sandwich	1240	56	156
#2. Blackened Chicken Sandwich	1090	43	147
#5. 3 Piece Tenders without sauce	1000	34	141

Popeye's® cont... (Oct '23)

Sandwiches & Wraps: *Each*	C	F	Cb
Classic or Spicy Chicken S'wich	700	42	50
Classic Bacon & Cheese Chkn S'wich	830	53	51
Seafood,			
Popcorn Shrimp, 4 oz	390	25	28
Sides: *Per Regular Size*			
Biscuit	205	13	20
Cajun Fries	270	14	33
Cole Slaw	140	10	12
Homestyle Mac &Cheese	280	21	16
Mashed Potatoes with Cajun Gravy	110	4	18
Red Beans & Rice	250	16	22
Kid's Meals: *includes 6 fl.oz Apple Juice & Apple Sauce*			
1 Piece Leg Meal	310	9	42
4 Piece Nuggets Meal	385	12	56
6 Piece Nuggets Meal	485	18	61
Mac & Cheese Meal	430	21	53
Desserts:			
Blueb. Lemon Cream Cheese Fried Pie	320	19	35
Cinnamon Apple Pie	240	16	35
Strawberry Biscuit	290	13	39

Port of Subs® (Oct '23)

Figures Based on West Coast Outlets	C	F	Cb
Classic Subs: *Per 8" White Sub with Standard Menu Components*			
#1 Ham, Salami, Capicolla, Pepperoni, Provolone	650	27	65
#2 Ham & Turkey, Provolone	550	15	66
#3 Salami & Turkey, Provolone	560	19	65
#4 Ham, Salami, Provolone	570	21	64
#5 Smoked Ham, Turkey, Cheddar	560	17	65
#6 Vegetarian, 3 Chse	670	34	68
#7 Roast Beef, Prov.	540	14	61
#8 Turkey, Provolone	540	14	66
#10 Rstd Chicken Breast, Provolone	550	14	64
#11 Ham, American Cheese	560	17	67
#12 Salami, Provolone	590	25	63
#13 Peppered Pastrami Turkey, Swiss	540	15	65
#15 Salami, Pepperoni, Provolone	600	27	63
#16 Chkn, Pepperoni, Pepper Jack	590	22	62
#17 Tuna, Provolone	700	29	65
#18 Roast Beef,Turkey, Provolone	540	14	64

Port of Subs® cont... (Oct '23)

Figures Based on West Coast Outlets

	C	F	Cb
***Hot Subs:** Per 8" White Sub with Provolone, without Additional Toppings*			
Melts: Grilled Buffalo Chicken	590	13	60
Grilled Chicken	590	13	60
Grilled Teriyaki Chicken	670	13	77
NY Steak	650	28	59
Pastrami	780	39	64
Ultimate BLT	690	36	61
***Wraps:** On Wheat Wrap w/ Standard Menu Compnents*			
Grilled: BBQ Chicken	730	22	75
Chicken Buffalo	650	22	59
Chicken Caesar	670	25	60
Gourmet Cheese	710	40	59
Pastrami Melt	850	47	62
Ultimate BLT	760	45	59
***Fresh Salads:** Standard Components without Dressing or Shakers*			
Caesar; Garden	70	3	9
Chef	260	15	13
Grilled Chicken; Gr. Chicken Spinach	280	7	11
Spinach	60	3	8
Tuna	350	20	12
***Salad Dressings:** Per 2 fl.oz*			
Caesar; Ranch, average	220	23	3
Honey Mustard	260	26	10
Mayo	150	16	0
***Sides:** Per Regular, 8 oz*			
Macaroni Salad	520	36	44
Potato Salad	380	21	47
***Soup:** Per Small Serving*			
Chicken Buffalo	190	12	13
Chicken Noodle	90	3	12
Cream of Broccoli	200	12	17
Tomato Bisque	120	6	14
***Breakfast Sub:** With American Cheese & Egg*			
5" White Bread:			
Bacon	450	22	39
Smoked Ham	390	14	39
Turkey Sausage	480	22	39
Wheat Wrap: Bacon	790	42	61
Smoked Ham	400	17	35
Turkey Sausage	840	55	61
Desserts:			
Chocolate Chunk Cookie, 4 oz	500	23	71
Jumbo Brownie	760	36	109
Oatmeal Raisin Cookie, 4 oz	480	20	69
White Choc. Macadamia Nut Cookie	530	26	67

Pret A Manger® (Oct '23)

East Coast Outlets.

	C	F	Cb
Baguettes:			
Chicken Banh Mi	620	23	78
Ham & Cheese	610	22	70
Pesto Caprese	690	36	70
Romesco Chicken & Mozzarella	670	30	71
Grain Bowl, Tikka Masala	400	14	36
***Salad Pots:** Per Pack*			
Cobb Shaker	160	12	4
Egg & Spinach	160	11	3
Elote Corn Shaker	170	11	14
***Sandwiches:** On Multigrain Bread Unless Indicated*			
Cheddar & Tomato	450	23	45
Chicken & Bacon	670	37	42
Egg Salad & Arugula	610	39	42
***Soups:** Per Small*			
Moroccan Lentil	260	11	30
Super Greens	140	4	20
***Salads:** With Set Dressing*			
Blackened Salmon, Avo & Quinoa	520	39	24
Chicken Avocado	510	39	21
Chicken Caesar	530	37	25
Mediterranean Mezze	590	44	40
Smoked Salmon Nicoise	450	37	10
***Wraps:** 7-Grain Wraps*			
Bang Bang Chicken	640	37	60
Crunchy Chipotle Chicken & Avocado	560	28	59
Falafel & Hummus	550	24	75
Mozzarella & Red Peppers	570	36	49
Breakfast:			
Baguette, Egg Salad & Bacon	490	31	38
Frittata, Shakshuka	310	12	16
Roll: Bacon, Egg & Cheddar	590	28	45
Egg & Cheddar	450	18	45
***Bakery:** Per Pack*			
Croissants: Almond	370	21	37
Chocolate	350	20	33
Pain au Raisin	390	20	46
Cookies: Chocolate Chunk, 2.5 oz	310	16	42
Harvest, 2.5 oz	280	12	40
Muffins: Blueberry, 4.5 oz	420	16	63
Cinnamon Kouign Amann	330	18	43
Desserts:			
Flourless Chocolte Fudge Cake	380	26	34
Keylime Cheesecake	310	20	27
Mango Coconut Rice Pudding	230	13	20
Raspberry Cheesecake	290	18	27
Strawberry Rhubarb Rice	180	8	21
Strawberry Rhubarb Yogurt Pot	110	4	10

Pretzelmaker® (Oct '23)

Pretzels: Per Small Serving	C	F	Cb
Bites: Salted, 6 oz	500	14	85
Cinnamon Sugar, 6 oz	530	14	90
Whole: Plain, 4 oz	310	3	66
Cinnamon Sugar, 5 oz	450	12	79
Garlic, 5 oz	430	12	74
Parmesan, 5 oz	450	15	66
Ranch, 5 oz	440	12	72
Pretzel Dogs: Regular	420	23	31
Mini (8)	430	29	33
Jalapeno (1), 6 oz	450	24	34
Sauces: *Per 2 oz*			
Caramel	100	1	22
Cheddar/Nacho Cheese, average	80	6	5
Cream Cheese	200	20	2
Pizza Sauce	30	1	6
Vanilla Glaze	170	0	42
Beverages: *Per 20 oz Unless Indicated*			
Blended Drinks:			
Cool Cappuccino	430	22	58
Mango Madness	500	16	90
Mocha Mania	580	22	94
Power Pomegranate	490	16	86
Strawberry Bananza	500	16	85
Fresh Lemonade: Original, 20 oz	140	0	38
Strawberry; Raspberry, 20 oz, av.	210	0	53

Qdoba® (Oct '23)

Entree Ingredients:	C	F	Cb
Meat: Bacon, 2 oz	230	17	2
Chorizo, 3 oz	260	20	5
Grilled: Adobo Chicken, 3.5	170	9	1
Steak, 3.5 oz	260	21	3
Ground Beef, 3.5 oz	190	12	4
Pulled Pork, 3.5 oz	110	5	0
Other Ingredients:			
Black Beans; Pinto Beans, av., 4 oz	135	1	24
Cilantro Lime Rice, 4 oz	190	3	38
Fajita Veggies, 2 oz	40	3	3
Hand Crafted Guac., 4 oz	170	15	9
Pico De Gallo, 2 oz	10	0	2
Romaine Lettuce for Salads, 3.5 oz	15	0	3
Salsa Roja/Verde, 1 oz, average	7	0	1
Seasoned Brown Rice, 4 oz	170	2	36
Shredded Cheese, 1 oz	110	9	1
Sour Cream, 1 oz	50	5	3
Tortilla Chips, 4 oz	560	26	75
Tortillas: Crispy Taco Shell	60	3	8
Crunchy Tortilla Shell	390	22	41
Soft Corn, 5.5"	60	1	11
Soft Flour: 5.5"	70	2	12
10"	210	5	36
12.5"	300	7	52
Whole Wheat Flour, 12.5"	280	7	45

Qdoba® cont...(Oct '23)

Signature Eats:	C	F	Cb
Bowls:			
Chicken Protein	670	32	39
Chicken Queso	740	30	74
Cholula Hot & Sweet Chicken	590	18	76
Fajita Vegan	530	17	79
Impossible Fajita	580	16	80
Burrito: Cholula Hot & Sweet Chicken	900	25	128
Southwest Steak	1110	47	133
Quesadilla, Quesabirria	1080	127	67
Salads: Citrus Lime Chicken	540	23	51
Impossible Taco	520	23	46
Street Style Tacos:			
Chicken:			
Corn Tacos (3)	490	22	43
Flour Tacos (3)	540	25	46
Desserts:			
Chocolate Chunk Cookie, 1.9 oz	280	14	36
Double Chocolate Brownie, 3.1 oz	360	16	52

Quiznos Subs® (Oct '23)

Subs: *Per 8" Regular Japaleno Cheddar Sub, with Standard Menu Toppings Unless Indicated*

Chicken:	C	F	Cb
Baja	800	32	76
Carbonara	890	42	73
Honey Mustard	850	36	80
Mesquite	800	33	73
Southwest Chicken	860	45	73
Classic:			
Chipotle Turkey	770	37	72
Honey Bacon Club	830	32	88
Spicy Monterey	600	15	81
Turkey Bacon Guacamole	840	37	79
Veggie Guacamole	810	44	81
Steak:			
Black Angus Steak,			
On Rosemary Parmesan	780	27	88
Chipotle Steak & Cheddar	840	44	73
French Dip	760	30	79
Peppercorn Steak	840	42	76
Salads: *Per Full Size With Set Dressing*			
Apple Harvest	520	29	48
Chef	590	46	13
Italian	700	57	18
Sides:			
Classic Tater Tots	210	11	25
Loaded	320	19	25
Side Salad with Red Wine Vinaigrette	270	26	9

Quiznos Subs® cont... (Oct '23)

Soups: Per Regular	C	F	Cb
Broccoli Cheese	220	14	18
Chicken Noodle	120	4	14
Chili	290	10	34
Tomato Basil Bisque	290	21	21
Breakfast:			
Biscuit: Egg & Cheddar	460	31	31
Sausage, Egg & Cheddar	630	48	31
Subs:			
Bacon, Egg & Cheddar	370	17	34
Ham, Egg & Cheddar	340	14	36
Sausage, Egg & Cheddar	550	37	35
Desserts: Chocolate Brownie, 3 oz	440	23	56
Chocolate Chunk Cookie, 3 oz	400	18	57
Cinnamon Sugar Cookie, 3 oz	400	17	58
Oatmeal Raisin Cookie, 3 oz	360	12	58

Rally's/Checkers® (Oct '23)

Burgers:	C	F	Cb
Baconzilla	960	75	41
Big Buford	770	57	41
Cheese Champ	530	37	40
Sandwiches: Crispy Fish	460	23	51
Spicy Chicken	580	49	38
Wings: Buffalo, medium, 5 pieces	360	23	3
Garlic Parmesan, 5 pieces	510	40	3
Sweet & Smokey BBQ, 5 pieces	430	23	19
Fries: Regular, medium	500	24	63
Chili Cheese Fries	540	37	43
Fully Loaded Fries	870	62	46

Ranch One® (Oct '23)

Sandwiches:	C	F	Cb
Chicken & Cheese	390	12	40
Chicken Philly, 9.3 oz	410	13	40
Grilled Classic Chicken, 9.4 oz	680	47	37
Original Crispy Chicken, 11.5 oz	640	31	60
Other Favorites:			
Chicken Fajitas, 10 oz	540	24	53
Chicken Teriyaki Bowl	530	7	86
Popcorn Chicken:			
Small, 5.5 oz	310	10	30
Large, 7.5 oz	420	14	40
Salads: *Completed*			
Grilled Chicken Caesar, 13.3 oz	430	30	14
Southwest Chicken, 17.5 oz	680	43	44
Fries:			
Medium, 5.8 oz	380	19	43
Large, 10.9 oz	530	27	58
Cheese Fries: Medium, 7.3 oz	490	27	46
Large, 11 oz	760	44	66

Red Hot & Blue® (Aug '22)

Starters:	C	F	Cb
Catfish Fingers	590	19	75
Nachos, with Chili	1005	51	103
Smokin Buffalo Wings	1045	85	28
BBQ Platters: Five Meat	935	63	15
Delta Double with Memphis Chkn	900	54	12
Pulled Pork	325	21	7
Smoked Sausage	965	68	36
Burgers:			
ALL IN	915	52	46
Classic Blues	665	32	44
Favorite Entrees: Delta Catfish	835	42	57
Delta Surf & Turf	1025	68	38
Southern Fried Chicken Crispers	760	35	50
Rib & Crispers Platter	1060	68	39
Ribs, Full Slab:			
Dry	1870	144	28
Sweet	1895	142	44
Sandwiches:			
Fried Delta Catfish	655	25	71
Grilled Chicken	360	6	40
Sides: BBQ Beans	255	2	48
Collard Greens	50	2	7
Fried Ocra	190	8	29
Mashed Potatoes, with gravy	310	14	44
Memphis Fries, 6 oz	345	19	38
Potato Salad	405	28	33
Sweet Potato	495	0	114
Sweet Potato Fries	375	19	49
Salads: Grilled Chicken Caesar	770	46	47
Southern Fried Chicken	710	31	60
Texas Smokehouse	670	36	36

Red Lobster® (Oct '23)

Appetizers: *As Served*	C	F	Cb
Cheddar Bay Shrimp	870	67	47
Lobster Pizza	700	35	59
Mozzarella Cheesesticks	730	40	58
Parrot Isle Jumbo Cocktail Shrimp	660	41	55
Signature Seafood Mushrooms	390	22	18
White Wine & Roasted Garlic Mussels	880	53	67
Pasta & Bowls: *Without Sides or Sauces*			
Bowl, Sesame-Soy Salmon	930	42	90
Pasta:			
Crispy Linguini Alfredo:			
with Cajun Chicken	1190	64	86
with Crab	1220	78	78
Lobster Linguini	1120	59	79

continued next page...

Red Lobster® cont... (Oct '23)

Handhelds: *Without Sides or Sauces*			
Crunch-fried Flounder Sandwich	1000	59	87
Dockside Cheddar Burger	660	29	42
Lobster & Shrimp Tacos	860	46	79
From The Sea: *Without Sides or Sauces*			
Fish & Chips	1230	65	117
Live Maine Lobster, stuffed	610	41	12
Parrot Isle Jumbo Coconut Shrimp	1040	64	82
Perfectly Grilled Atlantic Salmon	630	39	1
Perfectly Grilled Rainbow Trout	490	22	1
Salmon New Orleans, full	890	60	9
From The Land:			
6 oz Filet Mignon	250	12	2
7 oz Sirloin	260	11	1
10 oz New York Strip	580	35	2
Crispy Chicken Tenders	950	56	28
Maple Bacon Chicken	520	16	26
Seafood Combinations: *Without Sides or Sauces*			
Admirals Feast	1680	98	138
Caribbean Rock Lobster & Shrimp	920	63	47
Grilled Lobster, Shrimp & Salmon	930	50	5
Seaside Shrimp Trio	1430	87	104
Sides:			
Bacon, Mac & Cheese	600	34	46
Baked Potato, Plain	270	4	55
Caesar Side Salad	300	26	11
Crispy Brussels Sprouts	380	17	48
Crispy Green Beans	720	58	50
House Side Salad, without dressing	140	8	10
Loaded Baked Potato	520	26	57
Lobseter Topped Baked Potato	350	11	51
Mashed Potatoes	170	9	24
Orzo Rice	230	5	41
Sea Salted Fries	510	20	74
Sauces: 100% Pure Melted Butter	300	33	0
Cocktail Sauce	45	0	11
Marinara Sauce	35	2	4
Tartar Sauce	210	21	4
Desserts:			
Brownie Overboard	1020	57	121
Chocolate Wave	1110	62	134
Strawberry Vanilla Bean Cheesecake	470	26	56

For Complete Nutritional Data ~ see CalorieKing.com

Red Robin® (Oct '23)

Nutritional Information varies between restaurants. Please refer to Red Robin's website for further information.

Appetizers:	C	F	Cb
Fried Pickle Nickels	740	50	62
Pretzel Bites	780	39	91
The O-Ring Shorty	910	56	94
Towering Onion Rings	1290	57	179
Bar Wings & Yukon Chips: Plain	1080	70	21
with Banzai Sauce	1190	70	48
with Island Heat Sauce	1230	71	57
Boneless Wings: with Buzzard Sce	1010	57	70
with Island Heat Sauce	960	37	102
with Whisky River Sauce	1010	42	103
Burgers: *Without Fries or other Options*			
Classic: Bacon Cheeseburger	990	67	50
Guacamole Bacon	920	56	52
Keep It Simple, Beef	540	23	48
Monster	1220	76	62
Red Robin Gourmet Cheeseburger	810	46	60
Sauteed 'Shroom	770	40	53
Signature:			
Banzai	950	59	63
Royal Red Robin	1100	76	50
Scorpion	960	57	70
Smoke & Pepper	800	40	57
The MadLove	1060	57	71
The Southern Charm	1190	69	85
The Tycoon	870	50	61
Whiskey River BBQ	1140	74	75
Red's Throwback Doubles:			
Haystack	690	42	40
Pig Out	840	53	42
Red's	600	35	33
Veggie, Wedgie & More:			
Grilled Turkey	670	40	48
Impossible	760	40	70
Wedgie	520	33	17
Veggie	740	43	69
Veggie Vegan w/ Steamed Broccoli	260	11	35
Entrées:			
Arctic Cod Fish & Steak Fries	1560	90	135
Clucks & Fries	1330	82	104
Buffalo Style	1610	112	103
Ensenada Chicken Platter	390	14	12

Red Robin® cont... (Oct '23)

Sandwiches & Wraps: W/out Sides	C	F	Cb
BLTA Croissant	680	40	49
Crispy Chicken Wrap	930	57	70
Whiskey River BBQ Chicken Wrap	880	46	78
Soups:			
Chicken Tortilla: Cup	200	9	19
Bowl	390	19	37
Clam Chowder:			
Cup	210	15	12
Bowl	420	31	25
Red's Chili:			
Cup	210	9	18
Bowl	430	18	36
Salads: *Without Dressing Unless Indicated*			
Avo-Cobb-O	560	32	27
Crispy Chicken Tender	850	47	58
Simply Grilled Chicken	300	10	18
Southwest	790	51	47
Sides: Bottomless Steak Fries	360	16	49
Onions: Rings	280	1	61
Sauteed	25	2	2
Straws	200	14	16
Sauteed Mushrooms	120	6	11
Steamed Broccoli	30	1	6
Sweet Potato Fries	460	23	59
Yukon Chips	500	35	41
Yukon Chips	600	35	41
Desserts: Mountain High Mudd Pie	1340	59	188
Gooey Chocolate Brownie Cake	880	33	139

Roly Poly® (Oct '23)

Wraps: *Per 6" White Tortilla Unless Indicated*	C	F	Cb
Chicken: Basil Cashew Chicken	300	10	30
Chicken Caesar	310	11	30
Chicken Fajita	315	9	28
Santa Fe Chicken	305	11	28
Beef/Ham: Philly Melt	280	11	25
Ranch Roast	320	15	28
Tuna: Classic Tuna Melt	340	17	26
Popeyes Tuna on Wheat	305	10	31
Texas/Thai Hot Tuna, average	300	11	30
Turkey: Applejack	320	12	30
California	330	12	30
Veggie & Cheese:			
California Humer	305	13	32
Nutty Avocado on Wheat Tortilla	265	12	35
Salads: *Without Dressing*			
Alpine Chef	315	16	13
Chipotle Caesar	520	25	21
Just Veggies	95	0	19
Walnut Spinach	420	33	14

Round Table Pizza® (Oct '23)

Appetizers:	C	F	Cb
Boneless Wings, Oven Roasted:			
with BBQ Sauce (1)	100	2	13
with Buffalo Sauce (1)	90	4	8
Garlic Bread: 1 piece	70	4	9
with Cheese, 1 piece	110	6	9
Garlic Parmesan Twists, 1 twist	170	5	25
Burgers: Bleu Cheese	1220	81	66
Classic Cheeseburger	1280	91	57
Mushroom Swiss	1320	96	56
Smokehouse	1420	89	77
Pizzas: *Per 1⁄12 of Large 14" Pizza*			
Original Crust: Cheese	230	10	24
Gourmet Veggie	230	10	25
Guinevere's Garden Delight	220	8	26
Hawaiian	220	8	27
Italian Garlic Supreme	270	14	24
King Arthur Supreme	270	13	26
Maui Zaui Chicken	260	11	28
Montague's All Meat Marvel	290	15	24
Smokehouse Combo, Pepperoni	290	14	27
Triple Play Pepperoni	250	12	24
Pan Crust: BBQ Chicken	320	12	39
Gourmet: Chkn & Garlic	290	10	35
Veggie	280	10	35
Guinevere's Garden Delight	270	9	36
Hawaiian	280	8	37
Hearty Bacon Supreme	330	14	34
King Arthur Supreme	320	13	35
Montague's All Meat Marvel	340	16	35
Pepperoni	300	12	34
Triple Play Pepperoni	310	13	34
Stuffed Crust:			
BBQ Chicken	300	12	33
Cheese	270	12	25
Chicken Garlic Gourmet	280	11	30
Double Play Pepperoni	300	15	25
Gourmet Veggie	270	11	30
Hawaiian	270	9	31
King Arthur Supreme	300	13	31
Maui Zaui	290	11	32
Montague's All Meat Marvel	320	15	30
Pepperoni	280	12	30
Pasta: Chicken Bacon Alfredo, 3.5 oz	170	9	13
Macaroni & Cheese, 3.5 oz	230	14	16
Sandwiches: Chicken Club	670	27	58
Ham Club	670	30	59
Italian Meats	840	49	59

For Complete Nutritional Data ~ see CalorieKing.com

Rubio's Coastal Grill® (Oct '23)

Burritos: Flour Tortilla, As Served	C	F	Cb
Beef: All Natural Steak	930	39	103
California Steak	1120	63	88
Chicken, All Natural	880	34	105
Grilled Seafood:			
Ancho Citrus Shrimp	830	34	103
Beer Battered Fish	940	55	83
Classic Grilled Shrimp	880	35	101
Grilled Atlantic Salmon	920	46	93
Grilled Wild Mahi Mahi	830	36	93
Shrimp & Bacon	1010	52	93
***Tacos:** With Corn Tortilla Unless Indicated*			
Chicken: *Per One Taco*			
Classic All Natural	250	12	21
Grilled Gourmet	340	19	22
Natural Steak, Grilled: *Per One Taco*			
Classic	270	14	20
Gourmet	370	21	22
Street	120	5	9
Vegetarian: *Per One Taco*			
Classic Impossible	280	16	23
Gourmet: Grilled Impossible	350	20	24
Taco with Veggies	320	18	27
Street Impossible	130	6	12
Sides:			
Black Beans: Regular	100	2	15
Large	280	3	46
Cauli Rice: Regular	40	3	3
Large	120	8	10
Mexican Rice: Reg.	100	2	20
Large	270	4	53
No Fried Pinto Beans: Regular	110	1	17
Large	300	2	51
Quinoa & Brown Rice: Regular	80	1	14
Large	210	3	39
Tortilla Chips: Regular	210	3	43
Large	460	5	96
Salsas, average all varieties	10	0	3
***Salad & Bowls:** Entrée Size, Includes Dressing*			
Bowls: California Bowl	550	21	78
Cilantro Lime Quinoa	570	27	68
Mexican Street Corn	730	34	93
Salads: Avocado Corn	440	28	37
Chopped Salad	380	30	19
Mango Avocado	460	33	39

Ruby Tuesday® (Oct '23)

Appetizers: As Served	C	F	Cb
Blackened Chicken Quesadillas	980	62	44
Cheddar Cheese Queso & Chips	1130	66	99
Coconut Shrimp	360	10	59
Crispy Mozzarella Sticks (6)	600	28	57
Loaded Cheese Fries	1430	97	95
Loaded Potato Skins	1180	32	163
Onion Rings Appetizer	1390	96	115
Ruby's Signature Sampler	1400	72	126
Spinach Artichoke Dip	980	57	97
***Burgers:** Without Fries*			
Bacon Cheeseburger	800	47	37
Classic Burger	670	37	37
Impossible	590	30	46
Jalapeno Bacon Queso Burger	810	47	41
Ruby's Cheeseburger	720	41	38
Smokehouse Cheeseburger	960	53	63
Smashed: American	1080	66	38
Loaded Guac	1340	88	41
Mushroom Swiss	1510	91	46
***Cheesesteaks:** Without Sides*			
Five Cheese	850	46	50
Hickory Bourbon	910	44	60
Philly Hoagie	720	32	53
***Chicken:** Without Added Sides or Breadstick*			
Chicken Parmesan, single	1790	67	128
Crispy Chicken Tenders	390	19	20
Hickory Bourbon	250	5	18
***Pasta:** As Served*			
Blackened Shrimp & Sausage	1230	65	118
Crispy Chicken Mac 'n Cheese	1920	110	147
Parmesan Shrimp	1250	61	126
***Baby Back Ribs:** With Fries & Coleslaw*			
Classic BBQ Baby Back Ribs:			
Half Rack	1010	53	82
Full Rack	1480	77	103
***Sandwiches:** Without Sides*			
Grilled Chicken	540	22	36
Meatball Hoagie	1060	62	72
Ultimate Crispy Chicken	1070	51	98

Ruby Tuesday® cont... (Oct '23)

Seafood:	C	F	Cb
With Rice Pilaf & Grilled Zuchini			
Grilled Samon	540	25	36
Hickory Bourbon Salmon	620	25	54
Steak: *With Garlic Butter & Baked Potato*			
Ribeye: 12 oz	990	50	47
with Crispy Shrimp & Cocktail Sce	1310	68	74
with Grilled Shrimp	1090	52	48
with ½ Rack BBQ Baby Back Ribs	1460	73	68
with Hickory Bourbon Chicken	1240	55	66
Top Sirloin: 6 oz	550	10	49
with Crispy Shrimp & Cocktail Sce	870	28	75
with Grilled Shrimp	650	12	49
with ½ Rack BBQ Ribs	1020	34	70
with Hickory Bourbon Chicken	800	15	67
Sides: *Per Serving*			
Baked Potato	220	1	47
Coleslaw, ½ cup	240	18	16
French Fries	420	21	53
Grilled Zucchini	20	1	3
Onion Rings	340	19	37
Loaded: Baked Potato	600	31	50
French Fries	800	49	59
Tater Tots	790	48	59
Mac 'N Cheese	570	36	35
Mashed Potatoes	220	11	27
Rice Pilaf	190	3	33
Roasted Corn	190	10	24
Steamed Broccoli	70	1	5
Tater Tots	420	19	53
Salads: *With Menu Set Dressings*			
Rib Eye Steak	920	58	36
Ruby's Chicken Caesar:			
Crispy	890	59	50
Grilled	780	50	37
Salmon Ceasar Salad	930	67	36
Desserts: *As Served*			
Carrot Cake	630	36	69
Chocolate Chip Cookie Skillet	1350	71	174
New York Cheesecake	780	74	96
Ultimate Chocolate Cake	740	46	81

For Complete Menu ~ see CalorieKing.com

Runza® (June '23)

Burgers:	C	F	Cb
¼ Lb: Bacon Cheeseburger	440	25	25
Cheeseburger	400	21	25
Double	670	39	29
Hamburger	340	17	22
Double	550	31	22
Spicy Jack	510	32	25
Swiss Cheese Mushroom	450	27	25
Grilled Chicken Sandwiches:			
BBQ	360	11	30
Buffalo	340	11	25
Spicy Jack	450	22	25
Wraps: Buffalo Jr.	510	20	63
Ranch Jr.	500	20	63
Chicken Strips, 2 pieces	250	10	21
Runza Sandwiches: Original	490	16	64
Cheese Runza	550	21	67
Spicy Jack Runza	660	31	66
Swiss Cheese Mushroom Runza	560	23	65
Minis: Original	260	9	34
Cheese	290	11	36
Swiss Cheese & Mushroom	300	12	35
Sides: Chili	280	12	25
French Fries: Small	265	12	36
Large	475	22	64
French Onion Dip	100	7	6
Frings	670	33	85
Onion Rings	610	31	72
Salads: *Without Dressing*			
Southwest Chicken Salad, w/ Salsa	400	18	36
Sweet Berry Chicken	380	19	21
Dressings: Honey Mustard	290	27	13
SW Ranch	220	24	4
Soups: *Per Bowl*			
Boston Clam Chowder	280	15	29
Broccoli Cheese	240	16	20
Chicken Tortilla	150	6	16
Potato Bacon	260	14	30
Kids: *Without Beverage*			
Chicken Strip Meal w/ Small Fries	480	19	55
Junior: Cheeseburger, plain	300	16	20
Hamburger, plain	240	11	17
Swiss Cheese Mushroom Burger	310	18	19
Desserts:			
Chocolate Chip Cookie	490	23	70
Choc./Vanilla Ice Cream: Cones	215	5	32
Dish	190	5	27
Sundaes: Caramel; Chocolate	270	8	43
Turtle	330	14	44

7-Eleven® (Sept '18)

Breakfast Sandwiches: *Please visit Stores for latest menu items and nutritional information*	C	F	Cb
Biscuits:			
Sausage, 3.3 oz	330	22	28
Spicy Chicken, 4.5 oz	270	14	30
Croissants:			
Sausage, Egg & Cheese, 4.7 oz	450	32	23
English Muffin:			
Egg, Bacon & Chse, 4.5 oz	300	14	28
Egg, Cheese & Sausage, 5 oz	390	25	24
Salads: *Per Container*			
Balsamic Garden Salad, with Chicken, 6.5 oz	170	9	18
BLT, 8 oz	270	18	12
Caprese Salad, 4.5 oz	150	11	7
Chicken Caesar, 7.5 oz	390	28	17
Chicken Caesar Pasta Salad, 9 oz	540	24	61
Kale & Quinoa Salad, 6 oz	300	18	30
Mediterranean Pasta Salad, 8.5 oz	490	29	49
Side, 5 oz	30	0	7
Sandwiches/Melts:			
Chicken, Bacon Ranch Melt, 7.4 oz	560	22	56
Chicken Salad Sandwich, 6.6 oz	470	21	49
Double Cheeseburger, with American Cheese, 9.6 oz	800	54	35
Egg Salad Sandwich, 6.8 oz	480	24	50
Go!Smart Turkey Sandwich	300	3	48
Grilled Chicken Sandwich, w/ Honey Mustard BBQ Sauce, 6 oz	340	10	39
Italian Melt, 7.8 oz	610	39	38
Southwest Turkey Sandwich, 8 oz	560	28	48
Steak & Cheese Melt, 7.8 oz	680	35	57
Sides:			
Hash Brown (1), 2 oz	100	5	12
Potato Wedges (6), 0.7 oz	240	5	27
Taquitos,			
Chicken & Monterey Jack, (2), 5.3 oz	330	12	44
Drinks: Cappuccino, 8 fl.oz	180	4	36
Caramel Macchiato, 8 fl.oz	190	5	34
Cuban Coffee, with milk, 8 fl.oz	200	7	34
French Vanilla Cappuccino, 8 fl.oz	190	6	34
Skinny, 8 fl.oz	140	5	30
Hot Chocolate, 8 fl.oz	170	3	37
Peppermint Mocha, 8 fl.oz	180	4	36
Pumpkin Spice Late, 8 fl.oz	190	6	35
Slurpees, average all flavors:			
12 oz cup	95	0	26
22 oz cup	175	0	44
28 oz cup	220	0	56
Sugar Free, 12 oz cup	30	0	9

Saladworks® (Oct '23)

Salads: *W/out Dressing or Bread*	C	F	Cb
Asian Crispy Chicken	360	9	57
Avocado Cobb	450	28	15
Bently	350	18	11
Buffalo Bleu	290	13	16
Classic Greek	180	11	11
Grilled Chicken: Caesar	390	19	28
Mediterranean	230	10	16
Farmers Market	350	16	28
Roasted Turkey Club	340	9	40
Smokey BBQ Crispy Chicken	370	16	47
Sophie's	430	18	48
Soups: *Per Medium Serve, without Bread Roll*			
Baked Potato	340	24	28
Broccoli Cheddar	280	19	18
Chicken Noodle	180	5	18
Chicken Poblano	350	21	26
Chicken Tortilla	260	14	19
Lasagna w/ Turkey Ssg	230	11	21
Lobster Bisque	470	39	21
New England Clam Chowder	370	27	22
Warm Grain Bowls: *Without Dressing, Extras Or Bread*			
Asian Crispy Chicken	510	10	89
Avocado Cobb	520	23	42
Bently	490	19	42
Buffalo Bleu	430	14	47
Classic Greek	320	12	42
Farmers Market	500	18	59
Grilled Chicken Caesar	530	20	59
Roasted Turkey	330	9	40
Smoky BBQ Crispy Chicken	510	17	78
Southwest Chipotle Ranch	580	26	58
Wraps: *With Flour Tortilla W/out Dressing, Sides or Extras*			
Asian Crispy Chicken	670	17	105
Avocado Cobb	760	36	63
Bently	660	26	59
Buffalo Bleu	600	21	64
Classic Greek Salad	490	19	59
Farmers Market	660	24	76
Grilled Chicken Caesar	700	27	76
Roasted Turkey Club	650	17	88
Smokey BBQ Crispy Chicken	680	24	95
Sophie's Salad	740	26	96

Sandella's® (Oct '23)

Grilled Flatbread:	C	F	Cb
BBQ Cheese	430	9	67
Bacon & Cheddar	630	34	54
Chicken Fajita	500	18	52
Chicken Parmesan	560	20	55
El Paso	710	19	97
Ham & Cheddar	570	25	51
Meatball	630	29	56
Olympian	480	26	53
Pesto & Peppers	530	27	52
Philly Style	450	10	54
Spinach & Artichoke	610	33	54
Thai Chicken	630	24	66
Tomato Bacon	580	26	58
***Paninis:** With Standard Toppings*			
Americana	580	25	54
Arizona Chicken	660	23	78
Beef Fajita	630	27	58
Bistro Ham & Brie	560	19	70
Brazilian Beef, without cheese	500	6	86
Genoa	730	37	53
Napoli Chicken	440	17	49
Pastrami Melt	670	33	55
Philly Cheese	590	25	55
Spinach & Bacon	610	29	65
Toasted Caprese	380	14	50
***Quesadillas:** With Standard Toppings*			
Barbecue	570	18	66
Beef Fajita	570	22	55
Buffalo Chicken	510	20	49
Thai Veggie	570	27	60
***Salads:** With ½ Flatbread, without Dressing*			
Apple Walnut	370	13	60
Napa Valley	770	60	54
Panzanella	190	3	36
Siesta	310	15	44
Thai Chicken	330	13	35
***Rice Bowls:** Includes Flatbread & Standard Toppings*			
Asian Chicken & Broccoli	680	3	138
Mesquite BBQ	930	21	140
Southwest Veggie	810	20	126
Thai Peanut Saute	680	16	116
Wraps: *With Standard Toppings*			
California Turkey	410	10	55
Greek Salad	430	14	55
Nut & Honey	800	32	116
Seven Layer	570	23	66
Swiss Salad	500	20	62
Texas Beef	420	10	58
The Russian	400	7	60
Veggie & Cheese	450	19	52

Sarku Japan® (Oct '23)

Bento Box:	C	F	Cb
Fried Rice: Beef	830	32	98
Chicken	820	35	95
Shrimp	750	27	96
D'Lite Meals, Vegetables:			
with Fried Rice	430	10	79
with Noodles	640	14	109
with Steamed Rice	410	6	83
***Teriyaki Meals:** With Steamed Rice*			
Beef	580	16	80
Beef & Shrimp	690	21	85
Chicken	640	24	79
Chicken & Shrimp	750	29	85
Shrimp	530	12	80
Sushi Rolls: California	330	8	57
Chicken Teriyaki	360	11	53
Dancing Eel	430	13	61
Green Dragon	650	35	71
Philadelphia	430	18	49
Rainbow	360	7	51
Rock & Roll	550	21	66
Salmon	220	5	33
Tuna	190	0	33
Sauce, Teriyaki, 1.5 oz	45	0	9
Sides: Chicken Egg Roll	160	6	21
Dumplings (6)	260	12	29
Edamame	170	7	11
Miso Soup	50	2	6
Seaweed Salad	70	2	13
Shrimp Tempura (3)	390	30	23
Vegetable Spring Roll	190	9	15

Schlotzsky's® (Oct '23)

***Sandwiches:** Per Medium*	C	F	Cb
Albuquerque Turkey	1120	55	87
Beef Bacon Smokecheesy	1190	66	75
Chicken Bacon Smokecheesy	1090	57	73
Deluxe Original	950	42	79
Fiesta Chicken	990	50	75
Fiesta Turkey	990	50	82
French Dip	920	38	83
Fresh Veggie	590	24	75
Ham & Cheese, Original	830	31	79
Pastrami Reuben	940	43	85
Roast Beef & Cheese	920	41	79
Smoked Turkey Breast	530	9	81
The Original	860	40	77
Turkey Avocado	590	14	85
Turkey Bacon Club	990	45	82

continued next page...

Schlotzsky's® cont... (Oct '23)

Pizzas: Per 10" Pizza	C	F	Cb
BBQ Chicken & Jalapeno	970	22	143
Double Cheese	910	25	124
Pepperoni & Double Cheese	1070	38	125
Fresh Veggie	850	20	128
***#1 Salads:** Without Dressing*			
Chicken Avocado Cobb	370	16	21
Chicken Caesar	270	9	16
Greek Chicken	220	7	10
Strawberry Chicken	340	14	27
***Dressing:** Per 4 oz*			
Blue Cheese; Caesar	600	64	4
Italian	540	58	4
Ranch	440	44	4
Thousand Island	480	48	20
***Soup:** Per 10 oz Bowl*			
Broccoli Cheese	500	37	25
Chicken Noodle	110	2	16
Chicken Tortilla	160	6	22
Loaded Baked Potato	290	17	26
Timberline Chili	270	12	22
Tomato Basil	370	26	28
Chips:			
All varieties, average	230	14	24
***Kidz Meals:** Without Cookie or Drink*			
Cheese Pizza	450	9	74
Ham Sandwich	480	20	49
Pepperoni Pizza	510	13	74
Turkey Sandwich	480	20	50
Desserts:			
Brownie (1)	500	28	62
Cookies: Chocolate Chunk (1)	370	18	52
Sugar (1)	390	20	48
White Chocolate Macadamia (1)	400	22	47
***Breakfast:** Per Whole Burrito/Sandwich*			
Burritos: Bacon	460	22	41
Ham	490	21	44
Sausage	570	31	41
Veggie	430	19	44
Sandwiches: Bacon; Veggie	500	21	51
Ham	530	22	50
Sausage	650	32	49
Tacos: Bacon; Sausage, average	250	14	18
Ham	290	17	18
Veggie	220	10	21
Sides:			
Hash Brown, 1 piece	60	5	8
Mixed Fruit, 1 scoop	20	0	6

Second Cup® ~ *see CalorieKing.com*

Shake Shack® (Oct '23)

Burgers: Per Single Burger	C	F	Cb
Bacon Cheeseburger	500	29	25
Cheeseburger	440	24	25
Green Chile Cheddar Shack	470	26	28
Hamburger	370	18	24
Link	680	46	27
Lockhart Link	780	56	27
Shackburger	500	30	26
Shack Stack	770	45	50
SmokeShack	570	35	28
Veggie Shack: Regular	530	27	56
Vegan Style	390	22	50
Chicken: Bites (6)	300	19	15
Chicken Shack	550	31	34
Flat-Top Dogs:			
Garden Dog	180	3	27
Hot Dog	350	22	25
Shackmeister Cheddar Brat	690	51	33
Fries: Bacon Cheese	840	52	65
Cheese	710	44	64
Double Down	1910	117	164
Regular	470	22	63
Floats, Creamsicle	450	15	70
***Shakes:** Without Whipped Cream*			
Chocolate	750	45	76
Cookies & Cream	850	44	98
Vanilla	680	36	72
Add On, Whipped Cream	70	5	5
Breakfast:			
Single Sandwiches: Bacon	400	23	25
Egg & Cheese	340	19	25
Sausage	530	32	28

Shakey's® (Oct '23)

Pizzas: Per Slice, 1/10 12" Medium Size Pizza	C	F	Cb
Big Island: Pan Crust	210	6	30
Thin Crust	160	6	19
California Pizzarito: Pan Crust	265	12	30
Thin Crust	215	11	19
Cheese: Pan Crust	190	5	30
Thin Crust	135	5	17
Firehouse: Pan Crust	280	13	30
Thin Crust	230	12	20
Garden Veggie: Pan Crust	205	6	30
Thin Crust	150	6	19
Rustic Garlic Chicken: Pan Crust	215	6	30
Thin Crust	160	6	18
Shakey's Special: Pan Crust	255	11	30
Thin Crust	200	10	18
Texas BBQ Chicken: Pan Crust	220	6	32
Thin Crust	165	5	20
Ultimate Meat: Pan Crust	310	15	30
Thin Crust	260	14	20

Shakey's® cont... (Oct '23)

Golden Fried Chicken: Per Piece	C	F	Cb
Breast	360	11	16
Leg	175	10	6
Thigh	350	24	9
Wing	130	9	4
Rice: *Per ½ Cup*			
Mexican Fiesta	100	0	22
Pilaf	120	3	22
Sides & Extras: Enchilada	80	2	17
Garlic Bread, 1 piece	180	4	30
Macaroni & Cheese, 1 cup	350	17	33
Mashed Potatoes, ½ cup	65	1	13
Mojo Potatoes, 5 pieces	215	11	25
Penne Rigate	200	1	42
Pepperoni Pizza Twists	215	8	29

Shari's® (Oct '23)

Breakfast: *As Served*	C	F	Cb
Bacon & Eggs only	290	22	1
Buttermilk Pancakes	800	27	123
Country Sausage Benedict	1470	102	90
Double Smoked Sausage & Egg	450	32	6
French Toast, Traditional	960	62	82
Meat Lover's Skillet	1100	86	38
Sausage & Eggs Only	630	57	1
Shari's Sampler	1610	105	116
Ultimate Country Fried Steak	1060	72	67
Waffle	340	14	48
Lunch: *Without Side Choices*			
Chicken Strips	340	18	23
Salads: *Entrée Size, with Dressing*			
Caesar	460	40	15
Northwest Steak	890	50	65
Rustic Tuscan Chicken	510	32	21
Sandwiches: *Per Whole Sandwich*			
BLT on Texas Toast	540	26	51
Cajun Chicken Avocado Club	1360	74	115
Cuban on Ciabatta Roll	680	30	60
Grilled Ham & Four Cheese Melt, on Sourdough	1140	68	78
Hot Turkey on Whole Wheat	1040	31	129
Prime Rib Dip on French Roll	680	33	63
Traditional Club	1310	72	114
Dinner: *With Menu Set Sides*			
Beer Battered Fish & Chips	1600	119	104
Chopped Steak	930	50	50
Country Fried Steak	1010	63	83
Grilled Lemon Chicken	450	17	17
Slow Roasted Turkey	980	50	109
Wild Alaskan Salmon, grilled	470	28	19

Shari's® cont... (Oct '23)

Sides, Add-Ons:	C	F	Cb
Baked Potato: Plain	210	5	37
with Sour Cream & Butter	330	18	38
Broccoli	130	11	7
Coleslaw	140	10	11
French Fries	490	32	48
Loaded Baked Potato	330	15	38
Loaded Mashed Potatoes	410	21	42
Rice Pilaf	90	5	10
Shrimp Skewer	90	1	1
Stuffed Hash Browns	420	28	32
Tater Tots	370	26	33
Desserts:			
Pies:			
Banana Cream Dream	450	26	48
Chocolate Cream Supreme	510	30	54
Creamy Caramel Pecan Crunch	730	49	67
Peanut Butter Chocolate Silk	620	45	51
Tropical Coconut Cream	580	37	63

Sheetz® (Oct '23)

Breakfast Sandwiches:	C	F	Cb
Burrito, Bacon, Egg, Cheese & Salsa	280	12	30
Sandwiches:			
Farmhouse Cheddar Flatbread	310	11	32
Walker Breakfast Ranger	550	23	60
Wildwest Flatbread	290	10	32
Burgerz: Big Mozz	670	33	57
Boss Bacon	790	56	35
Cowboy	590	31	40
Twisted Swiss	760	45	50
Burritos: Cheese Chili & Totz	780	40	85
Screamin' Pork	750	29	87
Steak & Taters	810	40	83
Mac & Cheese Platter:			
Boom Chicka	650	39	43
Meatball	750	49	38
Morning	650	43	43
Sandwichez:			
Chicken: Big Mozz w/ Grilled Breast	600	19	60
Boss Bacon with Homestyle Breast	790	50	46
Grilled Cheese:			
American Cheese on Sourdough	440	23	47
Cheddar Cheese on Sourdough	450	24	46
Shwingz: with BBQ Sauce (6)	540	28	39
with Boom Boom Sauce	700	55	20
with Garlic Parmesan Sauce	660	50	18
with Spicy Asian Sauce	540	30	37

continued next page...

Sheetz® cont... (Oct '23)

Sliderz:	C	F	Cb
BL Tease	280	18	16
Boomin Onions & Cheddar Burger	160	9	17
Spicy Bacon Ranch Chicken	310	15	28
Sidez: *Without Sauce, Topping or Dipper*			
Cheesy Bacon Tator Bombs	290	19	20
Crispy Chicken Stripz:			
3 pieces	330	11	39
5 pieces	550	18	65
Curly Fryz, cup	450	23	55
Fryz, cup	390	13	64
Jalapeno Poppers	330	18	35
Loaded Fryz	600	20	97
Mac & Cheese	320	18	28
Mac & Cheese Bites	370	19	40
Mozzarella Cheese Sticks	410	14	52
Tater Totz, cup	460	28	48
Wisconsin Cheddar Bites, regular	440	36	8
Beverages: *With 2% Milk & Chocolate Sauce*			
Caramel Hot Chocolate, medium	700	23	109
Hot Chocolate, medium	730	22	118

Sizzler® (Oct '23)

Menus May Vary. Please Check Your Local Outlet For Menu Choices And Further Nutritional Information.

Burgers & Sandwiches:	C	F	Cb
Classic: ⅓lb Burger	830	57	44
⅓lb Cheeseburger	920	64	45
⅓ lb Bacon Cheeseburger	950	67	44
Grilled Chicken Avocado Sandwich	720	37	48
Malibu Melt	1840	155	69
Mega Bacon Burger	940	61	49
Double	1440	106	44
Smokey Bacon Burger	950	65	47
Entrees: *Without Sides, Condiments, Dipping Sauce or Optional Accompaniments*			
Chicken: *Small Plate*			
Italian Herb Chicken	230	6	1
Malibu Chicken	680	60	14
Combo Nation:			
Classic Steak Trio	1270	89	48
Steak & Jumbo Crispy Shrimp (8)	720	32	47
Steak & Lobster	720	51	2
Steak & Malibu Chicken	920	73	14

Sizzler® cont... (Oct '23)

Entrees (Cont): *Without Sides, Condiments, Dipping Sauce or Optional Accompaniments*	C	F	Cb
Ribs:			
BBQ: 6 bones	1870	145	32
3 Bones & BBQ Chicken, 7 oz	1170	70	34
Seafood:			
Atlantic Shrimp Skewers, peeled (2)	440	15	29
Grilled Salmon, 6 oz	370	23	3
Cilantro Lime Barramundi	470	17	34
Steaks:			
New York Strip, 12 oz	830	61	2
Ribeye, 14 oz	1100	88	3
Tri-Tip Sirloin, 8 oz	340	16	1
Steak Toppings: Grilled Onions	80	6	7
Sauteed Button Mushrooms	180	17	5
Sides: Cheese Toast	290	19	22
Cilantro Lime Rice	150	0	31
Garlic Mashed Potatoes	200	4	39
Rice Pilaf	170	4	31
Salted Baked Potato	510	30	55
Loaded	760	57	55
Street Fries	500	31	52
Vegetable Medley	80	5	8

Skyline Chili® (Oct '23

Burritos:	C	F	Cb
Chili Deluxe	610	33	38
Original	610	31	54
Coneys/Sandwiches:			
Coneys: Cheese, w/ onions & mstrd	350	23	25
Coney, plain	220	13	22
Sandwiches: Chili Cheese, with onions & mustard	290	17	24
Chili, with onions & mustard	180	8	23
Ways:			
Chili Spaghetti with Onion:			
Small	200	10	26
Regular	410	19	52
Large	540	25	70
Bowls: Black Beans & Rice	400	14	48
Chili	200	12	0
Loaded Chili	480	28	20
Steamed Potatoes:			
3-Way Potato	620	26	65
Cheddar Potato	630	33	65
Sour Cream Potato	460	19	65
Salads: *Without Dressing*			
Buffalo Chicken	220	11	12
Greek	210	12	17
Fries: Chili Cheese	840	53	61
Regular Fries	430	24	51

Smoothie King® (Oct '23)

Bowls:	C	F	Cb
Acai Cocoa Haze	610	21	105
Bee Berry Sting	440	7	90
Coco Pitaya -Yah	520	19	84
Go Go Goji Crunch	540	15	99
PB Delight	520	13	93
Fruit Smoothies: *Per 20 oz , with Standard Menu Components*			
Be Well Blends: *Without Turbinado*			
Blueberry Heaven	260	2	57
Vegan:			
Dark Choc. Banana	340	3	80
Pineapple Spinach	320	6	64
Enjoy A Treat Blends: *With Turbinado*			
Angel Food	350	1	82
Banana Boat	480	6	99
Caribbean Way	430	1	106
Muscle Punch	360	1	84
Passion Passport	430	0	105
Yogurt D-Lite	320	5	56
Get Fit Blends:			
High Intensity: Choc. Cinnamon	400	16	44
Veggie Mango	400	15	41
Original High Protein:			
Banana	340	12	34
Chocolate	390	12	43
Lemon	380	12	46
Pineapple	310	12	28
Peanut Power Plus: *With Turbinado*			
Chocolate	590	25	75
Strawberry	610	24	89
The Activator Recovery:			
Chocolate	200	3	22
Blueberry Strawberry	260	2	39
Pineapple	320	2	52
Strawberry Banana	270	2	37
The Hulk: With Turbinado			
Chocolate	640	22	104
Strawberry	890	34	146
Manage Weight Blends:			
Keto Champ: Berry	430	31	19
Chocolate	420	32	18
Metabolism Boost:			
Banana Passionfruit	270	3	51
Mango Ginger	280	3	49
Slim-N-Trim: With Stevia			
Chocolate	200	3	34
Strawberry	160	3	28
Vanilla	170	3	31
The Shredder: Strawberry	270	3	37
Vanilla	230	4	16

Snappy Tomato Pizza® (Oct '23)

Snappetizers:	C	F	Cb
Bone In Wings (6)	460	34	4
Flatbread, medium, ⅙ flatbread	270	12	33
Wedge Fries: Regular	220	10	28
Loaded	420	25	30
Hoagies: Chicken Ranch	910	44	75
Grilled Chicken	640	15	70
Ham & Cheese	570	15	71
Italian Combo	650	23	69
Steak & Cheese	760	35	73
Veggie Melt	490	11	74
Pasta, Plain Spaghetti/Rigatoni, av.	350	2	70
Sauce: Ranch	570	60	8
Snappy	80	2	8
Toppings: Bacon	120	8	1
Beef; Black or Green Olives, av.	50	4	2
Cheese	90	7	1
Chicken	120	3	1
Pepperoni	140	10	0
Peppers	5	0	1
Sausage	80	6	1
Tomatoes	5	0	1
Salads: Crispy Chkn, w/o dressing	280	9	24
Garden, without dressing	90	5	11
Grilled Chicken, w/out dressing	160	3	10
Dessert: Cinnabread, med., ⅙ slice	350	13	57
Raspberry Cinnabread, ⅙ slice	370	13	62

Sonic Drive-In® (Oct '23)

Burgers:	C	F	Cb
Bacon Cheeseburger with Mayo	860	54	54
Double	1140	77	52
Cheeseburger with Ketchup & Mayo	720	42	52
Double	1070	71	54
Veggie Burger with Ketchup & Mayo	500	17	70
Chicken:			
Sandwiches: Classic Crispy Chicken	550	30	48
Chicken Slinger	350	16	35
Boneless Wings: *6 Pieces*			
Asian Sweet Chili	470	24	32
Honey BBQ	470	24	33
Buffalo	440	28	17
Jumbo Popcorn: Small	330	19	24
Medium	490	28	36
Large	750	43	55
Tenders: Crispy, 3 pieces	260	12	16
5 pieces	430	20	27
Coneys: Chili Cheese	470	29	34
Footlong Quarter Pound	790	49	55

continued next page....

Sonic Drive-In® cont... (Oct '23)

6" Hot Dogs:	C	F	Cb
All American Dog	410	21	41
Cheesy Bacon Pretzel	430	29	27
Chicago Dog	400	20	41
Breakfast:			
Bagel Sandwich:			
Bacon	580	24	68
Sausage	730	39	68
Biscuit Sandwich: Bacon	530	29	40
Ham	510	24	43
Brioche Sandwich: Bacon	490	28	39
Ham	460	22	41
Burrito: Bacon	470	25	35
Ham	440	20	38
Stak & Egg	650	36	48
Cinnasnacks, w/out Frosting (3)	380	22	38
Croissonic: Bacon	480	32	31
Ham	460	27	34
French Toast Sticks, w/o syrup (4)	480	25	54
Toaster: Ham	500	24	45
Sausage	670	45	43
Sides: *Medium*			
Chedd 'R' Peppers (6)	490	48	56
Fries	290	13	38
with Cheese	380	22	39
with Chili & Cheese	450	26	42
Onion Rings	635	34	75
Ice Cream Sundaes: Caramel	490	22	61
Chocolate	430	22	51
Hot Fudge	520	26	65
Add Ons: Peanuts	40	4	2
Whipped Topping	70	5	5
Classic Shakes: *Per Medium*			
Caramel	830	41	97
Chocolate	810	43	95
Fresh Banana	850	41	108
Hot Fudge	940	48	113
Peanut Butter	940	59	87
Strawberry	790	41	92
Vanilla	820	45	89
Master Shakes: *Per Medium*			
Cheesecake	840	43	101
Oreo Cheesecake	1030	51	131
Oreo Chocolate	1000	51	125
Oreo Peanut Butter	1130	66	116
Strawberry Cheesecake	890	43	112
Sonic Blast: *Per Medium*			
Butterfingers Pieces	980	48	118
Choolate Chip Cookie Dough	920	45	118
M&M's Minis Choc. Candy	1060	54	127
Oreo Cookie Pieces	860	44	103
Reese's Peanut Butter Cups	990	55	110
Snickers Bars	890	46	103

Sonic Drive-In® cont... (Oct '23)

All Natural Lemonade:	C	F	Cb
Small	160	0	42
Medium	270	0	69
Large	400	0	105
Limeade Slush: Small	190	0	52
Medium	280	0	74
Large	430	0	116
Cold Brew Iced Coffee: *Per Medium*			
Original	260	13	32
French Vanilla	300	13	42

For Complete Nutritional Data ~ see CalorieKing.com

Southern Tsunami® (Oct '23)

Appetizers:	C	F	Cb
Calamari Salad, 4 oz	140	1	15
Edamame, 3 oz	120	5	10
Grilled Shrimp Dumplings, pkg	320	12	43
Seabreeze Salad, 4 oz	90	3	17
Premium Bowls:			
Chirashi: *With White Rice*			
Chicken	790	26	117
Kani Kama	780	25	124
Salmon, Tuna	810	29	115
Hawaiian Poke: *With White Rice*			
Tuna	660	18	96
Tuna, Salmon	710	24	96
Tuna, Salmon, Albacore	690	21	96
Ramen Noodle Salad,			
with Sesame Dressing	630	40	58
Rolls: *With White Rice*			
Classic Rolls: Calif. & Inari, 4 pcs	210	4	40
Cream Cheese: Imit. Crab, 15 pcs	530	15	83
Salmon, 15 pieces	580	22	76
Crunchy Shrimp, 6 pieces	250	9	35
Hawaiian, 5 pieces	240	9	34
Inari, 10 oz	510	8	97
Ocean Crab, 6 pieces	180	4	31
Hybrid:			
Berry Roll, 9 oz	400	13	64
Blueberry Roll, 5 pieces	240	9	29
Crunchy Tempura Roll, 10 oz	460	16	69
Done Deal Roll, 10.8 oz	520	22	64
Dynamite Roll, 5 pieces	290	10	34
Happy Mango Roll, Eel, 10 oz	490	18	69
Spicy Mango Roll, Unakaba, 9.9 oz	490	22	65

Southern Tsunami® cont... (Oct '23)

One Roll: *Ten Pieces, w/ White Rice*	C	F	Cb
California	310	6	58
California Salad Roll	340	9	57
Cream Cheese Roll:			
Imitation Crab	360	10	57
Salmon	400	15	53
Crunchy CA Rol	510	24	65
Crunchy Dragon:			
Orange	620	34	62
Red	570	27	62
White	550	25	70
Crunchy Shrimp Tempura	580	27	74
Dragon	480	22	65
Eel	360	8	58
Rainbow Roll:			
Albacore, Salmon, Tuna	440	13	57
Salmon, Shrimp, Tuna	430	13	57
Wraps: Berry , 4 pcs	80	4	12
California, 4 pieces	120	6	13
Smoked Salmon Roll, 3.5 oz	160	10	11
Spicy California Wrap, 4 pieces	150	10	13
Spicy Chkn Roll, 3.5 oz	120	6	11
Spicy Salmon, 4 pieces	140	9	11
Summer Roll 2, 1 piece, 3.5 oz	90	3	14
Teriyaki Chicken Roll, 1 piece, 3.5 oz	120	2	17
Vegetable Wrap, 4 pieces	80	4	11

Starbucks® (Oct '23)

Per Standard Ingredients. Please Check Instore Nutritional Information for Milk Varieties and Added Extas.

Brewed Coffee: *With 2% Milk Only*	C	F	Cb
Caffe Misto: Short, 8 fl.oz	50	2	5
Tall, 12 fl.oz	80	3	8
Grande, 16 fl.oz	110	4	10
Venti, 20 fl.oz	130	5	13
Hot Drinks: *With 2% Milk , Drizzle, Sauce & Wh. Cream*			
Chocolate:			
Kid's or Short, 8 fl.oz	190	9	21
Tall, 12 fl.oz	280	12	32
Grande, 16 fl.oz	370	16	43
Venti, 20 fl.oz	450	18	54
White Chocolate: *Without Drizzle*			
Kid's or Short, 8 fl.oz	240	11	28
Tall, 12 fl.oz	350	15	41
Grande, 16 fl.oz	440	19	55
Venti, 20 fl.oz	540	22	69

Starbucks® cont... (Oct'23)

Steamers:	C	F	Cb
Vanilla Creme: *With 2% Milk, Whipped Cream & Syrup*			
Kid's or Short, 8 fl.oz	180	9	20
Tall, 12 fl.oz	280	12	34
Grande, 16 fl.oz	350	14	44
Venti, 20 fl.oz	430	16	55
Hot Espresso Beverages: *With 2% Milk*			
Caffe Latte: *Without Toppings or Extras*			
Short, 8 fl.oz	100	4	10
Tall, 12 fl.oz	150	6	15
Grande, 16 fl.oz	190	7	19
Venti, 20 fl.oz	250	9	24
Caffe Mocha: *With Whipped Cream & Syrup*			
Short, 8 fl.oz	200	9	22
Tall, 12 fl.oz	290	13	33
Grande, 16 fl.oz	370	15	43
Venti, 20 fl.oz	450	18	54
Cappuccino: *Without Toppings or Extras*			
Short, 8 fl.oz	70	3	7
Tall, 12 fl.oz	100	4	10
Grande, 16 fl.oz	140	5	14
Venti, 20 fl.oz	200	8	20
Caramel Macchiato: *With Drizzle & Syrup*			
Short, 8 fl.oz	120	4	16
Tall, 12 fl.oz	190	6	26
Grande, 16 fl.oz	250	7	35
Venti, 20 fl.oz	310	9	44
Cinn. Dolce Latte: *W/ Toppings, Wh. Cream & Syrup*			
Short, 8 fl.oz	190	9	22
Tall, 12 fl.oz	270	12	33
Grande, 16 fl.oz	340	14	43
Venti, 20 fl.oz	420	16	54
Honey Almondmilk Flat White: *Without Toppings*			
Short, 8 fl.oz	80	3	15
Tall, 12 fl.oz	120	4	22
Grande, 16 fl.oz	170	5	30
Venti, 20 fl.oz	210	7	38
Cold Brew: *With Vanilla Sweetener & Chocolate Cream Cold Foam*			
Chocolate Cream:			
Tall, 12 fl.oz	190	12	20
Grande, 16 fl.oz	250	14	29
Venti, 20 fl.oz	300	16	36
Trenta, 30 fl.oz	320	16	40
Iced Shaken Espresso: *With Syrup & Cinn. Powder*			
Brown Sugar Oatmilk:			
Tall, 12 fl.oz	100	3	17
Grande, 16 fl.oz	120	3	22
Venti, 24 fl.oz	190	5	34

continued next page...

Starbucks® cont... (Oct '23)

Frappuccino Blended Coffee:	C	F	Cb
Per 16 fl.oz Grande, with Whole Milk, Standard Extras and Whipped Cream			
Caffe Vanilla	410	15	64
Caramel	380	16	55
Java Chip	440	19	64
Mocha Cookie Crumble	480	24	62
White Chocolate Mocha	420	17	61
Frappuccino Blended Creme: *Per 16 fl.oz Grande, with Whole Milk, Standard Extras and Whipped Cream*			
Chai	340	16	46
Double Chocolaty Chip	410	20	51
Vanilla Bean	380	16	53
White Chocolate	380	18	49
Refreshers: *Per 16 oz Grande*			
Draon Drink, Coconut Milk	130	3	26
Mango Dragonfruit	90	0	22
Pink Drink, Coconut Milk	140	3	28
Strawberry Acai Lemonade	140	0	35
Teas: *Per 16 fl.oz Grande*			
Hot Green Tea, Honey Citrus Mint	130	0	32
Lattes: *With 2% Milk, Standard Ingredients, w/out Extras*			
Chai	240	5	45
London Fog Latte	180	4	29
Matcha Green Tea Latte	240	7	34
Royal English B'fast, sweetened	150	4	21
Iced Latte: Chai	240	4	44
London Fog	140	3	25
Breakfast:			
Egg Bites, Kale & Mushroom, 1 piece	230	14	11
Sandwiches:			
Bacon, Gouda & Egg/Artisan Roll	360	18	35
Impossible/Sesame Ciabatta Bun	420	22	36
Wrap, Spinach, Feta & Egg White	290	8	34
Parfait, Berry Trio	240	3	39
Lunch:			
Sandwiches: Gr. Cheese, Sourdough	520	27	47
Ham & Swiss/Baguette	500	24	43
Tomato & Mozzarella/Focaccia	360	12	47
Turkey, Provolone & Pesto/Ciabatta	520	19	53

Starbucks® cont... (Oct '23)

Bakery: *Each*	C	F	Cb
Bagels: Everything	290	3	57
Plain	290	1	60
Brownie, Double Chocolate, 3.67 oz	480	28	55
Cake, cinnamon Coffee, 3.5 oz	380	15	57
Cookie, Chocolate Chip	370	19	47
Croissants: Butter	250	14	26
Chocolate	300	18	34
Danish, Cheese, 2.82 oz	290	14	33
Dessert Bar, Marshmallow Dream, gluten free	230	5	44
Glazed Doughnut	440	19	60
Muffin, Blueberry, 3.5 oz	330	14	47

Bottled Drinks ~ See Page 37

Steak Escape® (Oct '23)

Cheesesteaks: *Per Regular Size*	C	F	Cb
Bourbon & Bacon	1100	64	89
Grand Escape	690	28	66
Original Philly	710	30	68
Sriracha	790	34	73
Sandwiches: *Per Regular Size*			
Chicken Bacon Club	980	58	62
Crispy Buffalo Chicken	1020	48	90
Grandest Chicken	680	22	65
Ragin Cajun	700	27	63
Simply Chicken	550	13	60
Subs: *Per Regular Size*			
Black & Bleu	740	37	65
Cubano	910	47	66
Delerious Dagwood	1180	76	62
Hangover	890	39	76
Italian Hottie	920	48	66
Wraps:			
Bourbon & Bacon	1010	63	80
Smokin BBQ	700	32	68
Steakhouse Sirloin	950	63	65
Fries: Buffalo Chicken; Cajun Bleu	950	60	83
Loaded Cheese & Bacon, small	920	63	79
Naked, regular	650	34	78
Sriracha Steak	900	53	87
Potatoes: Bourbon & Bacon	1020	54	101
Delerious Dagwood	1100	66	74
Simply Chicken	460	4	72
Triple Cheesesteak	910	45	78
Salads: Bourbon & Bacon	720	54	33
Cubano	530	38	10
Hangover	630	29	50
Sriracha Cheesesteak	410	24	17

For Complete Nutritional Data ~ see CalorieKing.com

Steak 'n Shake® (Oct '23)

Steakburgers: Without Fries	C	F	Cb
Bacon 'n Cheese: Single	460	26	29
Double	600	38	29
Butter Steakburger	870	65	34
Garlic Double	730	50	33
Single Burger with Cheese	390	20	32
The Original Double	460	26	33
with cheese	530	32	32
Triple: with Cheese	750	50	32
without Cheese	610	38	32
The Original: Double	460	26	33
with Cheese	530	32	32
Western BBQ 'N Bacon	790	43	54
Chili: 3-way	710	21	98
5-way	1160	57	103
Chili Deluxe: Bowl	1000	56	71
Cup	500	28	36
Chili Mac, Regular	1200	61	112
Melts, Frisco	960	66	51
Sandwiches:			
Grilled Cheese	620	43	41
Gr. Cheese & Bacon	590	35	41
Steak Franks:			
Chili Cheese Frank	710	44	46
Steak Frank	390	23	32
Fries: *Per Regular*			
Cheese Fries	590	35	63
Chili Cheese Fries	760	39	83
French	450	24	54
Sides: Applesauce	90	0	22
Chicken Fingers (3)	330	18	22
Onion Rings, medium	330	17	39
Kid's:			
Chicken Fingers & Fries	380	25	25
Grilled Cheese Sandwich & Fries	780	56	51
Steakburger & Fries	460	27	39
Steakburger with Cheese & Fries	530	33	39
Steak Frank & Fries	540	36	40
Milk Shakes: *Per Regular*			
Banana	700	17	126
Birthday Cake	840	26	136
Butterfinger	760	22	128
Chocolate	600	17	101
M&M's	790	24	131
Oreo Red Velvet	960	30	157
Reese's Choc. Peanut Butter	980	47	118
Strawberry;Vanilla, average	615	17	104
White Chocolate	630	18	105

Subway® (Oct '23)

Build Your Own Sandwiches::	C	F	Cb
Per 6" with Set Menu Board Ingredients, w/o Dressing			
Black Forest Ham	280	4	42
Buffalo Chkn, grilled	380	12	42
Cold Cut Combo	320	10	41
Grilled Chicken	290	4	40
Italian BMT	400	16	43
Meatball Marinara	440	18	50
Oven Roasted Turkey	270	4	40
Roast Beef	310	5	42
Spicy Italian	470	24	42
Steak & American Cheese	360	10	40
Tuna	470	25	40
Veggie Delite	210	3	39
Series Sandwiches: *6" With Set Menu Board Ingredients*			
Cheeesesteaks: 1. The Philly	500	25	41
2. The Outlaw	490	22	40
3. The Monster	580	30	42
33. Teriyaki Blitz	450	14	53
Deli Heros: 15. Titan Turkey	490	23	40
17. Garlic Roast Beef	480	21	43
30. The Beast	730	44	45
99. Grand Slam Ham	500	24	43
Italianos: 4. Supreme Meats	590	32	44
6. The Boss	650	34	54
18. Ultimate BMT	560	30	43
23. Hotshot Italiano	620	38	43
Chicken:			
7. The Mexicali with Sliced Avocado	520	25	43
8. The Great Garlic	570	29	43
20. Elite Chicken & Bacon Ranch	570	29	43
Clubs: 10. All American Club	530	28	43
11. Subway Club	500	24	43
Wraps: *With Set Menu Board Ingredients, w/o Condiments*			
Build Your Own Plain Wrap:			
Black Forest Ham	440	11	58
Buffalo Chicken, grilled	560	19	56
Cold Cut Combo	530	23	55
Italian BMT	680	36	58
Meatball Marinara	780	38	76
Oven Roasted Turkey	430	10	54
Roast Beef	500	14	58
Rotisserie Style Chicken	500	15	54
Steak & American Cheese	570	20	55
Sweet Onion Chicken Teriyaki	590	11	83
Tuna	820	54	53
Veggie Delite	330	8	57

continued next page...

Subway® cont... (Oct '23)

Protein Bowls: *W/ Set Menu Board Ingredients*	C	F	Cb
Black Forest Ham	170	5	12
Buffalo Chicken, grilled	380	21	13
Cold Cut Combo	260	16	9
Grilled Chicken	200	4	9
Italian BMT	410	29	13
Meatball Marinara	530	32	33
Oven Roasted Turkey	150	3	8
Steak & American Cheese	380	19	12
Sweet Onion Chicken Teriyaki	350	5	46
Tuna	550	47	8
Salads: *Without Dressing*			
Black Forest Ham	120	3	12
Buffalo Chicken, grilled	300	19	13
Cold Cut Combo	160	9	10
Grilled Chicken	130	3	10
Italian BMT	240	15	12
Meatball Marinara	290	16	22
Oven Rstd. Turkey	110	2	10
Roast Beef	150	4	12
Rotisserie Style Chicken	150	5	10
Spicy Italian	310	23	12
Steak & Am. Cheese	210	9	12
Tuna	310	24	10
Breakfast: *With Set Menu Board Ingredients*			
Egg Patty on 6" Artisan Flatbread w/ Regular Egg:			
Bacon, Egg & Cheese	530	28	44
Black Forest Ham, Egg & Cheese	480	23	44
Egg & Cheese	450	22	43
Steak, Egg & Chse	520	25	44
Flatizza: Cheese	410	17	45
Pepperoni	470	22	45
Spicy Italian	510	26	46
Veggie	430	17	49
Pizzas, 8 Inch: Bacon	840	34	95
Cheese	720	24	94
Meatball	860	35	98
Pepperoni	850	35	95
Sliders:			
Ham & Jack Cheese	160	4	20
Italian Spice	250	15	20
Little Cheesesteak	180	7	20
Turkey & Pepper Jack	200	9	19

Swiss Chalet® (Oct '23)

Canadian Outlets	C	F	Cb
Starters:			
Cheese Perogies, 9.45 oz	450	12	79
Chicken Spring Rolls, 8 oz	570	22	65
Caesar Salad: no protein, 5 oz	340	6	13
with Bacon	400	11	14
Chicken Soup with crackers:			
Cup	130	3	15
Bowl	180	4	20
Crispy Wings: 5 pieces	840	43	60
10 pieces	1570	80	109
BBQ Ribs: *With Dinner Roll, Butter, Coleslaw & Sauce*			
½ Rack	980	57	75
with ¼ Chicken	1350	84	63
with ¼ Chicken White Meat	1260	70	63
with 5 Wings	1640	91	112
Full Rack	1600	103	90
Burgers: *With Mayo, Without Sides*			
Classic Hamburger	660	33	56
Veggie	460	15	57
Rotisserie Chicken: *W/ Dinner Roll, Butter & Chalet Sauce*			
¼ Dark Meat Chicken	610	33	31
¼ White Meat Chicken	540	19	31
½ Chicken	970	47	31
Double Leg	1040	60	31
Sandwiches/Wraps: *W/- Sauce & Pickle Unless Indicated*			
Chicken Pot Pie, with Dinner Roll			
Crispy Chicken Sandwich	680	33	68
Hot Rotisserie Chicken: Bun	590	20	47
White Meat Bun	500	10	47
Club Wrap	750	38	60
White Meat Wrap	700	32	60
Sandwich	680	21	65
White Meat Sandwich	600	11	65
Southern Canuck	840	28	90
White Meat Sandwich	800	25	90
Entree Salads: *As Served*			
Caesar: Without Chicken	270	13	27
with Crispy Chicken & Bacon	1170	42	49
with Rotisserie Chicken	1080	32	27

Swiss Chalet® cont... (Oct '23)

Sides: Per Serving	C	F	Cb
Baked Potato w/ Sour Crm & Chives	210	6	37
Creamy Mashed Potatoes	180	4	38
Garlic Green Beans	230	19	13
Market Vegetables, 8 oz	60	1	12
Poutine	800	47	76
with Rotisserie Chicken	940	51	76
Seasoned Rice Pilaf	300	4	59
Sweet Potato Fries	860	51	102
Fries:			
Crispy, 12 oz	660	27	100
Fresh Cut, 12 oz	580	31	73
Fresh Cut & Seasoned, 12.4 oz	620	33	78
Sauce: Chalet 4 oz	25	0	5
Chalet Dipping, 4 oz	20	1	3
Plum, 2 oz	120	0	27
Smoky BBQ, 4 oz	210	1	49
Wing: Hot, 2.25 oz	80	5	10
Medium, 2.4 oz	100	4	16
Mild, 2.45 oz	120	3	25
Desserts/Pies: *Oer Slice*			
Cheesecake with Caramel Topping	490	24	58
Chocolate Super Sundae	340	21	67
Coconut Cream Pie,	550	35	55
Fudge Cake	680	41	74
Lemon Meringue Pie	440	17	68

Taco Bell® (Oct '23)

Burritos: W/- Standard Components	C	F	Cb
Bean	350	9	55
Beefy 5-Layer	490	18	65
Cheesy Bean & Rice	420	16	55
Chili Cheese, regional	380	17	41
Chipotle Ranch Grilled Chicken	510	29	47
Supreme: Beef	390	14	51
Chicken; Steak	375	11	50
Steak, Bacon & Grilled Cheese	700	39	57
Fries: Nacho, regular	320	18	35
Large	460	26	51
Nachos: *With Standard Components*			
Nachos BellGrande:			
Beef	730	38	81
Chips & Nacho Cheese Sauce	220	13	24
Grilled Chicken	710	35	79
Steak	720	36	80
Power Bowls: *With Standard Components*			
Grilled Chicken	460	21	41
Steak	470	23	42
Veggie	420	20	47

Taco Bell® cont... (Oct '23)

Quesadillas: W/ Menu Set Sauce	C	F	Cb
Cheese	470	24	41
Chicken	520	26	41
Steak	520	26	41
Tacos: *Without Beans, Rice or Sauce*			
Chalupa Supreme: Beef	360	20	31
Black Bean Supreme	340	18	36
Grilled Chicken	340	17	29
Steak	350	18	30
Cheesy Gordita Crunch	490	28	41
Crunchy: Seasoned Beef	170	10	13
Steak	150	8	11
Nacho Cheese Doritos:			
Grilled Chicken	150	7	10
Steak	160	8	11
Soft: Grilled Chicken	160	5	16
Supreme	190	11	15
Supreme Soft: Grilled Chicken	190	7	18
Seasoned Beef	210	10	20
Sides: *Regular Size*			
Black Beans & Rice	160	5	25
Black Beans	50	2	7
Cheesy Fiesta Potatoes	240	13	28
Breakfast: *With Set Menu Board Ingredients, w/o Beans*			
Crunchwrap: *With Jalapeno Sauce*			
Bacon & Eggs	670	40	52
Sausage Patty	750	49	53
Steak	660	38	53
Cheesy Toasted Burrito: *With Nacho Cheese Sauce*			
Bacon & Egg	350	16	38
Sausage	350	17	38
Grande Toasted Burrito: *Without Sauce*			
Bacon & Eggs	570	30	52
Sausage Crumbles	450	22	50
Steak	450	18	51
Hash Brown Toasted Burrito: *Without Sauce*			
Bacon & Eggs	580	32	52
Sausage	570	31	51
Steak	570	28	52
Sweets:			
Cinnabon Delights, (2)	170	11	15
Cinnamon Twist	170	6	27
Freeze, Wild Cherry, 16 fl.oz	150	0	41

Note: Nutritional Information varies from state to state. Please refer to Taco Bell's Website

Taco Cabana® (Oct '23)

Cabana Burritos:	C	F	Cb
Includes Flour Tortilla, Rice, Refried Beans, Romaine, Meat, Shredded Cheese, Pico de Gallo & Sour Cream			
Chicken Fajita	660	25	74
Ground Beef	770	39	76
Shredded Chicken	730	33	76
Steak	680	29	74
***Cabana Bowls:** Includes Shell, Rice, Lettuce, Meat, Shredded Cheese, Pico de Gallo & Sour Cream*			
Chicken Breast Fajita	640	30	60
Ground Beef	750	44	61
Shredded Chicken	760	37	66
Steak Fajita	660	34	60
***Enchiladas:** Without Topping*			
Beef	250	18	15
Cheese	320	24	14
Chicken	230	14	15
***Flauta,** Chicken*	120	4	13
***Quesadillas:** Small, with Lettuce, Guac. & Sour Cream*			
Cheese	560	34	41
Chicken Fajita	710	40	52
Steak	630	38	43
Tacos:			
Crispy: Ground Beef	230	15	13
Shredded Chicken	210	12	13
Soft: Bean & Cheese	300	14	31
Carne Guisada	210	8	20
Chicken Fajita	210	6	21
Ground Beef	270	14	22
Mixed Fajita	220	7	21
Shredded Chicken	240	11	22
Steak Fajita	220	9	21
***Cabana Salads:** Includes Romaine Letuce, Shredded Cheese, Pico de Gallo, Black Beans & Tortilla Strips*			
Base Salad with Ranch Salsa	410	24	37
add Chicken Fajita	140	4	3
add Ground Beef	240	17	4
add Shredded Chicken	200	11	5
add Steak Fajita	170	9	3
Sides & Add-Ons:			
Black Beans, 8 oz	240	2	42
Chips: Small, 2.5 oz	340	18	41
Regular, 5.1 oz	680	35	81
Guacamole: Small, 4 oz	140	10	7
Regular Guacamole, 8 oz	290	24	18
Queso: Small, 4 oz	140	10	7
Regular Queso, 8 oz	290	20	13
Refried Beans with Cheese, 8 oz	530	29	49
Rice, 8 oz	310	6	58
Salsa, all flavors, 1 oz	5	0	1
Sour Cream, 3 oz	160	15	3
Table Tortillas, Corn, 0.9 oz	50	1	11

Taco Del Mar® (Oct '23)

***Burritos:** Includes Flour Tortilla, Rice, Refr. Beans, Protein, Cheese, Pico de Gallo & Sour Cream Unless Indicated*	C	F	Cb
Regular: Chicken	910	31	115
Ground Beef	950	37	116
Pork	900	31	115
Shredded Beef	910	31	116
Steak	870	27	117
Vegan with guacamole	680	15	115
Veggie with guac., without meat	840	29	119
***Burrito Bowls:** Per Regular Bowl, with Rice, Refried Beans, Protein, Cheese, Pico de Gallo & Sour Cream*			
Chicken	600	24	63
Pork	590	24	63
Shredded Beef	600	24	64
Steak	560	20	65
Vegan	370	8	63
Veggie with addeed guacamole	530	22	67
***Nachos:** Includes Chips , Refried Beans, Protein, Cheese, Pico de Gallo, Guacamole & Sour Cream*			
Beef: Ground	1210	78	90
Shredded	1160	71	90
Cheese	1040	66	88
Chicken; Pork, av.	1155	72	90
Fish	1200	74	100
***Enchilada Taco Platters:** Per 1 Corn & 1 Flour Tortilla, Protein, Cheese, Rice, Ench. Sauce, Refr. Beans,Lettuce, Pico de Gallo, Guacamole &, Sour Cream*			
Cheese	810	32	105
Chicken	850	31	105
Fish	880	33	116
Ground Beef	890	37	106
Pork	830	30	104
***Quesadillas:** Includes Flour Tortilla, Meat, Cheese & Pico*			
Cheese	590	29	57
Chicken	720	35	58
Fish	750	37	69
Ground Beef	760	41	59
Pork; Shredded Beef, average	705	34	58
***Taco Salads:** Includes Shell, Cheese, Refried Beans, Lettuce, Meat , Sour Cream & Pico de Gallo Unless Indicated*			
Chicken	710	38	59
Fish	730	41	70
Ground Beef	750	45	60
Pork	690	38	58
Vegan	670	25	97

Note: Nutritional Information varies from state to state. Please refer to Taco Del Mar Website

Taco John's® (Oct '23)

Burritos:	C	F	Cb
Bean	400	13	57
Boss, Chicken & Pico	800	27	107
Combination	430	18	50
Fried Chicken Grande Griller	740	39	80
Grilled Beef	690	41	56
Grilled Chicken	660	35	55
Meat & Potato: Beef	510	26	55
Chicken	490	22	54
Steak	500	25	54
Super, Beef	470	20	52
Super Nachos, beef, regular	800	41	84
Super Potato Oles,			
Beef, regular	1090	71	90
Quesadillas:			
Cheese	500	29	41
Chicken	560	30	43
Tacos: Crispy Beef	190	11	14
Softshell Taco: Beef	230	11	21
Chicken	210	7	21
Stuffed Grilled Beef	510	26	53
Taco Bravo Beef	350	15	41
Salads: *Without Dressing*			
Beef Taco Salad	710	45	57
Chicken Taco Salad	680	40	56
Steak Taco Saad	700	43	56
Sides:			
Black Beans	210	1	38
Chips & Nacho Cheese	380	19	45
Potato Oles: Small	460	30	43
Medium	650	42	61
Large	840	55	78
Refried Beans	360	8	52
Side Salad, without dressing	40	3	3
Condiments:			
Chipotle Lime Sauce, 1 fl.oz	140	14	3
Guacamole, 2.5 fl.oz	150	11	12
House Dressing, 1.5 oz	70	7	2
House Salsa, 1fl.oz	5	0	1
Nacho Cheese Sauce, 3 oz	110	9	5
Pico de Gallo, 1 oz	10	0	2
Sour Cream, 2.5 oz	140	13	4
Breakfast:			
Burritos: Bacon Scrambler	530	27	53
Sausage Meat & Potatoes	600	34	53
Sausage Scrambler,	600	34	54
Potato Ole Scrambler, Sausage	1100	71	89
Desserts: Churro	230	11	31
Mexican Donut Bites	330	7	53

Taco Mayo® (Oct '23)

Burritos:	C	F	Cb
Bean	450	14	63
Chicken Burrito Supreme	420	19	40
Double Smothered Dble Queso:			
Beef	930	43	88
Chicken	850	39	83
Mexicali Gr. Chicken	635	38	48
Super: Regular	525	21	56
Beef	525	21	56
Bowls: Chipotle Chicken	1225	71	91
Insalada Little Big	275	16	14
Mexicali Little Big	450	18	41
Queso Chicken	1035	48	92
Nachos:			
Classic: Beef Supreme	790	38	81
Cheese	370	20	44
Chicken Supreme	710	34	77
Ultimate Grande	990	51	93
Quesadillas: Beef Melt	655	35	45
Chicken Platter	690	40	45
Tacos: Crispy Beef	160	9	10
Fish	280	13	27
Soft Taco: Beef	230	10	19
Chicken	185	8	16
Taco Burger	360	15	32
Tamale Ole	715	38	64
Salads: *As Per Menu Description*			
Beef	665	33	55
Chicken	445	26	31
Sides: Cheddar & Chips	555	31	62
Guacamole	185	16	11
Guacamole & Chips	575	35	63
Mexicali Rice	180	9	17
Mixed Fruit Cup	60	0	16
Queso & Chips	575	29	62
Potato Locos, small	400	25	37
Refried Beans	225	4	34
Kids Meals:			
Burritos: with Fruit Cup	505	14	78
with Potato Loco	845	39	99
Quesadillas: with Fruit Cup	270	12	31
with Potato Loco	605	37	52
Tacos:			
Crispy: Beef with Fruit Cup	220	8	29
with Potato Loco	560	33	50
Soft: Beef w/ Fruit Cup	290	10	35
with Potato Loco	630	36	56

Taco Time® (Oct '23)

Burritos:	C	F	Cb
5 Alarm	420	15	58
Chicken B.L.T.	600	31	46
Sweet Pork	550	18	72
Big Juan: Chicken	590	16	79
Seasoned Beef	650	22	83
Casita: Chicken	450	16	44
Seasoned Beef	510	22	48
Crispy Burrito:			
Chicken	380	17	39
Meat	390	17	43
Pinto Bean	380	13	53
Soft Burrito: Pinto Bean	380	10	56
Seasoned Beef	420	16	46
Veggie	440	17	60
Nachos: Original	810	39	78
Chicken	880	40	78
Seasoned Beef	930	45	82
Optionals:			
Green Chili Pork Carnitas: Burrito	540	18	58
Chimichanga	590	21	65
Enchiladas	380	16	28
Soup, Enchilada, 8 oz	130	1	20
Quesadillas: Cheese	450	23	39
Chicken	520	24	42
Tacos:			
Soft Tacos: Chicken	360	10	42
Junior Seasoned Beef	300	13	29
Pork	440	16	43
Super Soft Tacos: Chicken	500	16	61
Pork	590	21	62
Seasoned Beef	560	21	65
Fries:			
Mexi: Small, 3.2 oz	190	12	19
Regular, 4.7 oz	300	19	29
Stuffed: Small, 4.5 oz	320	20	29
Regular, 6.6 oz	460	28	42
Salads: *Without Dressing*			
Fiesta, Chicken,12.3 oz	340	11	37
Taco: Chicken, 8 oz	310	14	26
Seasoned Beef , 7.5 oz	360	19	28
Breakfast:			
Burritos: *Regular Size*			
Bacon & Egg; Enchilada, average	480	21	50
Egg & Cheese	370	16	40
Sausage & Egg	520	26	50
Ultimate	720	44	51
Quesadilla	340	18	26
Taters & Gravy, regular	410	27	36
Desserts:			
Churros: Plain	210	16	15
Bavarian Cream	320	8	54
Cinnamon Crustos	320	5	64

TCBY® (Oct '23)

Soft Serve Frozen Yogurt: *Per 4 fl.oz*	C	F	Cb
Dairy Free/Sorbet:			
Chocolate Almond	100	1	28
Kiwi Strawberry Sorbet	90	0	22
Mango Sorbet	95	0	24
Orange Sorbet	90	0	23
Pink Lemonade	95	0	23
Watermelon Sorbet	100	0	25
No Sugar Added: Butter Pecan	90	0	19
Average other flavors	65	0	18
Super Fro Yo: Bananas Foster	90	0	23
Cake Batter; Golden Vanilla	105	2	22
Chocolate	100	2	22
Golden Vanilla	105	2	22
Graham Cracker	105	2	25
Greek Honey Vanilla	100	0	20
New York Cheesecake	115	2	23
Saalted Caramel, NSA	70	0	18
White Chocolate Mousse	120	2	24
Hand-Scooped Frozen Yogurt:			
Dairy Free, Psychedelic Sorbet	130	0	33
Gluten Free:			
Butter Pecan: Kid's, 4 fl.oz	220	10	27
Small, 6.4 fl.oz	350	16	43
Regular, 12.8 fl.oz	705	32	86
Chocolate Chocolate:			
Kid's, 4 fl.oz	120	3	20
Small, 6.4 fl.oz	190	4	38
Regular,12.8 fl.oz	385	8	76
Cookies & Cream:			
Kid's, 4 fl.oz	200	6	32
Small, 6.4 fl.oz	320	10	51
Regular, 12.8 fl.oz	640	19	102
Peanut Butter Delight:			
Kid's, 4 fl.oz	250	13	30
Small, 6.4 fl.oz	400	21	48
Regular, 12.8 fl.oz	800	42	96
Pralines & Cream: Kid's 4 fl.oz	210	6	27
Small, 6.4 fl.oz	335	10	43
Regular, 12.8 fl oz	670	19	86
Vanilla Bean:			
Kid's,4 fl.oz	170	5	27
Small, 6.4 fl.oz	270	7	43
Regular, 12.8 fl.oz	545	14	86

TGI Friday's® (Oct '23)

Appetizers/Snacks:	C	F	Cb
Boneless Wings:			
Apple Butter	880	42	83
Dragon-Glazed	900	43	82
Garlic Parm	1090	74	63
Whiskey Glazed	990	42	110
Chips & Salsa	240	10	29
Loaded Potato Skins, w/- Ranch Sour Cream	2120	92	283
Mozzarella Sticks, with Marinara	840	52	54
Pan Seared Potstickers, with Szechuan Sauce	590	25	72
Philly Cheesesteak Egg Rolls, with Beer Cheese Sauce	1070	61	82
Spinach Artichoke Dip	760	55	43
Traditional Wings:			
Apple Butter BBQ	740	55	29
Dragon-Glazed	750	56	28
Garlice Parm	940	87	9
Frank'sBuffalo	620	55	0
Whisley Gazed	840	55	56
Burgers: *With Regular Bun, without Sides*			
Bacon Cheeseburger	690	31	47
Beyond Meat Chseburger	860	53	52
Cheeseburger	770	52	41
Whiskey-Glazed	1140	56	117
Green Style, Beyond Cheeeseburger	580	40	16
Chicken & Seafood: *With Menut Set Sides*			
Crispy: Chicken Fingers, with Slaw, Fries & Honey Mustard	1030	67	74
Fried Shrimp (PB), with Fries, Coleslaw & Cocktail Sauce	930	45	82
Fish & Seasoned Fries, Coleslaw & Tartar Sauce	1180	72	97
Simply Gr. Salmon, with Jasmine Rice, & Lemon Butter Broccoli	830	41	81
Pasta: *Full Order, Fried*			
Cajun Shrimp & Chicken, with Breadstick	1390	60	132
Chicken & Broccoli Cheee Tortelloni with Breadstick, fried	1850	110	140
Chkn Parmesan, w/ Breadstick, fried	1630	75	161
Ribs: *With Crispy Fried Shrimp, Mashed Potatoes & Lemon-Butter Broccoli*			
Crispy Whisky: Half Rack (PB)	1170	49	154
Half Rack (HB)	1120	48	136

TGI Friday's® cont... (Oct '23)

Sandwiches: Without Sides	C	F	Cb
Bacon Ranch Chicken	690	31	47
Southern Fried Chicken	920	55	65
Whiskey Glazed Chicken	1160	56	107
Sizzling: *With Mashed Potatoes*			
Chicken & Shrimp	1030	71	41
Chicken & Cheese	930	60	37
Whiskey-Glazed Flat Iron Steak	1470	78	127
Salads:			
Caesar: with Grilled Chicken	790	59	21
without Protein	600	54	19
Million $ Cobb:			
Gr Chicken & Ranch	1000	86	21
without Protein	820	70	19
Soup,			
White Cheddar Broccoli Cheese	290	20	18
Sides: Fried Shrimp (PB)	210	9	21
Giant Onion Rings with Ranch	510	26	61
Jasmine Rice	370	10	63
Mashed Potatoes	130	4	23
Seasoned Fries	230	15	21
Desserts: *Per Whole Dish*			
Brownie Obsession	1180	58	154
Dessert Platter, small	3720	178	496
Oreo Madness, Stuffed	540	23	79

Thundercloud Subs® (Oct '23)

Subs: *Small, w/ Standard Toppings*	C	F	Cb
Classic: BLT	405	20	36
Genoa Salami	280	7	35
Roast Beef	290	4	35
Smoked Chicken	270	4	35
Turkey	255	4	36
Signature Subs:			
Club	445	19	38
California Club	475	23	40
NY Italian	540	30	37
Office Favorite	790	39	71
Texas Tuna	675	44	39
Veggie Delite, with Hummus	385	19	52

T.J. Cinnamons® (Oct '23)

Bakery:	C	F	Cb
Orig. Gourmet Cinn. Roll, 7.8 oz	840	42	106
Pecan Stick Bun, 8.3 oz	940	49	111

Tim Hortons® (Oct '23)

Breakfast:	C	F	Cb
Bagel BELT	560	24	62
Biscuit Sandwich:			
Angus Steak & Egg	400	20	34
Bacon, Egg & Cheese	415	23	33
Sausage, Egg & Cheese	530	34	33
Turkey Sausage, Egg & Cheese	425	23	34
Grilled Breakfast Wrap: Farmer's	680	42	54
Steak & Cheddar	440	21	40
Oatmeal, with Mixed Berries, reg.	210	3	44
Hash Brown, 1.9 oz	130	7	16
Lunch:			
Chili, small	330	18	18
Pasta, Mac & Cheese	490	27	48
Soup: *Per Small Size*			
Broccoli Cheddar	180	9	16
Chicken Noodle Soup	120	2	21
Hearty Vegetable Soup	80	0	14
Potato Bacon Cheddar Soup	260	15	22
Roasted Red Pepper & Gouda	220	14	17
Turkey & Wild Rice	130	2	25
Wraps:			
Grilled Chicken Fajita	430	19	39
Steak Fajita	430	20	40
Sides,			
Kettle Cooked Potato Chips, 1.4 oz	220	14	22
Cookies: Chocolate Chunk	210	9	32
Oatmeal Raisin Spice	210	8	32
Peanut Butter	250	15	24
White Chocolate Macadamia	220	11	29
Donuts: Apple Fritter	290	8	48
Boston Cream	220	6	35
Chocolate Dip	190	7	29
Football	230	8	34
Maple Dip	190	6	29
Old Fashion Dip	250	11	33
Muffins: Chocolate Caramel	410	15	64
Wild Blueberry	340	11	57
Whole Grain Pecan Banana Bread	350	11	60
Timbits: Apple Fritter (1)	50	2	9
Chocolate Glazed (1)	70	3	10
Honey Dip (1)	45	1	8
Old Fashioned Glazed (1)	70	3	10
Sour Cream Glazed (1)	90	5	12
Salted Caramel (1)	70	3	11

Tim Hortons® cont... (Oct '23)

Beverages:	C	F	Cb
Hot: Cappuccino, 15 fl.oz	100	0	15
Mocha Latte, 15 fl.oz	230	7	32
Iced: Coffee, cream & Sugar, 20 fl.oz	110	7	11
Latte, 20 fl.oz	240	7	35
Mocha Latte, 20 fl.oz	390	9	68

Togo's® (Oct '23)

California Outlet ~ Please check local outlet for menu items and nutritional information

	C	F	Cb
Cold Sandwiches: *Per Regular 6", with Menu Set Components on White Bread*			
#2: Ham & Swiss	650	28	58
#3:Turkey & Cheddar	650	29	56
#4: Turkey, Salami & Cheddar	820	46	56
#5: Turkey & Cranberry	610	18	76
#7: Roast Beef	630	20	57
#8: Roast Beef & Turkey	700	30	57
#16: The Italian	840	47	60
#20: Albacore Tuna	700	37	62
#23: Salami & Provolone	980	62	56
Hot Sandwiches: *Per Regular 6", with Menu Set Components on White Bread*			
#1: Chicken & Cheddar	820	43	59
#6: Meatball	840	39	73
#9: Pastrami	620	28	59
#31 Clubhouse Melt	860	49	57
#32: Pepperjack Melt	910	54	61
#37 Brewpub Chicken	880	45	65
#39 BBQ Chipotle Chicken	740	29	73
Wraps: *Per Whole 12" Spinach Tortilla Wrap, with Menu Set Components*			
Asian Chicken	650	28	70
Bacon Ranch Chicken	740	39	54
Chicken Caesar	580	22	60
Farmer's Market	500	24	61
Santa Fe Chicken	720	33	66
Salads: *Per Full Salad, with Dressing*			
Asian Chicken	670	43	42
Chicken Caesar	470	27	24
Farmer's Market	460	38	25
Santa Fe Chicken	790	55	37
Soups: *Per 10 oz*			
Broccoli Cheddar	220	14	16
Chicken Noodle	120	4	15
Chili with Beans	240	8	23
Brownie, Choc. Chunk, 3 oz	440	23	58
Cookies: Choc. Chunk, 3 oz	410	21	54
Peanut Butter, 3 oz	440	25	49

Tropical Smoothie Cafe® (Oct '23)

Menu & Nutrition Differ from Outlets to Outlet. Please Check Instore.

	C	F	Cb
Breakfast:			
All American Omelet Wrap	410	20	38
Peanut Butter Crunch Flatbread	580	23	79
Southwest Omelet Wrap	580	36	38
Flatbreads:			
Chicken Bacon Ranch	500	23	44
Chicken Pesto	430	16	43
Chipotle Chicken Club	490	24	42
Quesadillas: Santa Fe Chicken	600	28	50
Three Cheese Chicken	550	27	41
Sandwiches:			
Avocado Grilled Cheese	930	56	69
Chicken Caprese	660	26	62
with Bacon	720	31	62
Smoky Grilled Cheese	650	33	63
Turkey Bacon Ranch	560	20	59
Toasted Wraps: *In Flour Tortilla*			
Baja Chicken	640	24	67
Buffalo Chicken	510	21	44
Caribbean Jerk Chkn	590	17	74
Hummus Veggie	680	31	83
Supergreen Caesar Chicken	600	31	42
Thai Chicken	500	15	62
Classic Smoothies: *Per 24 oz with Turbinado*			
Bahama Mama	510	4	117
Beach Bum	550	4	131
Blimey Limey	480	0	119
Blueberry Bliss	340	5	86
Island Green	410	0	102
Lean Machine	490	0	124
Mango Magic	400	0	98
Mocha Madness	540	4	124
Paradise Point	430	0	110
Peanut Butter Cup	700	18	131
Peanut Paradise with Pea	730	17	109
Sunrise Sunset	400	0	97

Tubby's® (Oct '23)

Subs: *Per Regular 8" Sub, with Standard Ingredients, without Added Sauce or Dressing*

	C	F	Cb
Deli-Subs:			
Ham & Cheese	540	11	78
Turkey Breast	550	10	77
Turkey Club	630	17	77
Grilled Burger Subs:			
Cheeseburger Italiano	790	35	78
Pizza Burger	810	36	81
Taco	960	44	89

Tubby's® cont... (Oct '23)

Subs (Cont): *Per Reg. 8" Sub, with Standard Ingredients, without Added Sauce or Dressing*

	C	F	Cb
Grilled Chicken Subs: Gr. Chicken	450	5	75
Chicken & Broccoli	550	11	78
Chicken & Cheddar	540	11	75
Crispy Chicken	730	30	87
Grilled Steak Subs:			
Loaded Steak	650	18	82
Mushroom, Steak & Cheese	620	17	77
Pepper Steak & Cheese	630	17	77
Steak & Cheese	620	17	76
Specialty Subs: BLT	570	21	72
Cold Veggie	490	10	86
Tuna	570	11	76
Sides: Breaded Mushrooms	410	22	47
French Fries	390	24	39
Mac & Cheese Bites	350	22	29
Mozzarella Sticks	490	26	42
Seasoned Fries	370	28	30

Uno Pizzeria & Grill® (Oct '23)

	C	F	Cb
Appetizers: *Per Whole Dish*			
Mozzarella Sticks	1090	57	107
Muchos Nachos	1700	61	199
Shrimp & Crab Dip	1160	84	66
Burgers: *Without Friess*			
Bacon Cheddar	1350	99	35
Cheddar Burger, ½ lb	1110	81	35
Classic Beyond	560	32	42
Entrees:			
Chicken: *Without Sides or Breadstick*			
Chicken Tender Platter with Fries	1600	106	88
Mediterranean Chicken	560	21	43
Pasta: *With Housemade Bread*			
Chicken Spinoccoli	1260	62	105
Mac & Cheese	1740	103	140
Shrimp Scampi	1190	54	128
Steak & Seafood: *Without Sides or Breadstick*			
Grilled Shrimp & Sirloin	690	45	1
Lemon Basil Salmon	490	38	0
Sirloin, 10 oz	560	37	0
Sirloin Steak Tips	470	20	4
Deep Dish Individual Pizza: *Per Slice, ⅙ Pizza*			
Chicago Classic	360	26	19
Numero Uno	300	19	20
Prima Pepperoni	280	15	18
Sides: French Fries, 7.5 oz	450	33	35
Loaded Mashed Potatoes	420	26	37
Roasted Seasonal Vegetables	70	4	8
Sweet Potato Fries	430	25	47
Dessert:			
Awesome Chocolate Cake	1740	79	241
Uno Deep Dish Sundae	1520	74	206

Villa Italian Kitchen® (Aug '22)

Pizzas: Per Slice	C	F	Cb
Neapolitan: Buffalo	770	46	52
Deluxe	530	22	55
Sausage & Pepperoni	550	25	53
Stuffed: Baked Ziti	845	33	97
Spinach & Mushroom	735	33	79
Entrees:			
Chicken Pasta Primavera, 16 oz	505	20	58
Fettuccini Alfredo, 14 oz	765	38	85
Mac & Cheese, 14 oz	725	54	39
Pasta Primavera, 16 oz	495	21	66
Spaghetti & Meatballs, 18 oz	840	28	112
Sides: Caesar Salad, 4 oz	90	5	9
Garlic Roll	260	10	34
Garden Salad, 3 oz	15	0	3
Greek Salad, 6 oz	125	10	7
Roasted Potatoes, 6 oz	210	12	24
Sauteed Vegetables, 6oz	85	6	6

Vocelli Pizza® (Oct '23)

Pizzas: **Artisan:** *Per ⅛ of Medium Pizza, with Menu Set Components*	C	F	Cb
BBQ Chicken	290	10	35
Deluxe	260	11	29
Garlic Spinaci	230	9	27
Hawaiian	280	11	29
Mac'N'Cheese	280	12	30
Quattro Cheese	260	10	27
Spring Veggie	220	7	29
Linguini Pasta: *Single Serving*			
Chicken Alfredo	1200	54	129
Chicken Parmesan	960	26	144
Chicken Pesto	1230	57	128
House Baked Subs: *On Italian Bread*			
Buffalo Chicken	950	39	86
Chicken Parmesan	990	39	105
Meatball	1170	55	103
Vegetarian	880	42	93
Salads: *Per Regular Size, without Dressing*			
Garden Della Casa	200	10	21
Mediterranean	230	11	22
Tuscan Grilled Chicken	320	13	22
Desserts:			
Cannoli	150	7	17
Chocolate Chip Cookie	120	6	17
Cinnamon Sugar Breadsticks	1440	20	290

Wahoo's Fish Taco® (Oct '23)

Banzai Bowls: *With White Rice & Black Beans*	C	F	Cb
Blackened: Chicken	720	14	104
Fish	675	9	104
Carne Asada	795	24	102
Carnitas	890	26	105
Salmon	705	14	102
Burritos: *With Brown Rice & White Beans*			
Outer Reef: Blackened Chicken	765	32	79
Blackened Fish	725	28	79
Mushroom	700	32	81
Shrimp	705	28	79
Tofu	715	30	81
Side Kicks: Soft Corn Tortillas (3)	145	2	29
Flour Tortilla (1)	300	11	46
Shredder Sandwiches: *With White Rice & White Beans*			
Blackened or Charbroiled:			
Chicken, average	1045	36	140
Fish, average	1000	32	140
Carne Asada	1110	44	140
Wahoo Salads: Banzai Veggie	415	24	35
Carne Asada	690	48	22
Chicken, Blackned or Charbroiled, av	540	32	22
Salmon	550	32	22
Shrimp	460	26	24
Tofu	540	31	30
Soup, Chicken Tortilla	130	6	11

For Complete Nutritional Data ~ see CalorieKing.com

WAWA® (Oct '23)

Breakfast Sizzlis:	C	F	Cb
Bagels: Bacon, Egg & Cheese	450	21	45
Dble Bacon Dble Cheese	510	37	27
Pork Roll, Egg & Cheese	460	22	45
Sausage, Egg & Cheese	550	32	45
Biscuit, Chicken	500	25	55
Bowls: *W/ Starndard Components,, w/o Toppings or Extras*			
Bacon & Egg Omelet	260	20	3
Beef Steak & Scrambled Egg	610	42	13
Chicken Steak & Egg White Omelet	230	10	5
Pancake & Bacon	380	15	52
Pancake & Turkey Sausage	390	14	52
Burritos: *With Egg Omelet & Cheddar Cheese, without Toppings or Extras*			
Bacon	540	29	45
Sausage	640	40	45
Quesadillas: *With Egg Omelet, without any Extras*			
Black Bean & Egg Omelet	740	43	60
Chipotle Bacon Egg Omelet	730	44	51
Garlic Smoked Turkey & Egg Omelet	730	44	51
S'wich, Spinach, Tomato, Egg Omelet on Multigrain Bread	390	13	53

WAWA® cont... (Oct '23)

Hot Hoagies: On Classic Roll, without Cheese, Toppings or Spread	C	F	Cb
Beef Steak	620	21	68
Chicken Steak	620	12	71
Cuban	880	27	68
Meatball	1070	60	95
***Quesadillas:** Without Toppings*			
BBQ Chicken & Cheddar Cheese	650	22	64
Beef with Cheddar Cheese	560	28	44
***Soups:** Per Medium Serving without Toppings*			
Baked Potato with Cheddar & Bacon	400	27	26
Broccoli Cheddar Soup	280	21	14
Chicken Noodle	180	6	21
New Eng. Clam Chowder	310	20	23
Tomato Soup	330	22	28
***Sides:** Per Medium*			
Black Beans	300	7	46
Buffalo Mac & Cheese	520	27	49
Mashed Potatoes	470	27	47
Meatballs in a Cup	480	38	20
Rice & Beans	270	4	49
Rice	240	0	52
Bakery: Apple Fritter	640	26	96
Croissant	200	10	24
Muffins: Banana Nut	580	30	69
Blueberry	560	28	70
Coffee Roll	540	26	68
***Hot Beverages:** Per 16 oz, without Extras*			
Hot Cappuccino, with 2% milk	130	5	13
Mocha Latte, with 2% milk	350	6	64

Wendy's® (Oct '23)

Breakfast:	C	F	Cb
Biscuits:			
Bacon, Egg & Cheese	420	27	28
Honey Butter Chicken	500	29	44
Sausage, Egg & Cheese	580	43	28
Croissants: Bacon, Egg & Swiss	430	23	35
Maple Bacon Chicken	570	31	52
Sausage, Egg & Swiss	590	40	35
Hamburgers:			
Baconator	960	66	36
Bacon Double Stack	440	26	26
Big Bacon Classic: Single	650	41	38
Double	910	62	38
Daves: Single	590	37	37
Double	860	57	37
Triple	1160	81	38
Double Stack	410	24	26
Jr.: Bacon Cheeseburger	370	23	25
Cheeseburger Deluxe	340	20	27
Son of Baconator	630	40	36

Wendy's® cont... (Oct '23)

Sandwiches:	C	F	Cb
Asiago Ranch Chicken Club	600	28	50
Classic Chicken	490	21	49
Crispy: Chicken	330	16	33
Chicken BLT	420	23	35
Ghost Pepper Ranch Chicken	690	35	61
Loaded Nacho Chicken	670	30	66
Spicy:			
Asiago Ranch Chkn Club	600	28	51
Chicken	490	20	50
Wrap, Grilled Chicken	420	16	41
Crispy Chicken Nuggets: 4 pieces	180	12	9
6 pieces	270	17	14
Spicy Chicken Nuggets: 4 pieces	190	12	9
6 pieces	280	18	13
***Dipping Sauces:** Per 1 oz*			
Barbecue; Sweet & Sour, average	45	0	11
Buttermilk Ranch	120	12	2
Creamy Sriracha	120	12	3
Honey Mustard	90	7	7
***Fresh-Made Salads:** Full Size with Menu Set Dressing*			
Apple Pecan Grilled Chicken	540	28	44
Cobb	680	50	19
Parmesan Caesar Chicken	530	38	15
Taco	690	34	68
Sides: Apple Bites	35	0	8
Baked Potatoes: Plain	270	0	61
Bacon Cheese	440	13	64
Cheese	450	14	65
Chili & Cheese	520	27	53
Sour Cream & Chives	310	3	63
Chili: Small	240	11	22
Large	340	15	31
Fries: Baconator	460	26	43
Cheese Fries	470	27	44
Chili Cheese Fries	520	27	53
Natural Cut French Fries: Jr.	210	9	28
Small, 4 oz	260	12	35
Medium, 5 oz	350	16	47
Large, 6.5 oz	470	21	63
Bakery:			
Chocolate Chunk Cookie	330	16	43
Oatmeal Bar	280	10	45
Sugar Cookie	330	16	44
Frostys:			
Chocolate: Medium	390	11	61
Large	500	15	80
Strawberry: Medium	400	10	68
Large	520	14	89

For Complete Nutritional Data ~ see CalorieKing.com

Whataburger® (Oct '23)

Burgers & Sandwiches:	C	F	Cb
Whataburger:			
#1 Original	590	25	62
#2 Double Meat	830	44	62
#3 Triple Meat	1070	63	62
#4 Jalapeno & Cheese	680	32	63
#5 Bacon & Cheese	750	37	62
#6 Double Meat Jr.	420	20	37
#7 Whataburger Jr.	310	11	37
All Time Favorites:			
Honey BBQ Chicken Strip Sandwich	890	42	87
Mushroom Swiss Burger	1110	70	61
Patty Melt	940	61	45
Sweet & Spicy Bacon Burger	1080	62	69
Chicken:			
Grilled Chicken: Melt	390	11	39
Sandwich with Mayo	470	20	42
Whatachick'n Bites:			
6 pieces	390	19	25
9 pieces	580	28	37
Strips, 3 pieces	460	27	30
French Fries: Small	270	14	34
Medium	400	21	51
Large	530	28	68
Onion Rings: Medium	300	17	32
Large	450	25	49
Salad: *Without Dressing*			
Apple & Cranberry Grilled Chicken	380	12	38
Cobb with Spicy Chkn	550	32	21
Breakfast:			
Buttermilk Biscuit Sandwich:			
with Bacon	490	31	35
with Sausage	640	44	35
Honey Butter Chicken	580	36	52
Jalap. Cheddar Biscuit & Gravy	490	31	44
Taquitos: *With American Cheese*			
Bacon	400	23	29
Potato	440	25	28
Sausage	420	26	28
Desserts:			
Chocolate Chunk Cookie	230	11	31
Hot Apple Pie, 3 oz	270	14	34
Malts: Chocolate, 20 fl.oz	590	13	110
Vanilla, 20 fl.oz	540	14	94
Shake, Chocolate, 20 fl.oz	560	14	102

White Castle® (Oct '23)

Note: *Nutritional Information varies from state to state. Please check instore*

	C	F	Cb
Sliders:			
Bacon Cheese	220	14	15
Cheese	170	9	16
Crispy Chicken with Cheese	230	10	22
Chicken Ring with Cheese	200	10	18
Double Original	250	13	24
Double Smoked Cheddar Cheese	320	19	25
Impossible with Smoked Cheddar	230	13	17
without Cheese	190	10	18
Jalapeno Cheese	170	9	16
Panko Fish, plain	320	20	25
Panko Surf & Turf with Cheese	550	36	34
The Original	140	7	16
Veggie: Plain	190	10	22
with Honey Mustard	210	10	27
with Ranch	320	23	23
Sides: Chicken Rings, 6 p	320	20	12
Fish Nibblers: Small	320	16	28
Medium	590	29	51
Mozzarella Cheese Sticks (3)	460	33	26
Onion Chips, medium	930	65	73
Onion Rings, small, 4 oz	480	33	40
Fries:			
Cheese Fries	400	27	35
Fish Nibblers, medium	590	29	51
French Fries, medium	600	39	57
Loaded Fries, 5.7 oz	480	37	27
Mozzarella Cheese Sticks (5)	760	55	40
Onion rings, small	480	33	40
Breakfast: *With Cheddar Cheese*			
B'Fast Sliders: Bacon, Egg & Cheese	260	17	15
Bologna, Egg & Cheese	250	16	15
Egg & Jalapeno Cheese	210	13	15
Sausage, Egg & Chse	350	26	15
Original Slider, with Egg & Cheese	270	18	16
Toasted Sandwiches:			
Bacon, Egg & Chse	380	23	29
Egg & Cheese	270	13	29
Sausage, Egg & Chse	420	27	29
Waffle Sliders:			
with Bacon, Egg & Cheese	390	26	27
with Sausage, Egg & Cheese	490	36	28
Hash Round Nibblers:			
Small	360	28	25
Medium	720	55	51
Dessert:			
On A Stick: Fudge Dipped Brownie	240	12	34
Gooey Butter Cake	220	9	31

Wienerschnitzel® (Oct '23)

Hot Dogs: On Hot Dog Bun	C	F	Cb
Chicago Dog	330	15	37
Chili Dog	300	15	30
Chili Cheese Dog	350	20	30
Junkyard Dog	430	24	42
Kraut Dog	280	14	29
Mustard Dog	280	14	28
Veggie: Backyard	320	13	39
BBQ	300	9	43
Chicago	290	9	41
Hot Dog Substitute, add to any Dogs:			
All Beef Dog	100	10	1
Pretzel Bun Substitute,			
add to any Dog	140	4	23
Burgers:			
Cheeseburger	350	14	31
Double	760	45	31
Chili Cheeseburger	450	24	27
Double	770	45	30
Corn Dog	230	13	21
Sandwich, Polish Sausage	500	34	36
Sides: *Per Regular*			
Chili Cheese Fries	530	29	53
Bacon Ranch	630	39	54
French Fries: Small	310	16	38
Medium	440	23	54
Large	640	33	79
Breakfast:			
Biscuits: Egg, Bacon, Cheese	490	30	36
Egg, Sausage, Cheese	580	39	40
Biscuit & Gravy	390	21	42
Burritos:			
Chili Cheese Egg	350	14	39
Egg, Bacon, Cheese	410	20	38
Egg, Sausage, Cheese	510	29	42
Croissant:			
Egg, Bacon & Cheese	530	31	40
Egg, Sausage & Cheese	620	40	44
Hash Brown Po'Taters	330	23	28
Desserts:			
Classic Banana Split	670	17	129
Cones: Chocolate Dipped	350	21	40
Froot Loop Dipped	390	22	47
Sundaes:			
Caramel; Choc;olate, av.	395	14	65
Strawberry	370	14	59

Winchell's® (Oct '23)

Donuts: Per Donut	C	F	Cb
Buttermillk Bars, Choc Iced/Glazed	420	19	61
Chocolate Cake Donuts:			
Chocolate Iced	210	9	33
Plain	170	9	22
White Cake Donuts: Cherry Iced	270	12	40
Cinnamon Crumb	330	16	45
Maple Iced	270	12	40
French, Glazed; Maple/Vanilla Iced	270	14	32
Holes: Chocolate Sprinkles (1)	140	6	21
Cinnamon Crumb (1)	130	6	17
Glazed (1)	90	5	12
Jelly Filled:			
Apple with Cinnamon Crumb	370	15	53
Raspberry with Glaze	390	13	61
Strawberry with Sugar	380	13	60
Old Fashioned, Glazed; Maple Iced	410	17	60
Raised Ring: Chocolate Iced	270	10	41
Coconut	240	12	30
Fancy: Apple Fritter	600	23	93
Bear Claw (1)	700	38	75
Butterfly (1)	530	23	74
Cinnamon Roll (1)	630	31	80

WingStreet (Oct '23)

Chicken: *Without Dipping Sauce*

Bone Out Wings: *Per Wing*	C	F	Cb
Buffalo, Mild	90	4	10
Cajun rub	80	4	6
Garlic Parmesan	130	9	6
Honey BBQ	100	4	11
Lemon Pepper Rub; Ranch Rub	80	4	6
Naked	80	4	6
Spicy Garlic	110	6	8
Sweet Chili	100	5	10
Traditional Bone In Wings: *Per Wing*			
Buffalo, Mild	100	5	5
Cajun Rub	80	5	1
Garlic Parmesan	140	11	1
Honey BBQ	110	5	7
Lemon Pepper Rub	80	5	1
Naked	80	5	0
Spicy Garlic	120	8	3
Sweet Chili	100	5	4
Sauces:			
Blue Cheese	220	23	2
Ranch	210	22	2

Yard House® (Oct '23)

Appetizers: With Sides & Sauce	C	F	Cb
Blackened Ahi Sashimi	450	13	16
Chicken Lettuce Wraps	750	37	64
Chicken Nachos	2630	168	164
Chili Garlic Edamame	490	36	29
Four Cheese Spinach Dip	800	63	41
Fried Calamari	990	70	55
Guac & Chips	800	53	77
Parmesan Truffle Fries	500	24	63
Poke Nachos	880	60	51
Shitake Garlic Noodles	780	49	17
Sweet Potato Fries	650	26	98
Wings:			
Boneless: BBQ	980	48	55
Lemon Pepper	770	41	54
Whiskey Black Pepper	810	27	54
Crispy Traditional: Buffalo	1120	82	85
Korean Chili Garlic	1230	79	86
Lemon Pepper	940	64	83
Whiskey Black Pepper	1070	51	83
Gardein: Buffalo	900	57	53
Lemon Pepper	750	43	51
Whiskey Black Pepper	800	29	51
Grilled Burgers: *Without Fries*			
BBQ Bacon Cheddar Burger	1370	91	68
Beyond with side salad	1000	61	77
Bleu Cheese & Bacon	1070	67	55
Kurobuta Pork Burger	1170	74	65
Truffle Cheeseburger	1280	89	57
Fries: French	360	14	52
Sweet Potato	400	22	47
Truffle	410	20	53
Chicken: *With Menu Set Sides*			
Cilantro Lime	590	18	30
Fontina Vodka Penne	1460	70	99
Maui Pineapple	1320	38	147
Nashville Hot with Pancakes	1610	83	162
Orange	1730	67	221
Pizza:			
BBQ Chicken	1400	51	150
Gardein, BBQ Chicken	1350	45	88
Margherita	1140	52	120
Pepperoni &Mushroom	1100	48	112
The Carnivore	1520	81	111
Three Cheese	1040	43	109

Yard House® cont... (Oct '23)

Sandwiches: Without Fries	C	F	Cb
Double-Decker BLT	1140	78	70
Gardein: Grilled Chicken & Avocado	1040	72	57
Nashville Hot Chicken	1110	72	75
Korean: BBQ Beef Cheesesteak	1310	67	100
BBQ Chicken Cheesesteak	1190	64	94
Stacked Turkey Club	1360	85	81
Seafood: *As Served*			
Beer-Battered Fish & Chips	1920	139	104
Mediterranean Salmon	630	38	50
Noodles: Lobster Garlic Noodles	1230	54	110
Sesame Shrimp	530	15	37
Sesame Crusted Ahi Tuna	670	38	54
Whiskey Glazed Salmon	920	37	51
Steaks: *With Menu Set Sides*			
8 oz Filet Mignon	900	51	52
Bone-In Ribeye: 20 oz	1420	81	110
with Shrimp	1530	83	132
Korean Ribeye	2000	106	149
Thai Grilled Pork Chop	660	30	56
Salads: *Regular Entree Size*			
Cobb with Chicken	940	66	25
Kale & Romaine, Caesar w/- Shrimp	750	49	36
Tacos: *With Flour Tortilla*			
Baja Shrimp (1)	320	12	16
Carne Asada (1)	240	12	16
Grilled Korean Beef (1)	340	20	16
Dessert: Mini Cheesecake Brulee	400	24	43
Bread Pudding with Creme Anglaise	820	39	102
Chocolate Lava Cake	750	40	87

For Complete Nutritional Data ~ see CalorieKing.com

Yoshinoya® (Oct '23)

Appetizers:	C	F	Cb
Clam Chowder, 8 oz	180	12	16
Spring Rolls (2)	280	12	27
Regular Bowls: *With White Rice & Mixed & Vegetables*			
Grilled Chicken:			
Habanero	620	11	90
Hanabi Hot	510	11	87
Sweet Chili Shrimp	710	18	112
Kid's Meal: *With White Rice & Mixed Veggies*			
Tempura Orange Chicken	520	18	55
Dessert: Cheesecake	360	22	35
Chocolate Chip Cookie (1)	170	7	26
Flan	270	9	38

Zero Subs ~ see CalorieKing.com

Notes on Cholesterol

- **Cholesterol** is a white waxy substance produced mainly by our liver. It is also found in animal food products. Plant foods have no cholesterol.
- **Cholesterol is essential to life.** It is a structural part of every body cell wall and is the building block for vitamin D, sex hormones, and bile acids which help in the digestion of dietary fats. **Cholesterol is also vital for a healthy brain** (which contains some 20% of total body cholesterol).
- **The body makes sufficient cholesterol** for its needs and does not rely on cholesterol in the diet. Dietary fats have a major influence on blood cholesterol levels. (See next page)
- **A high blood cholesterol level may increase** the risk of atherosclerosis — the thickening of arteries that can reduce or block blood flow to the heart, brain, eyes, kidneys, sex organs and other body parts.

  This in turn increases the risk of heart attack, stroke, blindness, kidney failure, impotence and other blood circulatory problems.

  Other risk factors which increase the risk of atherosclerosis include high blood pressure, smoking, obesity and uncontrolled diabetes.

Heart Attack Warning Signals

Many victims die before reaching the hospital by ignoring warning signals and delaying medical help.

Symptoms vary and commonly include:

- **Chest pain,** vice-like squeezing or burning sensation in center of the chest or between the shoulder blades, or in the mid-back. Pain may even feel like severe indigestion.
- **Pain** may be felt in the arms, shoulders, neck or jaw.
- **Shortness of breath** often occurs with or before chest discomfort.
- **Other signs,** with or without pain, include a cold sweat, nausea or light-headedness.

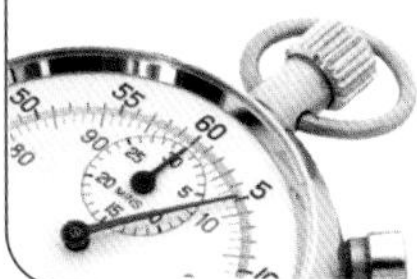

If you experience any of the above symptoms call IMMEDIATELY for medical help. Every minute counts.

***Call 9-1-1** or your emergency number*

Blood Cholesterol

CHECK YOUR RISK!

Total Cholesterol Level (mg/dl)		Risk of Heart Attack
240 and above	~	High Risk
200 - 239	~	Borderline/High
Below 200	~	Desirable

- **Know your cholesterol level, particularly if there is a family history of heart disease or stroke.**
- **Blood triglyceride levels are also important to check.**
- **All adults should have their cholesterol, HDL and triglycerides tested at least every 5 years.**

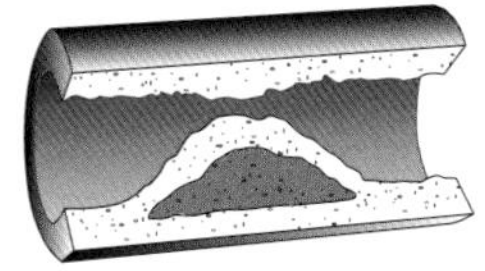

▲ **Atherosclerosis can clog arteries and impede blood flow to the heart or other body organs.**

▼ **A thrombus (blood clot) can form on unstable, festering athero-sclerotic plaque and rapidly block blood flow. A heart attack or stroke can result.**

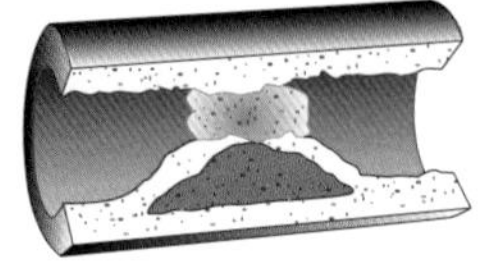

Fats & Cholesterol Guide

The amount and type of dietary fat has the greatest influence on blood cholesterol levels.

Fats in food are a mixture of 3 basic types: saturated, monounsaturated, and polyunsaturated. Animal fats are mainly saturated while plant oils and fish oils are mainly mono- and polyunsaturated.

Saturated fats have subgroups known as long-chain, medium-chain, and short-chain fats. Most of the long-chain fats raise blood cholesterol.

Long-chain saturated fats are found mainly in full-cream milk, cheese, butter, cream, fatty meats and sausages, and processed foods.

Medium-chain fats (MCT) have little effect on LDL-cholesterol but may raise 'good' HDL. 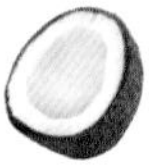
***Note: Coconut oil** has some MCT but is mainly saturated fat – so limit use.*

Monounsaturated fats tend to more selectively lower LDL-cholesterol and maintain the protective 'good' HDL-cholesterol in the bloodstream – but only if they replace saturated fats in the diet. Foods rich in monounsaturates include avocados, olives and olive oil, peanuts and macadamia nuts.

Polyunsaturated fats consist of two main classes. **Omega-6** polyunsaturates tend to lower blood cholesterol. Wholefood sources include soybeans, eggs, avocados, nuts and seeds. Minimize use of safflower, sunflower and corn oils which can oxidize very easily.

Omega-3 polyunsaturated fats can significantly lower blood triglycerides; and reduce the risk of thrombosis, heart arrythmmia, and artery spasm.

Best practical omega-3 sources include fish (salmon, sadines, tuna), fish oil, omega-3 algae oil (vegan), omega-3 enriched eggs, flaxseed and walnuts.

A balanced intake of the two omega classes is important for optimal health. For most Americans, increasing omega-3 intake would help attain a more ideal balance.

Trans fats from hydrogenated vegetable oils and shortenings should also be avoided. They are common in commercial baked and fried food products such as cakes, muffins, pastries, doughnuts, fried snacks and french fries.

DIETARY FATS COMPARISON

■ Saturated Fat ■ Monounsaturated Fat

Polyunsaturated Fats:

□ Linoleic (Omega-6) ■ Alpha-Linolenic (Omega-3)

OILS	PERCENTAGE CONTENT			
CANOLA OIL	7	63	20	10
LINSEED/FLAX OIL	9	19	17	55
SAFFLOWER OIL	9	14	77	
GRAPESEED OIL	10	22	68	
SUNFLOWER OIL	11	23	66	
CORN OIL	14	32	52	2
OLIVE OIL	14	76		10
SOYBEAN OIL	15	23	54	8
PEANUT OIL	19	45	34	2
COTTONSEED OIL	26	16	58	
PALM OIL	51	39		10

SPREADS & FATS
Saturated Fat includes 'Trans Fats' ❑ WATER CONTENT

SPREADS & FATS					
LIGHT MARGARINE	14	14	21		51
CANOLA MARGARINE	18	45	12	6	19
POLYUNSATURATED MARG	24	20	36		20
BUTTER	57	18		2	24
LARD	41	47			12
BEEF FAT	44	37		4	15

GOOD SOURCES OF OMEGA-3 FATS

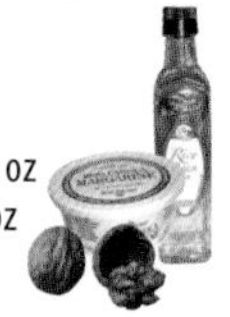

Plant Sources	Omega-3 Fats (Grams)
Canola Oil, 1 Tbsp, ½ fl.oz	1.5g
Flaxseed Oil, 1 Tbsp	8g
Soybean Oil, 1 Tbsp	1.2g
Canola Margarine, 1 Tbsp, ½ oz	1g
Soybeans, cooked, ½ cup, 4 oz	0.5g
Walnuts, ½ oz	0.5g

FISH - *Per 4 oz Serving*

High Content: Salmon (Chinook), Tuna, 3g
Trout (Lake), Sardines, Herring, Mackerel 3g

Medium Content:
Salmon, (Pink/Red/Coho), 4 oz 2g

Fair Content: *Per 4 oz Serving* 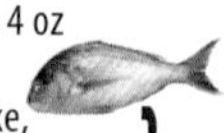
Bass, Catfish, Cod, Grouper, Hake, Halibut, Kingfish, Perch, Pollock, Shark, Trout (Rainbow), Tuna, Crab, Oysters, Blue Mussels, Shrimp, Squid } 0.5-1g

How Much Is Needed?

As little as 1-2 grams daily of omega-3 fats may benefit general health. High doses of fish-oil supplements should only be taken as directed by your Healthcare provider.

Dietary Cholesterol

Cholesterol in food varies in its effect on blood cholesterol level (BCL) from person to person. Much depends on the amount and type of fat and fiber eaten at the same meal.

Any elevating effect of dietary cholesterol on BCL is more likely to occur when the diet is high in saturated fat. Little elevation, if any, generally occurs when dietary fats are balanced in favor of mono- and poly-unsaturated fats (including omega-3 fats).

Example: While fish does contain cholesterol, the omega-3 fats can prevent any increase in BCL. Conversely, a meal containing no cholesterol but rich in saturated fat may result in a significant increase in BCL - as well as impairing artery wall functions.

Consequently, the need to be overly concerned about dietary cholesterol is being de-emphasized in favor of simply limiting total fat, saturated fat, and trans fat in particular – and substituting unsaturated fats (including omega-3 fats).

Note: Persons with familial (genetic) hyper-cholesterolemia should limit cholesterol; and ideally follow a plant-based diet.

The liver usually cuts back its own cholesterol production in response to cholesterol in the diet. Many people can consume high-cholesterol foods without concern.

However, it is difficult to identify just who is at risk - the so-called 'hyper-responders'. Because over 50% of Americans have a BCL above ideal levels, it may be prudent to limit cholesterol intake to less than 300mg daily, as well as to adopt a heart-healthy diet.

This limitation still allows the inclusion of most foods that are regularly eaten – even the overly maligned egg.

Avocados (like all plant foods) contain no cholesterol. Their fats are mainly monounsaturated and can lower blood cholesterol.

CHOLESTEROL COUNTER

Cholesterol is found only in foods of animal origin. Plant foods contain no cholesterol.

	Cholesterol mg
Meat - Average all types:	
Lean Meat, cooked, 120g	100
Fatty Meat, cooked, 120g	100
Fat, thick strip, 60g	40

Note: While lean meat and fat have similar amounts of cholesterol, choose lean meat to limit fat intake.

	Cholesterol mg
Chicken/Turkey, average, 120g	100
Organ Meats: Liver, fried, 4 oz	500
Brains, beef, pan fried, 3 oz	1700
Sausages: Frankfurter, 40g	25
Salami, 2 slices, 55g	40
Bacon: 3 slices, cooked, 30g	20
Fish: Fish fillets, average, ckd, 120g	70
Tuna/Salmon, canned, 100g	50
Scallops, 9 medium, 3 oz	30
Prawns, raw, 100g	110
Oysters, raw, 6 medium, 85g	45
Crayfish, Crab, cooked, 100g	70
Eggs (Chicken), 1 large	210
1 medium	180
Egg White, *Scramblers*	0
Milk/Yoghurt: Whole, 1 cup, 250ml	30
Light/low-fat Milk (1%), 1 cup	10
Skim/Non-fat, 1 cup	10
Soy Milk, Tofu, Tempeh	0
Cheese: Natural/Hard/Cream, 30g	30
Cottage, low-fat, 2 Tbsp, 40g	5
Cream Cheese, 30g	25
Fats: Butter, 1 Tbsp, 20g	45
Margarine, Oils (vegetable)	0
Mayonnaise, 1 Tbsp	10
Cream: Heavy, whipping, 2 Tbsp, 40g	40
Light/Sour, 2 Tbsp	10
Ice Cream: Full-fat (10-11%), 100ml/50g	20
Low-fat (less than 4%), 50g	5
Fruit, Vegetables, Avocados	0
Nuts, Seeds, Grains	0
Coffee, Tea, Beer, Wine	0

For Comprehensive Food Listings ~ see www.CalorieKing.com

DIETARY TIPS TO LOWER BLOOD CHOLESTEROL

1. **Maintain a healthy weight.**
If overweight, lose weight with a sensible, low-fat meal plan and daily exercise.

2. **Reduce saturated fat intake by:**

(a) eating less dairy fat. Choose low-fat or fat-reduced milk, yogurt, soy drinks, and cheese.

(b) replacing saturated fats with whole foods rich in monounsaturated and polyunsaturated fats – such as fish, nuts, seeds, avocado and olives.

Limit vegetable oils but choose mainly extra virgin olive oil and black seed oil. Avoid frying which can oxidize fats and harm health.

(c) eating less fat from meat and poultry. Choose lean cuts of meat and skinless chicken. Go easy on lunch meats, salami and fatty sausages.

Eat more fish, particularly higher fat fish such as salmon, herring, albacore tuna and sardines. They contain omega-3 fats that benefit the heart and all body cells.

(d) eating less saturated and trans fats from baked and fried fast-foods. Avoid deep-fried foods. Avoid donuts, cakes, pastries and cookies unless made with healthier fats and oils.

3. **Increase your soluble fiber intake.**
Foods rich in soluble fiber include beans, lentils, chickpeas, hummus, nuts, seeds, psyllium-seed husks and psyllium-fiber supplements. Oat bran, rice bran and barley are also good sources; as are fruit, vegetables, nopales (cactus leaves) and avocados. *(See Fiber Guide - Page 264-269)*

4. **Eat more soy bean foods such as:**
soy drinks, tofu, tempeh (cultured soy beans), soy flour, soy vegetarian foods and edamame (fresh green soybeans).

Soy protein in place of animal protein can significantly decrease high blood cholesterol levels, LDL cholesterol and blood triglycerides while maintaining 'good' HDL cholesterol.

5. **Eat more fruit, vegetables, and whole grains** in place of high-fat foods.
Aim for 2 fruits and 5 servings of vegetables per day. They also contain valuable antioxidants. The fat of avocados (and most nuts) is mainly unsaturated and can lower blood cholesterol levels.

6. **Limit cholesterol to 300mg per day.**
(Extra Notes ~ See Previous Page)

7. **Avoid brewed unfiltered coffee**
(espresso; plunger-style). Several cups per day may raise blood cholesterol. Filtered coffee is fine.

8. **Spread your food intake over the day.**
Have 3-4 smaller meals per day rather than just 1-2 very large meals. Nibbling, versus gorging, favors lower blood cholesterol.

Eat most food during the day and less at night.

ALCOHOL – WINE

Alcohol is a mixed bag. Moderate amounts of 1-2 drinks daily appear to reduce the risk of heart attack and ischemic stroke in older persons.

However, larger amounts increase the risk of high blood pressure, obesity, heart failure and hemorrhagic stroke, and can aggravate hypertriglyceridemia: as well as many other health hazards. *(See Alcohol Guide – Page 23)*

The speculative benefits of moderate alcohol intake have been overstated in the media. The overriding harmful effects of excess alcohol do not allow its recommendation for any aspects of health promotion.

Fruit, Vegetables & Tea Also Protect:

Red wine and red grapes (more so than white) contain antioxidants which may help protect cholesterol in the blood from becoming oxidized.

Most fruits, vegetables, whole-grains, nuts and tea also contain protective antioxidants.

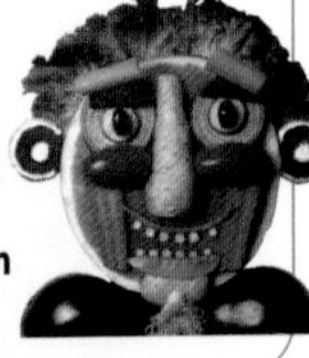

How Fats Affect Blood Flow

Fats in the diet affect more than blood cholesterol levels. They can also strongly influence blood clot formation and thrombosis, as well as blood flow and ultimate oxygen delivery to body parts and organs. While advanced atherosclerosis can impede blood flow to the heart and other organs, it is thrombosis (complete blockage by blood clots) or arterial spasm which commonly results in a heart attack or stroke.

Plant and fish oils rich in omega-3 fats lessen the risk of blood clots, thrombus formation, and artery spasm by reducing platelet stickiness and adhesion to artery walls. This also reduces inflammation of the artery wall lining. This in turn reduces the risk of atherosclerotic plaque becoming unstable and reactive.

Omega-3 fats also improve blood flow by reducing blood viscosity and increasing the flexibility of red blood cells that need to flex and twist on themselves in order to squeeze through tiny narrow capillaries often half their diameter.

A diet high in saturated fats (longer chain) has the opposite effect by stiffening red blood cell membranes and increasing blood viscosity, thereby hindering blood flow.

Stiff red blood cells may also form aggregates that resemble coin stacks. In narrow blood vessels, this further impedes blood flow and impairs oxygen release through the much-lessened surface area of red blood cell membranes exposed to blood.

Note: Smoking, lack of exercise, and stress can have similar adverse effects on thrombosis, red blood cell flexibility, and blood flow.

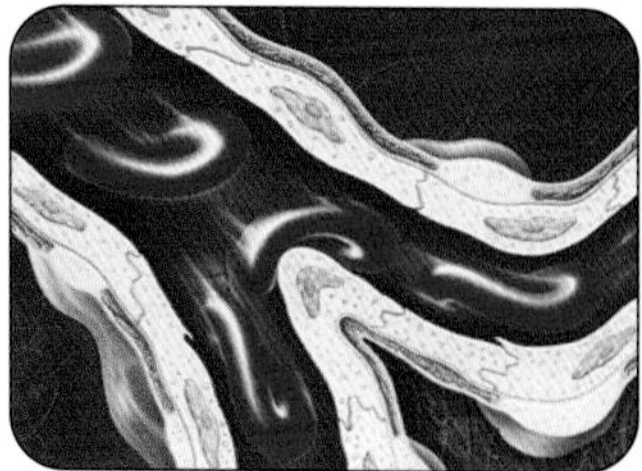

▲ *Picture of Healthy Blood Flow*

Flexible red blood cells twist and slide through tiny capillaries - often half the diameter of red blood cells.

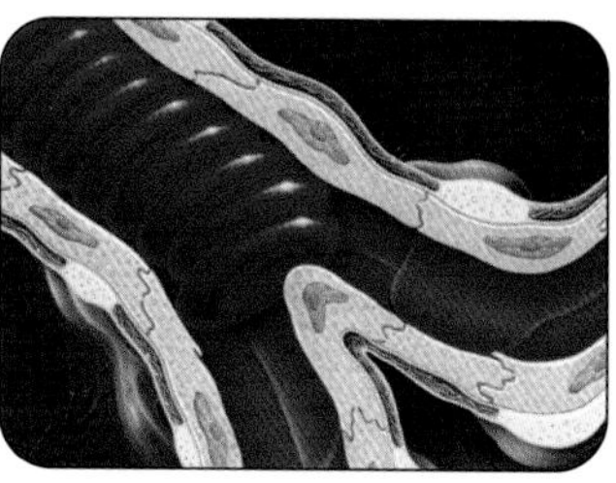

▲ *A Not-So-Healthy Picture!*

Red blood cells have lost their flexibility and ability to twist and slip through capillaries. They are stacked up, thereby impeding blood flow.

A diet high in saturated fats can contribute to this picture - as can smoking, lack of exercise, and stress.

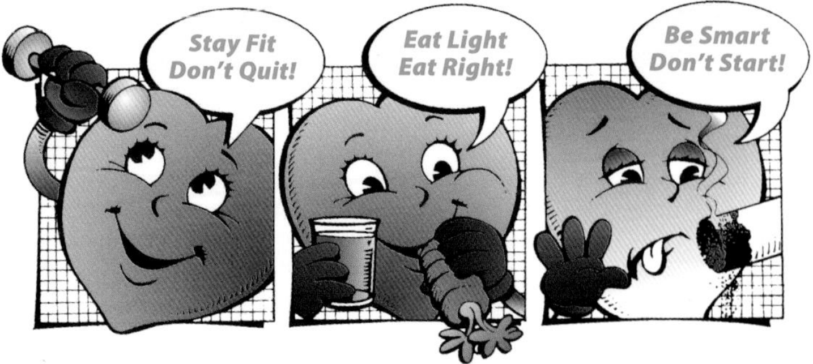
Stay Fit
Don't Quit!
Eat Light
Eat Right!
Be Smart
Don't Start!

Fiber Guide

Introduction

Fiber

Fiber is the general term for those parts of plant food that we cannot digest (although bacteria in the large bowel partly digests fiber through fermentation). It is not found in foods of animal origin (meats, dairy products).

Fiber promotes intestinal health, bowel regularity, can benefit diabetes and blood cholesterol levels, and may help prevent colon cancer. High-fiber foods also assist weight control.

Most Americans don't eat enough fiber – less than 20 grams/day – instead of a healthier 25 to 35 grams/day.

A fiber-rich diet assists the growth of friendly gut microbes that can benefit our metabolism, weight and blood glucose levels – as well as hunger, mood and our immune system.

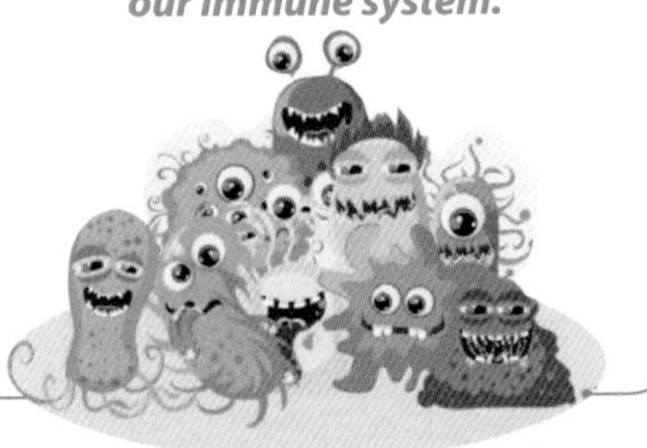

Types of Fiber

Plant foods contain a mixture of different fibers in varying proportions. Insoluble and soluble fiber categories are based on their solubility in water. All types of fiber are beneficial to the body.

- **Insoluble fibers** (cellulose, hemi-celluloses, lignin) make up the structural parts of plant cell walls.

  Best food sources are wheat bran, corn bran, rice bran, wholegrain cereals and breads, beans and peas, nuts, seeds, and the skins of fruits and vegetables.

These fibers absorb many times their own weight in water. They create a soft bulk and hasten the passage of waste products through the intestines.

They promote bowel regularity, and aid in the prevention and treatment of uncomplicated forms of **constipation, diverticulosis and hemorrhoids.**

The risk of colon cancer may also be reduced by fiber's diluting effect on potentially harmful substances.

- **Soluble fibers (pectin, gums, mucilages)** are found mainly within plant cells, soy milk (whole bean) and products.

Best Sources of Soluble Fiber:

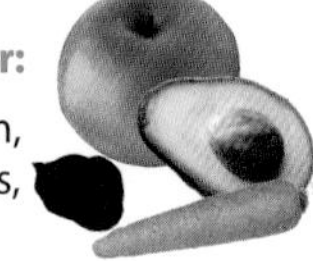

Fruits and vegetables, oat bran, barley, beans and peas, prunes, psyllium and flax seed.

These fibers form a gel which slows both stomach emptying and the absorption of sugars from the intestines. **This helps to control blood sugar levels.**

Weight control is also aided by the slower emptying of the stomach and the feeling of **fullness provided by soluble fiber.**

Soluble fiber can also lower blood cholesterol by binding bile acids and excreting them. More body cholesterol must then be broken down to supply bile acids for emulsification of dietary fats. **Rice bran, while not high in soluble fiber, can also lower blood cholesterol.**

- **Resistant starch** is that part of starchy foods (approx. 10%) which is tightly bound by fiber and resists normal digestion. Friendly bacteria in the large bowel ferment and change the resistant starch into short-chain fatty acids, which are important to bowel health and may protect against colon cancer.

Starchy foods include bread, cereals, rice, pasta, potatoes and legumes.

Fiber & Weight Control

Fiber can assist weight control in several ways. Fiber-rich foods such as fresh fruit and vegetables, potatoes and wholegrain bread contain few calories for their large volume (due to their low-fat, high-water content).

Their bulk fills the stomach and satisfies the appetite much sooner than fiber-depleted foods. The extra chewing time also contributes to satiety, and gives the stomach time to register a feeling of fullness. Excessive calories are less likely to be consumed.

Fiber-depleted foods and drinks are more concentrated in calories; e.g. fats, sugar, candy, soft drinks, fruit juices, alcohol. They require little or no chewing. Large amounts with excessive calories can be consumed before the appetite is satisfied.

Example: Whereas one fresh apple might satisfy the appetite, an apple juice drink with the equivalent sugars and calories of 2-3 apples only minimally satisfies the appetite. (See illustration below.)

High-fiber foods fill the stomach. Fewer calories are consumed.

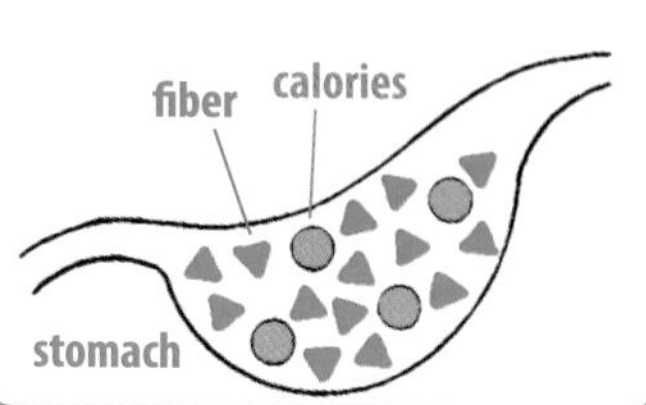

Low-fiber foods are more concentrated in calories. More food must be eaten to fill the stomach.

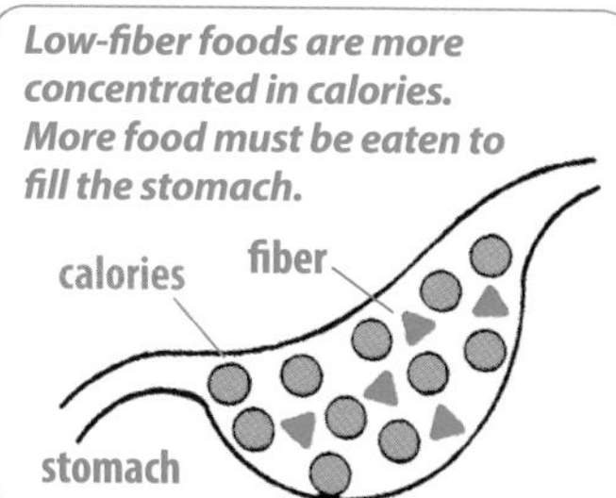

EFFECTS OF REMOVING FIBER FROM FOOD

2-3 pieces of fresh fruit produces 1 glass of fruit juice. The removal of fiber concentrates the sugars and calories.

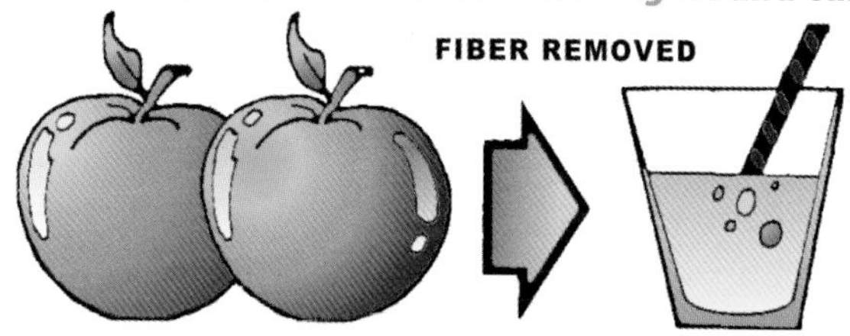

FRESH FRUIT	(Comparison)	FRUIT JUICE
Higher Fiber	✦	Negligible Fiber
Low Calorie Density	✦	High Calorie Density
Long Eating Time	✦	No Eating Time (Drink)
Satisfies Hunger	✦	Does Not Satisfy Hunger
Sugars Slowly Absorbed	✦	Sugars More Quickly Absorbed
Less Insulin Required	✦	More Insulin Required
Supports Gut Microbes	✦	Fewer Benefits to Microbes

Fiber Guide ~ Constipation

Constipation

Constipation can reasonably be defined as a failure to have a bowel movement at least every second day – and just as importantly, without straining or pain.

Typically, constipated stools are too hard, too narrow and too small.

The **main cause** is simply a lack of dietary fiber. Other contributing factors include insufficient fluids, too little exercise, emotional stress, gastrointestinal disease, lack of proper dentition to chew high-fiber foods, and some medications (e.g. some antacids, antidepressants, pain medications).

Note: Check with your doctor to rule out any underlying medical problem – especially if you have a change in bowel habits in middle-age or later years.

DESIRABLE FIBER INTAKE

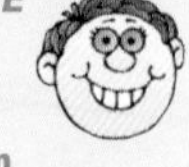
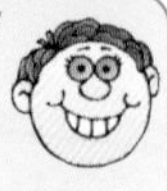

Adults: 25-35gm per day
Children (under 18): Age + 5gm
Example: 6-year old (6 + 5)= 11gm

SAMPLE FOOD QUANTITIES
For 35 Grams of Fiber/Day

		Fiber
	Breakfast Cereal (higher-fiber)	5g
plus	4 slices wholegrain Bread	6g
plus	3 servings fresh Fruit	9g
plus	1 medium Potato (w. skin)	4g
or	1 cup Brown Rice	
or	½ cup wholegrain Pasta	
plus	3-4 servings Veggies/Salad	6g
plus	1 cup Bean Soup	5g
or	¼ cup Baked/Soy Beans	
or	½ cup Corn/Peas/Lentils	
or	1¼ oz Almonds (natural)	
or	3 medium Figs	

HINTS TO INCREASE FIBER AND AVOID CONSTIPATION

1. **Breakfast is an important** contributor to daily fiber intake. Eat high-fiber breakfast cereals (bran-based cereals, oatmeal etc.). Add 1-2 tablespoons of unprocessed bran.

   Dried fruits, chopped nuts, soy grits, and seeds are also excellent additions to cereals.

   Note: A gradual increase in fiber will prevent bloating, gas or pain. People intolerant to bran may benefit from psyllium-based fiber supplements and cereals.

2. **Drink adequate water daily.** Fiber works by absorbing many times its own weight in water.

3. **Eat wholegrain breads,** or fiber-enriched breads. They have over double the fiber of regular white bread.

4. **Enjoy fruit as fresh fruit** with skin rather than as fruit juice. Enjoy wholegrain pasta, barley, brown rice, nuts and seeds.

5. **Eat more vegetables,** salads and legumes – especially cooked beans, lentils, potatoes with skins, avocado, broccoli, brussels sprouts, cabbage, carrots, celery, and peas.

6. **Add bran** (barley/rice/wheat) or soy grits to soups, casseroles, yogurt, desserts, cookies, cakes. Also use whole-meal flour or soy flour in place of white flour. Use nuts, seeds, and ground linseed.

7. **Snack** on fresh or dried fruits, carrot or celery sticks, popcorn, nuts or seeds, wholegrain crackers, high-fiber bars (low-fat). Limit amounts if overweight.

8. **Exercise regularly** to strengthen abdominal muscles and stimulate the gut. Keep up water intake, especially in warm weather.

9. **Avoid** indiscriminate and regular use of harsh laxatives. They can overstimulate the intestinal muscles and may make normal bowel activity impossible. It may take several weeks to restore normal bowel function.

FOODS WITH ZERO FIBER

- **Dairy Products (Milk, Cheese, etc.)**
- **Meats, Poultry, Fish, Eggs**
- **Fats/Oils, Sugar/Syrups**

(Only foods of plant origin contain fiber.)

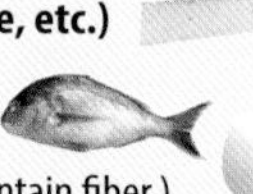

Fiber ~ Fiber (grams)

Breakfast Cereals

	Fiber
General Mills:	
Basic 4, 1 cup, 2 oz	3
Cheerios (Honey Nut; Multigrain), 1⅓ cups, 1 oz	4
Chex, Rice, cup	2
Cinnamon Toast Crunch, 1 cup, 1.4 oz	2
Fiber One, Original Bran, ⅔ cups, 1.4 oz	18
Kix, 1½ cups, 1.4 oz	3
Lucky Charms, 1 cup, 1.3 oz	2
Oatmeal Crisp Almond, 1 cup, 2 oz	6
Raisin Nut Bran, ¾ cup, 1.7 oz	6
Total, Whole Grain, 0.875 oz	2
Trix, 1¼ cups, 1.4 oz	1
Wheat Chex, 1 cup, 2 oz	8
Wheaties, 1 cup, 1.26 oz	4
Kellogg's:	
All-Bran, Buds, ½ cup, 1.58 oz	17
Corn Flakes, 1½ cups, 1.4 oz	1
Frosted Flakes, 1 cuo, 1.4 oz	0.5
Frosted Mini Wheats, 2 oz	6
Krave, Chocolate, 1 pkg, 1.87 oz	3
Mueslix, 1 cup, 2.4 oz	5
Raisin Bran, 1 cup, 2 oz	7
Rice Krispies, 1½ cups, 1.4 oz	0
Special K, 1 cup, 1.4 oz	3
Kashi:	
Kashi Go: Crunch, ¾ cup, 1.8 oz	9
Coconut Almond Cr., ¾ cup, 1.9 oz	6
P'nut Butter Cr., ¾ cup, 1.9 oz	6
Honey Alm. Flax Cr., ¾ cup, 1.7 oz	8
Original, 1 cup , 1.9 oz	10
Organic: Blueb. Clusters, 1 cup 1.9 oz	3
Honey Toasted Oat , 1 cup, 1.4 oz	5
Maple Waffle Crisp, 1 cup, 1.4 oz	4
Whole Wheat Biscuits, avg all flavors, 2 oz	6

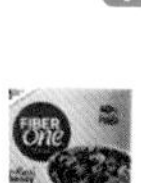

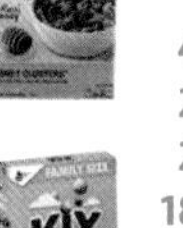

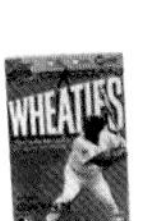

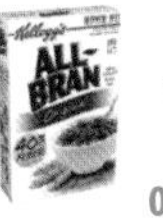

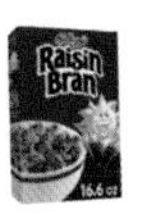

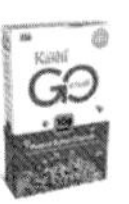

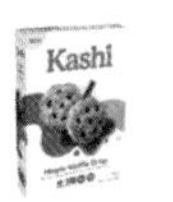

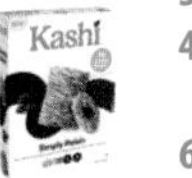

Breakfast Cereals (Cont)

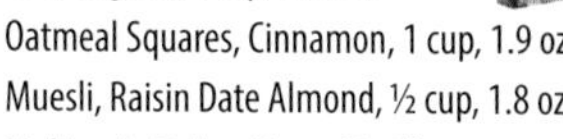

	Fiber
Quaker:	
Corn Crunch, 1 cup, 1.3 oz	5
Life, Original, 1 cup, 1.45 oz	3
Oatmeal Squares, Cinnamon, 1 cup, 1.9 oz	5
Muesli, Raisin Date Almond, ½ cup, 1.8 oz	5
Multigrain Flakes, Honey Vanilla, ¾ cup, 2.2 oz	3
Quisp, 1¼ cups, 1.45 oz	0.5
Real Medleys, Multigrain, Cherry, ¾ cup, 1.9 oz	4
Simply Granola, Oats, Honey, Raisins & Alm., 2.4 oz	7
Post:	
Alpha Bits, 1 cup, 1 oz	2
Better Oats, Maple & Br. Sugar, 1 oz pouch	3
Bran Flakes, 1 cup, 1.34 oz	7
Dunkin', Mocha Latte, 1⅓ cups, 1.34 oz	0
Grape Nuts, Original, ½ cup, 2 oz	7
Great Grains, Blueberry Morning, 1 cup, 2 oz	4
Honey Bunches of Oats, Vanilla, 1 cup, 0.95 oz	4
Raisin Bran, 1¼ cups, 2.1 oz	9
Shredded Wheat, Original, Spoon, 1⅓ cups, 2 oz	8

Brans & Supplements, Metamucil

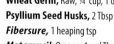

	Fiber
Oat Bran: 1 Tbsp (level)	1
⅓ cup, (5⅓ Tbsp), 1 oz	5
Rice Bran, raw, ⅓ cup, 1 oz	6
Wheat Bran, Unprocessed:	
Raw, 1 Tbsp	1.5
2 Tbsp (level), ¼ oz	3
¼ cup, (4 Tbsp), ½ oz	6
Wheat Germ, Raw, ¼ cup, 1 oz	4
Psyllium Seed Husks, 2 Tbsp	8
Fibersure, 1 heaping tsp	5
Metamucil: Orange, 1 rnd Tbsp, 11g	3
Fiber Wafers (2)	6

Hot Cereals, Oatmeal

	Fiber
Bulgur (Cracked Wheat), ckd, 1 cup	8
Corn/Hominy Grits, dry, 3 Tbsp, 1 oz	0.5
Cream of Wheat, cooked, 1 oz	1
Oatmeal, cooked ⅔ cup	3

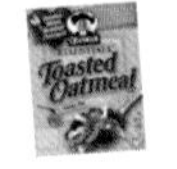

Fiber Counter

Breads & Crackers

	Fiber
Bread: White, 1 slice, 1 oz	0.6
Whole-wheat, 1 slice, 1 oz	1.5
Wholegrain, 1 slice, 1 oz	2
Rye, Pumpernickel, 1 oz	1.5
Bagel/Roll/Bun, 1 medium, 2 oz	1.5
Pita, whole wheat, 6.5″ pocket	4.5
Crackers: Graham, average, 2	0.4
Saltine, 4 crackers	0.4
Crispbreads, average, 2	4
Matzo, 1 board, 1 oz	1
Rice Cakes, average, 1 cake	0.3
Tortilla: Regular, 6″	0.5
Whole-wheat, 6″	1.3

Barley, Pasta, Rice & Flours

Barley, pearled, raw, 1/4 cup, 1.7 oz	8
Rice:	
White, cooked, 1 cup	0.6
Brown, cooked, 1 cup	3.5
Rice-A-Roni, average, 1 cup, prepared	1.5
Spaghetti/Noodles: Cooked, 1 cup	2
Whole-Wheat, cooked, 1 cup	4
Flour: Wheat, All-purpose, 1 cup, 4.5 oz	3.5
Whole-Wheat, 1 cup, 4.5 oz	15
Cornmeal, stone ground, 1 cup, 4.5 oz	13
Carob Flour, 1 cup, 3.5 oz	41
Hemp Wholemeal Flour, 1 cup, 3.5 oz	41
Rye Flour, 1 cup, 3.5 oz	15
Soy Flour: Defatted, 1 cup, 3.5 oz	17
Full-fat, raw, 1 cup, 3 oz	8
Soy Meal, defatted, 1 cup, 4.5 oz	14

Frozen Entrees & Dinners

***Average All Brands**: Per Serving*	
Beans/Chili base, average	6-10
Potato/Pasta base, average	4-6
Vegetable base, average	3
Meat/Chicken base, average	2-3
Pizzas, 1/4 large, average	3
Vegetarian Soy Burgers, 1 pattie	4

Soups

Chicken Noodle, 1 cup	0.5
Tomato Soup, average, 1 cup	0.5
Vegetable Soup, average, 1 cup	3
***Health Valley:** Per 1 Cup*	
Chicken & Rice	1
Minestrone	6
Split Pea	13
Tomato	5
Vegetable	4
Progresso, Tomato	6

Fast Foods & Restaurants

	Fiber
Hamburgers: Small, average	1.5
Large/Whopper, average	2.5
Hot Dog, Regular	1.5
French Fries: Small serving, 2.5 oz	2.5
Regular/Medium, 3.5 oz	3.5
Chicken Nuggets, 6 pack	0.5
Chicken Sandwich, average	2
Taco, average	4
Sundaes, Shakes, Soft Drinks	0
Arby's, Classic Roast Beef Sandwich	2
Burger King: Whopper	2
Impossible Whopper	4
Del Taco, Beyond 8 Layer Burrito	9
Denny's: House Salad, no dressing	3
Bacon Avocado Cheeseburger	5
Club Sandwich	8
Super Bird Sandwich	2
Domino's: 12″ Thin Crust, 1 slice	0.5
12″ Handmade Pan Crust, 1 slice	0.5
12″ Deluxe, Hand Tossed, 1 slice	1
McDonald's: Big Mac	3
Hamburger	1
Egg McMuffin	2
Quarter Pounder with Cheese	2
***Pizza Hut:** Per 1 Slice, Medium*	
Original Pan Pizza: Cheese, Pepp.	2
Supreme	2
Thin 'n Crispy, Supreme	2
Hand-Tossed, average all varieties	2
Subway: 6″ 9 Grain Honey Oat Roll	4
6″ 9 Grain Wheat Roll	4
Habanero Wrap	2
Taco Bell: Bean Burrito, vegan	11
Power Menu Bowl, Veggie	10

Cakes, Cookies, Snack Bars

Apple/Fruit Pie, 1 serving, 4 oz	2
Cake: With plain flour, 1 serving, 3.4 oz	1.5
With whole-wheat flour, 1 serving	3
Carrot Cake, 4 oz	4
Cookies, oatmeal, (3 small/1 large)	1
Donuts, medium, 1.7 oz	0.7
Fruit Cake, 1 serving, 1.5 oz	2
Fig Bars, 1 cookie, 0.5 oz	0.7
Muffins, Oat Bran (2 small, 1 large), 4 oz	5
Granola Bars, average, 1 bar	2
Atkins Advantage Bars, av.	7
Clif Bars, 2.5 oz	4
Fiber One (Gen. Mills):	
Oats & Chocolate, 0.8 oz	9
Other Bars, 0.8oz	6
Fiber Plus, Chewy, 1.27 oz	9
Health Valley, Cereal Bars	0.5
Luna Bars, avg., 1.7 oz	3
Special K, Chocolate Protein Meal Bar, 1.6 oz	3

Chocolate, Chips, Popcorn

	Fiber
Cheese Balls/Curls/Twists	1
Chocolate, Hard Candy, 1 oz	0
Chocolate with nuts/fruit, 2 oz bar	1.5
Mars Bar, 1.8 oz	1
Potato Chips; corn chips, 1 oz	1
Popcorn, 3 cups	3
Pretzels, Twists (6)	1

Nuts, Seeds

	Fiber
Almonds: Natural, 25 nuts, 1 oz	3.5
Blanched (skins removed), 1 oz	3
Cashews, Filberts, Pecans, 1 oz	1.7
Hepm Seeds, 3 Tbsp, 1 oz	9
Peanuts, Mixed Nuts, Coconut, 1 oz	2.5
Peanut Butter, 2 Tbsp, 1 oz	2
Pistachio Nuts, dried, shelled, 1 oz	3
Walnuts, Black/English, dried, 1 oz	2
Seeds: Amaranth, 2½ Tbsp, 1 oz	3.5
Flax Seeds, 3 Tbsp, 1 oz	7
Psyllium Seed Husks, 5 Tbsp, 1 oz	20
Quinoa Seeds, 3 Tbsp, 1 oz	1.7
Sesame Seeds, whole, 1 oz	3.4
Sesame Butter/Tahini, 2 Tbsp, 1.1 oz	1.4
Sunflower Kernels, ¼ cup, 1 oz	3.8

Fruit – Fresh

	Fiber
Apples: 1 medium, 5½ oz (whole)	
with skin + core	3.7
with skin, no core	3.2
without skin, no core	1.7
Apricots, 2 medium, 4 oz	1.5
Avocado, average, ½ medium	6
Banana, 1 medium, 6 oz (w. skin)	3
Blueberries, raw, ½ cup, 2.5 oz	1.7
Cherries, sweet, raw, 8 fruits, 1.6 oz	1
Grapefruit, average, ½ fruit, 10 oz	1.4
Grapes, 1 medium bunch, seedless, 7 oz	2
Kiwifruit, 1 medium, 2.7 oz	2.3
Mango, 1 medium, 11 oz (whole)	1.6
Melons, Cantaloupe, 4 oz (edible)	1
Nectarine, 1 medium, 4 oz	1.9
Olives, average all types, 7 jumbo, 2 oz	1.5
Oranges, 1 medium (7-8 oz w. skin)	
5½ oz (peeled)	3.8
Passionfruit, 2 medium, 2.5 oz	5
Peaches, 1 large, 6 oz	2
Pears, raw, 1 medium, 6 oz	4.5
Pineapple, 1 slice, 3 oz	1.2
Plums, 2 medium, 6 oz	1.8
Strawberries, 6 medium/3 large, 2 oz	1
Watermelon, 4 oz (edible)	0.5

Fruit – Dried, Juice

	Fiber
Dried Fruit: Apricots, 8 halves, 1 oz	2.2
Dates (3 med); Raisins (2 Tbsp), 1 oz	1.5
Figs, 3 medium, 1½ oz	5
Prunes, 4 medium, 1 oz	2
Fruit Juice: Orange/Apple etc, 1 glass	<0.5
Prune Juice, 5 oz	1.4
Carrot Juice, 8 oz	1.8

Vegetables

	Fiber
Asparagus, 4 medium spears	1.3
Bean Sprouts, ½ cup, 2 oz	1
Beans: Snap/Green, ½ cup, 2 oz	2
Baked Beans in Tom Sce, ½ c, 4.5 oz	5
Dried Beans, cooked, average, ½ cup	7
Beets, ckd, slices, ½ cup, 3 oz	1.7
Broccoli, cooked, ½ cup, 3 oz	2.4
Brussels Sprouts, ckd, ½ cup, 3 oz	3.5
Cabbage: White, ckd, ½ cup, 2.5 oz	1
Red, ckd, ½ cup, 2.5 oz	2
Carrots, 1 medium (7½"), ½ cup, 3 oz	2.5
Cauliflower, cooked, 3 flowerets, 2 oz	1.5
Celery, raw, diced, 1 cup, 3.5 oz	1.6
Chickpeas (Garbanzos), ckd, ½ c., 3 oz	6.5
Corn: Kernels, cooked, ½ cup, 2½ oz	2.5
Corn on the Cob, 1 ear, 5 oz	4
Cucumber/Lettuce/Mushrooms, 2 oz	0.5
Eggplant, raw, sliced, ½ cup, 1.5 oz	2
Lentils, cooked, ½ cup, 3.5 oz	8
Mixed Vegetables, frozen, cooked, ½ cup	3
Onions: Raw, 1 medium, 4 oz	1.5
Spring Onions, chop., ¼ cup, 1 oz	0.7
Peas: Green, raw, ½ cup, 2.5 oz	3.7
Cowpeas (Black-eyed), ckd, ½ cup	10
Split Peas, cooked, ½ cup, 3.5 oz	8
Peppers, sweet, raw, 1 large, 6 oz	3
Potatoes: 1 medium, with skin, 5 oz	4
1 medium, without skin	2.5
½ cup mashed, 3.5 oz	1.5
French Fries, small, 2.6 oz	3
Spinach, cooked, ½ cup, 3 oz	2.2
Squash: Summer, cooked, ½ cup, 3 oz	2.5
Winter, cooked, ½ cup, 3.5 oz	2.4
Tomatoes: 1 medium, 4.5 oz	1.5
Tomato Sauce, 1 cup	0.3
Soybean Products: Miso, ½ c., 5 oz	7.4
Tempeh, cooked, 1 piece, 3 oz	2
Tofu, ½ cup, 4.4 oz	0.4

Salads:

	Fiber
Side Salad, average	1
Bean Salad, ½ cup	5
Coleslaw, ½ cup	1
Potato Salad, ½ cup	2

Protein Guide

General Notes

- **Protein has many important body functions.** It builds and repairs muscle, and is the basis of our body's organs, hormones, enzymes, and antibodies to fight infection.
- **Inadequate protein leads to a drop in immune response** with greater susceptibility to illness and infections. Muscle stength and muscle mass also drops
- **Protein is also an emergency fuel** in the absence of sufficient carbohydrate and fats. For this reason, weight loss should be gradual so as to preserve protein levels in muscle, the heart and other body organs.
- **When changing to a vegetarian diet,** include legume beans (soy, chickpeas etc.), lentils, nuts, seeds, tofu, tempeh; as well as wholegrain cereals and flours. Also try nutritional yeast flakes, and plant-based meat substitutes (*Beyond Meat; Impossible* burgers). Dairy products (lower fat) and eggs can enhance nutrient intake.
- **Vegan Diets:** Elderly persons and children with smaller appetites may struggle to obtain sufficient protein on vegan diets. To boost protein, add more concentrated protein foods such as tofu, tempeh, yogurt, eggs, milk, fish, or protein powder supplements.

Protein & Muscle

- Although muscles are built of protein, protein is not a special fuel for working muscle cells – carbohydrates and fats are.
- In fact, a diet high in protein (and fat) and low in carbohydrate can significantly reduce the performance of endurance sports athletes. **Carbohydrates** are the best fuel for muscles exercised for long periods.
- Any **extra protein** required by athletes and body-builders can easily be obtained from the extra food eaten to satisfy hunger and energy needs.

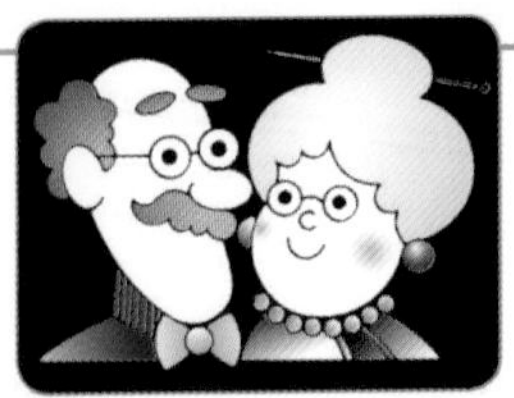

Elderly people (and dieters) must eat sufficient food to ensure adequate protein intake

Aim for 3 meals daily with at least 25-30 grams of protein per meal – rather than a large amount of protein at just one meal (which cannot be fully used by the body).

RECOMMENDED DAILY PROTEIN INTAKE ~ HEALTHY RANGE ~
(Lower figure is RDA)

		PROTEIN
Children:	1-3 yrs	13g-26g
	4-8 yrs	19g-38g
	9-13 yrs	34g-64g
Males:	14-18 yrs	52g-120g
	19+	56g-120g
Females:	14+	46g-110g
Pregnancy:		71g-120g
Breastfeeding:		71g-120g

Note: On lower-calorie diets, aim for higher amounts of protein within the Healthy Range.

Pro ~ Protein (grams)

Meats, Sausages

	Pro
Bacon, 3 medium slices	6
Ground Beef Patty, lean, cooked, 3 oz	21
Ham: Luncheon, 2 slices, 1½ oz	7
Roasted, 2 pieces, 3 oz	18
Lamb chop, broiled, 3 oz	22
Liver, cooked, 3 oz	23
Pastrami, 3 slices, 1¾ oz	10
Pork, cooked, lean, 3 oz	24
Roast Beef, lean, 2 slices, 3 oz	24
Sausages: Bologna, 2 sl., 2 oz	7
Braunschweiger, 2 sl., 2 oz	8
Pork link, thick, 2 oz	6
Frankfurter, 1⅓ oz	5
Salami, hard, 3 slices, 1 oz	7
Steak: Average all cuts, lean (no fat)	
Small (4 oz raw/3 oz cooked)	23
Medium (6 oz raw/4¼ oz cooked)	34
Large (10 oz raw/7¼ oz cooked)	57

Meat Substitutes (Vegan)

	Pro
Beyond Meat: Beef/Burger, 4 oz	20
Sausages, 2 patties, 2 oz	11
Impossible, 4 oz Patty	19
Vegetarian Patties, av., 4 oz	13

Chicken/Turkey: *Without Skin*

	Pro
Chicken, cooked: Breast, Roasted, 4 oz	36
Leg/Thigh,Roasted, 2 oz	14
½ Whole Chicken	60
Drumstick, Rstd, 1 med., 3 oz	13
Turkey: Light meat, cooked, 3 oz	28
Dark meat, lean, 3 oz	24

Fish

	Pro
Fresh Fish: *Per 4 oz, cooked*	
Cod, Flounder/Sole, Pollock	28
Catfish, Haddock, Halibut, M/Mahi	28
Ocean Perch, Swordfish, Orange Roughy	28
Canned Fish: Tuna, av., 3 oz	25
Salmon, pink, 3 oz	17
Salmon, red, 3 oz	17
Sardines, 3 whole (3"), 1¼ oz	9
Shellfish: Crabmeat, 3 oz	17.5
Clams, raw, 4 large/9 sml, 3 oz	11
Crayfish, cooked, 3 oz	20
Lobster, cooked, 3 oz	17
Oysters, raw, 6 medium, 3 oz	7
Scallops, 2 lge/5 small, 1 oz	5
Shrimp, raw, 6 large, 1½ oz	8.5
Fish Products: Fish Sticks, 4 sticks	10
Fish Portions, in batter, 4 oz	13
Gefilte Fish, 1 medium ball, 2 oz	8

Eggs

	Pro
1 Large Egg, whole	6
Egg Yolk	3
Egg White	3
Omelet: Plain, 2 eggs	13
Ham & cheese	17
Egg Substitutes, (liquid):	
Egg Beaters, ¼ cup, 2 oz	4.5
Better 'n Eggs/Scramblers, ¼ cup, 2 oz	6

Milk, Yogurt, Ice Cream

	Pro
Milk: Whole: 2%, 1 cup	8
Low-Fat (1%); Fat-Free, 1 cup	8.5
Chocolate Milk, 1 cup	8
Thick Shake: Chocolate, 10 oz	9
Vanilla, 10 oz	11
Soymilk, (fortified), average, 1 cup	7
Soy Dream, Enriched, shelf-stable, 1 cup	7
Yogurt, average all brands:	
Plain, 6 oz	8
Fruit flavors, 6 oz	7
Chobani, Greek, Plain, 6 oz	14
Soy, fruit flavors, 6 oz	7
Ice Cream: Rich, ½ cup	2
Regular, Vanilla, ½ cup	2.5
Sherbet, ½ cup	1
Custard, baked, ½ cup	7

Cheese

	Pro
Hard Cheeses, average, 1 oz	7
Cottage Cheese, ½ cup	13
Cream Cheese, avg., 1 oz	2
Ricotta, part skim, ½ cup	14

Bread, Bagels, Biscuits

	Pro
Bread: *With enriched flour*	
1 slice, 1 oz	2
4 thin slices, 4 oz	8
4 thick slices, 6 oz	12
Bagel, plain 2 oz	6
Biscuits, 1 oz	2
Pita Bread, 1 pita, 1½ oz	4
Pumpernickel, 1 slice, 1 oz	3

Infant/Baby Foods

	Pro
Infant Formula Milk:	
Enfamil/Gerber/Similac, Regular/Low Iron , 5 fl.oz	2.2
Isomil/Nursoy/ProSobee,	3
Baby Cereals: *Average all brands*	
Dry, 4 Tbsp, ½ oz	1
Jars, with fruit, 4½ oz	1

Protein Counter

Breakfast Cereals

	Pro
Hot Cereals ~ *Cooked:*	
Bulgur, cooked, 1 cup, 5 oz	9
Oatmeal: Reg., non-fortified, 1 cup	6
Instant, fortified, avg., 1 pkt	4
Quaker, all flavors, 1/2 cup	5
Corn/Hominy Grits: 1 cup	3
Quaker: Reg., 3 Tbsp, 1 oz	3
Instant White, 1 packet	2
Cream of Wheat, 1 cup	4
Brands ~ *Ready-To-Eat*	
General Mills:	
Cheerios, Original, 1¼ cups, 1.4 oz	5
Chex, Corn, 1¼ cups, 1.4 oz	3
Kix, Original,1½ cupss, 1.4 oz	3
Lucky Charms, Original, 3/4 cup, 1 oz	2
Total, Raisin Bran, 1¼ cups, 2.3 oz	4
Wheaties, 1 cup, 1.3 oz	3
Kashi:	
7 Whole Grain Flakes, 1¼ cups, 2.1 oz	7
GO: Love, Chocolate Crunch, ¾ cup, 1.83 oz	10
Rise, Original, 1¼ cups, 2 oz	12
Honey Toasted Oat, 1 cup, 1.41 oz	4
Super Loops, 1 cup, 1.35 oz	4
Warm Cinnamon Oat, 1 cup, 1.41 oz	4
Whole Wheat Biscuits, Autumn, 2 oz	7
Kellogg's:	
All-Bran, Original, 1.83 oz pkg	6
Apple Jacks, Original, 1⅓ cups, 1.4 oz	2
Corn Flakes, 1½ cups, 1.41 oz	3
Product 19, 1 cup, 1 oz	3
Rice Krispies, 1 1/4 cup, 1.2 oz	2
Special K: Original, 1.27 oz	7
Granola, Touch of Honey, ½ cup, 1.83 oz	6
Prottein, 1⅓ cups, 2 oz	15
Post:	
Grape Nuts, Original, 1/2 cup, 2 oz	6
Raisin Bran, 1¼ cups, 2.1 oz	5
Quaker:	
Corn Bran Crunch, 1 cup, 1.35 oz	2
Life, Vanilla, 1 cup, 1.45 oz	4
Multigrain Flakes, Honey Vanilla, ¾ cup, 2.2 oz	7
Simply Granola, Oats, Honey & Alm., ⅔ cup, 2.2 oz	7

Brans & Wheatgerm

	Pro
Oat Bran, raw, 1 Tbsp	2
Rice Bran, raw, 2 Tbsp	1
Wheat Bran, unprocessed, 2 T.	1
Wheat Germ, 2 Tbsp, 1/2 oz	4

Grains & Flours, Yeast

	Pro
Amaranth grain, cooked, 1/2 cup, 4.5 oz	5
Barley, 1/2 cup, 3.2 oz	12
Buckwheat Flour, Whole-groat, 1 cup	15
Carob Flour, 1 cup, 3.6 oz	5
Corn Flour, 1 cup, 4 oz	11
Corn Meal, 1 cup, 4 1/2 oz	8
Flour: White, 1 cup, 5.6 oz	9
Wholegrain, 1 cup, 4¼ oz	16
Hemp Wholemeal Flour, 1 cup, 3.5 oz	30
Millet, wholegrain, 1 cup, 3½ oz	12
Quinoa, raw, ⅓ cup, 1.5 oz	6
Rye Flour: Dark, 1 cup, 4 1/2 oz	18
Light, 1 cup, 3 1/2 oz	9
Soy Flour, full fat, 1 cup, 3 oz	29
Yeast: Brewers, 2 Tbsp, 1/2 oz	8
Nutritional Yeast Flakes *(Red Star),* 1 heaping Tbsp, 1/2 oz	8

Rice, Spaghetti, Macaroni

	Pro
Rice: Brown/White, average 1 cup cooked, 6 1/2 oz	5
Spaghetti/Macaroni/Noodles (enriched):	
Cooked, 1 cup, 4 1/2 oz	7
Canned: in Tomato Sce, 1/2 cup	2
with Meatballs, 1 cup, 8 oz	10
Macaroni & Cheese, 1 cup, 9 oz	8

Soups

	Pro
With Noodles/Vegetables, 1 cup	3
With Meat/Beans/Peas, 1 cup	8

Fruit

	Pro
Fresh/Canned:	
Average, all types, 1 medium/2 small fruit	1
Avocado, 1/2 medium	2
Dried Fruit: Apricots, 8 halves, 1 oz	1
Dates, 6 dates, 2 oz	1.5
Figs, 4 medium figs, 2 oz	2
Prunes, 5 medium, 1 1/2 oz	1
Raisins, 1 oz	1
Fruit Juice: Average, 1 cup	0.5
Prune Juice, 6 fl.oz	1
Tomato Juice, 1 cup, 8 fl.oz	1.5

Vegetables

	Pro
Beans: Snap/green, 1/2 cup, 2 oz	1
Dried: Average all types, cooked, 1/2 cup	7
Baked Beans, 1/2 cup 4 1/2 oz	5
Bean Sprouts, mung, 1 c., 4 oz	3
Broccoli, raw, 1/2 cup, 1 1/2 oz	1.5
Cabbage; Cauliflower, raw, 1 c. 3 oz	1.5
Chickpeas, cooked, ½ cup, 3 oz	8
Corn: Raw, 1/2 cup kernels, 3 oz	2.5
1 ear trimmed to 3 1/2"	2
Lentils, cooked, 1/2 cup 3 1/2 oz	9
Mushrooms, raw, 1/2 c., sliced	1
Peas: Green, raw, 1/2 c., 2 1/2 oz	4
Split Peas, cooked, 1 cup, 7 oz	16
Potatoes: *Cooked:*	
1 medium, with skin, 5 oz	3.3
without skin, 4 oz	2.3
French Fries, small, 2.6 oz	2
Potato Salad, 1/2 cup, 4 oz	3.5
Pumpkin, 1/2 cup mashed, 4.3 oz	1
Seaweed, kelp, 1 oz	<1
Spinach, cooked, 1/2 cup, 3 oz	2.7
Squash, ckd, all types, 1/2 cup	1
Tomatoes, 1 medium, 4 1/2 oz	1
Vegetables, mixed, ckd, 1 cup	2.5
Soybeans, cooked, 1/2 cup, 3 oz	14

Tofu, Tempeh, Miso

	Pro
Tofu, raw, firm, 1/2 cup, 4 1/2 oz	10
Tempeh, 1/2 cup, 3 oz	16
Miso, 1/2 cup, 5 oz	16
Miso Soup, 1 cup	3
Soybean Protein *(TVP)*, 1 oz	18

Cakes, Pastries, Pies

	Pro
Banana Nut Bread, 4 oz	6
Carrot w. cream cheese frosting, 4 oz	4
Cheesecake, 1 piece, 4 oz	6
Chocolate, 1 piece, 2 oz	2
Fruitcake, 1 piece, 3 oz	4
Croissant, plain, small, 2 oz	5
Danish Pastry, 1 pastry, 2 1/4 oz	4
Donuts, average, 2 oz	4
Muffins, average, 1 med., 1 1/2 oz	3
Pancakes, 4" diam., two, 2 oz	4
Pies: Fruit, 1 piece, 5 1/2 oz	4
Pecan, 1 piece, 5 oz	7
Puddings, average, 1/2 cup, 4 1/2 oz	4
Waffles, 1 large, 2 1/2 oz	7

Peanut Butter

	Pro
Regular: 2 Tbsp, 1.1 oz	8
Peter Pan Plus, 2 Tbsp, 1.1 oz	8

Sugar, Honey, Jam

	Pro
Sugar: White	0
Brown, 1 Tbsp	0
Molasses: Light/Med., 1 Tbsp	0
Blackstrap, 1 Tbsp, 3/4 oz	0
Corn Syrup, 1 Tbsp, 3/4 oz	0
Honey, Jams, Jelly	0

Candy, Chocolate, Carob

	Pro
Candy, sugar-based	0
Chocolate: Plain, 2 oz bar	4
with nuts, 2 oz bar	6
Carob, plain, 2 oz	6

Cookies, Crackers, Chips

	Pro
Cookies, average, 4 cookies	2
Crackers, Graham, 2 1/2" sq., (2)	1
Rice Cakes, average, one	1
Corn/Potato Chips, 1 oz	2

Nuts:

	Pro
Almonds, shelled, 20-25 nuts	6
Brazil Nuts, 7-8 medium nuts, 1 oz	4
Cashews, 12-16 nuts, 1 oz	5
Hemp Seeds, 3 tbsp, 1 oz	9
Macadamias, 1 oz	2
Peanuts, dry rsted, 40 nuts, 1 oz	6
Pecans, 24 halves, 1 oz	2
Walnuts, 15 halves, 1 oz	4

Seeds:

	Pro
Chia Seeds, raw, 2 Tbsp, 1.1 oz	5
Flax Seeds, 3 Tbsp, 1 oz	6
Sesame Seeds, dry, 1 Tbsp	2
Pumpkin Kernels, dry, hulled, 1 oz	7
Sunflower Seeds, dried, hulled, 1 oz	6

Granola & Food/Protein Bars

	Pro
Granola Bars, average, 1 bar, 2 oz	2
Bariatrix, Proti-Bars (1), 1.4 oz	15
Cliff, Builder's Protein, av., 1 bar	20
GeniSoy, Protein Bars, 1.6 oz	15
Jenny Craig, Bars, av., 1 oz	10
Luna Protein, av., 1 bar	12
Met-Rx, "Big 100", av., 3.5 oz	31
Myoplex 30, all flavors, 3 oz	30
Optifast 800, all flavors, 1.72 oz	14
PowerBar, Protein Plus	20
Slim-Fast: Protein Meal Bars, 1.7 oz	10
Keto Meal Bar, 1.48 oz	7
Special K: Keto Meal Bars, 2.2 oz	7
Protein Meal Bars, 1.5 oz	7

High Protein Drinks & Powders — Pro

Atkins, Shakes, 11 fl.oz — 15
Bob's Red Mill, Protein Powders:
- Chia Protein, 1/3 cup, 1.45 oz — 20
- Pea Protein, ¼ cup, 1oz — 21
- Soy Protein, ¼ cup, 0.75 oz — 17
- Whey/Hemp Protein, ¼ cup, 0.75 oz — 15

Boost, High Protein, 8 fl.oz bottle — 20
- Plus Protein Shake, 8 fl oz — 14

Carnation, B'fast Essentials, 11 fl.oz — 10
Ensure, Plus, 8 fl.oz bottle — 13
Gatorade, Protein Recovery Shake, 11 oz — 20
GNC, Lean Shake, 14 fl oz — 25
Hemp Protein Powder, ¼ cup, 1 oz — 14
Met-Rx Meal Replacement, RTD:
- High Protein; 51, 15 fl.oz — 51

Myoplex, Original Nutrition Shake, 1 pkt — 42
Optifast 800, prepared, 8 fl oz — 16
Premier Protein, Chocolate, 11 fl.oz — 20
Pure Protein Shake, 11 fl.oz — 35
Slim-Fast Shakes: Keto, 11 fl.oz — 8
- Advanced Energy, 11 fl.oz — 20

Special K, Protein Shakes, 10 fl.oz — 15
Weider, Mass 1000, 4 scoops, 7 oz — 34
Pumpkin Protein Powder, 2 Tbsp, ½ oz — 9
Whey Protein Powder: 100%, plain, 1 oz — 24
- Choc Flavor, 1 scoop, 0.8 oz — 18

Coffee, Tea, Soda

Coffee, Coffee Substitutes, 1 cup, 8 fl.oz — 0
Coffee, with 2 oz milk, 1 cup, 8 fl.oz — 2
Caffe latte, large, 16 fl.oz — 12
Cappuccino, large, 16 fl.oz — 8
Frappuccino, average, 16 fl.oz — 6
Hot Chocolate, with milk, 1 cup, 8 fl.oz — 8
Soft Drinks/Soda, Tea, all types — 0

Beer, Wine, Spirits

Beer, 12 fl.oz — 1
Wines, red/white, 1 glass — 0
Spirits/Liquor — 0

Fast-Foods/Burgers

Pancakes, average all outlets, 3 — 8
Shakes, Chocolate, 16 fl.oz — 12
Sundaes, Average all outlets — 7
Arby's:
- Buffalo Chicken Slider — 12
- Buttermilk Crispy Chicken S'wich — 24
- Classic Roast Beef Sandwich — 23
- Fire-Roasted Philly — 34

Burger King: Cheeseburger — 15
- Double Bacon Cheeseburger — 24
- Double Stacker King — 61
- Impossible Whopper — 25
- Whopper Sandwich — 28

Fast Foods/Burgers (Cont) — Pro

Carl's Jr: Beyond Famous Star with Cheese — 33
- Charbroiled Chicken Club Sandwich — 44
- Famous Star Burger with Cheese — 28
- Super Star Burger with Cheese — 48

Del Taco: Beyond 8 Layer Burrito — 27
- Beyond Avocado Taco — 12
- Beyond Taco — 19
- Epic Beyond Original Mex — 44

Domino's Pizza: *Hand Tossed (12")*
- Buffalo Chicken, 1 slice — 12
- Honolulu Hawaiian, 1 slice — 10
- Ultimate Pepperoni, 1 slice — 11

KFC: Original Breast — 39
- Extra Crispy Chicken Tender — 19
- Kentucky Grilled, Breast — 38

McDonald's: Big Mac — 25
- Buttermilk Crispy Chicken S'wch — 27
- Cheeseburger — 15
- Chicken McNuggets (4) — 9
- Filet-O-Fish — 16
- Hamburger — 12
- Quarter Pounder with Cheese — 30
- French Fries: Small, 2.5 oz — 3
  - Large, 5.4 oz — 7
- Shakes, medium — 14
- Breakfast: Egg McMuffin — 17
  - Bacon, Egg & Cheese McGriddles — 18
  - Sausage Burrito — 13
  - Sausage McMuffin with Egg — 21

Pizza Hut: *Per Medium, 1 slice, 1/8 Pizza*
- Thin 'n Crispy, Supreme — 10
- Pan Pizzas, Hawaiian Chicken — 11
- Hand Tossed: Pepperoni Lover's — 12
  - Ultimate Cheese Lover's — 11

Red Robin, Veggie Burger — 24
Subway: *6" Subs with standard toppings, no oil*
- Black Forest Ham — 15
- Meatball Marinara — 20
- Spicy Italian — 20
- Subway Club — 20
- Turkey Breast — 15

Taco Bell: Bean Burrito, vegan — 13
- Burrito Supreme, Beef — 16
- Cheesy Gordita Crunch — 21
- Chicken Chalupa — 16
- Grilled Soft Beef Taco — 9
- Steak Chalupa — 15

Wendy's:
- Grilled Asiago Ranch Chkn Club — 42
- Dave's Double Burger — 49
- Homestyle Chicken Sandwich — 27
- Jr Cheeseburger — 19

White Castle, Impossible Burger w/o Chse Slider — 9

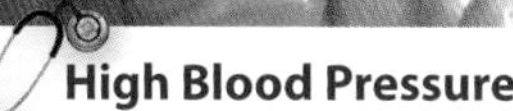

High Blood Pressure

Many American adults have hypertension (high blood pressure), and are unaware of it. It is generally symptomless, so **have your blood pressure checked annually** – particularly if it runs in the family.

Untreated hypertension overworks the heart, damages arteries and promotes atherosclerosis. This in turn greatly increases the risk of heart disease, stroke, blindness, kidney disease and impotence. The earlier hypertension is detected, the sooner it can be brought under control.

BLOOD PRESSURE CLASSIFICATION

For Adults Age 18 & Older ~ Not Acutely ill or on Medication (American Heart Association)

	DIASTOLIC		SYSTOLIC
Normal ➤	Below 80	and	Below 120
Prehypertension ➤	80-89	or	120-139
Hypertension:			
Stage 1 ➤	90-99	or	140-159
Stage 2 ➤	100 or more	or	160 or more

Treating Hypertension

Prehypertension (in the chart above) means you don't have high blood pressure now but are likely to develop it in the future.

You can take steps to lessen the risk by adopting healthy lifestyle habits such as:

- reducing sodium intake
- eating adequate fruit and vegetables
- losing weight if overweight
- limiting alcohol to 2 drinks or less daily
- quitting smoking
- exercising regularly, managing stress.

Stage 1 hypertension can often be treated with the above lifestyle changes.

Stage 2 hypertension usually requires drug therapy. However, salt restriction, abstaining from alcohol, and the above lifestyle changes will improve the success of drug therapy, and enable smaller drug doses to be prescribed.

HYPERTENSION DAMAGES ARTERIES & PROMOTES ATHEROSCLEROSIS

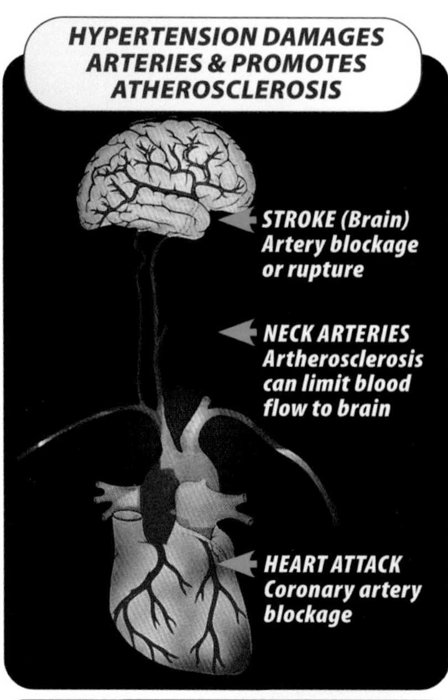

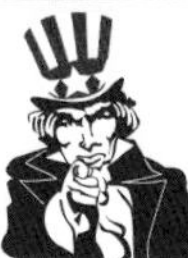

STROKE
KNOW THE WARNING SIGNS

Stroke is a medical emergency!
If you notice one or more of these signs, call 9-1-1 or your doctor immediately.

These signs may be signalling a possible stroke or transient ischemic attack:

- **Sudden weakness** or numbness in your face, arm, or leg on one side of your body.
- **Sudden confusion,** trouble speaking or understanding. Slurred speech.
- **Sudden trouble seeing,** in one or both eyes
- **Sudden trouble walking,** dizziness, loss of balance or coordination.
- **Sudden severe headache** - 'a bolt out of the blue' – with no apparent cause.

Extra Info: www.stroke.org

Salt & Sodium Guide

Salt & Sodium

- **Sodium is a mineral element** most commonly found in salt (sodium chloride). It also occurs naturally in much smaller amounts in animal and plant foods, and water – normally sufficient for our needs without having to add salt to our diet.
- **Sodium is required** for nerve and muscle function, as well as to balance the amount of fluid in our tissues and blood. Sodium acts like a sponge to attract and hold fluids in body tissues.
- **Excess sodium** can cause water retention, and increase the risk of developing hypertension. Very high salt intake may also increase the risk of stomach cancer.
- **Too little sodium** may cause low blood pressure (hypotension), and decrease blood flow to the heart, brain and kidneys – especially during exercise. (A certain blood volume is required to sustain the blood pressure needed for adequate blood flow in the capillaries).

Salt-Sensitive Persons

- **Normally, our kidneys** excrete excess dietary sodium. The thirst we feel after a salty meal is the body calling for water to dilute the sodium, and enable the kidneys to flush out excess sodium.
- **However, 'salt - sensitive'** persons (up to 70% of adults) tend to retain excess sodium (above approximately 3000mg daily) instead of excreting it. Such persons are more likely to develop hypertension and would benefit most from sodium restriction. Assume you are susceptible if there is a family history of hypertension.
- **Although not everyone will benefit, all Americans are being asked to moderate their salt and sodium intake** as a public health measure – particularly because so many do not know whether or not they have hypertension, and also because we do not know just who is salt-sensitive.

SAFE SODIUM LEVELS

The American Heart Association recommends a **maximum sodium intake of 1500mg per day** for adults with normal blood pressure.

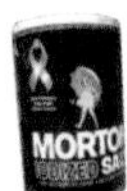

Persons with hypertension and kidney ailments are usually restricted to as little as **1000mg sodium per day**. Your doctor will discuss the correct sodium level for you.

FINDING HIDDEN SODIUM

On average, **less than one third of our sodium intake comes from the salt shaker.**
The rest is hidden in processed foods that have salt added during manufacture.

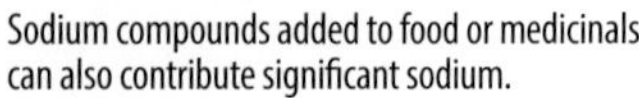

Sodium compounds added to food or medicinals can also contribute significant sodium.

Sodium bicarbonate in particular is widely used in antacid tablets (such as *Alka Seltzer*) and powders. Sodium bicarbonate contains 27% sodium by weight. Each gram has 270mg of sodium. Large amounts of sodium can be unwittingly consumed – up to 600mg per tablet. (See Antacids ~ Page 280)

Example: 2 *Alka-Seltzer* Tablets = 1000mg sodium

Other sodium compounds include monosodium glutamate (MSG), sodium ascorbate, sodium nitrite, and sodium citrate.

POTASSIUM BALANCES SODIUM

Potassium helps to balance sodium by helping the kidneys to excrete excess sodium. Fruit and vegetables are rich sources of potassium - another reason to ensure you have your 5-7 servings every day.

Nuts also provide potassium as well as magnesium and other heart-healthy nutrients and anti-oxidants. Eat them unsalted.

Note: This info is only for people with normal kidney function. Also not for persons on potassium-sparing diuretics.

ALCOHOL DANGER

Excessive alcohol intake contributes to hypertension. Susceptible persons should avoid or limit alcohol intake to 1-2 drinks per day.

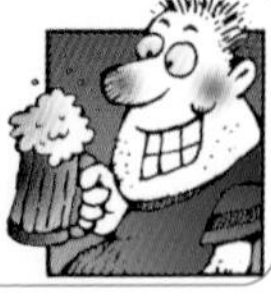

Sodium accounts for only 40% of the weight of salt (sodium chloride). Examples:
1 gram (1000mg) Salt has 400mg Sodium
1 teaspoon (5g) Salt has 2000mg Sodium

HINTS TO REDUCE SODIUM

- **Cut down use of the salt shaker.** Start with an easy 50% cut in sodium by using Lite Salt (*Morton*) or *Cardia* Salt. Then gradually cut back until you can leave the salt shaker off the table. Sea salt is still high in sodium.
- **Use fresh herbs,** and salt-free seasonings to add flavor to food.
- **Choose low-sodium,** sodium-free, and reduced-sodium products in place of regular, salted products.
- **Check food labels for sodium levels.** FDA Guidelines for sodium descriptors are:
  - **Reduced Sodium:** At least 25% less sodium than the original product
  - **Low Sodium:** 140 mg or less/serving
  - **Very Low Sodium:** 35mg or less/serving
  - **Sodium Free:** Less than 5mg/serving
  - **No Salt Added:** Made without the salt normally added, but still contains the sodium that is a natural part of the food
- **Use reduced-sodium breads,** butter and margarine. Regular varieties are considered high in sodium in view of their significant contribution to our diet.
- **Go easy on salty condiments and sauces** such as ketchup, mustard, soy sauce, spaghetti sauces, and salad dressings. Use low-sodium varieties.
- **Limit pizzas and salty fast-foods.** Check the *CalorieKing.com* food database.
- **Avoid salty snack foods** such as potato chips, corn chips, salted nuts, pretzels and cheesy-flavored snacks. **Choose unsalted** popcorn, nuts or seeds. Eat more fruit.
- **Don't salt children's food** to your taste.
- **Avoid antacids with** sodium bicarbonate (such as *Alka-Seltzer*). They are high in sodium. Look for low-sodium alternatives.

FOODS HIGH IN SODIUM

- Bread (4 slices/day), Bagels, Biscuits
- Cheese, Butter, Margarine
- Pickles, Sauerkraut, Olives
- Condiments, Sauces
- Salad Dressings
- Canned vegetables/salads/beans

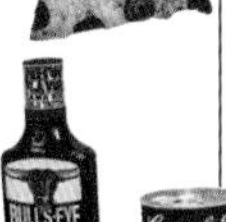

- Deli Salads (with dressing)
- Frozen/Packaged Meals/Entrees
- Soups: Canned/dry; bouillon cubes

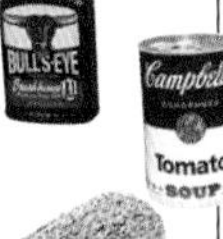

- Meats: Ham, bacon, sausage, luncheon meats, smoked meats
- Canned Fish (in brine/salt)
- Sea Salt, Garlic/Celery Salt
- Snack Foods (potato chips, pretzels)
- Tomato Juice (Canned), V8 Vegetable Juice

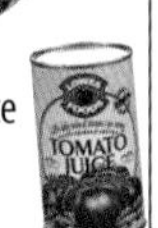

- Fast Foods: Pizza, Burgers, Chicken
- *Alka-Seltzer* Antacid

MODERATE SODIUM

- Meat, Fish, Poultry - Unprocessed
- Milk, Yogurt, Soy Drinks, Eggs
- Peanut Butter
- Breakfast Cereals (less than 200mg/serving)
- Chocolate Candy, Fruit/Nut Bars
- *Reduced Sodium & Low Sodium* Products

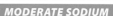

FOODS LOW IN SODIUM

- Products labelled *Very Low Sodium*, or *Sodium Free*
- Bread (No Salt Added)
- Fresh fruits and vegetables
- Canned and Dried Fruits
- Potatoes, Rice, Pasta
- Dried Beans & Lentils, Tofu
- Nuts & Seeds (unsalted)
- Corn & Popcorn (unsalted)
- Pepper, Spices, Herbs
- Jam, Honey, Syrup
- Candy, Gum
- Hard & Jelly Candy
- Coffee, Tea, Alcohol
- Fresh Fruit Juices, Water

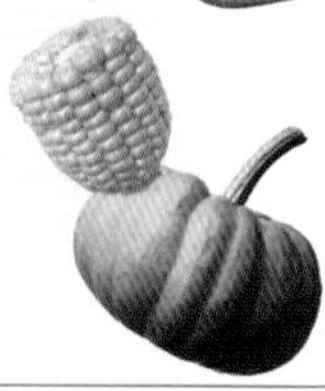

Sodium Counter

The American Heart Association recommends a sodium intake of less than 1500mg/day

Milk & Dairy Products

Item	Sodium
Milk: Whole/lowfat/skim, average 1 glass, 8 fl.oz	120
Whole, low sodium, 1 cup	5
Choc Milk, 1 cup	130
Soy Milk, 8 fl.oz	30
Buttermilk, cultured, 8 fl.oz	250
Dry/Powder, skim, 1/4 cup, 1 oz	110
Yogurt, with fruit average, 8 oz	130
Cheese: Bleu, 1 oz	330
Cottage Cheese, Creamed, ½ cup, 4 oz	450
Kraft: American, Singles, 1 sl., 0.7 oz	240
American, Deli Deluxe, 2 slices, 0.9 oz	400
Philadelphia Cream Cheese, Tub, Orig.,1.1 oz	125
Parmesan, 1 oz	435
Ricotta Cheese, ½ cup, 4 oz	110
Swiss, Shredded Natural, 1oz	55
Triple Cheddar, 1 oz	170

Ice Cream, Frozen Yogurt

Item	Sodium
Ice Cream, average, 1/2 cup	50
Frozen Yogurt, 1/2 cup	50

Fats/Oils

Item	Sodium
Butter/Margarine:	
Regular, 2 Tbsp, 1 oz	230
Unsalted, reg., 2 Tbsp, 1 oz	5
Mayonnaise, avg., 2 Tbsp, 1 oz	160
Oils/Lard/Drippings	0
Cream, average, 1 Tbsp	5
Coffee-Mate: Powdered, Original, 1 tsp	5
Liquid, all flavors	0-5

Eggs

Item	Sodium
Whole, 1 large	70
Omelet: 2 egg, plain	220
With 1 oz Cheddar Cheese	400
Egg Beaters: Original, 3 Tbsp	90
Flavors, average, 3 Tbsp	140

Meats

Item	Sodium
Meat, average all types, cooked Beef/Lamb/Veal/Pork, 4 oz	80
Corned Beef, cooked, 3 oz	800
Bacon, cooked, 2 slices, 0.5 oz	270
Ham, 3 oz	1100

Meat Substitutes (Vegan)

Item	Sodium
Beyond Meat: Beef/Burger, 4 oz	350
Sausage, cooked, 1 link	500

Sodium ~ Sodium (mg)

Sausages & Deli Meats

Item	Sodium
Bologna, 1 oz	280
Frankfurter, 2 oz	640
Ham, chopped, 0.8 oz slice	290
Liverwurst (Braunschweiger), 1 oz	320
Pepperoni, 5 slices, 1 oz	570
Salami: Cooked, 1 oz	350
dry/hard, 1 oz	600
Sausage, 1 oz link	220
Pork, 2 oz patty	260
Spam: Classic, 2 oz	790
25% Less Sodium, 2 oz	580
Turkey Roll, 1 oz	160

Chicken & Turkey

Item	Sodium
Chicken/Turkey, cooked, unsalted, 4 oz	80
Stuffing Mixes, average., ½ cup	500

Fish:

Item	Sodium
Fresh Fish: average, plain	
Cooked, 4 oz, without bone	60
Broiled w. butter, 4 oz	150
Breaded & fried, 4 oz	320
Fish fillets, batter-dipped 3 oz	350
Fish sticks, 1 oz stick	160
Gefilte Fish, with broth, 1 pce, 1.5 oz	220
Herring, pickled, 2 pces, 1 oz	260
Lobster, meat only, 4 oz	180
Oysters, fresh, 6 med., 3 oz	95
Salmon: Canned, 3 oz	460
No Salt Added, 3 oz	65
Smoked fish, average, 3 oz	650
Tuna: Canned, drained, 3 oz	160
Light, drained, 3 oz	200
No Added Salt, 3 oz	40
Spicy Flavored, 5 oz	260

Entrees & Meals

Item	Sodium
Frozen Meals, average	600-1300
Lean Cuisine, Favorites	500-800
Stouffer's, Meat Lovers Lasagna	750
Dinners, average	900-1200
Side Dishes, average	400-600
Pizza, frozen, 1/4 large, 6 oz	800-1200
Microwave, Cup Meals	900-1200
Cup Noodles, average	1050-1280

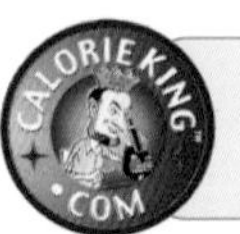

More Sodium Counts: www.CalorieKing.com

Soups

	Sodium
Condensed: Average, 1 cup, 8 oz	800-1000
Low Sodium, average	70
Chicken Noodle, average, 1 cup	900
Bouillon Cube, average	950
Top Ramen Noodle Soup, 3 oz pkg, av.	1600
Soup Cups, average	850
Soup Mixes, average, 1 cup	900

Condiments, Sauces, Dressings

	Sodium
A-1 Sauce, 1 Tbsp	280
Barbecue Sauce, 1 Tbsp	130
Bragg's Liquid Aminos, 1 tsp	350
Chili Sauce, 1 Tbsp	230
Ketchup: Tomato, 1 Tbsp	180
Low Sodium, 1 Tbsp	20
Mayonnaise, 1 Tbsp	80
Mustard, 1 tsp	70
Pizza Sauce, 1/2 cup	700
Salad Dressings, 2 Tbsp, 1 oz	160-400
Spaghetti Sauce, 1/2 cup	500
Soy Sauce: 1 Tbsp	900
Lite, 1 Tbsp	600
Sweet & Sour, 1/2 cup	250
Tabasco, 1 tsp	25
Vinegar, Lemon Juice	0
Worcestershire, 1 Tbsp	65
Tomato: Sauce, 1 cup	1200
Paste/Puree (salted), 1/2 cup	1000
No Salt Added, 1/2 cup	75

Salt & Salt Substitutes

	Sodium
Table Salt: 1 teaspoon, 6g	2400
Single Serve package, 1 g	400
Cardia Salt, 1 teaspoon	1080
Lite Salt, 1 teaspoon, 6g	1200
Morton, No Salt Substitute, 1 tsp	5
Garlic/Onion/Seasoned Salt, 1 tsp, 4g	1350
Garlic/Seasoned Salt 1 teaspoon, 4g	1300
Sea Salt, 1 teaspoon, 5g	2250

Seasonings, Herbs & Spices

	Sodium
Baking Powder, 1 tsp, 3g	340
Baking Soda (Sodium bicarb), 1 tsp, 3g	810
Accent, Flavor Enhancer, ¼ tsp	160
Chili Powder, 1 tsp, 3g	25
Curry Powder	0
Lemon Pepper 1 tsp	340
Meat Tenderizer, 1 tsp, 5g	1750
MSG (Monosodium Glutamate), 5g	500
Mrs Dash, Blends/Marinades	0
Old Bay: Seasoning, 1 tsp, 2.4 oz	560
Seasoning, Less Sodium, 1 tsp, 2.4 oz	360
Pepper, Mustard (dry), 1 tsp	1
Yeast, Nutritional, 1 Tbsp	10

Breakfast Cereals

	Sodium
Kellogg's:	
All-Bran, Original, ⅔ cup, 1 oz	95
Special K, Original, 1¼ cups, 1.4 oz	270
Corn Flakes, 1½ cup,s 1 oz	300
Raisin Bran, 1 cup, 2 oz	200
Quaker:	
Corn Crunch, 1 cup, 1.3 oz	220
Multigrain Flakes, av., ¾ c., 2.2 oz	40
Real Medleys, ⅔ cup, 1.83 oz	15-45
Simply Granola, average, 1/2 cup	30-35
General Mills, Total, 1 cup, 1.4 oz	190
Oatmeal: Regular, 3/4 cup	1
Quaker, Instant Maple & Brown Sugar (1 pkt)	260

Breads, Bagels, Crackers

	Sodium
Bread: Thin Slice, average 1 oz	140
Thick Slice, 1.5 oz	210
Low Sodium, 1 oz	10
Bagels: Plain, medium, 2 oz	200
Large, take-out, average, 4 oz	550
Panera Bread, 3.8 oz	410
Biscuits, average, 1 oz	180
Bun/Roll: 1 medium, 1.5 oz	200
Large, 4 oz	560
Crackers: Saltine, 2 crackers	70
Low Salt, 2	25
Graham, 2 regular	50
Croissant, Plain, average, 2 oz	280
Rice Cakes, average	25
Ritz Crackers, Hint of Salt, 1 oz	60
RyVita, Original Crispbread, 2 slices	30

Cookies, Cakes, Desserts

	Sodium
Cookies: Average, 2-3 cookies, 1 oz	100
Average, 1 cookie, 2.5 oz	180
Baked Custard, 1/2 cup	100
Brownie, 1.5 oz	130
Carrot Cake, 8 oz	650
Cheesecake, 7 oz	350
Cinnamon Sweet Roll, 2 oz	250
Danish, Apple/Fruit	250
Donut, average	150
Muffins: 1 medium, 2 oz	150
1 extra large, 4 oz	300
Pancakes, (4"), x 3	360
Fruit Pies, average, 7 oz	600
Pudding: Average, 1/2 cup	160
Jell-O Instant Pudding Mix, 1/4 pkg	350
Waffles: Home-made, 7", 2.5 oz	350
Frozen: Average, 1.2 oz	260
Aunt Jemima, Homestyle, 3 pancakes	460

Sodium Counter

Fruit & Juices

	Sodium
Fresh Fruit, average all types, 1 serving	1
Dried/Canned Fruit, ½ cup	1
Fruit Juice: Fresh, squeezed, 6 fl.oz	1
Commercial, aver., 6 fl.oz	20
Tomato Juice *(Campbell's)*, 8 fl.oz	680
Low Sodium (No Salt Added), 8 fl.oz	140
V8 Vegetable *(Campbell's)*:	
11.5 fl.oz bottle	920
Low Sodium, 5.5 fl.oz can	95

Vegetables

Fresh/Frozen (No Salt Added): Per ½ Cup	
Asparagus, Bean Sprouts, Corn	3
Beets, Carrots, Celery, ½ cup	40
Broccoli, Cabbage, Cauliflower	10
Cucumber, Green Beans, Mushroom, Okra	3
Onions, Peas, Potato, Pumpkin, Squash	3
Peppers, Hot Chili, raw, each	3
Spinach, Turnips, ½ cup, cooked	40
Tomato, 1 medium, 5 oz	10
Canned: Asparagus, 4 spears	300
Beans, baked in tomato sauce	450
Beets, ½ cup, 3 oz	240
Corn Kernels, ½ cup, 3 oz	190
Creamed, ½ cup, 4.5 oz	330
Mushrooms w. butter sce, 2oz	550
Peas, ½ cup, 3 oz	250
Sauerkraut, ½ cup, 4 oz	750

Pickles, Olives

Olives: pickled: Green, 1 large	90
Ripe/black, 1 large	40
Pickles: Bread & Butter, 4 slices, 1 oz	200
Dill, 1 pickle, 2.5oz	900
Sweet, 1 gherkin, 0.5 oz	130

Soybean Products

Miso (Soy Paste), ¼ c., 2.5 oz	2500
Soybean Protein Isolate, 1 oz	280
Tempeh, Natural, ½ cup, 3 oz	5
Tofu, average, ½ cup, 4 oz	5

Jam, Honey, Syrups

Jam/Jelly, 1 Tbsp	2
Honey/Maple Syrup, 1 Tbsp	1
Log Cabin, Maple Syrup,2 Tbsp, 1 fl.oz	55
Syrup, Lite, 2 Tbsp, 1 fl.oz	95

Peanut Butter

Peanut Butter: Regular, 2 Tbsp, 0.5 oz	190
Jif, Low Sodium, 2 Tbsp	65
Trader Joe's, Unsalted, 2 Tbsp	0

Snacks, Nuts

	Sodium
Cheese Balls/Curls, 1 oz	280
Cheetos, Cheddar Popcorn, 1 oz	260
Corn/Tortilla Chips: average, 1 oz	220
Fritos, Lightly Salted, 1 oz	80
Granola bars, average, 1 bar	80
Nuts: Plain, unsalted, 1 oz	1
Lightly salted, 1 oz	80
Salted or Honey Roasted, 1 oz	160
Popcorn: Plain (unsalted), 1 cup	1
Flavored, average, 1 cup	60
Salt added, 1 cup	180
Potato Chips: Plain, 1 oz	160
Lay's, Lightly Salted, 1 oz	65
Flavored, average, 1 oz	200
Pretzels: Regular, 3, 1 oz	450
Soft, salted, large	1000

Candy, Chocolate

Chocolate, milk, 1 oz	30
Fudge, chocolate, 1 oz	55
Candy Bars, average, 1.5 oz	60
Hard Candy, 1 oz	10
Licorice, 1 oz	30

Beverages, Alcohol

Coffee or Tea, 1 cup	1
Cocoa: Dry, plain, 1 Tbsp	0
Mix, average, 1 envelope	120
Quik, 2 tsp	35
Soft Drinks, average, 8 fl.oz	20
Mineral Water: Perrier, 8 fl.oz	5
Gatorade, Thirst Quencher, 8 fl.oz	110
Red Bull: 8.4 fl.oz can	105
Sugar Free, 8.4 fl.oz	105
Water, Average, 1 cup, 8 fl.oz	5
Alcohol: Beer, average, 12 fl.oz	15
Wines, average, 4 fl.oz	10
Spirits (distilled), 1.5 fl.oz	1

Antacids ~ Alka-Seltzer

	Sodium
Alka-Seltzer: *Per Tablet*	
Original; Heartburn	570
Extra Strength	590
Lemon Lime	500
Gold	310
Alka-Mints, chewable	0
Bromo Seltzer, 3/4 capful	760
Picot, 1 packet, 5g	670
Rolaids, All types	0
Tums, Regular/Extra Strength	0

Cold & Flu ~ Alka-Seltzer Plus

Effervescents, average, 1 tablet	480
Fast Crystal Packs; Liquid Gels	0

Fast-Foods & Restaurants	Sodium
Burger King:	
Bacon Double Cheeseburger	670
Cheeseburger	560
Double Stacker King	1871
Hamburger	385
Whoppers: Original	980
Triple with Cheesse	1475
Whopper Jr.	390
Impossible Whopper	1080
Chicken Sandwich, Original	1170
Sides: French Fries, medium, salted	570
Onion Rings, medium	1315
Breakfast, Ham, Egg & Cheese Croissan'wich	1000
Carl's Jr.:	
Burgers: Famous Star w/ Cheese	1270
Beyond Famous Star w/ Cheese	1600
The Big Carl	1380
Denny's:	
Burgers: Bacon Avocado Cheeseburger	1650
Slamburger	1780
Sandwiches: Club	2060
Mega Philly Cheese Melt	2120
Dinner: Brooklyn Spaghetti & Meatballs	2510
Premium Chicken Tenders	2360
Sides: Broccoli	110
Seasoned Fries	1110
Red-Skinned Potatoes	580
Breakfast: BlueberyPancakes (2)	1400
Moons Over My Hammy Omelette, w/ Hash	2200
Santa Fe Skillet	1700
Sides: Hash Browns, 1 serving	360
Sausages (2)	300
Jack In The Box:	
Burgers: Bacon Ultimate Cheeseburger	1590
Jumbo Jack	580
Jumbo Jack Cheeseburger	990
Sandwiches: H'style Ranch Chicken Club	1869
Sourdough Grilled Chicken Club	1500
KFC:	
Chicken Breast: Original	1190
Extra Crispy	1150
Kentucky Grilled	710
Popcorn Nuggets, Large	1820
Sandwich, Crispy Twister	1260
Tenders, Extra Crispy Tenders, each	610
Wings, Nashville HotSpicy Crispy (1)	450
Sides: Macaroni & Cheese	590
Mashed Potatoes with Gravy	520
Potato Wedges	700

Fast-Foods & Restaurants	Sodium
McDonalds:	
Burgers: Big Mac	1010
Cheeseburger	720
Double	1180
Hamburger	510
Quarter Pounder with Cheese	1150
Chicken McNuggets, 4 pieces	330
McChicken, Sandwich	560
French Fries: Small, 2.6 oz	180
Medium, 3.9 oz	260
Large, 5.9 oz	400
Ketchup, 1 package, 10g	90
Breakfast: Egg McMuffin	760
Big Breakfast	1490
Hash Browns, 2 oz	310
Hotcakes & Sausage	880
Sausage Burrito	800
Sausage McGriddles	990
Desserts/Shakes: Hot Fudge Sundae	180
Strawberry Banana Smoothie, medium	50
Pizza Hut:	
Original Pan Pizza: *Per Slice, Medium 12"*	
Meat Lovers	660
Cheese	450
Pepperoni Lover's	580
Supreme	500
Subway: *On 9 Grain Wheat Bread*	
6" Sandwiches: *With Set Menu Toppings*	
Chicken Bacon Ranch Melt	1100
Meatball Marinara	1040
Spicy Italian	1240
6" Breakfast Flatbread S'wich: *With Set Menu Toppings*	
Bacon, Egg & Cheese	1200
Black Forest Ham, Egg & Chse	1180
Egg & Cheese	950
Steak, Egg & Cheese	1270
Taco Bell:	
Burritos: Beefy 5-Layer	1250
Supreme, Chicken	1110
Chalupa Supreme, Chicken/Steak, av	545
Nachos: BellGrande, Chicken	1050
Steak	1030
Specialties, Cheese Quesadillas	990
Tacos: Soft Chicken	450
Crunchy Supreme	340

Index A - C

FAST-FOODS INDEX
~ PAGE 175 ~

Index E - K

FAST-FOODS INDEX ~ PAGE 175 ~

FAST-FOODS INDEX ~ PAGE 175 ~